OUTPATIENT
MEDICINE

....

OUTPATIENT
MEDICINE *second edition*

STEPHAN D. FIHN, MD, MPH

Head, Division of General Internal Medicine
Professor of Medicine
Professor of Health Services
University of Washington School of Medicine
Director, Northwest Field Program Health Services Research
  and Development
VA Puget Sound Health Care System
Seattle, Washington

DAWN E. DeWITT, MD, MSc

Assistant Professor of Medicine
University of Washington School of Medicine
Attending Physician, University of Washington Medical Center
  and Roosevelt Clinic
Seattle, Washington

W.B. SAUNDERS COMPANY
A Division of Harcourt Brace & Company
Philadelphia   London   Toronto   Montreal   Sydney   Tokyo

10/2001

W.B. SAUNDERS COMPANY
A Division of Harcourt Brace & Company

The Curtis Center
Independence Square West
Philadelphia, Pennsylvania 19106

Library of Congress Cataloging-in-Publication Data

Outpatient medicine / [edited by] Stephan D. Fihn, Dawn E. DeWitt.—2nd ed.

p.   cm.

Includes bibliographical references and index.

ISBN 0–7216–6257–9

1. Ambulatory medical care—Handbooks, manuals, etc.   I. Fihn, Stephan D.
   II. DeWitt, Dawn E.   [DNLM: 1. Ambulatory Care.   2. Primary Health
   Care.   WX 205   0942   1998]

RC55.088 1998   616—dc21

DNLM/DLC   96–46544

OUTPATIENT MEDICINE   ISBN 0–7216–6257–9

Printed in the United States of America.

Last digit is the print number: 9   8   7   6   5   4   3   2   1

*To **Alan** and **Judy**,*
who made this book possible.

Material in the chapters listed below is in the public domain:

Chapter 1 Role of the Ambulatory Provider, *Chapter 3* Ethics in Outpatient Medicine, *Chapter 7* Principles of Screening, *Chapter 8* Periodic Health Assessment, *Chapter 10* Alcohol Problems, *Chapter 11* Adult Immunizations, *Chapter 16* Fever, *Chapter 20* Dizziness, *Chapter 22* Principles of Dermatologic Diagnosis and Therapy, *Chapter 23* Pruritus, *Chapter 24* Corns and Calluses, *Chapter 25* Warts, *Chapter 26* Superficial Fungal Infections, *Chapter 27* Scabies and Lice, *Chapter 28* Eczema, *Chapter 29* Seborrheic Dermatitis, *Chapter 30* Herpes Zoster, *Chapter 31* Acne, *Chapter 32* Psoriasis, *Chapter 33* Malignant Melanoma, *Chapter 34* Urticaria, *Chapter 57* Sinusitis, *Chapter 58* Cerumen Removal, *Chapter 64* Sleep Apnea Syndromes, *Chapter 66* Upper Respiratory Infection, *Chapter 67* Lower Respiratory Infection, *Chapter 68* Asthma and Chronic Obstructive Pulmonary Disease, *Chapter 69* Pulmonary Function Testing, *Chapter 70* Thoracentesis, *Chapter 71* Arterial Blood Sampling, *Chapter 77* Edema, *Chapter 88* Exercise Tolerance Testing, *Chapter 90* Colorectal Cancer Screening, *Chapter 99* Cirrhosis and Chronic Liver Failure, *Chapter 100* Viral Hepatitis, *Chapter 103* Hemorrhoids and Anal Fissures, *Chapter 108* Shoulder Pain, *Chapter 113* Restless Legs Syndrome, *Chapter 114* Muscle Cramps, *Chapter 115* Paget's Disease, *Chapter 116* Osteporosis, *Chapter 127* Injection of the Subacromial Bursa, *Chapter 130* Painful and Swollen Calf, *Chapter 131* Raynaud's Syndrome, *Chapter 133* Leg Ulcers, *Chapter 134* Local Care of Diabetic Foot Lesions, *Chapter 142* Alcohol Withdrawal, *Chapter 143* Idiopathic Facial Palsy, *Chapter 156* Male Infertility, *Chapter 169* Erectile Dysfunction, *Chapter 170* Dysuria, *Chapter 171* Scrotal Pain, *Chapter 174* Nephrolithiasis, *Chapter 175* Urinary Tract Infections in Women, *Chapter 177* Urinary Tract Infections in Men, *Chapter 178* Bacteriuria in the Elderly, *Chapter 180* Hematuria, *Chapter 183* Scrotal Mass, *Chapter 187* Insomnia, *Chapter 188* Somatization, *Chapter 193* Psychological Assessment, *Chapter 195* Bleeding, *Chapter 201* Chronic Anticoagulation, *Chapter 206* Altered Mentation in the Patient with Cancer, *Chapter 207* Management of Pain in Patients with Cancer, *Chapter 208* Dyspnea in Patients with Cancer, *Chapter 209* End-of-Life Care for Patients with Cancer, *Chapter 211* Bacteriuria in Pregnancy

Contributors

William Abernethy, MD
Fellow, Division of Cardiology,
Department of Medicine,
Massachusetts General Hospital,
Boston, Massachusetts
> *Acute Chest Pain; Recurrent Chest Pain*

Jessie H. Ahroni, PhD, ARNP, CDE
Project Manager, Seattle Diabetic
Foot Study, VA Puget Sound Health
Care System, Seattle, Washington
> *Diabetic Foot Care Education; Local Care of Diabetic Foot Lesions*

Bradley D. Anawalt, MD
Assistant Professor of Medicine,
University of Washington School of
Medicine; Director of Resident
Ambulatory Care Training, VA Puget
Sound Health Care System, Seattle,
Washington
> *Male Infertility; Erectile Dysfunction*

Dennis L. Andress, MD
Associate Professor of Medicine,
University of Washington School of
Medicine; Staff Physician, VA Puget
Sound Health Care System, Seattle,
Washington
> *Paget's Disease; Osteoporosis*

Anthony L. Back, MD
Assistant Professor, Division of
Oncology, University of Washington
School of Medicine; Attending
Physician, VA Puget Sound Health
Care System, Seattle, Washington
> *Altered Mentation in the Patient with Cancer; Management of Pain*

in Patients with Cancer; Dyspnea in Patients with Cancer; End-of-Life Care for Patients with Cancer

Howard J. Barnebey, MD
Clinical Assistant Professor of
Ophthalmology, University of
Washington School of Medicine,
Seattle, Washington
> *Screening for Glaucoma; Glaucoma*

Ernie-Paul Barrette, BS, MA, MD
Assistant Professor, Division of
General Internal Medicine,
Department of Medicine, University
of Washington School of Medicine
and Medical Center, Seattle,
Washington
> *Unintentional Weight Loss; HIV Infection: Disease Prevention and Antiretroviral Therapy; HIV Infection: Office Evaluation; HIV Infection: Evaluation of Common Symptoms*

Paul B. Bascom, MD
Assistant Professor and Director,
Comfort Care Team, Oregon Health
Sciences University, Portland,
Oregon
> *Death of Clinic Patients*

Donald W. Belcher, MD
Associate Professor of Medicine,
University of Washington School of
Medicine; Staff Physician, VA Puget
Sound Health Care System, Seattle,
Washington
> *Periodic Health Assessment; Insomnia*

Joshua Benditt, MD
Associate Professor of Medicine,
University of Washington School of
Medicine; Medical Director of
Respiratory Care Services, University
of Washington Medical Center,
Seattle, Washington
> *Pleuritic Chest Pain; Hemoptysis;
> Pleural Effusion*

Thomas D. Bird, MD
Professor, Neurology, University of
Washington School of Medicine;
Chief, Neurology, VA Puget Sound
Health Care System, Seattle,
Washington
> *Tremor*

Griffith M. Blackmon, MD, MPH
Acting Instructor, University of
Washington School of Medicine,
Seattle, Washington
> *Screening for Occupational and
> Environmental Lung Disease*

Edward J. Boyko, MD, MPH
Associate Professor, Department of
Medicine, University of Washington
School of Medicine; Chief, Section
of General Internal Medicine, VA
Puget Sound Health Care System,
Seattle, Washington
> *Inflammatory Bowel Disease*

Clarence H. Braddock, III, MD, MPH
Assistant Professor, Department of
Medicine and Medical History and
Ethics (Adjunct), University of
Washington School of Medicine;
Associate Chief of Staff, Education,
VA Puget Sound Health Care
System, Seattle, Washington
> *Ethics in Outpatient Medicine*

Katharine A. Bradley, MD, MPH
Assistant Professor, Department of
Medicine, University of Washington
School of Medicine; Director,

Women's Clinic, and Investigator,
Health Services Research and
Development, VA Puget Sound
Health Care System, Seattle,
Washington
> *Alcohol Problems*

Michael K. Brawer, MD
Professor, Department of Urology,
University of Washington School of
Medicine; Attending Physician,
University Hospital; Chief, Section of
Urology, VA Puget Sound Health
Care System, Seattle, Washington
> *Cancer of the Genitourinary Tract;
> Prostate Cancer*

Diana D. Cardenas, MD, MS
Professor, Department of
Rehabilitation Medicine, University
of Washington School of Medicine;
Director, Rehabilitation Medicine
Clinic, University of Washington
Medical Center, Seattle, Washington
> *Chronic Nonspecific Pain Syndrome*

Robert M. Centor, MD
Professor and Chief, Division of
General Internal Medicine, and
Associate Dean, Primary Care,
University of Alabama at
Birmingham and Medical Center,
Birmingham, Alabama
> *Pharyngitis*

Edmund Chaney, PhD
Associate Professor, Department of
Psychiatry and Behavioral Sciences,
University of Washington School of
Medicine; Staff Psychologist,
Consult/Liaison Team, Mental
Health Service, VA Puget Sound
Health Care System, Seattle,
Washington
> *Psychological Assessment*

James J. Coatsworth, MD
Clinical Associate Professor,
University of Washington School of
Medicine; Staff Neurologist, Virginia
Mason Medical Center, Seattle,
Washington
Seizures; Electroencephalography

Craig V. Comiter, MD
Chief Urology Resident, Veterans
Affairs Medical Center; Chief
Resident, Harvard Program in
Urology, Harvard Medical School,
Boston, Massachusetts
Urinary Incontinence

Mindy A. Cooper, MD
Assistant Professor of Medicine,
Division of Nephrology, University of
Washington School of Medicine;
Attending Physician, Harborview
Medical Center, Seattle, Washington
Chronic Renal Failure; Proteinuria

David C. Dale, MD
Professor of Medicine, University of
Washington School of Medicine,
Seattle, Washington
Lymphadenopathy

Feroza Daroowalla, MD, MPH
Fellow, Pulmonary and Critical Care
Medicine and Occupational
Medicine, University of Washington
School of Medicine, Seattle,
Washington
Pleural Effusion

Julie F. DeLeo, MD
Clinical Instructor of Medicine,
Brown University School of
Medicine; Fellow in Women's
Health, Division of General Internal
Medicine, Rhode Island Hospital,
Providence, Rhode Island
Cervical Cancer Screening

Dawn E. DeWitt, MD, MSc
Assistant Professor of Medicine,
University of Washington School of
Medicine; Attending Physician,
University of Washington Medical
Center and Roosevelt Clinic, Seattle,
Washington
*Diagnosis and Management of
Drug Abuse; Congestive Heart
Failure; Echocardiographic and
Nuclear Assessment of Cardiac
Function; Diabetes Mellitus*

Richard A. Deyo, MD, MPH
Professor, Department of Medicine
and Department of Health Services,
University of Washington School of
Medicine; Seattle, Washington
Low Back Pain

Andrew K. Diehl, MD, MSc
Professor of Medicine and Chief,
Division of General Medicine,
University of Texas Health Science
Center at San Antonio, San Antonio,
Texas
Biliary Tract Disease

Mariann J. Drucker, MD
Acting Assistant Professor in
Radiology, University of Washington
School of Medicine, Seattle,
Washington
Mammography and Breast Imaging

David C. Dugdale, MD
Associate Professor, Department of
Medicine, University of Washington
School of Medicine, Seattle,
Washington
*Dyspepsia; Sigmoidoscopy and
Colonoscopy*

Susan A. Egaas, MD
Resident, Emergency Medicine,
Denver Health and Hospitals,
Denver, Colorado
Dysphagia and Heartburn

Diane L. Elliot, MD
Professor of Medicine, Division of
Health Promotion and Sports
Medicine, Oregon Health Sciences
University, Portland, Oregon

*Diagnosis of Pregnancy; Diabetes
Mellitus in Pregnancy; Gestational
Diabetes Mellitus; Pregnancy and
Hypertension; Asthma in
Pregnancy; Thyroid Disorders in
Pregnancy*

Stephan D. Fihn, MD, MPH
Head, Division of General Internal
Medicine, Professor of Medicine,
Professor of Health Services,
University of Washington School of
Medicine; Director, Northwest Field
Program Health Services Research
and Development, VA Puget Sound
Health Care System, Seattle,
Washington

*Role of the Ambulatory Provider;
Redness of the Eye; Colorectal
Cancer Screening; Shoulder Pain;
Injection of the Subacromial Bursa;
Dysuria; Nephrolithiasis; Urinary
Tract Infections in Women; Chronic
Anticoagulation; Bacteriuria in
Pregnancy*

David G. Fryer, MD
Associate Clinical Professor of
Medicine, University of Washington
School of Medicine; Neurologist,
Virginia Mason Clinic, Seattle,
Washington

Dementia

Neal D. Futran, MD, DMD
Assistant Professor, Department of
Otolaryngology—Head and Neck
Surgery, University of Washington
School of Medicine and Medical
Center, Seattle, Washington

*Detection and Initial Management
of Oral Cancer*

Gregory C. Gardner, MD
Associate Professor, Division of
Rheumatology, University of
Washington School of Medicine,
Seattle, Washington

*Hip Pain; Wrist and Hand Pain;
Knee Pain; Ankle and Foot Pain;
Polymyalgia Rheumatica and
Temporal Arteritis; Osteoarthritis*

Barak Gaster, MD
Chief Medical Resident, Providence
Seattle Medical Center, University of
Washington Medicine Residency
Program, Seattle, Washington

Benign Prostatic Hyperplasia

Michael G. Glenn, MD
Clinical Associate Professor,
University of Washington School of
Medicine; Section Chief,
Otolaryngology, Virginia Mason
Medical Center, Seattle, Washington

Epistaxis

Marye J. Gleva, MD
Assistant Professor of Medicine,
Department of Medicine,
Cardiovascular Division, Washington
University School of Medicine, St.
Louis, Missouri

*Chronic Ventricular Arrhythmias;
Supraventricular Arrhythmias*

Erika Goldstein, MD, MPH
Associate Professor, Internal
Medicine, University of Washington
School of Medicine; Attending
Physician, Harborview Medical
Center, Seattle, Washington

Hyperventilation Syndrome

Geoffrey H. Gordon, MD
Associate Professor of Medicine and
Psychiatry, Oregon Health Sciences
University; Staff Physician, Veterans
Affairs Medical Center, Portland,
Oregon

Somatization

Richard E. Green, MPA
VA Puget Sound Health Care
System, Seattle, Washington
*Cancer of the Genitourinary Tract;
Prostate Cancer*

Deborah L. Greenberg, MD
Assistant Professor of Medicine,
University of Washington School of
Medicine, Seattle, Washington
Obesity; Anorexia; Diarrhea

Diane Greenberg, PhD
Clinical Faculty, Psychiatry and
Behavioral Sciences, University of
Washington School of Medicine;
Clinical Psychologist in General
Internal Medicine Clinic, VA Puget
Sound Health Care System, Seattle,
Washington
Psychological Assessment

Kenneth E. Hamrick, OD
Adjunct Clinical Instructor, Pacific
University College of Optometry,
Forest Grove, Oregon; Staff
Optometrist, VA Puget Sound
Health Care System, Seattle,
Washington
Visual Impairment

Jodie K. Haselkorn, MD, MPH
Associate Professor, Department of
Rehabilitation Medicine, and
Adjunct Associate Professor,
Department of Epidemiology,
University of Washington School of
Medicine; Staff Physician, VA Puget
Sound Health Care System, Seattle,
Washington
Chronic Nonspecific Pain Syndrome

Lonny M. Hecker, MD
Clinical Assistant Professor of
Medicine, University of Washington
School of Medicine;
Gastroenterologist, Pacific Medical
Center, Seattle, Washington
Upper Gastrointestinal Endoscopy

David H. Hickam, MD, MPH
Professor, Department of Medicine,
Oregon Health Sciences University;
Coordinator, Health Services
Research and Development,
Veterans Affairs Medical Center,
Portland, Oregon
*Acute Chest Pain; Recurrent Chest
Pain; Angina*

Allan D. Hillel, MD
Associate Professor, Department of
Otolaryngology—Head and Neck
Surgery, University of Washington
School of Medicine and Medical
Center, Seattle, Washington
*Detection and Initial Management
of Oral Cancer*

Jan V. Hirschmann, MD
Professor of Medicine, University of
Washington School of Medicine;
Assistant Chief, Medical Service, VA
Puget Sound Health Care System,
Seattle, Washington
*Principles of Dermatologic Diagnosis
and Therapy; Pruritus; Corns and
Calluses; Warts; Superficial Fungal
Infections; Scabies and Lice;
Eczema; Seborrheic Dermatitis;
Herpes Zoster; Acne; Psoriasis;
Malignant Melanoma; Urticaria*

Richard M. Hoffman, MD, MPH
Assistant Professor, University of New
Mexico School of Medicine; Staff
Physician, Albuquerque VA Medical
Center, Albuquerque, New Mexico
*Assessment of Physical Activity;
Cancer of the Genitourinary Tract;
Prostate Cancer*

Thomas M. Hooton, MD
Associate Professor, University of
Washington School of Medicine;
Medical Director, Harborview
Medical Center Madison Clinic,
Seattle, Washington
Sexually Transmitted Diseases

Hugh F. Huizenga, MD
Acting Instructor, University of
Washington School of Medicine;
Staff Physician, VA Puget Sound
Health Care System, Seattle,
Washington
Sleep Apnea Syndromes

Andrew F. Inglis, Jr, MD
Associate Professor, University of
Washington School of Medicine;
Attending Physician, Division of
Otolaryngology, Children's Hospital
and Medical Center, Seattle,
Washington
Otitis Media and Externa

Sarah Jackins, PT
Clinical Assistant Professor
Orthopaedics/Rehabilitation
Medicine, University of Washington
School of Medicine; Manager,
Physical Therapy and the Exercise
Training Center, University of
Washington Medical Center, Seattle,
Washington
*Physical Therapy Care of
Outpatients*

Kathleen Jobe, MD
Assistant Professor of Medicine,
University of Washington School of
Medicine; Attending Physician,
Emergency Services; Associate
Residency Director, Emergency
Medicine, University of Washington
Medical Center, Seattle, Washington
Dyspnea

Kaj Johansen, MD, PhD
Professor of Surgery, University of
Washington School of Medicine;
Director, Surgical Education,
Providence Seattle Medical Center,
Seattle, Washington
*Peripheral Arterial Disease; Doppler
Measurement of Ankle Pressures*

Elaine C. Jong, MD
Clinical Professor of Medicine,
University of Washington School of
Medicine; Co-Director, Travel and
Tropical Medicine Service, and
Director, Hall Health Primary Care
Center, University of Washington
Medical Center, Seattle, Washington
Travel Medicine

Howard J. Kaplan, MD
Westchester-Bronx Retina Group,
Yonkers, New York
Diabetic Retinopathy

Wishwa N. Kapoor, MD
Professor of Medicine, University of
Pittsburgh School of Medicine;
Chief, Division of General Internal
Medicine, and Vice-Chairman,
Department of Medicine, University
of Pittsburgh Medical Center,
Pittsburgh, Pennsylvania
*Syncope; Palpitations; Ambulatory
Cardiac Monitoring*

Michael B. Kimmey, MD
Associate Professor of Medicine,
Division of Gastroenterology,
University of Washington School of
Medicine; Section Chief of
Gastroenterology and Director,
Gastrointestinal Endoscopy,
University of Washington Medical
Center, Seattle, Washington
Peptic Ulcer Disease

James L. Kinyoun, MD
Professor of Ophthalmology,
University of Washington School of
Medicine, Seattle, Washington
Diabetic Retinopathy

Shoba Krishnamurthy, MBBS
Clinical Professor of Medicine,
University of Washington School of
Medicine; Gastroenterologist, Pacific
Medical Center, Seattle, Washington
Constipation

Mary B. Laya, MD, MPH
Assistant Professor of Medicine,
University of Washington School of
Medicine, Seattle, Washington
>   *Breast Cancer Screening; Initial*
>   *Evaluation of a Breast Mass; Breast*
>   *Pain in Nonlactating Women*

Wendy Levinson, MD
Professor of Medicine and Chief,
Section of General Internal
Medicine, University of Chicago,
Chicago, Illinois
>   *Effective Communication in the*
>   *Ambulatory Care Setting*

Thomas D. Lindquist, MD, PhD
Clinical Professor, Department of
Ophthalmology, University of
Washington School of Medicine;
Director, Cornea and External
Disease Service, Department of
Ophthalmology, Virginia Mason
Medical Center, Seattle, Washington
>   *Dry Eyes and Excessive Tearing;*
>   *Cataracts; Foreign Bodies and*
>   *Corneal Abrasions; Conjunctivitis;*
>   *Foreign Body Removal*

Benjamin A. Lipsky, MD
Associate Professor, University of
Washington School of Medicine;
Hospital Epidemiologist and
Director, General Internal Medicine
Clinic, VA Puget Sound Health Care
System, Seattle, Washington
>   *Adult Immunizations; Fever;*
>   *Urinary Tract Infections in Men;*
>   *Bacteriuria in the Elderly*

Deborah J. Lium, PhD
Research Assistant, Department of
Medicine, University of New Mexico
School of Medicine, Albuquerque,
New Mexico
>   *Assessment of Physical Activity*

James B. Maclean, MD
Clinical Associate Professor of
Medicine, University of Washington
School of Medicine; Neurologist,
Virginia Mason Medical Center,
Seattle, Washington
>   *Multiple Sclerosis*

Kathleen H. Makielski, MD, FACS
Associate Professor, Department of
Otolaryngology, University of
Washington School of Medicine;
Chief, Otolaryngology—Head and
Neck Surgery, Pacific Medical
Center, Seattle, Washington
>   *Hiccough (Singultus)*

Steven R. McGee, MD
Associate Professor of Medicine,
University of Washington School of
Medicine; Attending Physician, VA
Puget Sound Health Care System,
Seattle, Washington
>   *Anorexia; Dizziness; Fatigue;*
>   *Cerumen Removal; Edema;*
>   *Congestive Heart Failure; Exercise*
>   *Tolerance Testing; Dysphagia and*
>   *Heartburn; Hemorrhoids and Anal*
>   *Fissures; Restless Legs Syndrome;*
>   *Muscle Cramps; Painful and*
>   *Swollen Calf; Raynaud's Syndrome;*
>   *Leg Ulcers; Alcohol Withdrawal;*
>   *Idiopathic Facial Palsy; Scrotal*
>   *Pain; Scrotal Mass*

Marguerite J. McNeely, MD, MPH
Clinical Professor, Division of
General Internal Medicine,
University of Washington School of
Medicine; Physician, Hall Health
Primary Care Center, Seattle,
Washington
>   *Fatigue*

Terrie Mendelson, MD
Associate Professor of Medicine and
Director of Housestaff Education
and Program Director, University of

California, San Francisco; Director,
Evidence-Based Medicine Program,
VA Medical Center, San Francisco,
California

Female Infertility

Ravi Moonka, MD
Acting Instructor, University of
Washington School of Medicine;
Staff Surgeon, VA Puget Sound
Health Care System, Seattle,
Washington

Diverticulitis

Marc W. Mora, MD
Consultant and Internist, Group
Health Cooperative of Puget Sound,
Tacoma Specialty Center, Tacoma,
Washington

*Preoperative Hematologic Problems;
Preoperative Infectious Disease
Problems*

M. Connie Morantes, MD
Acting Instructor, Division of
General Internal Medicine,
University of Washington School of
Medicine; Attending Physician, VA
Puget Sound Health Care System,
Seattle, Washington

*Cirrhosis and Chronic Liver Failure;
Viral Hepatitis*

Anne W. Moulton, MD
Associate Professor of Medicine,
Brown University School of
Medicine; Associate Physician,
Division of General Internal
Medicine, Rhode Island Hospital,
Providence, Rhode Island

Cervical Cancer Screening

Cynthia D. Mulrow, MD, MSc
Professor of Medicine, The
University of Texas Health Science
Center at San Antonio; Senior
Research Associate, Department of
Veterans Affairs, South Texas

Veterans Health Care System, Audie
L. Murphy Memorial Veterans
Hospital Division, San Antonio,
Texas

Screening for Hearing Impairment

James C. Orcutt, MD, PhD
Professor of Ophthalmology,
University of Washington School of
Medicine; Chief of Ophthalmology
Section, VA Puget Sound Health
Care System, Seattle, Washington

Eye Pain

Catherine M. Otto, MD
Associate Professor of Medicine and
Director, Training Program in
Cardiovascular Disease, University of
Washington School of Medicine;
Associate Director,
Echocardiography Laboratory,
University of Washington Medical
Center, Seattle, Washington

*Aortic Stenosis; Other Valvular
Disease; Echocardiography*

Douglas S. Paauw, MD
Associate Professor of Medicine and
Coordinator of Student Teaching,
Department of Medicine, University
of Washington School of Medicine,
Seattle, Washington

*Diagnosis and Management of
Drug Abuse; Gout/Hyperuricemia;
Gynecomastia*

Laird G. Patterson, MD
Clinical Professor, Department of
Neurology, University of Washington
School of Medicine; Staff
Neurologist, Virginia Mason Medical
Center, Seattle, Washington

*Seizures; Dementia; Entrapment
Neuropathies; Parkinsonism*

David R. Perera, MD, MPH
Clinical Professor of Medicine and
Gastroenterology, University of

Washington School of Medicine;
Consulting Gastroenterologist,
Group Health of Puget Sound,
Seattle, Washington

Inflammatory Bowel Disease

Stephen H. Petersdorf, MD
Assistant Professor, Medical
Oncology, University of Washington
School of Medicine; Acting Clinical
Director, High Dose Chemotherapy
Service, University of Washington
Medical Center, Seattle, Washington

*Thrombocytopenia; Polycythemia;
Anemia; Sickle Cell Disease*

Linda E. Pinsky, MD
Assistant Professor; Director,
Resident Ambulatory Education,
Roosevelt General Internal Medicine
Clinic, University of Washington
School of Medicine, Seattle,
Washington

*Cholesterol Screening;
Hyperlipidemia; Common Thyroid
Disorders*

Charles E. Pope, II, MD
Professor Emeritus, Medicine,
University of Washington School of
Medicine; Attending Physician,
University of Washington Medical
Center, Seattle, Washington

Abdominal Pain

Heidi Powell, MD
Acting Instructor, Department of
Medicine, Division of General
Internal Medicine, University of
Washington School of Medicine,
Seattle, Washington

Hoarseness

Hubert N. Radke, MD
Associate Professor, University of
Washington School of Medicine;

Division Chief of General Surgery,
VA Puget Sound Health Care
System, Seattle, Washington

Diverticulitis

John Ravits, MD
Assistant Clinical Professor of
Medicine, University of Washington
School of Medicine; Attending
Physician, Section of Neurology,
Virginia Mason Medical Center,
Seattle, Washington

*Muscular Weakness;
Electromyography and Nerve
Conduction Studies*

Dominic Reilly, MD
Assistant Professor, Medicine,
University of Washington School of
Medicine; Director, Medicine
Consultation Service, University of
Washington Medical Center, Seattle,
Washington

*Preoperative Evaluation;
Preoperative Cardiovascular
Problems; Preoperative Pulmonary
Problems*

James R. Revenaugh
Assistant Professor, Division of
Cardiology, and Director, Cardiac
Catheterization Laboratory,
University of Utah School of
Medicine, Salt Lake City, Utah

*Echocardiographic and Nuclear
Assessment of Cardiac Function*

**Nancy J. Roben, ARNP, BSN
(Retired)**
Adult Nurse Practitioner, VA Puget
Sound Health Care System, Seattle,
Washington

Chronic Anticoagulation

Gerald J. Roth, MD
Professor of Medicine, University of
Washington School of Medicine;
Chief, Hematology Section, VA

Puget Sound Health Care System, Seattle, Washington

Bleeding; Transfusion Therapy

Mark M. Schubert, MD, DDS, MSD
Associate Professor, Oral Medicine, School of Dentistry, University of Washington; Adjunct Assistant Professor, Otolaryngology and Head and Neck Surgery, University of Washington School of Medicine; Attending Physician, University of Washington Medical Center, Fred Hutchinson Cancer Center, Swedish Hospital, Seattle, Washington

Dental Disease

Jane Schwebke, MD
Assistant Professor of Medicine, University of Alabama at Birmingham; Medical Director, Sexually Transmitted Disease Clinic, Jefferson County Health Department, Birmingham, Alabama

Vaginitis

John Sekijima, MD
Gastroenterologist, Pacific Medical Clinic, Seattle, Washington

Jaundice

Donald J. Sherrard, MD
Professor of Medicine, University of Washington School of Medicine; Chief of Nephrology, VA Puget Sound Health Care System, Seattle, Washington

Nephrolithiasis

Kirk K. Shy, MD, MPH
Professor, Department of Obstetrics and Gynecology, University of Washington School of Medicine; Chief, Obstetrics and Gynecology, Harborview Medical Center, Seattle, Washington

Contraception

Kathleen C. Y. Sie, MD
Assistant Professor, Otolaryngology–Head and Neck Surgery, University of Washington School of Medicine; Division of Pediatric Otolaryngology–Head and Neck Surgery, Children's Hospital & Medical Center, Seattle, Washington

Tinnitus

David L. Simel, MD, MHS
Associate Professor, Duke University School of Medicine; Associate Chief of Staff for Ambulatory Care, Durham Veterans Affairs Medical Center, Durham, North Carolina

Principles of Screening

Gregory E. Simon, MD, MPH
Investigator, Center for Health Studies, and Psychiatrist, Mental Health Service, Group Health Cooperative, Research Assistant Professor of Psychiatry and Behavioral Sciences, University of Washington School of Medicine, Seattle, Washington

Screening for Depression; Generalized Anxiety; Management of Depression; Psychosis; Panic Disorder; The Difficult Patient

Shawn J. Skerrett, MD
Assistant Professor of Medicine, Pulmonary and Critical Care Medicine, University of Washington School of Medicine; Attending Physician, University of Washington Medical Center and VA Puget Sound Health Care System, Seattle, Washington

Cough and Sputum; Upper Respiratory Infection; Lower Respiratory Infection; Asthma and Chronic Obstructive Pulmonary Disease; Pulmonary Function Testing; Thoracentesis; Arterial Blood Sampling

Beth Skrypzak, MD
Section Head, Department of
Obstetrics/Gynecology, Virginia
Mason Medical Center, Seattle,
Washington
  *Abnormal Uterine Bleeding; Pelvic
  Pain in Women*

C. Scott Smith, MD
Assistant Professor of Medicine and
Adjunct Assistant Professor of
Medical Education, University of
Washington School of Medicine,
Seattle, Washington; Staff Internist,
VA Medical Center, Boise, Idaho
  *Preoperative Endocrine Problems;
  Preoperative Pulmonary Problems*

David L. Smith, MD
Associate Professor of Medicine,
Oregon Health Sciences University;
Staff Physician, Internal Medicine/
Rheumatology, Veterans Affairs
Medical Center, Portland, Oregon
  Prepatellar and Olecranon Bursitis

Thomas Staiger, MD
Acting Instructor and Attending
Physician, General Internal Medicine
Center, University of Washington
Medical Center and Roosevelt Clinic,
Seattle, Washington
  Smoking Cessation

John F. Steiner, MD, MPH
Associate Professor of Medicine,
Preventive Medicine, and Biometrics,
University of Colorado Health
Sciences Center; Attending
Physician, University Hospital,
Denver, Colorado
  Compliance; Essential Hypertension

John B. Stimson, MD
Clinical Associate Professor of
Medicine, University of Washington
School of Medicine; Physician, The
Polyclinic, Seattle, Washington

  *Abnormal Taste and Smell;
  Fibromyalgia; Myofascial Pain
  Syndromes; Trigger Point Injection;
  Benign Prostatic Hyperplasia*

Maryrose P. Sullivan, MD
Instructor of Surgery, Harvard
Medical School, Boston; BioMedical
Engineer in Urology, VA Medical
Center, West Roxbury, Massachusetts
  Urinary Incontinence

Eliza Sutton, MD
Internist, General Internal Medicine,
Providence Health Care Center,
Everett, Washington
  Menopausal Symptoms

Lynne P. Taylor, MD
Clinical Assistant Professor,
University of Washington School of
Medicine; Attending Neurologist,
Virginia Mason Medical Center,
Seattle, Washington
  Cerebrovascular Disease

Susan W. Tolle, MD
Professor of Medicine and Director,
Center for Ethics in Health Care,
Oregon Health Sciences University,
Portland, Oregon
  Death of Clinic Patients

Shin-Ping Tu, MD, MPH
Acting Instructor, University of
Washington School of Medicine,
Seattle, Washington
  Hematuria

Asher A. Tulsky, MD
Assistant Professor of Medicine,
University of Rochester School of
Medicine and Dentistry; Attending
Physician, St. Mary's Hospital,
Rochester, New York
  *Determining Disability: The Primary
  Care Physician's Role*

Barbara E. Weber, MD, MPH
Assistant Professor of Medicine,
University of Rochester School of
Medicine and Dentistry; General
Medicine Unit Chief, St. Mary's
Hospital, Rochester, New York
   Palpitations

Craig G. Wells, MD
Assistant Clinical Professor of
Ophthalmology, University of
Washington School of Medicine;
Ophthalmologist, Vitreoretinal
Associates, Seattle, Washington
   Ophthalmoscopy

Richard H. White, MD
Professor of Medicine, University of
California, Davis, School of
Medicine; Chief, Soft-Tissue
Rheumatic Disease Clinic, University
of California, Davis, Medical Center,
Sacramento, California
   *General Approach to Arthritic
   Symptoms; Interpretation of Serologic
   Tests; Injection of the Trochanteric
   Bursa; Aspiration/Injection of the
   Knee*

John W. Williams, Jr, MD, MHS
Associate Professor, University of
Texas Health Science Center at San
Antonio; Director, Continuity of
Care Clinic, Audie L. Murphy
Memorial Veterans Hospital, San
Antonio, Texas
   Sinusitis

Joyce E. Wipf, MD
Assistant Professor of Medicine and
Associate Director, Medicine
Residency Program, University of
Washington School of Medicine;
Staff Physician, VA Puget Sound
Health Care System, Seattle,
Washington
   *Redness of the Eye; Tuberculosis
   Screening; Atrial Fibrillation;
   Headache; Peripheral Neuropathy*

Emily Y. Wong, MD
Acting Instructor, University of
Washington School of Medicine;
Attending Physician, University of
Washington Women's Health Care
Center, Seattle, Washington
   Pelvic Inflammatory Disease

Subbarao V. Yalla, MD
Associate Professor of Surgery
(Urology), Harvard Medical School,
Boston; Chief, Urology Section, VA
Medical Center, West Roxbury,
Massachusetts
   Urinary Incontinence

Bessie A. Young, MD
Acting Clinical Instructor, University
of Washington School of Medicine;
Staff Nephrologist, Group Health
Cooperative, Seattle, Washington
   Electrolyte Abnormalities

Acknowledgments

. . . .

We would like to acknowledge several people who made important contributions to this edition of *Outpatient Medicine*. The influence on this book of first edition co-editor Steve McGee remains considerable both in substance and in spirit. Pat Tulip's tireless help in typing and tracking manuscripts was invaluable. Several pharmacists provided greatly appreciated assistance in compiling drug information. They include Susan E. Comes, PharmD, at the University of Washington, and Debra Redman, RPh, Amanda Pitts, RPh, and Eric Chantelois, RPh, at the VA Puget Sound Health Care System.

Foreword

....

The direction of patient care has progressed inexorably from the inpatient to the outpatient setting. This has been occurring since the first edition of this book was published, and the end is not in sight. It has certainly influenced the way in which students learn, and in which faculty teach. In fact, some of us old-timers who cut our clinical teeth on the wards have had more than a little difficulty adapting to the outpatient paradigm. Indeed, the first edition of this book fell short only when some of the authors forgot that they were in the clinic rather than at the bedside.

This is a minor quibble, however, because this book has many virtues. First, its chapters are clear, concise, and to the point. They provide the essential information without indulging in the mechanistic speculations and in the arcana of differential diagnosis in which we internists so often revel. Moreover, the tables and charts are readily understandable and helpful. Second, it deals with the mundane as well as the cataclysmic. For example, the chapter on hemorrhoids is full of pearls. Third, it delves into "paramedical" phenomena like pregnancy, pre- and postop care, and disorders that internists have traditionally referred to specialists such as gynecologists, ophthalmologists, and orthopedic surgeons. At the same time it makes quite clear when such referrals are indicated. Fourth, it places screening and prevention in perspective. In my view, preventive medicine has often overpromised, or, worse, has been used as an excuse for achieving cost-savings. Fifth, for the most part, it points out that outpatient medicine deals with chronic diseases and that it is no tragedy not to solve a problem on the first visit, but permissible to solve it on the second, third, or fourth, and even to watch it disappear without a clear answer. There is no sin in that as long as the patient gets well.

The editors have, by and large, chosen authors who are not household names, but who are very active patient-oriented doctors. The ones I know see patients daily or at least several times a week. For that judgment we readers should be grateful. We should also know that this book is not the sole instrument for providing knowledge in depth (the excellent, often comprehensive references make this point explicit) or for cramming for the certifying examination of the American Board of Internal Medicine. What you see in this book is what you get: a companion for the doctor (in post-training) who sees outpatients in a generalist setting. For that purpose alone it should sit on every generalist's office or clinic desk.

ROBERT G. PETERSDORF, MD
VA Puget Sound Health Care System
Seattle, Washington

Foreword _To The First Edition_

∎ ∎

Having had the privilege of browsing through this book in manuscript form, my impression is that the editors and contributors have assembled a novel, helpful collection of concise articles that will be of assistance to all physicians who deal with ambulatory adult patients. The intended readership includes not only general internists and family practitioners, but also physicians whose principal interests lie in other fields: the medical subspecialties, obstetrics, and various branches of surgery. Thus its subjects include some minor, early manifestations which tend to be categorized as belonging within the provinces of organized specialties but which actually do not require specialized skills and technologies.

The work recognizes the realities of a new era, in which medical practice has shifted from a preponderance of acute infectious processes afflicting younger patients to today's medicine, in which we deal largely with an older patient population, presenting chronic problems related to more than one disease and more than one organ system.

The authors and editors also recognize the obligation of today's health care providers to limit costs, avoid expensive hospital care, and enable patients to continue their regular activities in normal life settings. Thus we frequently find the statement that a certain diagnostic or therapeutic procedure is _not_ warranted. Also there is information about relative costs of medicines which could be prescribed for the same complaint.

I am acquainted with the editors, as well as many of the contributors, and I know their dedication to ambulatory medical care. It has been gratifying to observe their success in teaching this branch of medicine, and to see how warmly it is esteemed by medical students and house officers.

PAUL B. BEESON

Preface

. . . .

In the preface to the first edition we remarked that during the prior decade, the delivery of medical care in the United States had changed radically, including a myriad of new technologies for diagnosis and treatment, striking transformations in the way the medical care was funded, and new demands for physician accountability and patient autonomy. We also commented that while the process of medical care had become increasingly complex, there had been a paradoxical shift in the primary site of care from the hospital to the clinic. In the 5 years since the first edition was published, this metamorphosis has continued and even accelerated. Other innovations have emerged as well. There is a growing recognition that medical practice in all settings must be based on scientific evidence rather than simple clinical experience. Clinical guidelines are proliferating at an astounding rate. Computerized information systems are being installed widely, and the paperless office is no longer a novelty. Most physicians have at least a portion of the patients in their clinical practice covered by some type of managed care plan, and a substantial proportion work exclusively in managed care environments.

It might be asked whether a textbook is still relevant in our rapidly evolving field when timely access to concise and accurate information is critical, but often all too difficult. Based on the comments received about the first edition, we think so. Despite advances in information technology, the lowly book remains an inexpensive and useful random access device for students and residents as well as harried practitioners.

With these circumstances in mind, we have striven to make *Outpatient Medicine* comprehensive enough to be helpful but brief enough to be consulted on the spot when information is needed. As in the first edition, the book contains concise reviews that address the most common clinical questions encountered in outpatient medicine. We do not intend for *Outpatient Medicine* to substitute for a comprehensive ambulatory medicine textbook, of which there are several superb examples.

After introductory sections that survey general aspects of ambulatory care and preventive medicine, the book is divided into sections by organ systems. Chapters within each organ system section discuss one of four areas: 1) screening for disease, 2) approach to common symptoms, 3) approach to specific problems and syndromes, and 4) procedures. Much of the information is condensed into tables and, if appropriate, diagnostic or therapeutic algorithms. To avoid unnecessary repetition of information, the chapters are extensively cross-referenced. Each chapter concludes with a few key references, annotated to guide further reading. All chapters have been updated, and new chapters on ethics, travel medicine, chest pain, HIV infection, and cancer have been added.

We hope the busy student, house officer, and practicing generalist will continue to carry this book to clinic and refer to it when direction is needed during encounters with patients. We very much appreciated constructive criticisms from readers of the first edition and look forward to your comments on this edition as well.

STEPHAN D. FIHN
DAWN E. DEWITT

Contents

SECTION IV
Disorders of the Skin

SECTION V
Disorders of the Eye

SECTION X
Musculoskeletal Disorders

SECTION XV
Genitourinary and Renal Disorders

SECTION XVI
Psychiatric and Psychosomatic Disorders

SECTION XVII
Hematologic Disorders

SECTION I
General Aspects of Ambulatory Care

• •

1 Role of the Ambulatory Provider

STEPHAN D. FIHN

Life is short, and the Art long; the occasion fleeting; experience fallacious and judgment difficult. The physician must not only be prepared to do what is right himself, but also to make the patient, the attendants, and externals cooperate.

Hippocrates, from the *Aphorisms*

Until recently, the primary setting of adult medical care and of medical education has been the hospital ward. The bulk of expenditures for medical care traditionally has been consumed in the inpatient setting. Medical students and internal medicine residents have spent the overwhelming majority of their clinical rotations addressing the needs of hospitalized patients.

Today, for a variety of reasons, medical care is being delivered more often in the office or clinic than in the hospital. The enormous expense of hospitalization has compelled both payers and patients to seek alternatives, especially outpatient treatment. As a result, inpatient days have declined dramatically over the past decade; and in many communities, hospitals have reduced their operational beds or have closed. Many problems that a few years ago would have mandated hospital admission are now routinely treated in the clinic. This trend has been hastened by the development of sophisticated diagnostic and therapeutic interventions that can be safely and effectively used in the outpatient setting. Patients usually prefer the lower cost and morbidity associated with outpatient treatment. Those patients who need hospitalization are now discharged sooner, in part because of systems of reimbursement that create strong disincentives to hospitalization. Early outpatient follow-up is typically an integral part of the discharge plan.

The transfer of care to the outpatient setting has made the hospital ward a less attractive site of practice for many physicians and trainees. Most hospital admissions are now for previously diagnosed conditions or complications occurring in severely compromised patients. Many types of clinical disorders, such as endocrinologic, rheumatologic, and dermatologic diseases, are seldom encountered in the hospital. There is little opportunity to observe the evolution of disease or understand its effect on the patient's daily life. Dealing exclusively with hospitalized patients can produce a narrow perspective about strategies for medical care that may disregard the complexity and importance of continuity of care in the outpatient setting. Pressure to reduce the length of hospital stays, an emphasis on technical procedures, and the use of predetermined therapeutic protocols limit opportunities for reflection about complex disorders and time for teaching.

In this rapidly changing environment, the evolving role of the ambulatory care provider is a demanding one. Coincident with the escalating sophistication and specialization of medical care, there has been a paradoxically increasing demand for primary care providers who can deliver comprehensive longitudinal care. Patients expect these clinicians to take a broad perspective on their medical condition, rather than to focus exclusively on a single organ system. Patients with complex problems also want their primary physician to serve as an advocate and advisor and to coordinate the care delivered by specialists. Health care purchasers such as insurers, large corporations, governmental agencies, and health maintenance organizations also look to the primary care provider to plan and coordinate care and, in the process, to control costs. As the coordinator of care, the ambulatory care provider is expected to address the full spectrum of problems that arise, not only medical problems but also social and emotional problems. In addition to dealing with diagnostic and therapeutic issues, the practitioner is often asked to assist patients with financial and living arrangements.

Some clinicians view this array of responsibilities as too demanding or as extending unnecessarily beyond the bounds of traditional medical practice. This opinion is prevalent among trainees who have grown accustomed to the inpatient environment, where most attention is typically directed toward reversing acute problems and correcting physiologic derangements. The goals of outpatient treatment, however, are often substantially different from those of inpatient treatment and mandate a broader definition of the provider's role. Many patients may be elderly and suffering from a number of different disorders. Established chronic diseases often cannot be eradicated or reversed, and the primary aims of therapy are to lessen symptoms, improve function, and prevent further deterioration. To achieve these ends, it is essential to understand the patient's activities, resources, and support systems. In the process, the provider often develops an intimate bond with the patient and the patient's family—one of the uniquely satisfying experiences of providing continuous care.

However, practice in the outpatient setting also presents a number of unique and sometimes difficult issues. Unlike inpatients, who are often highly dependent medically and under almost continuous observation, outpatients are independent and have their own agendas and responsibilities. Busy clinic schedules may not allow time to address all of the issues in complete depth, requiring that problems be prioritized and dealt with selectively. Orders cannot simply be written with the assurance that the patient will actually take a medication or undergo a procedure. Patients may be unable or unwilling to make frequent follow-up visits. They want to be involved in decisions about their care, making negotiation between the patient and provider a common occurrence.

In recent years, several large-scale clinical trials have addressed issues in the management of common outpatient problems. Nonetheless, randomized trials dealing with a number of common outpatient topics are lacking, and much of practice remains based largely on experience and opinion. Recognizing this fact, the practitioner should remain flexible and be willing to seek imaginative solutions to thorny problems. For a variety of reasons, it is often impossible to adhere to textbook recommendations. It is usually advisable to involve the patient in developing compromise solutions. Partial solutions, although less satisfying, are usually preferable to impractical solutions and many times achieve a successful clinical outcome. Confrontation is rarely effective.

The experienced ambulatory practitioner becomes adept at operating effectively and efficiently in this complicated environment. Involving patients in the process of care is often the most successful strategy. Patients are usually cognizant of time pressures and are eager to forge a successful working partnership with their provider. They appreciate the provider's attempts to tailor diagnostic and treatment plans to meet their own special needs. They endorse efforts to educate them about the nature of their condition and about beneficial measures they can adopt on their own. Patients often avidly accept responsibility for aspects of their own care, such as monitoring parameters and adjusting therapy. Well-timed feedback reinforces these positive behaviors.

The deft outpatient clinician also learns to use time effectively as an important diagnostic and therapeutic agent. Simply observing a patient to glean more data before making a decision to intervene is often more informative than any laboratory or imaging test. The therapeutic qualities of "tincture of time" are hackneyed but nonetheless genuine. Most patients are grateful for efforts to limit the time and expense required by numerous clinic visits and extensive diagnostic evaluations. Astute clinicians develop a sense for the tempo of a patient's illness and plan follow-up intervals accordingly. Longer intervals between visits are often possible by scheduling interim telephone contact.

Because imaging tests are often inconvenient and must be scheduled in the future, the outpatient provider must rely heavily on the physical examination. Routine, complete physical examinations are rarely warranted, whereas the careful, directed examination is essential.

One of the more time-consuming tasks is maintaining medical records. Because of the frequent complexity of outpatient management and involvement of multiple providers, the record of care must be clear and adequately detailed. Yet, to keep pace, the practitioner must also make notes concise. A modified SOAP (Subjective/Objective Assessment and Plan) format is often a useful way to organize data. An entry for each category of each problem is not necessary at every visit. The advantage of this approach is that it helps to maintain an active problem list, which is essential for tracking patients with complicated problems over time. Tabular or graphic records (flow sheets) greatly aid in the care of outpatients and save time. Flow sheets can be used to record preventive services provided and to track important clinical data such as blood pressure, weight, and blood glucose levels in diabetics. Used in this manner, a flow sheet can be a valuable reminder to perform indicated procedures and can save the time otherwise spent reviewing a thick record to determine when a given procedure was last performed. Flow sheets can also be used to update medication profiles, obviating the need to list them anew after each visit.

Increasingly, however, paper records are being replaced by computerized systems. Computers have obvious advantages in that clinical data are universally available in a variety of locations (unless the system is down), can readily be present in tabular or graphic formats, and are more easily searched for specific findings or abnormalities. Moreover, several studies have now shown that computerized reminders can improve the quality of care and reduce cost. Another major benefit of computers is the potential to have all sorts of reference material, such as digital textbooks, journal articles, and clinical guidelines, immediately at hand. Unfortunately, many clinicians are poorly trained in the use of computers and many medical computing systems are cumbersome, are slow, and make impractical demands on clinicians. Nevertheless, it is inevitable that computers will play an increasingly prominent role in medicine, and the efficient clinician must become adept in their use.

The clinician must judiciously manage not only time but other resources as well. An increasing number of patients are insured under capitative care arrangements in which a fixed amount is allotted for each patient. Some insurance plans require substantial copayments or deductibles and do not cover drugs or special outpatient services, resulting in substantial out-of-pocket expenses for patients. Frequent office visits and multiple prescriptions are a financial burden for many families. Providing high-quality care requires sensitivity to the cost of care and making every effort to balance expense against expected benefit. All too often patients are asked to undertake difficult or costly treatment programs for which evidence of effectiveness is absent or marginal. Even some treatments of known efficacy may be of dubious value if other, more serious illnesses are present. Therapies that seem trivial to the provider may be quite vexing to patients. Each time the patient is seen, it is worthwhile to reexamine the therapeutic regimen and reconsider the risks and cost-benefit ratio.

A sensible approach to providing preventive care is also important. A number of screening tests and interventions have been conclusively shown to reduce morbidity and improve survival. The outpatient provider should aggressively implement these procedures whenever indicated. Many other commonly performed procedures, even some vigorously advocated by professional organizations, lack convincing evidence of efficacy. The clinician should apply preventive interventions with the same thoughtfulness that all other types of care are given.

In the hectic clinic atmosphere, clinicians occasionally forget the important role they play in their patients' lives. Even though patients may recognize the inability of medical care to halt or completely palliate an irreversible decline in their health, many derive consolation and comfort from visits with their regular practitioner. The salutary effects of simply listening and caring should never be dismissed.

As society comes to recognize the limits of technology, there is a resurgence of respect and enthusiasm for the central role of the primary care provider. It is an exacting role that is intellectually challenging and emotionally rewarding. Medical care is now being reorganized around outpatient facilities, with the emergence of new tests and treatments for use in this setting. The astute clinician will master these advances but will continue to recognize that effective practice requires applying this knowledge in an individualized manner guided by a meaningful, personal relationship with the patient.

2 Effective Communication in the Ambulatory Care Setting

WENDY LEVINSON

Rationale. During the medical interview, the clinician must efficiently accomplish three tasks: (1) gather necessary medical information; (2) develop rapport and trust; and (3) educate, instruct, and motivate the patient. Specific communication skills can make the interview more effective and efficient. A successful interview promotes diagnostic accuracy, patient compliance, patient satisfaction, clinician satisfaction, and optimal health outcomes. Good communication also helps prevent patient dissatisfaction and malpractice litigation.

Information Gathering. The clinician needs information to formulate diagnostic hypotheses, test them, and reformulate new ones. Patients need to inform the physician about symptoms, the experience of being ill, and how the problem is affecting their life. Helpful techniques to collect data effectively are listed below:

1. *Use open-ended questions.* Use of open-ended questions early in the interview provides the interviewer with a broad view of what the patient considers to be important. Clinicians should follow open-ended inquiries with more specific questions to gather missing details. Not only does this approach give a more comprehensive picture of the patient's problem but it also is a more efficient strategy than the traditional use of multiple focused questions.

2. *Permit the patient to speak without interruption.* On average, physicians first interrupt patients 18 seconds into their opening statement about the purpose of the visit. Early interruptions can disrupt the development of trust and the flow of the interview. The efficient interviewer gathers

information in the sequence and organization provided by the patient, rather than forcing the patient to conform to a framework.

3. *Survey the breadth of problems early in the interview.* A problem recognized by all clinicians occurs when the patient mentions a new problem as the interview seems to be concluding. This often occurs when the patient has not expressed his or her real agenda early in the interview. To avoid this the clinician should ask the patient "What else?" after the statement of the initial problem and should continue asking "What else?" until all the problems that the patient wants to discuss have been set forth. Although it may not be possible to cover all the topics during one visit, the provider and patient can negotiate what will be covered that day.

4. *Facilitate the patient's story.* To help patients tell the story of their illness, clinicians may use statements like "Go on" and "Tell me more" and indicate nonverbally to the patient that more detail is desirable. This is particularly useful during the initial part of the history when using open-ended questions.

5. *Summarize and check.* Summarizing or repeating parts of the history provides opportunities to correct inaccurate data and allows patients to know that the clinician listens attentively. This can be done briefly following natural breaks in the interview, before moving to a different line of inquiry.

Rapport Building and Addressing Patients' Feelings. Each patient comes to an appointment with real concerns about a problem that interferes with his or her life. The patient has usually thought about the appointment for several days and has often formulated ideas about the cause of the problem and possible treatments. Frequently the problem affects the patient's work, relationships, or sense of well-being. Patients frequently are anxious or distressed when they arrive at the office. Addressing the patient's feelings helps build an alliance between the patient and the clinician and makes the interaction more satisfying for both. Often clinicians think they are "opening a can of worms" by asking about patients' feelings and are worried that this will take too much time in the interview. In fact, addressing the patient's feelings improves the quality of diagnostic information and the therapeutic alliance and makes the interview more efficient. Communication skills to build rapport and deal with patient feelings include the following:

1. *Express empathy.* The practitioner should name the feeling that the patient is experiencing. Examples of statements that recognize the patient's emotional experience are "It sounds as though you are really frustrated" or "You seem sad." Such comments indicate concern for the patient's emotional experience.

2. *Express understanding or reassurance about the feeling.* Clinicians should indicate that they genuinely believe that the patient's feelings are legitimate. For example, the clinician may say, "Many patients feel anxious when they come to the doctor. That's normal." Although clinicians may not always agree that the emotional reaction is appropriate, they can still understand that it is a real feeling for the patient.

3. *Demonstrate respect.* There are many ways, verbal and nonverbal, to dem-

onstrate respect for the patient. Specific strategies include interviewing the patient when he or she is dressed, especially in an initial interview; providing privacy and expressing concern for the patient's comfort; and asking the patient's opinion about the cause of the problem and ideas about treatment. Understanding patient beliefs about the nature of the illness or treatment options is essential to patient compliance.

4. *Prepare for the interview.* Most patients recognize the clinician's busy schedule and wish to use time to maximum advantage. They also want to feel that the clinician has a special interest in and understanding of their concerns. This concern can be readily conveyed by spending a few minutes reviewing the medical record *before* the visit. Even if the physician is behind schedule, it is worth taking time to review the record after notifying the patient that appointments are running late.

Education and Motivation. To realize the benefit of a therapeutic plan, the clinician and patient need to agree on what the problem is and what to do about it. Negotiation is particularly important when helping patients with lifestyle changes (e.g., smoking or dietary change). The key to motivating patients is actively involving them in the development of treatment plans rather than prescribing a treatment regimen. The clinician can use simple questions to actively involve the patient and promote compliance:

1. *What do you know about . . . ?* This question allows the clinician to explore the patient's knowledge and beliefs about the illness or treatment. For example, a clinician might ask, "What do you know about diets to manage diabetes mellitus?" During this discussion information about the treatment can be corrected or added.

2. *How do you feel about . . . ?* This allows the clinician to understand the patient's emotional reaction to a particular illness or treatment option. For example, a patient might say that she feels overwhelmed by having to make the dietary changes necessary. The clinician can then express empathy and understanding about the patient's feelings and incorporate this information into modifications of the treatment plan.

3. *What are you willing to do?* Once the patient has the appropriate information about treatment options, it is essential to find out what part of the proposed treatment the patient is willing to implement. Again, this asks the patient to be an active decision-maker instead of blindly following the clinician's plan.

4. *What help might you need?* This asks the patient to anticipate the type of assistance that might be necessary to carry out the plan. For example, the patient with diabetes might need the help of the spouse with the dietary changes; an appointment for both with a nutritionist might be appropriate.

5. *What problems might arise?* It is helpful to ask the patient to anticipate potential barriers to implementing the therapy and allow an opportunity to plan strategies to address these difficulties. If unmentioned, these barriers might lead to noncompliance.

6. *Now what is your plan?* With this question the clinician asks the patient to reiterate in detail the treatment plan. The clinician can check what the patient has heard and probe any discrepancies between the patient's

and the clinician's understanding of the plan. The review also reinforces the patient's responsibility for implementing the treatment plan.

Cross-Reference: Compliance (Chapter 4).

REFERENCES

1. Beckman HB, Frankel RM. The effect of physician behavior on the collection of data. Ann Intern Med 1984;101:692–696.

   The average patient has three reasons for a visit and gets interrupted within an average of 18 seconds of starting to tell his or her story. Few patients are allowed to tell their story fully. How these interviewing errors interfere with collection of adequate data and alter the physician–patient relationship is discussed.

2. Bird J, Cohen-Cole SA, Mance R. The three function model of the medical interview. In Lipkin M, Putnam S, Lazare A, eds. The Medical Interview. New York, Springer-Verlag, 1991.

   Three functions of the clinical interview are data gathering, emotion handling, and behavior management. A set of basic interviewing skills is described.

3. Lipkin M. The medical interview and related skills. In Branch WT, ed. The Office Practice of Medicine. Philadelphia, WB Saunders, 1987:1287–1306.

   Stepwise guidance and insight into the opening of the interview is provided; and practical advice is given about the physical environment, preparing oneself to listen, and how to structure the opening.

4. Lipkin M, Putman S, Lazare A. The Medical Interview, Clinical Care, Education, and Research. New York, Springer-Verlag, 1995.

   All aspects of the medical interview and physician–patient relationships are explored in this comprehensive textbook.

· ·

3   Ethics in Outpatient Medicine

CLARENCE H. BRADDOCK, III

Outpatient providers, like clinicians on the inpatient wards or in the intensive care unit, face a variety of ethical dilemmas. Although the concerns may seem less dramatic or urgent, they represent a much broader array of issues, such as compliance with medical treatments, confidentiality, and advance care planning.

As compared with the inpatient setting, interactions between patients and primary care practitioners develop over a longer period of time, permitting a richer and more complex relationship. Providers have the opportunity to see their patients in both good and poor health, and often on more equal footing when the patient is clothed, active, and independent. These are opportunities to glimpse the patient's personhood in a manner that is different from the hurried inpatient care environment.

Decision-making in the outpatient setting often occurs over an extended period of time, allowing patients to consider carefully any proposed diagnostic tests or treatments. Their reflection about treatment preferences is less often clouded or pressured by the effects of acute illness, allowing them to play a more active role in decision-making.

The frequency of ethical issues in outpatient visits differs from inpatient practice. The most common category of ethical problems involves patients' preferences. Questions about psychological influences on patients' expressed preferences, truth-telling, and compliance accounted for 59% of all ethical problems observed in one study. Cost of care, the most frequent single ethical issue, accounts for almost 9% of ethical problems.

A proposed taxonomy of outpatient ethical issues divides them into three categories: problems of dual loyalty, problems of communication, and problems of professional and social responsibility (Table 3–1). Many of these problems also occur in the inpatient setting, but their frequency in the outpatient setting mandates special awareness.

THE APPROACH TO ETHICAL PROBLEM SOLVING

Maintaining and fostering an atmosphere of mutual respect, open communication, and shared decision-making is essential. The variety of ethical issues that arise in outpatient medicine necessitates a problem-solving approach that is applicable to a wide range of ethical dilemmas. One approach that has gained wide use involves consideration of topics in four categories: medical indications, patient preferences, quality of life, and contextual features. This approach

Table 3–1. TAXONOMY OF OUTPATIENT ETHICAL ISSUES

Problems of Dual Loyalty	*Problems of Professional and Social Responsibility*
Financial conflicts of interest	Ambulatory education
Legal obligations	Pharmaceutical representatives
Demanding families	For-profit care and research
Referral and consultation	Impaired colleagues
Personal time	Community health
Problems of Communication	
Psychological factors	
Difficult patients	
Noncompliance	
Treatment refusals	
Lifestyle interventions	
Alternative health care	
Competency	
Advance directives	
Assisted suicide	

From LaPuma J, Schiedermayer D. Outpatient clinical ethics. J Gen Intern Med 1989;4:413–420.

emphasizes a consistent and structured method for gathering of relevant facts, analogous to the use of history taking and physical examination as the basis for clinical problem solving. These facts are used to generate hypotheses about the central ethical issue and draw potential parallels to similar cases. The approach is practical in its orientation, seeking to resolve cases with a concrete plan of action rather than abstract deliberation.

In the medical indications category, each medical condition and its proposed management is evaluated for the extent to which it fulfills any of the goals of medicine, such as improvement in function or relief of symptoms. The likelihood of achieving those goals is also considered. For example, if the dilemma involves compliance with antihypertensive medications, the practitioner should review the intent of the intervention and the relevant data about the potential benefits and risks associated with treatment or the alternative, nontreatment.

The patient preferences category involves consideration of the patient's desires in conjunction with his or her mental capacity to make health care decisions. Lacking such capacity, a surrogate decision-maker should be sought to address the patient's wishes for various interventions. This category reminds outpatient clinicians to discuss advance care planning and advance directives for decisions and decision-makers with their patients. These discussions often provide insights about patients' wishes that can be extremely valuable during later hospitalization for acute illness.

In evaluating quality of life, the clinician should discuss with the patient the potential impact of various interventions. By considering their likely effect on quality of life, the clinician can provide the patient an opportunity to make informed decisions about these alternatives. These discussions often prompt further discussion with family members about the value they place on quality of life in different health states.

The contextual features category allows for consideration of social, legal, economic, and institutional circumstances that can influence the decision or be influenced by the decision. For instance, when seeing a patient with a communicable disease, the clinician's willingness to keep the illness confidential is influenced by state law governing the reporting of communicable diseases. Often contextual features modify rather than dictate the practical solution, although this example shows how contextual features may be decisive in some circumstances.

This approach to ethical problems solving in the outpatient setting prompts the clinician to undertake meaningful discussions with patients about the nature of their condition and their views and preferences. The nature of outpatient practice and the long-standing relationships between physician and patient can make ethical discussions easier and more substantive.

REFERENCES

1. Braddock CH, Fihn SD, Levinson W, Jonsen AR, Pearlman RA. How doctors and patients discuss clinical decisions. J Gen Intern Med 1997 *(In press)*.

   By applying a new taxonomy to audiotaped physician-patient encounters in the office setting, the authors describe the range and types of issues discussed and judge how well these discussions adhere to principles of joint decision-making and informed consent.

2. Connelly JE, DalleMura S. Ethical problems in the medical office. JAMA 1988;260:812–815.

   This is a study of the range of ethical issues that occurred in office visits for one of the authors.

3. Jonsen AR, Siegler M, Winslade WJ. Clinical Ethics: A Practical Approach to Ethical Decisions in Clinical Medicine, 3rd ed. New York, McGraw-Hill Book Company, 1992.

Classic yet readable, this book describes a practical approach to ethical problem solving, with extensive references to other materials.

4. LaPuma J, Schiedermayer D. Outpatient clinical ethics. J Gen Intern Med 1989;4:413–420.

A taxonomy is proposed to categorize clinical ethical issues in the outpatient setting, noting important differences from inpatient practice.

4 Compliance

JOHN F. STEINER

Compliance with therapy is defined as the extent to which a patient's behavior (e.g., in keeping appointments, modifying lifestyle, taking medications) conforms to medical advice. Compliance is a crucial link between the *process* of medical care (the interaction between physician and patient) and the *outcomes* of care (the physiologic and functional consequences of treatment). Clinicians often distinguish patients who are "compliant" with treatment from those who are "noncompliant." In fact, many patients take their medications intermittently; these patients are better viewed as partially compliant rather than as absolutely noncompliant with therapy. For most chronic diseases, rates of partial compliance with medications range from 30% to 50%; lack of adherence to recommended behavioral changes is even more common. Partial compliance has long been identified as a barrier to successful treatment; over 30 years ago, patients with a history of rheumatic fever who failed to take sufficient antibiotic prophylaxis were found to have higher rates of recurrent streptococcal infections. More recent work has confirmed the link between partial compliance and poor therapeutic outcomes. For example, reduced compliance is the most common reason for inadequate blood pressure control in hypertensive patients, a common reason for rehospitalization in patients with congestive heart failure and hypertension, and a predictor of poor seizure control in patients with epilepsy.

Physicians often regard partial compliance simplistically, as the patient's defiance of the physician's orders. Research in the social sciences suggests that variations in compliance are better understood as a component of the patient's attempt to control or regulate the illness, based on his or her understanding of the disease and its treatment. A clinician who understands the reasons for such medication "experiments" can better assist the patient in reaching their common goal of treating the disease.

Diagnosis of Partial Compliance with Medications. Identification of partially compliant patients is difficult. Physicians cannot predict accurately which patients are taking their medications as prescribed. Moreover, attainment of a therapeutic goal, such as a controlled blood pressure, is not always an accurate measure of compliance, because many factors other than drug therapy, such as regression to the mean, concurrent nonpharmacologic treatment, or the natural history of the disease, also influence treatment outcomes. Serum drug levels or physiologic effects of drugs (resting pulse in patients on β-adrenergic blockers, prothrombin times in patients receiving warfarin) are also imperfect compliance measures because of pharmacokinetic and pharmacodynamic variability among individuals. Compliance measures used in clinical trials, such as pill counts and electronic medication monitors, are too cumbersome or expensive for routine use. Measures of medication refill rates from centralized pharmacies in managed health care systems may be helpful in assessing pill acquisition, the first stage in compliance. The best screening test for reduced compliance in clinical care is to ask the patient, directly but nonjudgmentally: "Most people have trouble taking their medicine. Do you ever have trouble taking yours?" In response to this question, about 55% of patients who are partially compliant will acknowledge the fact (i.e., the sensitivity of self-report is about 55%), and reports of reduced compliance are generally accurate (positive predictive value of 80% to 90%). However, even those who acknowledge partial compliance generally report being more compliant than they actually are.

Improvement of Compliance. On recognizing partial compliance, the physician should consider whether the patient would benefit from improved adherence. In their efforts at self-regulation, some patients correctly discover that their medications are unnecessary or are prescribed in excessive doses. If the patient has attained the desired outcome despite partial compliance, it may be possible to stop or reduce the medication.

To improve compliance, the clinician should explore the patient's view of the illness and its treatment. Although attempts to educate the patient about the disease and its consequences are useful, such efforts alone rarely improve compliance. Simple treatment regimens lead to better compliance; patients are most likely to comply with once-a-day drugs. Strategies for behavior modification can also enhance compliance in several ways:

1. The physician can identify and reschedule patients who drop out of care.
2. The individual can learn to monitor the illness through techniques such as home blood pressure measurement or glucose testing.
3. The patient can link the taking of medication to other routine activities. For example, the patient can store pills next to the coffeepot or hairbrush, where they will be seen every morning.
4. Family members or home health care workers can be enlisted to monitor the disease or assist the patient in taking pills.
5. The clinician can establish contracts with the patient to provide rewards for adherence, such as credit toward the purchase of a blood pressure cuff for home use.

Combinations of these behavioral strategies work best, but require continuous reinforcement.

REFERENCES

1. Cramer JA, Mattson RH, Prevey ML, Scheyer RD, Ouellette VL. How often is medication taken as prescribed? A novel assessment technique. JAMA 1989;261:3273–3277.

This study demonstrates the insights that electronic medication monitors can offer in compliance research, proves the clinical adage that adherence improves with simpler medication regimens, and links compliance to outcomes (seizure control) in a group of epileptic patients.

2. Haynes RB, Taylor DW, Sackett DL, eds. Compliance in Health Care. Baltimore, Johns Hopkins University Press, 1979.

   The standard textbook in the field, this work includes the epidemiology, measurement, and implications of compliance for medical practice and clinical research.

3. Haynes RB, Wang E, Gomes MD. A critical review of interventions to improve compliance with prescribed medications. Patient Ed Counseling 1987;10:155–166.

   This comprehensive literature synthesis emphasizes the need for practitioners to learn and employ techniques of behavior modification to improve adherence.

4. Leventhal H, Cameron L. Behavioral therapies and the problem of compliance. Patient Ed Counseling 1987;10:117–138.

   A view of compliance from the perspective of the social sciences summarizes the most common theories of compliance behavior.

5. Stephenson BJ, Rowe BH, Haynes RB, Macharia WM, Leon G. Is the patient taking the treatment as prescribed? JAMA 1993;269:2779–2781.

   A discussion of clinically applicable methods for detecting reduced compliance emphasizes the identification of two "at-risk" groups: individuals who do not keep appointments and those who do not respond to treatment and report lapses in adherence.

■ ■

5 Determining Disability: The Primary Care Physician's Role

ASHER A. TULSKY

Conducting a disability evaluation is a confusing and often frustrating process for most primary care physicians. This is mainly due to three factors: (1) the number of different private and governmental disability programs; (2) a lack of understanding, by providers and patients alike, of what the process entails; and (3) the ambiguity physicians often feel when simultaneously providing primary care and assessing an applicant for disability. The situation is aggravated by the marked increase in applicants over the past decade. In 1995, 3.6 million initial disability claims for Social Security were filed, representing an 86% increase since 1990. Recent changes in welfare legislation will likely lead to an even greater increase in applications. By understanding the disability evaluation process and their role in the process, primary care physicians can be more effective and will find the experience less distressing.

In the United States, there are two major governmental programs that provide redress for work incapacity: Social Security Disability and workers' compensation. There are, in addition, hundreds of private disability programs administered by commercial insurance companies. The Social Security Disability Program is the world's largest nationally administered program with uniform regulations and well-outlined definitions of medical impairment. Workers' compensation, however, is a state-based system, and procedures vary from state to state. Private insurers also have different medical, vocational, and economic eligibility criteria for applicants to receive cash benefits. Although the focus of this discussion is on Social Security Disability Insurance (SSDI), many of the principles also apply to other programs.

The Social Security Disability Process. The Social Security Administration (SSA) regulates two distinct disability programs that provide for cash benefits if eligibility criteria are met. Title II, or SSDI, provides coverage for those disabled workers and their dependents who have contributed to the trust fund through a payroll tax on their earnings. Title XVI, or Supplemental Security Income (SSI), is a needs-based entitlement program that provides a minimum income level for the aged, blind, and disabled who have not contributed to the trust fund. These two programs differ only in their economic and vocational eligibility criteria; they share the same medical criteria for benefits eligibility. Knowledge of several SSA definitions (from the SSA's handbook for physicians entitled *Disability Evaluation Under Social Security*) is important in understanding how the disability determination process works.

Disability is "the inability to engage in any substantial gainful activity by reason of any medically determinable physical or mental impairment which can be expected to result in death or has lasted, or can be expected to last, for a continuous period of not less than 12 months." It refers to the incapacity of an individual to meet certain standards of physical efficacy and/or economic responsibility and is assessed by an administrative agency.

Impairment is "a physical or mental limitation in function resulting from a disease process. The impairment must manifest as signs or laboratory findings apart from symptoms." Abnormalities that manifest themselves only as symptoms are not medically determinable (e.g., pain or fatigue). Impairment reflects the organic pathophysiologic characteristics of the disease. Physicians document impairment only, not disability.

Medical evidence is information supplied by physicians; it includes findings of the history and physical examination and supporting laboratory data. Although the medical evidence provides the cornerstone in the application process, it is not the sole determining factor.

The claimant initiates the process at a local SSA office, where an administrative worker takes a medical history, occupational history, and detailed income history. Medical evidence is obtained from the treating physician and other sources such as hospital discharge summaries. A consultative examination may be purchased by the SSA when medical evidence is missing. At this time the physician is expected only to document the patient's medical impairment, *not* to render an opinion on the applicant's ability to work. A physician-administrator panel employed by the agency then renders an initial determination based on a composite of determined medical impairment(s), age, education, and past work experience.

If the applicant disagrees with an unfavorable initial administrative decision, the applicant must request reconsideration within 60 days. Another physician-administrator panel reconsiders the application; and if the decision is again unfavorable, the applicant may appeal to an administrative law judge (a specially trained administrator who adjudicates cases within the Social Security system). Further appeals go to the Social Security Appeals Council and finally US District Court. For these latter stages of the appeals process, claimants often secure the services of an attorney on a contingency basis, or in SSI cases, a free legal services attorney. It is at the appeals stage that the physician may render an opinion on the patient's employability. Before this, he or she only provides the medical evidence. Updated medical evidence is presented at each of these levels, which is one reason physicians get recurrent requests for medical evidence.

The appeals process can be protracted, with processing times in 1995 estimated to be 154 days for the decision of an initial disability claim and 342 days between an appeal to an administrative law judge hearing and a decision. Because of these prolonged turn-around times, the SSA is planning changes, including streamlining the appeals process, providing uniform medical evidence forms (currently different among states), offering better reimbursement to physicians for earlier return of medical evidence forms, and assigning a disability claim manager to handle most aspects of the claim at the initial level. In addition, SSA plans to develop standard training materials for physicians and consultation examiners.

The Role of the Primary Care Physician. The principal role of the physician in the initial disability application is to provide medical evidence for the administrative agency by documenting medical impairment. Misperceptions of this role by physicians and patients alike may lead to anger and anxiety, straining the physician–patient relationship. If physicians have a clear concept of their role and are knowledgeable about the disability determination process, they can play an important role in the outcome.

At the initiation of the application process, the primary care provider should discuss the reasons a patient feels the need to apply for disability income and what alternatives exist to discontinuing employment. This is a good time to elicit the patient's ideas, concerns, and expectations about living with a disability and the effect that leaving the work force might have on a patient's self-image. It is also a good time to clarify with the patient the disability determination process and the role the physician will play in it. The patient should clearly be told that the physician only documents impairment in the initial application and is not expected to make a statement regarding the patient's employability. The patient should also be aware of the potentially lengthy course of the determination process. It is best to avoid predicting the chances of the patient's receiving disability benefits.

The medical evidence forms supplied by the Social Security Determinations Agency should be completed by addressing specific medical criteria described in the SSA's handbook for physicians. These criteria are broken down by organ system. The handbook is available free of charge from the US Department of Health and Human Services or at any local SSA office.

Based on these defined criteria, the physician completes the medical evidence form by documenting the diagnosis, including history, physical examination, laboratory tests, and assessment as to severity. The physician also forwards copies of key diagnostic studies with the initial request for information. Dictating the medical summary, with appropriate copies of relevant laboratory reports, studies, and hospital discharge summaries, can streamline the paperwork. A toll-free dictation service is listed on the medical evidence forms for this purpose. Copies of these summaries are returned to the physician for the patient's record and may also be used to respond to requests for information from private insurance companies. An alternative method of providing medical evidence and perhaps most time efficient for the practitioner is to photocopy appropriate portions of the medical record and forward these to the administrative office.

Applicants who are denied benefits and who appeal may face lengthy delays. Periodic updated reports may be requested from the primary care provider. If there has been no change in clinical status since the time of the initial assessment, this is all that needs to be documented. Copies of all forms and summaries should be kept with the patient's medical record in a separate section for easy reference.

During the appeals process, the physician may be asked for an opinion regarding the patient's ability to work. At this time, letters and personal statements are not only accepted but also welcomed and can have an impact on the final determination.

The timely submission of the medical evidence forms is important. Delays by physicians due to perceived lack of time, aversion to the paperwork, and minimal reimbursement contribute in part to the prolonged time to final determination. Patients unable to work may undergo undue hardship until benefits begin, with delays sometimes lasting a year or more. Anticipated changes in the determination process will tie improved physician reimbursement to the promptness of forms completed and returned.

Impact on the Physician–Patient Relationship. Practitioners often believe that one of the major challenges they experience in performing disability assessments is the intrusion of a bureaucratic agency into the physician–patient relationship. Tension develops when it is not clear to either the patient or the practitioner whether the physician is playing the role of advocate or adjudicator. It is further complicated by the requirement for objective evidence of impairment, that is, physical evidence of organic disease as a cause of impairment. Physicians know that much of disability consists of illness behavior that cannot be objectively documented. When patients experience distress that limits their ability to work, it is often more a psychosocial than a pathophysiologic process that is involved. Studies have shown a strong relationship between psychosocial work environment and musculoskeletal pain disorders, whereas physical findings are less predictive of these disorders. Conflict may arise between the physician and patient when there is discordance between the physical findings and a patient's perception of his or her disability.

Several communication strategies may help to avoid conflict. First, it is important to clarify to the patient the disability process and the physician's role in reporting objective, laboratory-based evidence of impairment. Second, the physician should avoid confusing the disability evaluation process with the delivery of good primary care. It is recommended that providers:

1. Find out what other stresses, conflicts, and demands the patient is experiencing, because this may provide insight into the illness behavior.
2. Be empathic. When a provider responds in a supportive manner to the distress that accompanies illness, loss of livelihood, and the vagaries of a bureaucratic system, this empathy can help forge a collaborative relationship without sacrificing the physician's integrity.
3. Set clear boundaries and limits, making clear to patients that the provider's care and the requirements for disability evaluation are different. Effective limit setting is the key to avoiding getting "caught in the middle" between the patient's experience of illness and the very specific responsibilities physicians have in the evaluation process.
4. Be aware of different perceptions of illness that patients and providers may have and at the same time strive to remain nonjudgmental. Whereas many physicians tend to be compulsive and driven, rarely missing a day of work for personal illness, many patients may not be able to function effectively with similar limitations.

REFERENCES

1. Carey TS, Hadler NM. The role of the primary physician in disability determination for Social Security insurance and workers' compensation. Ann Intern Med 1986;104:706–710.

    This is still the best description of the process of evaluation of disability claims and when the primary care physician should be involved.

2. Deyo RA, Diehl AK. Psychosocial predictors of disability in patients with low back pain. J Rheumatol 1988;15:1557–1564

    A prospective study of 179 patients with low back pain found that psychosocial characteristics predicted functional disability better than physical findings.

3. Disability Evaluation Under Social Security. Social Security Administration publication No. 64-039. Washington, DC, US Department of Health and Human Services, 1995.

    The most recently updated version of the comprehensive listing of clinical findings that fulfill the Social Security Administration's definition of impairment, this edition has revised respiratory, cardiovascular, and immune system listings and should be in every primary care provider's office.

4. Linton SJ, Kamwendo K. Risk factors in the psychosocial work environment for neck and shoulder pain in secretaries. J Occup Med 1989;31:7:609–613.

    This descriptive study of 420 secretaries at a large medical center suggests a relationship between neck and shoulder pain and psychosocial work environment factors. Work content and social aspects of work were found to be most influential.

5. Plan for a New Disability Claim Process. Social Security Administration publication No. 01-005. Washington, DC, US Department of Health and Human Services, 1994.

    An overview of the current problems in processing disability claims is provided along with an outline of anticipated changes in this process.

6 Death of Clinic Patients

SUSAN W. TOLLE and PAUL B. BASCOM

Advance Directives. Approximately 80% of deaths occur in hospitals or long-term care facilities, and 70% are under circumstances in which a decision is made to withhold medical intervention. It is increasingly important that families and physicians have previously discussed and understood a patient's preferences regarding life-sustaining treatment. When those discussions occur in the clinic, before death is imminent, admission to the hospital for terminal care may be prevented. The patient is still capable of making thoughtful decisions, and the family and the physician can be confident that they understand the patient's preferences. Communication both respects the patient's values and facilitates the adjustment of survivors. In one study of surviving spouses a year after a loved one's death, those who made decisions about withholding or withdrawing life-sustaining treatment without the benefit of a prior directive from the patient had many continuing anxieties. They continued to wonder whether they had made the right decision, whereas spouses who clearly understood their loved one's wishes were more often at peace with their decisions.

Even though most patients wish their physicians would talk with them about advance planning for serious illness, initiating these conversations can be uncomfortable for the physician and the patient. Patients' anxieties often increase when they fear their physician is encouraging advanced planning for medical reasons. Patients find it reassuring to know that the physician talks with all of his or her patients about these issues and that a serious health problem has not prompted the discussion because the physician has serious concerns about the patient's health. A helpful approach is to open the conversation with: "I like to talk with all of my patients about advance planning for serious illness. I do not expect any sudden change in your health in the near future, but an accident could happen to any of us at any time. There have been some recent changes in the law that clarify a patient's rights to set limits on his or her health care. Many of my patients want to talk about these laws and share their values and goals. I am open to talking with you about these issues."

Two types of advance directives are commonly available. One is the living will, which is more prevalent and allows patients the right to refuse life-sustaining treatment when death is imminent. The newer and more flexible document, the power of attorney for health care, allows patients to appoint someone else to act as their health care representative should they be unable to speak for themselves. Although advance directives are often completed in the outpatient setting, the Patient Self-Determination Act requires that all adult patients admitted to hospitals, nursing homes, or hospice programs be informed of their right to refuse life-sustaining treatment and offered the opportunity to sign an advance directive. Because state statutes vary, the organization

18

Choice in Dying offers current state specific forms and information on advance directives. It can be reached at 1-800-989-WILL or 212-366-5540.

Terminal Illness. Most deaths are anticipated. It is important to discuss several issues with the patient and family before the patient's death.

1. Tell patients specifically what to expect regarding their illness.
2. Reassure patients that everything will be done to keep them comfortable.
3. Help patients share the diagnosis with friends or family so they can provide support and help with advance planning and legal issues.
4. Discuss advance directives.
5. Encourage conversations about organ donation and autopsy.

Family members take particular comfort in knowing they have followed the patient's wishes.

HOME HOSPICE CARE. Since enactment of the Medicare Hospice Benefit a decade ago, an increasing number of dying patients are being cared for at home with the help of home hospice agencies. Eligibility for home hospice care includes the presence of an illness likely to cause death within 6 months in the usual course of the illness and the availability of a caregiver, family member, or other to provide care on a 24-hour basis. Of equal importance is the recognition, by patient, family, and physician, that the disease is terminal and that the focus of treatment is amelioration of symptoms and not prolongation of life.

Enrolling patients in home hospice provides access to an array of benefits through the skills of a multidisciplinary team. Regular visits by a nurse skilled at pain assessment and titration of opioid analgesics assist physicians to maintain good pain control even as symptoms worsen. Nurses can teach patients and families how to use opioids and recognize side effects. Physical therapists select appropriate assistive equipment for the home and teach families caregiving skills in the presence of declining functional status. Social workers aid families in obtaining financial assistance and other community resources and begin discussions about post-death planning needs, such as selection of funeral homes. If further spiritual support is desired, a chaplain from the team may visit the home.

At the time of death, the nurse should immediately go to the home to confirm the death and to provide emotional support to family members. Home hospice programs also provide bereavement services to surviving family members for up to 1 year after the death.

Notification of a Patient's Death. After a patient's death, the needs of the survivors are influenced by the duration of the patient's illness, whether the death was expected, the patient's age, the amount of advanced planning and guidance the patient has provided, whether family members were present at the time of death, and the strength of the physician–family relationship. After a long terminal illness, death may be a relief for the family and physician. Conversely, sudden and unexpected death in a healthy person can be catastrophic for survivors.

EXPECTED DEATH. As death approaches, advance planning with families about notification of death may be helpful. When death is long expected, some families believe they have said their good-byes and ask to be notified by phone when the death occurs. They may want the opportunity to return to the patient's bedside. Others may request that another individual, family friend, or clergy be notified first. Some families strongly wish to be present at the bedside at the time of death and deeply appreciate notification that the patient's death appears imminent. These families desire privacy (i.e., a room where they can grieve together without interruption) and the extra time physicians may spend with them. Predictable questions may arise: Did the patient suffer? What was the immediate cause of death? Was the patient aware of the family members' presence? Was there anything the family could have done to prevent the patient's death? What does the family do next? Religious preferences should be considered; and, if appropriate, specific denominational representatives should be summoned.

The physician should understand the hospital's administrative procedures regarding completion of forms, return of personal effects, autopsy, and organ donation. Federal legislation requires that family members be offered the opportunity to consent to an anatomic gift if the patient is medically eligible as a donor. Before these discussions take place, however, the physician should determine the patient's eligibility to avoid offering the opportunity to donate only to realize later that the organs or tissues cannot be used. Consent for organ donation and autopsy is the exclusive prerogative of the next of kin or legal guardian; the physician can only advise, explaining potential benefits to the family while respecting their right to accept or refuse.

The physician's support of the family does not end with the patient's death. For close family members, the bereavement period is characterized by depressive symptoms and somatic complaints and, for some, increased rates of hospitalization and even death. Table 6–1 lists different avenues of subsequent contact between survivors and primary physicians; these options provide knowledge and comfort and tend to reduce the survivor's anxiety.

UNEXPECTED DEATH. The unexpected death of a clinic patient creates special needs both for family members, who have little opportunity for advanced planning, and for physicians, who often experience concern about personal inadequacy. Families are often the first to learn of a patient's death when it occurs outside the hospital; the physician, once notified, should telephone the family to provide emotional support and, if possible, clarify the cause of death.

When an unexpected death occurs in the hospital, physicians are frequently apprehensive about conveying the news to the family. In general, revealing an unexpected death by telephone should be avoided. Most families

Table 6–1. OPTIONS IN PROVIDING BEREAVEMENT SUPPORT

Send a sympathy card
Call the family
Attend the funeral
Mail bereavement information*: pamphlets on grief and a community support list
Provide a lay explanation of the autopsy findings
Schedule a family conference
Cultivate a network to facilitate your own support

*Contact the hospital social worker or chaplain.

prefer to be called and asked to come to the hospital, where they can be notified of the death in person. Some consider this practice deceptive and prefer to be told during the initial phone conversation. It is usually easy to separate these two groups. Some survivors, when asked to come to the hospital, will ask the physician directly if the patient has died. They should be told the truth. Those who do not ask probably prefer to be told at the hospital because it allows direct contact with the physician, offers the opportunity for family members and close friends to be notified together for mutual support, and allows family members an opportunity to see the deceased. Viewing the body directly confirms the reality of death and helps family members overcome denial and begin the grieving process.

Maintaining open communication with the patient's loved ones is important, though often difficult after an unexpected death (see Table 6–1). Survivors often appreciate written information about the normal grieving process. The optimal timing for bereavement information varies; some prefer to receive it after the memorial service, whereas most others find it most helpful 2 weeks to 3 months after an unexpected death. After an unexpected death, families often need longer to adjust and are more likely to benefit from a bereavement support group, although many are unable to attend support groups for at least 3 months. Support is even more valuable for families with a limited social support system and for survivors of patients who have committed suicide.

The Physician's Emotional Needs. Physicians commonly believe that their own outward expression of grief over a patient's death somehow falls short of personal, professional, or societal expectations. Usually family members do not find it offensive when physicians express emotion after a patient's death. Physicians cannot help having feelings about the death of a long-standing clinic patient. These feelings may include sadness, fear of inadequacy, a sense of loss, and even a sense of relief. To ignore these feelings or to allow them to go unaddressed is unhealthy. Physicians also benefit from sharing their fears of inadequacy and feelings of loss with a colleague or a support group. Attending a patient's funeral not only may help physicians express and resolve their own feelings but shows respect for the patient and family.

REFERENCES

1. Creagan ET. How to break bad news and not devastate the patient. Mayo Clin Proc 1994; 69:1015–1017.

   Strategies are given for delivering bad news both before and after a patient's death.

2. Gordon GH, Tolle SW. Discussing life-sustaining treatment: A teaching program for residents. Arch Intern Med 1991;151:567–570.

   An educational program is outlined for residents to practice their skills in discussing advance directives.

3. Irvine P. The attending at the funeral. N Engl J Med 1985;312:1704–1705.

   This article suggests that physicians often benefit from attending the funeral of their patient.

4. Tilden VP, Tolle SW, et al. Decisions about life-sustaining treatment: Impact of physicians' behaviors on the family. Arch Intern Med 1995;155:633–638.

Through family interviews specific behaviors of health care providers are identified that increased or reduced the family's burden in making the decision to withdraw life support.

5. Tolle SW, Bascom PB, Hickam DH, et al. Communication between physicians and surviving spouses following patient deaths. J Gen Intern Med 1986;1:309–314.

Data are provided about unmet needs from interviews with 105 surviving spouses.

Preventive Services

● ●

7 Principles of Screening

DAVID L. SIMEL

Definition. Screening is the process of detecting disease early, before it causes symptoms. Several factors must be present for effective screening programs:

1. The target disease is an important clinical problem.
2. The screening test is accurate, widely available, and acceptable to patients and physicians.
3. The natural history of the target disease is understood, and there is a presymptomatic stage.
4. Treatment for the target condition is available, acceptable, and efficacious.

Principle 1. *The target disease is an important clinical problem.* To be "important," the disease must be common enough that many patients benefit from early detection. In addition, the disease should be associated with significant morbidity or mortality. Examples of common important diseases include hypertension, breast carcinoma, and gestational diabetes.

Prevalence describes the proportion of patients who have disease in a given population (Fig. 7–1):

$$\text{Prevalence} = \frac{(A + C)}{(A + B + C + D)}$$

Prevalence describes the prior odds that a disease is present before a screening test is performed. Thus,

$$\text{Prior odds} = \frac{\text{Prevalence}}{1 - \text{Prevalence}}$$

		Disease	
		Present	Absent
Test Result	Positive	*A*	*B*
	Negative	*C*	*D*

Figure 7–1. 2 × 2 Table (see text).

All of the material in Chapter 7 is in the public domain, with the exception of any borrowed figures and tables.

For example, if the prevalence of disease is 5%, the prior odds = (0.05)/
(0.95) = 0.053.

When reading medical literature, the physician must understand the population used to describe test performance. Because the prevalence of disease
may depend on geography and on the sex and age of the patient, the
physician's patient population may differ from published study populations.

Principle 2. *The screening test is accurate, widely available, and acceptable.* Screening
tests must be acceptable and available (e.g., reasonable cost and little discomfort for patients; easy to perform or order for the physician). However, to
decide whether a screening test works the clinician uses the operating characteristics of a test, *sensitivity* and *specificity,* together with the prior odds.

$$\text{Sensitivity} = \frac{\text{No. of diseased patients with a positive screening test}}{\text{No. of all patients with the disease}} = \frac{A}{A + C}$$

$$\text{Specificity} = \frac{\text{No. of normal patients with a negative screening test}}{\text{No. of all normal patients}} = \frac{D}{B + D}$$

These values define the odds favoring disease if the test result is positive (also
called the positive likelihood ratio [LR+]):

$$\text{LR}+ \ = \frac{\text{Sensitivity}}{1 - \text{Specificity}}$$

or the odds favoring disease if the test result is negative (also called the negative
likelihood ratio [LR−]):

$$\text{LR}- \ = \frac{1 - \text{Sensitivity}}{\text{Specificity}}$$

For example, a test with sensitivity of 80% and specificity of 80% has an LR+
of 4.0 and an LR− of 0.25.

The prior odds are multiplied by the appropriate likelihood ratio to yield
the odds of disease after performing the test:

$$\text{Posterior odds} = \text{Prior odds} \times \text{LR}$$

The likelihood ratio is represented by LR+ for a positive screening test result
and LR− for a negative screening test. Thus, the posterior odds depends on
the prevalence of disease in the population under study and on the operating
characteristics of the test. If a test with a sensitivity of 80% and a specificity of
80% yields positive results in a patient from the population described in
principle 1, the odds that disease is actually present increases from the prior
odds of 0.053 to the posterior odds 0.053 × 4.0 = 0.212.

Because it is sometimes easier to think of the probability of an event than
the odds of an event, the odds ratio can be converted back to probability
estimates by the equation:

$$\text{Probability} = \frac{\text{Odds}}{1 + \text{Odds}}$$

Therefore, a positive test result increases the prior probability of disease (prevalence) from 5% to the posterior probability of 17.5% for this example [0.212/ (1 + 0.212)].

To assess the likelihood of disease when a test result is negative, multiply the prior odds by LR− to get the posterior odds (e.g., 0.053 × 0.25). In this example, a negative test result decreases the probability of disease from 5% to 1.3%.

Some clinicians prefer to use predictive values rather than likelihood ratios to describe the diagnostic impact of test results. The positive predictive value is figured as the proportion of patients with positive screening tests who actually have disease; the negative predictive value is figured as the proportion of patients with negative tests who actually do not have disease. Predictive values have limited diagnostic utility unless the population prevalence is well described.

Principle 3. *The natural history of the target disease is understood, and there is a presymptomatic stage.* This simple statement is extremely important. If there is no presymptomatic stage of a disease, the disease cannot be detected before it causes symptoms. Thus, for such disease (e.g., impotence, appendicitis, or pneumonia) there will be no effective screening test.

Principle 4. *Treatment for the target condition is acceptable, available, and efficacious.* This final principle suggests that we should screen only for diseases that can be affected positively by treatment. Although this may seem obvious, determining whether treatment is acceptable, available, and efficacious may be difficult. This decision requires a clear understanding of the individual patient's medical, psychological, and socioeconomic conditions and requires the physician to know the best available medical information. For many diseases for which evidence of treatment efficacy from randomized clinical trials is lacking, decision analysis may suggest appropriate strategies that can be considered for individual patients. Screening for cervical carcinoma is a strategy that meets these requirements. Screening for lung carcinoma does not meet these requirements because current evidence suggests that screening has no impact on outcomes.

REFERENCES

1. Sackett DL., Haynes RB, Guyatt G, Tugwell P. Clinical Epidemiology: A Basic Science for Clinical Medicine. Boston, Little, Brown & Co, 1991.

   This is the single best reference to learn methods for critically appraising evidence of efficacy from the medical literature.

2. Sox HC, Blatt MA, Higgins MC, Marton KI. Medical Decision Making. Boston, Butterworths, 1988.

   This is an excellent introductory text regarding the tools of decision and cost-effectiveness analysis. The appendix lists likelihood ratios for commonly performed tests.

3. US Department of Health and Human Services. Clinician's Handbook of Preventive Services. Baltimore, Williams & Wilkins, 1996.

   This is a superb and readable text with recommendations for screening that are supported with evidence from the literature.

8 Periodic Health Assessment

DONALD W. BELCHER

Preventive Services. In selecting general preventive services for adult patients, it is important to distinguish between a test's usefulness for diagnostic versus its usefulness for screening purposes. Many tests of proven value in the diagnosis of symptomatic adults (e.g., glucose and hemoglobin determinations, thyroid studies, chest radiography) perform poorly as screening measures in asymptomatic adults. This discussion is largely based on an authoritative review, the *Guide to Clinical Preventive Services*, by the US Preventive Services Task Force, which uses explicit criteria of efficacy and effectiveness to evaluate preventive activities (see Chapter 7, Principles of Screening) and compares its recommendations with those published by other authorities.

Because the prevalence of a target condition or of related risk factors determines a screening test's predictive value, general preventive services are most effective when directed at subgroups with certain age, sex, or behavioral factors (Table 8–1). Patients at higher risk because of a family medical history, environmental hazards, or other risk factors need special preventive services (Table 8–2). Health maintenance flow sheets that list recommended prevention activities, attributes of target groups, and frequency of testing are helpful aids for practitioners. Over 75% of Americans see a physician each year—far more than are likely to volunteer for separate screening programs. Patient visits for management of chronic or episodic illnesses should serve as opportunities to provide preventive services. Rapport and familiarity with an individual patient's health status assist in the appropriate delivery of prevention services. Preventable behaviors lead to a heavy burden of illness and death. Special attention should be given to smoking cessation strategies (see Chapter 12, Smoking Cessation) and how to identify and manage alcohol and substance abuse (see Chapter 9, Diagnosis and Management of Drug Abuse, and Chapter 10, Alcohol Problems), areas where physicians express difficulty in intervening. To avoid overlooking adult immunizations, practitioners need to understand the rationale for immunizing general and high-risk patients (see Chapter 11, Adult Immunizations). Despite incomplete evidence and conflicting recommendations, physicians must make prevention decisions for individual patients and should update these recommendations as additional information becomes available.

The Periodic Health Assessment. The periodic health assessment is more than an examination. It is a set of recommended prevention activities to be conducted at specified intervals for various age groups. It includes risk factor assessment, immunization, disease screening (physical examination, laboratory tests, or other procedures), and patient health education (i.e., the acronym

Table 8–1. **PREVENTION RECOMMENDATIONS FOR GENERAL ADULT POPULATION**

Procedure	Target Condition	Target Group	Recommendation
Smoking cessation	Cardiovascular and pulmonary disease; some cancers	Smokers	Annual counseling
Alcohol moderation	Medical conditions; accidents, violence	General	Annual counseling
Diet change	Obesity; medical	General	Periodic assessment
Exercise schedule	Coronary heart disease; various	General	Individualize to needs
Blood pressure measurement	Hypertension	General	At 1- to 2-yr intervals
Breast examination	Breast cancer	Women 40+ yr	Annual
Papanicolaou smear	Cervical cancer	Women 20–65 yr	3-yr intervals or less
Influenza vaccine	Influenza	Elderly: patients with chronic disease	Annual vaccination
Pneumococcal vaccine	Pneumonia	Elderly: patients with chronic disease	Vaccinate once; may repeat in very elderly after 5 years
Tetanus/diphtheria toxoid	Infections	General	10-yr intervals
Cholesterol (total; low density lipoprotein)	Coronary heart disease	Men (35–64 yr) and women (45–64 yr)	5-yr intervals
Mammography	Breast cancer	Women 50–69 yr	At 1- to 2-yr intervals
Fecal occult blood test	Colorectal cancer	Men and women 50–74 yr	1- to 2-yr intervals
Sigmoidoscopy	Colorectal cancer	Men and women 50–74 yr	Frequency unclear

RISE). It is more selective and individualized than a routine medical checkup and has a higher yield and a lower cost. The purpose of the periodic health assessment is to prevent certain target diseases (primary prevention) or to detect disease at an early stage and improve outcome (secondary prevention).

A consensus on the content or frequency of the adult periodic health assessment is elusive, with authorities often differing in their interpretation of published evidence or recommendations. There may be insufficient information about a disease's natural course (e.g., prostate cancer), the estimated cost-benefit ratio for different screening intervals (e.g., mammography), or the appropriateness of applying trial results to age groups other than those studied (e.g., cholesterol screening). Much remains to be learned about disease prevention in adults older than age 65, the group at highest risk for many diseases such as coronary heart disease, most cancers, and strokes. Screening activities for vision, hearing, falls, foot problems, and osteoporosis—important concerns for the elderly—are generally not listed among recommendations because test effectiveness is unknown.

Recommendations. Table 8–1 lists recommended adult preventive care activities, the target group, and the frequency of testing.

Table 8–2. PREVENTION RECOMMENDATIONS FOR HIGH-RISK INDIVIDUALS

Procedure	Target Condition	Target Group	Recommendation
Estrogen counseling	Osteoporosis	Women, perimenopausal smokers	At menopause
Aspirin counseling	Coronary heart disease	Men aged 50+ with cardiovascular risk factors	Periodically
Skin review	Skin cancer	Family history; history of excess sun, cancer precursors*	Special surveillance, annual examination
Oral cavity examination	Oropharyngeal cancer	Smokers, drinkers	Annual
Thyroid examination	Thyroid cancer	History of upper body irradiation	2- to 3-yr intervals
Papanicolaou smear	Cervical cancer	Women aged 65+ with irregular screening history	Annual × two negatives
Testes examination	Testicular cancer	Men < 40 years; history of cryptorchidism	Periodic
Vaccination (influenza; pneumococcal)	Pneumonia, complications	Resident of nursing home or extended care facility	Annual influenza; pneumococcal—may repeat in very elderly after 5 yr
Human immuno-deficiency virus (HIV), hepatitis B	Acquired immunodeficiency syndrome, hepatitis	Possible HIV exposure	Individualized testing: safe sex counseling
VDRL	Syphilis	Multiple sexual partners	Individualized testing
Mammography	Breast cancer	Family history of premenopausal breast cancer	Start at age 35
Colonoscopy	Colorectal cancer	Family history	Persons aged 50+: every 3–5 yr

*Dysplastic nevi, some congenital nevi.
VDRL, Venereal Disease Research Laboratory.

Preventive Cardiology. Because cardiovascular disease dominates disease patterns in the United States and because effective early detection techniques are lacking, primary prevention is an important goal. Epidemiologic studies, such as the Framingham Study, link smoking, hypertension, and elevated cholesterol levels to the development of coronary heart disease, stroke, and peripheral vascular disease. Half of coronary heart disease is attributable to smoking, hypertension, and elevated cholesterol, with 30% of cases being due to cigarette smoking.

Whereas smoking cessation and control of hypertension reduce complications of coronary heart disease by 50% per year and 25% per year, respectively, lowering elevated cholesterol reduces such events by about 19% per year. Smoking cessation also reduces lung disease and deaths from cancer, improves pregnancy outcome, and reduces illness in family members (from passive exposure to smoking). Widespread public acceptance that smoking cessation is beneficial, an increasing awareness of risk from passive exposure, and smoke-free policies in hospitals, domestic airlines, and many job sites help motivate smokers to change. Strategies to individualize smoking interventions are discussed in Chapter 12.

Treatment of moderate to severe hypertension (diastolic blood pressure of 105 mm Hg or higher) clearly reduces the rates of stroke, congestive heart failure, and hypertensive renal failure. Trials indicate that all hypertensive adults, whose diagnoses are based on three separate blood pressure measurements, benefit from treatment. The benefits of treating mild hypertension are probably modest.

Because about 60% of hypertensive patients are overweight—twice the rate as in the general population—it is prudent to include advice about weight control, sodium restriction, and adequate exercise. Recent studies indicate that minority groups experience more complications from hypertension, in part because of lower compliance with medication and a belief in nonmedical models to explain hypertension. The treatment of systolic hypertension, more prevalent in the elderly, has similar benefits (see Chapter 85, Essential Hypertension).

In the United States, cholesterol levels tend to rise with age. The evidence for an epidemiologic association of cholesterol levels with coronary heart disease is clear, but the exact benefits of intervention trials are debated. Treatment has well-established benefits for individuals with known coronary artery disease. Cholesterol reduction also benefits asymptomatic middle-aged adults with high levels. Most physicians tell patients with high cholesterol levels to reduce their fat intake, lose weight, and exercise more. In the trials usually cited, diet was tested not alone but in combination with other interventions, such as smoking cessation, the treatment of hypertension, or the administration of cholestyramine or an HMG-CoA reductase inhibitor. Persons who consistently comply with dietary advice may lower their cholesterol levels about 5%, but responses vary considerably and relapse is common. Consequently, a decision to intervene usually involves the prescription of a lipid-lowering medication and regular testing (see Chapter 152, Hyperlipidemia). Many physicians do not have the time, nutritional information, or behavior modification skills necessary to counsel patients regarding diet; these physicians are encouraged to involve dietitians and to refer patients to selected community nutrition education programs.

The total cholesterol level, measured without fasting, was the value used in epidemiologic studies and all primary prevention trials and remains the starting point for assessing an individual's risk. Recent food intake does not affect values. The National Cholesterol Education Program (NCEP) recommends that all adults be tested at 5-year intervals. High-risk persons, defined as those having a total cholesterol level of 240 mg/dL or higher, should also undergo lipoprotein analysis to determine high density lipoprotein (HDL) and low density lipoprotein (LDL) values before diet modification or selection of a lipid-lowering medication. Persons with borderline cholesterol levels (200–239 mg/dL) and two or more risk factors (including male sex) or known coronary heart disease are managed as high-risk individuals. Although the NCEP guidelines are valuable as a structured screening approach, there is concern that they may overstate the potential benefit of cholesterol reduction for low-risk individuals with only modest cholesterol elevations. Women and older persons with coronary heart disease benefit from drug treatment, but evidence that asymptomatic women and elderly persons should be screened is not yet available. Until future trials in men and women of all ages demonstrate the feasibility and benefits of lowering cholesterol levels, it seems prudent to direct screening efforts toward high-risk groups, including persons with known coronary heart disease, those with a relevant family history (i.e., history of hyperlipidemia, heart attack, or sudden death before age 55), or patients who smoke, are hypertensive, or have diabetes mellitus. An optional group to screen might be other adults younger than age 65, beginning in men at age 35. Because women have a later onset of hypercholesterolemia and coronary disease, routine screening in women should begin around age 45.

Cancer Risk Reduction and Screening. Cancer, the second leading cause of death in the United States, was the focus of the earliest risk reduction and screening studies. Few cancers are amenable to early detection and treatment. Screening trials for lung cancer in male smokers, for example, have been uniformly unsuccessful, which emphasizes the need to dissuade new smokers and to encourage smokers to quit. Research on the causative and protective roles of dietary factors in cancer development is expanding. Available information is retrospective, with diet trials now underway. The Office of the Surgeon General has published diet recommendations consistent with good nutritional practices and aimed at reducing the risk of developing certain cancers. These recommendations include reducing fat intake to 30% of total diet calories; including fruit (especially citrus), vegetables (carotene-rich and cruciferous— e.g., broccoli, cauliflower), and adequate fiber (e.g., whole wheat) in the diet; and consuming minimal amounts of salt-cured, smoked, or nitrite-containing foods.

Several cancers with long presymptomatic stages that are amenable to early detection and intervention have shown improved outcomes with screening. The three modalities used to screen women for breast cancer are physical examination, breast self-examination (BSE), and mammography. Annual clinical breast examination is recommended for all women aged 40 and older. As generally practiced, breast examination by physicians fails to detect early-stage breast cancer (without node involvement) in about half of women later diagnosed to have breast cancer. Although physician performance might be improved with better training and monitoring compliance, supplementary tactics are needed.

The effectiveness of BSE remains unclear because it has low sensitivity and uncertain specificity and it has not been shown to reduce cancer-associated mortality. Efficacy is hindered by poor proficiency and irregular compliance. There appears to be decreased BSE sensitivity with increasing patient age, when breast cancer has its highest incidence.

Mammography is the only screening technique proven to lower breast cancer deaths. It demonstrates small, nonpalpable tumors with little risk of radiation side effects. The cost of screening mammography (currently about $100) is a major deterrent to its wider use, although increasing coverage by health insurance should help women for whom cost is an obstacle. Authorities disagree about the age at which a baseline mammogram should be obtained and the intervals for repeat screening in low-risk women. Mammography is recommended starting at age 50 and repeated every 1 to 2 years until about age 75. For high-risk women with a family history of premenopausal breast cancer in first-degree relatives, clinical breast examination and mammography should be started at age 35 (see Chapter 158, Breast Cancer Screening).

The marked fall in cervical cancer deaths in the past three decades is attributed to the widespread use of the Papanicolaou smear, a long presymptomatic period, and effective treatment. Based on a large population database and assumptions about test performance, Papanicolaou smears are recommended for women from ages 20 to 65, at intervals of 3 years or less. Some individuals have high-risk behavior or inadequate long-term testing. Sexually active teenagers and women with multiple sexual partners warrant earlier and perhaps more frequent testing. Elderly women who have not had regular or recent Papanicolaou tests should have two annual consecutive tests (with negative results) before discontinuation of Pap testing (see Chapter 157, Cervical Cancer Screening).

Indirect evidence based on the natural history of colorectal cancer and a small set of studies suggest that screening may reduce the mortality from colorectal cancer. Several screening methods have been proposed to detect asymptomatic colorectal cancer when it is potentially curable. These methods include endoscopy, which may be used to identify and remove adenomatous polyps before they progress to cancer. Although relatively inexpensive and easy to perform, digital rectal examination assesses only the last 4 inches of the large bowel and has not reduced cancer rates. Because bowel lesions bleed intermittently, the fecal occult blood test has limited sensitivity. Taking two test samples on 3 different days, for a total of six samples, is recommended. Various fecal occult blood tests, including the Hemoccult II, are available, but all have low specificity for cancer and low predictive power because other gastrointestinal causes of bleeding might exist. One trial showing annual fecal occult blood testing to be effective in persons aged 50 to 74 used rehydrated specimens and frequent colonoscopies because of the frequency of positive occult blood tests.

Sigmoidoscopy is more sensitive than the fecal occult blood test. Its regular use is associated with reduced mortality from cancers within reach of sigmoidoscopy. However, it is unacceptable to many patients. The flexible 65-cm sigmoidoscope is more comfortable and detects two to three times the number of cancers identified with the rigid 25-cm instrument. However, flexible sigmoidoscopy requires patient preparation before endoscopy and an experienced operator and costs $100 or more. Consequently, endoscopy is often used as a diagnostic procedure in persons with a positive fecal occult blood test. A reasonable screening approach for an average-risk patient between the ages of 50 and 75 years might be a fecal occult blood test every 1 to 2 years. The addition of flexible sigmoidoscopy (performed with a 65-cm scope) every 3 to 5 years would improve screening sensitivity. If a first-degree relative had colorectal cancer (see Table 8–2), a barium enema examination to assess the entire colon can be substituted for sigmoidoscopy every 3 to 5 years.

Few of the common cancers are amenable to early detection and treatment. Available tests are too insensitive (e.g., prostate and bladder cancer), the cancer develops rapidly (e.g., ovarian cancer), or treatment is ineffective (e.g., lung cancer). If the cancer is slow growing and usually localized at diagnosis, as is true for 75% of endometrial cancers, patient education (e.g., to report unusual vaginal bleeding) is more beneficial than screening.

Other Prevention Activities. Alcohol abuse, although highly prevalent in a patient population, is generally unrecognized at early stages and even after symptoms develop. Physicians do not screen for alcohol abuse for several reasons. In a society with a high consumption of alcohol, definitions such as "harmful," "hazardous," or "problem drinking" need to be considered. Practitioners may feel uncomfortable with the topic, ineffectual in counseling, or pessimistic about patient compliance with advice; or they may believe that referral services are inaccessible. Patients frequently deny that their problems may be related to alcohol consumption. Increased public awareness of alcohol-related hazards (vehicle accidents, risk during pregnancy, medication effects) may make asking questions about alcohol use more acceptable.

Several questions are recommended to screen for possible alcohol abuse, such as "Are you currently drinking?" and details of type, frequency, and circumstances. Clinicians are becoming aware of hazardous drinking patterns (heavy drinking or drinking before driving) that are linked to future complications. Additionally, a positive response to any of the CAGE questions ("Have you tried to *C*ut down? Are you *A*nnoyed when questioned about drinking? Do you ever feel *G*uilty about your drinking? Do you have an *E*ye-opener early in the day?") suggests a problem with alcohol. Once a potential candidate for referral is identified, the physician's interpersonal skills, rapport, and persistence are valuable assets to motivate the patient to accept further diagnostic evaluation at an alcohol rehabilitation program (see Chapter 10, Alcohol Problems).

Infectious Disease. Adult infectious disease screening and immunization practice received little attention until the recent epidemics of sexually transmitted diseases and the acquired immunodeficiency syndrome (AIDS) occurred and the aging US population's susceptibility to respiratory tract infection was recognized. Immunization recommendations are described in detail in Chapter 11.

High-Risk Factors. Certain behavioral or exposure factors or a family history places an individual at higher risk of becoming ill than those individuals without such risk factors. Table 8–2 is a list of prevention activities for persons with predisposing risk factors for skin, oropharyngeal, testicular, or thyroid cancer. Aspirin chemoprophylaxis can be prescribed for men aged 50 years and older who have cardiovascular risk factors such as hypertension, smoking, diabetes, or elevated cholesterol levels. A discussion of estrogen replacement therapy with perimenopausal women at greater risk of developing osteoporosis (e.g., smokers) is recommended (see Chapter 161, Menopausal Symptoms). For persons whose residence or behavior constitutes additional health hazards, immunization or certain tests should be provided.

Cross-References: Principles of Screening (Chapter 7), Diagnosis and Input of Drug Abuse (Chapter 9), Alcohol Problems (Chapter 10), Adult Immunizations (Chapter 11), Smoking Cessation (Chapter 12), Assessment of Physical Activity (Chapter 72), Colorectal Cancer Screening (Chapter 90), Sigmoidoscopy and Colonoscopy (Chapter 104), Cholesterol Screening (Chapter 150), Cervical Cancer Screening (Chapter 157), Breast Cancer Screening (Chapter 158), Menopausal Symptoms (Chapter 161).

REFERENCES

1. Bradley KA, Donovan DM, Larson EB. How much is too much? Advising patients about safe levels of alcohol consumption. Arch Intern Med 1993;153:2734–2740.

In addition to screening for alcohol-related problems, physicians should recommend that all nonpregnant persons limit themselves to three drinks on any occasion and avoid hazardous activities after drinking.

2. Kerlikowske K, Grady D, Kutin SM, et al. Efficacy of screening mammography: A meta-analysis. JAMA 1995;273:149–154.
   This very careful analysis suggests that benefits from screening 50- to 74-year-old women appear after 7 to 9 years of follow-up.

3. Krahn M, Naylor C, Basinski A, Detsky A. Comparison of an aggressive (U.S.) and a less aggressive (Canadian) policy for cholesterol screening and treatment. Ann Intern Med 1991;115:248–255.
   Similiar quality-adjusted life-year results were calculated for a theoretical cohort of middle-age men in a comparison of NCEP ("aggressive") and Canadian guidelines (age 35–59; total cholesterol 265+).

4. McGinnis JM, Foege WH. Actual causes of death in the United States. JAMA 1993;270:2207–2212.
   According to these authors about half of all US deaths in 1990 could be attributed to preventable conditions.

5. Office of Disease Prevention and Health Promotion, Public Health Service, Department of Health and Human Services. Clinician's Handbook of Preventive Services. Washington, DC, U.S. Government Printing Office, 1996.
   This volume describes valuable tactics for implementing clinical preventive care.

6. U.S. Preventive Services Task Force. Guide to Clinical Preventive Services, 2nd ed. Baltimore, Williams & Wilkins, 1996.
   This is an outstanding overview of current prevention information, including a comparison of recommendations by the US Preventive Services Task Force with those of other authorities.

■ ■

9   Diagnosis and Management of Drug Abuse

DAWN E. DeWITT and DOUGLAS S. PAAUW

Epidemiology. In the United States 11 to 13 million people use illicit drugs regularly and meet the criteria for abuse or dependence. Approximately half of all children try illicit drugs before leaving high school. Cocaine use has grown from an estimated 5.4 million people in 1974 to 22.2 million users in 1985 to 20 to 30 million users in 1994, with 4 million of those using cocaine regularly. Cocaine is third only to alcohol and marijuana (10 million regular users) in popularity. Two million people use heroin regularly, and 500,000 users are addicted. Fifteen percent to 25% of ambulatory patients have problems related to substance abuse. Approximately 25% of human immunodeficiency virus (HIV) is related to needle sharing, and in some cities 50% of heroin addicts are HIV positive. Mortality among heroin users is 10 per 1000 annually from causes including overdose, suicide, violence, hepatitis, endocarditis, and HIV infection. Each year, approximately 20,000 deaths result from illicit drug use. Among adolescents, half of all deaths are related to substance abuse.

Symptoms and Signs. A high index of suspicion must be maintained regarding drug use because only 10% of problems are recognized by primary caregivers. All patients should be asked direct questions regarding substance use as part of the routine history. Patients who have a family history of drug use, who have a history of sexual abuse, and who "doctor shop" or who request pain medications by name should be screened with direct questions. Behaviors that should raise suspicion include frequent missed appointments, "lost" prescriptions, requests for letters for disability or sick days, agitation, or depression. Screening for HIV risk factors should be routine and explicit. If the patient has a history of drug use, the history should focus on types and frequency of drugs used, first use, duration, most recent use, withdrawal symptoms, past and current treatment, methods used to support drug use, medical illnesses related to use including sexually transmitted diseases, psychiatric history, and current supports and consequences of use. Information specific to injection drug use, which includes intravenous drug use and "skin popping," should include needle sharing, skin and needle cleansing techniques, use of substances to "cut" or dilute drugs, and use of street antibiotics. All histories should include specific questions regarding depression (present in 70%), trauma, domestic violence, sexual abuse, suicide, or thoughts of harming others.

The general physical examination should note abnormal vital signs, appearance including trauma, weight, and personal hygiene. Specific findings related to injection drug use should be sought, including "tracks," abscesses, and trauma. Table 9–1 lists specific findings by type of drug use.

Infectious complications of injecting drugs include hepatitis B and hepatitis C, HIV, infectious endocarditis, septic pulmonary embolism, cellulitis, abscesses, osteomyelitis, septic arthritis, and septic thrombophlebitis. Tetanus occurs more frequently in injection drug users than in others of similar age. Botulism has been reported as a rare complication. Injection drug use–related infections often differ from infections in the general population. Infectious endocarditis is more often right-sided and due to *Staphylococcus aureus* rather than left-sided disease due to streptococci, as seen in those who are not injection drug users. *S. aureus* is the most common organism seen in infectious endocarditis and skin infections in injection drug users, and most of these individuals are colonized by *S. aureus*, including methicillin-resistant *S. aureus*. Other organisms seen in injection drug users with infectious endocarditis include enterococci, *Streptococcus viridans, Serratia, Pseudomonas* (from tap water), *Candida,* and *Neisseria sicca* (from licking needles). Cellulitis, arthritis, and osteomyelitis are more often due to gram-negative organisms, anaerobes, or multiple bacteria. Injection drug users are more likely to have osteomyelitis of the vertebrae (50%) or pelvic or sternoclavicular joints (30%) than the extremities (20%). A febrile injection drug user is more likely to have a local infection or minor illness than infectious endocarditis (≤ 10%), but studies have shown that physicians are unable to predict who will have infectious endocarditis, especially because right-sided infectious endocarditis is more common in injection drug users, and therefore patients often do not have physical signs commonly seen in left-sided infectious endocarditis such as Janeway's lesions or Osler's nodes.

Noninfectious complications of injection drug use include talc granulomas; interstitial lung diseases; panlobular emphysema in intravenous amphetamine

Table 9-1. SUMMARY OF DRUG USE FINDINGS AND COMPLICATIONS

Drug (Route of Use)	Complications	Examination Findings	Withdrawal Syndrome
Marijuana (oral or smoked)	Motor vehicle accidents Pulmonary disease Amotivational syndrome Physical dependence Decreased male fertility Impotence	Reddened conjunctivae Swollen eyelids Tearing Horizontal nystagmus Tachycardia	Irritability Sleep disturbance
Benzodiazepines (oral)	Physical dependence Motor vehicle accidents	↓ Pupillary constriction Horizontal nystagmus Nonconvergence	Tachycardia Hypertension Nervousness Sweating Increased reflexes
Hallucinogens (oral) PCP (phencyclidine MDMA (ecstasy) LSD	Weight loss Nervousness Hallucinations	Nystagmus (horizontal or vertical) Decreased corneal reflex Retracted upper lid Swollen eyelids	
Amphetamines (speed) (oral or injected)	Weight loss Nervousness	Tachycardia Hypertension	Depression Fatigue
Cocaine (90% nasal, 30% freebase or crack, 10% injected)	Transient ischemic attack/stroke Seizures Chest pain/myocardial infarction Arrhythmias Paranoia Rhabdomyolysis Pneumomediastinum	Cachexia Dilated pupils ↓ Pupillary constriction ↓ Corneal reflex Perforated nasal septum Excoriations Burned thumb (lighter) Hyperreflexia	Fatigue Depression Anxiety Craving
Anabolic steroids (injected)	Stroke Hypertension Abnormal results of liver function tests (43%) Abnormal creatinine Decreased high-density lipoproteins	Jaundice Gynecomastia Testicular atrophy ↑ Muscle bulk	
Heroin (injected)	Pulmonary edema Respiratory arrest Lung talc granulomas	Constricted pupil Nonreactive pupil Ptosis ↓ Corneal reflex	Piloerection Tachycardia Hypertension Fever Tearing Rhinorrhea Yawning Dilated pupils Craving Vomiting, diarrhea

users; pneumothorax; digital ischemia from arterial injection of cocaine; and pulmonary embolization of needle fragments. Renal failure may be seen as a complication of hepatitis, amyloidosis, or rhabdomyolysis.

Clinical Approach. Laboratory screens for drug use are easily available, but practitioners should be aware that 5% to 30% of positive results are false positives. If the cause of fever is not immediately apparent, admission should be strongly considered in all febrile injection drug users. Routine evaluation of patients should include tuberculosis testing, serologic tests for hepatitis, and examination for sexually transmitted diseases. On the East Coast, 30% of injection drug users are tuberculin positive and 27% of crack users have positive results of serologic testing for syphilis. All patients should have current tetanus immunization.

Management. Patients should be referred to groups such as Narcotics or Cocaine Anonymous or to treatment centers. The department of public health usually provides information on available inpatient or outpatient resources. Patients who are addicted to cocaine are at very high risk of relapse (50% vs. 30% of other addicts). Desipramine has been shown to decrease cocaine use and craving during withdrawal. Patients addicted to heroin should be enrolled in methadone maintenance if possible. Higher doses of methadone (i.e., 50 mg/d vs. 20 mg/d) have been associated with less heroin use by patients. Abstinence has been associated with increased employment, enhanced social stability, and improved mental health. Clonidine has also been used to treat patients with heroin withdrawal.

Counseling and testing for HIV infection should be made available. The provider should discuss safe sex practices, the risk of needle sharing, and methods to obtain clean needles and syringes. If the patient is sharing needles, consistent use of bleach should be encouraged. Full-strength bleach should be in contact with equipment twice for at least 30 seconds, followed by two water rinses. Used bleach and water should be discarded.

Follow-Up. Physicians should see patients regularly during early abstinence and reinforce the goals of treatment. Counseling of family members when appropriate should be encouraged. Physicians should be aware of the abuse potential of prescribed medications and the complications of abuse. Medications with potential for abuse should be kept in locked cabinets, and Drug Enforcement Agency (DEA) numbers should not be printed on prescriptions except when necessary. Quantities of medication should be spelled out to prevent changes by the patient. A flow chart record of doses and prescriptions should be maintained and a single physician chosen to prescribe controlled substances to each patient.

Cross-References: Principles of Screening (Chapter 7), Periodic Health Assessment (Chapter 8), Alcohol Problems (Chapter 10).

REFERENCES

1. Caulker-Burnette I. Primary care screening for substance abuse. Nurse Pract 1994;19(6):42–48.
   Key areas in history taking, physical examinations, and laboratory data are identified as indications for screening. Concrete information regarding consequences of drug use is discussed.

2. Cherubin CE, Sapira JD. The medical complications of drug addiction and the medical assessment of intravenous drug users: 25 years later. Ann Intern Med 1993;119:1017–1028.
   This is a comprehensive review of medical problems that occur in injection drug users.

3. Coleman P. Overview of substance abuse. Prim Care 1993;20(1):1–18.
   Historical and epidemiologic data are provided including criteria for abuse and dependence.

4. Screening for alcohol and other drug abuse. US Preventive Services Task Force. Am Fam Physician 1989;40:137–146.

   Principles of screening and use of laboratory testing are discussed with recommendations of national organizations.

5. Warner EA. Cocaine abuse. Ann Intern Med 1993;119:226–235.

   A complete review including a discussion of complications is presented.

■ ■

10 Alcohol Problems

KATHARINE A. BRADLEY

SCREENING

The goal of alcohol-related screening in primary care settings is to identify a spectrum of problem and at-risk drinkers. Problem drinkers include patients with alcohol abuse and dependence, as well as those who do not meet diagnostic criteria for abuse and dependence but have experienced adverse consequences due to drinking. At-risk drinkers are those who have not yet developed problems due to drinking but are at increased risk as a result of their drinking practices. Alcohol-related problems may be medical, psychosocial, legal, or financial and can result from daily or episodic heavy drinking (Table 10–1).

The lifetime prevalence of alcohol abuse or dependence in primary care populations ranges from 11% to 36%; only 5% to 12% of patients meet criteria for current alcohol abuse and dependence. The prevalence of current alcohol abuse and dependence is highest among men, younger individuals, and whites (Table 10–2). Younger age, male gender, Northern European descent, and a family history of alcohol problems are risk factors for alcohol abuse and dependence. Although alcohol abuse and dependence are three times more common in men than women, women develop medical consequences due to drinking at lower levels of consumption.

Rationale. Although no single treatment program has been proven universally effective, a variety of treatments have been shown to be superior to no treatment. Randomized controlled trials of brief interventions with at-risk drinkers have resulted in decreased alcohol consumption, blood pressure, serum γ-glutamyltransferase, and days hospitalized among men. Referral of problem drinkers to alcohol treatment has also been shown to decrease alcohol consumption and alcohol-related problems at 18 months, irrespective of whether the patient accepted and completed the referral.

Screening using questionnaires (such as the CAGE, AUDIT, or TWEAK; see Table 10–4) is more sensitive and specific for alcohol abuse and dependence than laboratory testing. The four-question CAGE performs well in men and black women, whereas the AUDIT or TWEAK may perform better in white

Table 10–1. DEFINITIONS OF ALCOHOL-RELATED PROBLEMS

DSM-IV criteria for alcohol dependence*:

A maladaptive pattern of alcohol use leading to clinically significant impairment or distress as manifested by 3 or more of the following in the same 12-month period:

1. Tolerance to alcohol (need for markedly increased amounts of alcohol to achieve the desired effect or markedly diminished effect with continued use of the same amount).
2. Alcohol withdrawal or use of alcohol or a similar substance (i.e., benzodiazepine) to avoid withdrawal.
3. Alcohol often consumed in greater amounts or over a longer period than intended.
4. Persistent desire or unsuccessful efforts to cut down or control alcohol use.
5. A great deal of time spent obtaining, drinking, or recovering from the effects of alcohol.
6. Important social, occupational, or recreational activities are given up because of alcohol use.
7. Drinking is continued despite knowledge of having a persistent or recurrent physical or psychological problem that is likely caused or exacerbated by alcohol use.

DSM-IV criteria for alcohol abuse*:

A maladaptive pattern of alcohol use leading to clinically significant impairment or distress as manifested by 1 or more of the following in the same 12-month period:

1. Recurrent drinking resulting in a failure to fulfill major obligations at work, school, or home.
2. Recurrent drinking in situations in which it is physically hazardous (e.g., driving when impaired by alcohol).
3. Recurrent alcohol-related legal problems.
4. Continued drinking despite having persistent or recurrent social or interpersonal problems caused or exacerbated by drinking (e.g., arguments, physical fights).

At-risk drinking†:

Men	5 or more drinks per occasion
	Over 17 drinks a week
Women	4 or more drinks per occasion
	Over 12 drinks a week

*Reprinted with permission from the Diagnostic and Statistical Manual of Mental Disorders, Fourth Edition. Copyright 1994 American Psychiatric Association. Washington, DC.

†Definitions of at-risk drinking vary; these are derived from empirical data (Sanchez-Craig et al., 1995, and Wechsler et al., 1995).

Table 10–2. PREVALENCE OF ALCOHOL ABUSE OR DEPENDENCE DURING THE PAST YEAR IN THE UNITED STATES

	Prevalence (%)			
	Women		Men	
Age (Yr)	BLACK	NONBLACK	BLACK	NONBLACK
< 30	3.3	11.0	12.3	23.5
30–44	4.2	3.9	8.8	10.9
45–64	1.9	1.5	5.2	5.6
≥ 65	0.0	0.3	0.8	1.2

Adapted from Grant BF, Hartford TC, Dawson DA, Chou P, Dufour M, Pickering R. Prevalence of DSM-IV alcohol abuse and dependence, United States, 1992; Epidemiologic bulletin. Washington, DC, National Institute on Alcohol Abuse and Alcoholism, 1994:243–248.

women. Two or more "yes" responses on the CAGE are usually considered a positive screen. The probability of a screen-positive patient's having an alcohol problem is dependent on the prevalence of alcohol problems in the screened population (Table 10–3).

The AUDIT was designed to screen for at-risk drinking, in addition to alcohol problems. If the CAGE or TWEAK questionnaire is used to screen for alcohol problems, patients who have had a drink in the past year should be asked further questions to clarify their typical drinking pattern (Table 10–4). Although typical quantity and frequency questions such as those in Table 10–4 are quick and easy to use, a strategy of asking patients separately about their consumption of beer, wine, and liquor improves recognition of at-risk drinkers. In addition, asking patients how often they drink six or more drinks on a single occasion identifies many at-risk drinkers who would otherwise be missed.

Strategy. All patients should be screened by physicians, nurses, or other health care professionals annually. Screening is more effective if allied health care professionals and routine surveys are employed to supplement the activities of primary providers. Patients who have evidence of current alcohol-related problems or who drink heavily should be evaluated further by the primary care provider. This assessment should include a detailed evaluation of a patient's drinking and related psychosocial, employment, financial, or legal problems. Inquiring further about the patient's positive responses to specific screening questions can provide a comfortable opening (see Table 10–4). Knowledge about where, when, and with whom the patient drinks; the patient's assessment of his or her own drinking; and any past or current consideration of change can help to select appropriate interventions. For instance, a partner who drinks heavily may be an important obstacle to a patient's changing his or her drinking habits. Similarly, evidence of tolerance, blackouts, driving, or arguments after drinking can be used as feedback.

With patients who drink heavily, the interview and examination should also identify medical problems linked to heavy alcohol use. The screening examination can identify hypertension, oropharyngeal tumors, congestive heart failure, liver disease, muscle weakness, peripheral neuropathy, and malnutrition. Laboratory tests may include a complete blood cell count, including measurement of the mean corpuscular volume (MCV), and liver function tests, including determination of the serum γ-glutamyltransferase level (GGT). Although the physical examination and laboratory testing are not sensitive

Table 10–3. SENSITIVITY AND SPECIFICITY OF THE CAGE FOR A LIFETIME HISTORY OF ALCOHOL ABUSE AND DEPENDENCE

CAGE Score	Sensitivity	Specificity	Postscreening Probability*		
			10%	20%	30%
0	—	—	0.02	0.03	0.19
1	0.89	0.81	0.14	0.27	0.72
2	0.74	0.91	0.33	0.53	0.88
3	0.44	0.98	0.59	0.76	0.96
4	0.25	0.100	0.92	0.96	0.99

*Prevalence of alcohol abuse/dependence in screened population.

Adapted from Buchsbaum DG, Buchanan RG, Centor RM, Schnoll SH, Lawton MJ. Screening for alcohol abuse using CAGE scores and likelihood ratios. Ann Intern Med 1991; 115:774–777.

Table 10–4. RECOMMENDED SCREENING STRATEGY

All Patients

1. Do you drink alcohol?
2. When was the last time you had a drink containing alcohol?

CAGE Questions:

3. Have you ever felt you ought to *C*ut down on your drinking?
4. Have people *A*nnoyed you by criticizing your drinking?
5. Have you ever felt bad or *G*uilty about your drinking?
6. Have you ever had a drink first thing in the morning (*E*ye-opener) to steady your nerves or get rid of a hangover?

For Patients Who Have Had a Drink in the Past Year:

1. How often have you had a drink containing alcohol in the past year? Consider a drink to be a can or bottle of beer, a glass of wine, a wine cooler, or one cocktail or shot of hard liquor (such as scotch, gin, vodka).†
2. How many drinks containing alcohol did you have on a typical day when you were drinking in the past year?†
3. How often did you have 5 or more drinks on one occasion in the past year? (For women: use "4 or more")†

Optional Questions About Common Alcohol-Related Problems:

1. How many drinks does it take before you feel the first effects of the alcohol? (Tolerance is often defined in terms of 3 or more drinks)*
2. How often in the past year have you been unable to remember what you said or did after drinking (blackouts)?†
3. How often in the past year have you been in arguments or fights after drinking? (most common consequence of heavy drinking)

Helpful Questions for Further Assessment of Drinking Practices:

1. You mentioned you had once ___ (cut down on your drinking, felt bad or guilty about your drinking, etc.). Can you tell me more about that?
2. In order to understand if your drinking could be affecting your ___ (health or some more specific aspect of the patient's health that you know he/she cares about, e.g., sleep problems, depression, fatigue, high blood pressure, abnormal laboratory tests), I'd like to ask you more questions about your drinking practices. What alcoholic beverage do you usually drink? On your heaviest drinking day, how much ___ do you drink? (Repeat for beer, wine, and liquor.)
3. Do you think you drink more than you should? Are you interested in drinking less? What would it be like to stop drinking any alcohol?

*Adapted from the TWEAK questionnaire screen (Tolerance, Worried, Eye-opener, Amnesia, Kut-down).

†Adapted from the AUDIT questionnaire screen (Alcohol Use Disorders Identification Test).

screens for at-risk and problem drinking (i.e., less than 40% sensitive), abnormal physical and laboratory findings suggestive of harm due to drinking can help motivate patients to change their drinking habits.

Based on a thorough assessment, the provider can place each patient on a spectrum from non–problem drinkers to dependent drinkers. This knowledge, combined with an understanding of how alcohol use fits into the patient's life and recognition of potential obstacles to change, will guide subsequent management.

MANAGEMENT

Clinical Approach. Brief primary care interventions can benefit a spectrum of patients from at-risk drinkers to patients with alcohol dependence. Patients with alcohol dependence typically have evidence of impaired control over drinking, tolerance to alcohol, or withdrawal; they often need to abstain to manage their drinking problems and should be offered referral to abstinence-oriented treatment or self-help programs (Table 10–5). Patients who suffer from adverse consequences of drinking but do not have evidence of alcohol dependence may be able to learn to reduce their drinking to safe levels. These patients should be offered referral, but brief interventions alone have been shown to decrease alcohol consumption and related problems. Patients who have no evidence of adverse consequences due to drinking but who drink more than the recommended amounts should be advised to decrease consumption. All patients should be advised against driving after drinking. Women should be advised to stop drinking before becoming pregnant.

Primary care physicians can perform brief 5- to 15-minute interventions that decrease alcohol consumption and improve liver function tests and blood pressure in males who are heavy or problem drinkers. *Simply making a comprehensive assessment* of patients' drinking patterns and problems may motivate some patients to reduce alcohol consumption, especially women. Assessing a patient's readiness to change may identify those patients contemplating change, who may be most likely to change their drinking habits.

Feedback of relevant information, linking the patient's drinking and health, is an important component of effective interventions. Patients may decide to change the way they drink when they see the connection between their drinking and problems they are experiencing (e.g., interpersonal, employment, financial, or legal difficulties or medical problems such as indigestion or hypertension). As mentioned above, although laboratory tests are an insensitive screen for alcohol problems, using them for feedback when they are abnormal may motivate patients to change their drinking habits.

Table 10–5. MANAGEMENT OF PROBLEM DRINKERS

1. Assess withdrawal in alcohol-dependent patients.
2. Assess previous attempts at change, reasons the patient may be interested in changing, and obstacles to change.
3. Provide nonjudgmental feedback linking drinking to problems the patient cares about. Avoid introducing the label "alcoholic" unless the patient self-identifies.
4. If a heavy-drinking patient does not have overt problems due to drinking, explain that research has shown that his or her pattern of drinking is associated with increased health risks. Daily consumption over three drinks is associated with increased risk of hypertension and cirrhosis. Consumption over four drinks in a single day has been associated with arguments and physical fights.
5. Advise alcohol-dependent patients to abstain. If a patient is not initially willing to abstain, recommend decreased consumption and not driving after drinking (harm reduction).
6. Offer referral to a specialized alcohol treatment program, Alcoholics Anonymous (AA), or both to all alcohol-dependent patients and patients with milder alcohol problems who are willing to abstain.
7. Be optimistic regarding the benefits of treatment, indicating to the patient that there is a cumulative benefit of repeated efforts at behavior change.
8. Follow-up with the patient at 1 month to discuss the patient's experience with treatment, self-help, or attempted controlled drinking. Encourage the patient to return irrespective of continued drinking.
9. Empathize regarding the difficulty of behavioral change while firmly maintaining advice to change.

Table 10–6. OUTPATIENT MANAGEMENT OF WITHDRAWAL

1. Establish a recent decrease or cessation of alcohol consumption and motivation to abstain.
2. Assess symptoms and signs of withdrawal (see Table 10–7), coexisting medical or psychiatric conditions, recent seizure, and concurrent drug use.
3. Patients with serious concurrent psychiatric or medical conditions, recent seizure, or impending delirium tremens (autonomic hyperactivity and delirium) should be admitted for inpatient management of withdrawal.
4. If the patient has mild to moderate withdrawal symptoms (see Table 10–7), has no serious concomitant disease, and can be evaluated daily for evidence of withdrawal and continued abstinence, consider outpatient benzodiazepine treatment.
5. Document vital signs, symptoms and signs of withdrawal, blood alcohol level, and blood glucose.
6. Various fixed-dose regimens of benzodiazepines are used, including oxazepan, 30 mg as needed depending on withdrawal symptoms, up to four times a day and at bedtime, or chlordiazepoxide, 50 mg every 6 hours for four doses, followed by 25 mg every 6 hours for eight doses. Benzodiazepines should *not* be taken if the patient is somnolent, is sleeping, or has signs of benzodiazepine intoxication. (Hourly symptom-triggered regimens have some proven benefits for inpatient management of withdrawal but have not been adequately evaluated in outpatient settings.)
7. Encourage the patient to take oral fluids and carbohydrates, and prescribe thiamine and a multivitamin.
8. Refer patients to specialized alcohol treatment programs (if available) for rehabilitation and relapse prevention.

Explicit advice should be given to either abstain or decrease consumption depending on the presence or absence of dependence as outlined earlier. For patients who do not wish to abstain from alcohol consumption, advice should include an explicit recommendation for a maximum number of standard-sized drinks per drinking day (1 to 2 drinks per day for women; 2 to 3 drinks per day for men) and a maximum number of drinks per week (8 to 12 for women; 12 to 17 for men).

When patients do not accept that their drinking is excessive, the primary care provider can communicate relevant information linking the patients' drinking and health (feedback) followed by simple advice. When patients express interest in changing their drinking, interventions should focus on advice, strategies, and referral. Strategies that can help patients drink moderately include drinking for quality rather than quantity (e.g., drinking less, but drinking only a favorite, probably higher quality beer or wine), drinking alcoholic beverages with food (to decrease absorption), alternating nonalcoholic and alcoholic beverages, and abstaining for a period of several weeks before attempting moderate drinking (to decrease tolerance).

No single type of treatment program has been shown to be effective for all patients with alcohol dependence, but patients who receive some treatment are likely to do better than those who receive none. The specific treatment services available to any individual patient will vary somewhat depending on the setting and the patient's insurance coverage or ability to pay. Because of economic pressures, treatment is increasingly being provided in the outpatient setting. Alcoholics Anonymous (AA) offers free self-help groups throughout the United States. These groups provide daily meetings to help patients abstain "one day at a time." Many alcohol-dependent and alcohol-abusing patients find that attending daily or weekly AA meetings helps them remain sober.

Withdrawal. Primary care patients with alcohol dependence who wish to abstain will often ask for help with alcohol withdrawal. Mild to moderate alcohol withdrawal can be safely managed on an outpatient basis. Primary care providers can manage alcohol withdrawal safely if they can see patients daily for evaluation of withdrawal and, when necessary, for prescription of benzodiazepines (Tables 10–6 and 10–7).

Follow-Up. Because behavioral change takes time and alcohol abuse and dependence are often chronic, recurring conditions, primary care providers should arrange follow-up appointments for all patients who drink heavily or have a history of alcohol problems. New evidence of harm due to a patient's alcohol use should be continually sought and used as feedback regarding the adverse effects of drinking in repeated brief interventions. Patients should be evaluated and treated for coexisting psychiatric disorders such as depression, anxiety,

---

Table 10–7. THE CLINICAL INSTITUTE WITHDRAWAL ASSESSMENT FOR ALCOHOL—REVISED (CIWA-AR)*

1. NAUSEA/VOMITING: Ask "Do you feel sick to your stomach? Have you vomited?" (scores ranging from 0 = "no nausea with no vomiting" to 7 = "constant nausea, frequent dry heaves and vomiting")
2. TREMOR: Arms extended and fingers spread apart (from 0 = "no tremor" to 7 = "severe, even with arms at side")
3. PAROXYSMAL SWEATS: (from 0 = "no sweat visible" to 7 = "drenching sweats")
4. ANXIETY: Ask "Do you feel nervous?" (from 0 = "no anxiety, at ease" to 7 = "equivalent to panic states or as seen in delirium or psychosis")
5. AGITATION: (from 0 = "normal activity" to 7 = "paces back and forth, constant movement, thrashing about")
6. TACTILE DISTURBANCES: Ask "Have you had any itching, pins and needles, burning numbness, or do you feel bugs crawling on your skin?" (from 0 = "none" to 7 = "extreme")
7. AUDITORY DISTURBANCES: Ask "Are you more aware of sounds around you? Do they frighten you? Are you hearing anything that disturbs you or that you know is not there?" (0 = no "none" to 7 = "extreme")
8. VISUAL DISTURBANCES: Ask "Does the light appear to be too bright? Is its color different? Are you seeing anything that disturbs you or that you know is not there?" (from 0 = "none" to 7 = "extreme")
9. HEADACHE OR FULLNESS IN HEAD: Ask "Does your head feel different? Does it feel like there is a band around your head?" Do not rate dizziness. (from 0 = "not present" to 7 = "extremely severe (worst ever)")
10. ORIENTATION AND CLOUDING OF SENSORIUM: (from 0 = "oriented and can do serial 3s" to 4 = "disoriented to place/person"). Reorient if necessary.

---

*This instrument (requiring 2–5 minutes to administer) can be used as an adjunct to a baseline medical evaluation, and to follow symptoms and signs over the course of withdrawal. Many acute medical conditions, aside from alcohol withdrawal, can produce both the mental status changes and autonomic hyperactivity measured by this scale.

Less than 10 points reflects minimal or absent withdrawal; no benzodiazepines are needed. Scores of 10–19 represent mild to moderate withdrawal; benzodiazepines are advised, but withdrawal can be managed safely as an outpatient if no other complications are present. Over 19 points indicates severe withdrawal for which inpatient management is recommended.

From Wartenberg AA, Nirenberg TD, Liepman MR, Silvia LY, et al. Detoxification of alcoholics: improving care by symptom triggered sedation. Alcohol Clin Exp Res 1990;14:71–75.

eating disorders, and abuse of other psychoactive drugs. Patients should also be cautioned against excessive use of acetaminophen and the hazards of driving or participating in water sports after drinking.

Attitude. Many experts believe empathy and optimism are important parts of a therapeutic relationship that can enhance brief interventions. Showing respect for the patient by seeking to understand where drinking fits into his or her life can help forge this therapeutic relationship. Patients often change their drinking pattern when they believe it threatens something they value (e.g., their health, relationships, jobs). But drinking also often benefits them. Patients will therefore have ambivalence about changing the way they drink. Accepting and exploring this ambivalence can be helpful. Ultimately, understanding what a patient values and how drinking relates to those values may allow a provider to help a patient move toward behavioral change.

Cross-References: Diagnosis and Management of Drug Abuse (Chapter 9), Alcohol Withdrawal (Chapter 142), Screening for Depression (Chapter 185).

REFERENCES

1. Barnes HN, Aronson MD, Delbanco TL. Alcoholism—a Guide for the Primary Care Physician. New York, Springer, 1987:1–231.

   This text is an outstanding and thorough primer on alcohol problems in the primary care setting even though it was published before brief interventions aimed at abstinence or moderate drinking were demonstrated to be useful in primary care settings.

2. Bien TH, Miller WR, Tonigan S. Brief interventions for alcohol problems: A review. Addiction 1993;88:315–336.

   This good review of the literature on brief interventions includes a discussion of the potential "active ingredients."

3. Buchsbaum DG, Buchanan RG, Centor RM, Schnoll SH, Lawton MJ. Screening for alcohol abuse using CAGE scores and likelihood ratios. Ann Intern Med 1991;115:774–777.

   This paper validated the CAGE questionnaire in a primary care setting.

4. Fuller RK. Refining the treatment of alcohol withdrawal. JAMA 1994;272:557–558.

   This article contains a good, brief review of the literature on the treatment of alcohol withdrawal.

5. Hayashida M, Alterman AI, McLellan T, et al. Comparative effectiveness of inpatient and outpatient detoxification of patients with mild to moderate alcohol withdrawal syndrome. N Engl J Med 1989;320:358–365.

   This study demonstrated the safety and efficacy of outpatient management of alcohol withdrawal.

6. Sanchez-Craig M, Wilkinson A, Davila R. Empirically based guidelines for moderate drinking: 1 year from three studies with problem drinkers. Am J Public Health 1995;85:823–828.

   This reference and the one below are studies demonstrating levels of alcohol consumption at which psychosocial problems develop.

7. Wechsler H, Dowdall GW, Davenport A, Rimm EB. A gender specific measure of binge drinking among college students. Am J Public Health 1995;85:982–985.

8. Connors, GJ. Screening for alcohol problems. In Assessing Alcohol Problems: A Guide for Clinicians and Researchers. NIH Publication No. 95-3745. 1995;17–29.

   This is a complete summary of currently available screening questionnaires.

11 Adult Immunizations

BENJAMIN A. LIPSKY

Epidemiology. Immunizations are extremely cost-effective but are often neglected in adults because of a lack of established tradition or because of broad legal requirements. Only 58% of elderly Americans received influenza vaccine in 1994 and only 30% received pneumococcal vaccine, despite the fact that these vaccinations are reimbursed by Medicare. The three major target groups for inoculation against vaccine-preventable diseases are (1) healthy individuals who are susceptible because they lack previous immunization or infection; (2) persons who are at risk from these diseases because of their occupation or lifestyle; and (3) patients whose age or medical conditions increase the risk of morbidity or mortality from these diseases. Interest in immunizations for adults has increased with the recognition that some vaccine-preventable diseases now occur primarily in persons older than 20, yet the majority of adults at risk are not protected against most of these diseases (Table 11–1). Vaccines against selected uncommon diseases (e.g., rabies, plague, anthrax, yellow fever, typhoid, cholera, meningococci) are available for those at risk because of lifestyle, occupation, or travel.

Clinical Approach. Table 11–2 is a summary of the current recommendations for vaccinations of adults in various groups. Contraindications to adult immuni-

Table 11–1. REPORTED CASES OF VACCINE-PREVENTABLE CHILDHOOD DISEASES IN THE UNITED STATES

Disease	Maximal No. of Cases (y)	1993 Cases*	Reduction (%)
Diphtheria	206,939 (1921)	0	−100.0
Pertussis	265,269 (1934)	6,132	−97.7
Tetanus†	1,560 (1923)	9	−99.4
Poliomyelitis (paralytic)	21,269 (1952)	0‡	−100.0
Measles	894,143 (1941)	277	−99.9
Rubella§	57,686 (1969)	188	−99.7
Congenital rubella syndrome	20,000 (1964–1965)	7	−99.9
Mumps‖	152,209 (1968)	1,630	−98.9

*Provisional data that may change because of late reporting.

†Data from the CDC on tetanus refer to deaths, not cases; CDC does not have information on the numbers of reported tetanus cases before 1947. The number of reported deaths refers to 1992. Mortality data for 1993 are not available. The provisional number of tetanus cases reported for 1993 is 42.

‡Excludes an estimated four cases of vaccine-associated paralysis.

§Rubella first became a reportable disease in 1966.

‖Mumps first became a reportable disease in 1968.

Data from the National Immunization Program, Centers for Disease Control and Prevention, Atlanta, GA.

Table 11–2. VACCINE RECOMMENDATIONS FOR SELECTED POPULATIONS IN THE UNITED STATES*

Patients	TD	MMR	Polio	Flu	Pneu.	Hep. B	Hep. A	Varicella
Vaccines								
General Use								
18–64 y old	V B	(V)	S			†		(V)
≥ 65 y old	V B		S	V	V			(V)
Special Uses								
Pregnancy‡		X				S		X
Occupational exposure								
College students		(V)						(V)
Health care workers		(V)		V		S	S	
Day care personnel		(V)	(V)	V			V	
Lifestyles								
Homosexual men and heterosexuals						V	V	
with multiple partners						V	V	
Injection drug users	V					V	V	
Travelers to endemic areas								
Environmental situations								
Prison inmates						V		
Mentally retarded (institutionalized)						V	V	
persons				V	S			
Nursing home residents								
Compromised hosts§								
Chronic organ system or systemic				V	V	S		
disease								
Immunosuppressed persons		X		V±	V±	V±		X

*Special considerations may apply for travelers. There is good evidence from at least one properly randomized controlled trial to support all of these recommendations (except for pneumococcal vaccine).

†Vaccination now recommended for all infants and for previously unvaccinated adolescents.

‡Pregnant patients:
1. Live virus vaccines (measles, mumps, rubella, rubeola, varicella) should generally be avoided because of theoretic risks to the fetus, although there are no clinical data to support this risk.
2. Hepatitis A, Hepatitis B, pneumococcal, and influenza vaccines are neither specifically indicated nor contraindicated.
3. Tetanus-diphtheria vaccine should be administered to those not previously immunized.
4. Polio immunization is not indicated unless traveling to highly endemic areas, in which case inactivated vaccine (IPV) should be given.

§HIV-infected patients:
1. May receive all appropriate vaccines during asymptomatic stages but should not take certain live virus vaccines (e.g., oral polio vaccine, varicella vaccine) or bacille Calmette-Guérin vaccine.
2. Efficacy of vaccines is best when vaccination is given as early in the course of the HIV infection as possible.

TD, tetanus-diphtheria; MMR, mumps-measles-rubella; Flu, influenza; Pneu., pneumococcal; Hep. B, hepatitis B; Hep. A, hepatitis A; V, routine administration; (V), administer if not previously infected or vaccinated; B, boosters every 10 years; S, selected high-risk individuals; X, contraindicated; ±, variable immunogenicity.

Table 11–3. ESTIMATED EFFECT OF FULL USE OF VACCINES RECOMMENDED FOR ADULTS

Disease	Estimated No. of Annual Deaths	Estimated Vaccine Efficacy (%)*	Current Vaccine Utilization (%)†	Additional No. of Preventable Deaths per Year‡
Influenza	20,000§	70	41	8,260
Pneumococcal infection	40,000	60	20	19,200
Hepatitis B	5,000	90	10‖	4,050
Tetanus-diphtheria	< 25	99	40¶	< 15
Measles, mumps, and rubella	< 30	95	Variable	< 30

*Indicates efficacy in immunocompetent adults.

†The percentage of targeted groups who have been immunized.

‡Calculated as potential additional vaccine utilization × estimated vaccine efficacy × estimated annual deaths.

§Variable (range, 0 to 40,000).

‖Highly variable (range, 1% to 60%) among different targeted groups.

¶This estimate is based on seroprevalence data.

Table 11–4. KEY INFORMATION ON RECOMMENDED VACCINES

Disease	Vaccine	Dose/Route	Indications	Precautions	Frequency	Special Considerations	Approximate Cost*
Measles	Measles live virus† (Attenuvax)	0.5 mL SQ	All children and adults born after 1956 without previous live virus vaccination or evidence of previous infection	Pregnancy; immunosuppression; egg or neomycin allergy	Once; second dose for young adults entering college or health care professions or traveling abroad	Persons vaccinated from 1963–1967 may need revaccination	$16
Mumps	Mumps live virus‡ (Mumpsvax II)	0.5 mL SQ	All children and susceptible adults (particularly men)	Same as measles	Once; no booster	MMR is vaccine of choice if all three needed	$31 (MMR) $12 (Mumpsvax)
Rubella	Rubella live virus† (Meruvax II)	0.5 mL SQ	All children and susceptible adults (particularly women of childbearing age and those working in congregate situations)	Same as measles	Once; no booster	Pregnancy within 3 mo of vaccination may damage fetus; vaccine may cause arthralgias, paresthesias	$14 (R) $21 (MR)
Tetanus/ Diphtheria	Adsorbed tetanus and diphtheria toxins (TD)	0.5 mL IM	All children and adults	History of allergy or neurologic reaction from previous dose	Two doses 1–2 mo apart; third dose 6–12 mo later; booster every 10 years	See reference 5. Boosters at 10-y intervals may increase adverse reactions	$1 (TD) $13 (DTP)
Pneumococcal	Polyvalent pneumococcal polysaccharide (Pneumovax 23); Pnu-Imune 23)	0.5 mL SQ or IM	Children and adults at increased risk, especially those with asplenia; ≥ 65 y old; chronic cardiac, pulmonary, and perhaps other disorders	Local soreness may occur, especially with revaccination	Once; repeat vaccination recommended for those at highest risk who were vaccinated > 6 y ago	Efficacy is poor in immunocompromised hosts; data to support use in high-risk US populations are limited	$12 (Medicare part B coverage)
Influenza	Inactivated virus (Fluogen; influenza virus vaccine)	0.5 mL SQ	Persons ≥ 65 y old or with high-risk conditions or residing in chronic care facilities; also essential public and health care workers	Egg allergy; local soreness, fever, myalgias may occur	Annually (before December)	Vaccine changes annually; efficacy in high-risk US population is well established (decreases risk of pneumonia, hospitalization, and death)	$5 (free to Medicare beneficiaries)

Table continued on following page

47

Table 11–4. KEY INFORMATION ON RECOMMENDED VACCINES *Continued*

Disease	Vaccine	Dose/Route	Indications	Precautions	Frequency	Special Considerations	Approximate Cost*
Polio	Live oral polio virus (Orimune) (IPOL)	OPV: 0.5 mL PO; IPV: 1 mL SQ	All children; routine vaccination for adults is unnecessary; vaccinate those at high risk because of travel or occupation, preferably with IPV	OPV: pregnancy, immunosuppression; IPV: streptomycin or neomycin allergy	OPV: three doses ≥ 6 wk apart; fourth dose ≥ 6 mo later; IPV: four doses per package insert	Rare instances of paralysis in recipients of OPV and their close contacts	$15/dose (OPV) $25/dose (IPV)
Hepatitis B	Recombinant HBsAg vaccine (Recombivax-HB, Engerix-B)	1 mL IM (in deltoid)	Multiple sex partners; all infants and unvaccinated adolescents; intravenous drug abusers; hemophiliacs; health care workers; staff and patients in mental institutions	None	Two doses 4 wk apart; third dose 5 mo later	Effectiveness decreased with increased age or obesity or injection in buttock	$173 (for 3 doses; Medicare coverage in renal failure)
Hepatitis A	Inactivated virus (Havrix)	1 mL IM (in deltoid)	Persons > 2 y old at risk because of travel, lifestyle, occupation	None	Once, with a booster dose 6–12 mo later	May be administered concomitantly with IG	$45
Varicella	Varicella attenuated live virus (Varivax)	0.5 mL SQ	Susceptible persons ≥ 1 y old	Pregnancy; defer for ≥ 5 mo after transfusions or VZIG; avoid salicylates for 6 wk	2 doses, 4–8 wk apart	Recipients should avoid close association with susceptible high-risk patients	AWP–$50

*Wholesale cost to pharmacist, from 1995 *Drug Topics Red Book*; Varivax 1997 AWP price.
†Also available in measles-rubella live virus (M-R-VAX II) and measles-mumps-rubella live virus (M-M-R II).
‡Also available in rubella-mumps live virus (Bivax II)
Vaccinations should not be given to persons with a febrile illness (> 38° C)
Do not give live virus vaccines to immunocompromised patients.
Measles, mumps, rubella, DTP, and OPV can be given simultaneously.
MMR, measles-mumps-rubella; MR, mumps-rubella; TD, tetanus-diphtheria; DTP, diphtheria-tetanus-pertussis; OPV, oral polio vaccine; IPV, inactivated polio vaccine; IG, immune globulin; VZIG, varicella-zoster immune globulin.

zation are commonly misunderstood. The following are *not* generally contraindications to vaccination:

1. A previous vaccination that produced local tenderness, redness, or swelling or fever less than 40.5°C (104.9°F)
2. Mild acute upper respiratory or gastrointestinal illness accompanied by fever less than 38°C (100.4°F)
3. Current antimicrobial therapy, convalescence from a recent illness, or exposure to an infectious disease
4. Pregnancy in another household member
5. Breast feeding
6. Personal history of "allergies," *excluding* anaphylactic reactions to neomycin (for combined measles, mumps, and rubella vaccine) or streptomycin (for oral polio vaccine) or to eggs (for influenza vaccine)
7. Family history of "allergies," adverse reactions to vaccination, or seizures

Key information on selected vaccines is listed in Tables 11–3 and 11–4. Up-to-date immunization recommendations can be obtained by calling the Centers for Disease Control and Prevention hot line at (404) 639-1610 and following the automated instructions.

Cross-Reference: Periodic Health Assessment (Chapter 8).

REFERENCES

1. American College of Physicians Task Force on Adult Immunization and Infectious Diseases Society of America: Guide for Adult Immunization, 3rd ed. Philadelphia, American College of Physicians, 1994.

   This is the most recent revision of the most thorough guidelines in this field.

2. Gardner P, Schaffner W. Immunization of adults. N Engl J Med 1993;328:1252–1258.

   A thorough review is presented including information on all available vaccines.

3. Fedson DS. Adult immunization: Summary of the National Vaccine Advisory Committee Report. JAMA 1994;272:1133–1137.

   This report outlines five goals and 18 recommendations for improving adult immunization.

4. Poland GA, Love KR, Hughes CE. Routine immunization of the HIV-positive asymptomatic patient. J Gen Intern Med 1990;5:147–152.

   This is a review of the risk of vaccine-preventable diseases and the safety and efficacy of vaccination in patients infected with human immunodeficiency virus.

5. Update on Adult Immunization. Recommendations of the ACIP. MMWR 1991;40(No RR-12):1–94.

   This is a thorough and up-to-date overview of recommendations for all aspects of immunization.

12 Smoking Cessation

THOMAS STAIGER

Epidemiology. Cigarette smoking is the primary cause of preventable premature death in the United States, accounting for nearly 20% of deaths in 1990. Smokers are roughly twice as likely as nonsmokers to die at any given age. Twenty-six percent of US residents are smokers, and 70% of these want to quit. Forty-five percent of the US population who have ever smoked have quit.

Rationale. Smokers and their families experience substantial health benefits when a patient quits smoking. A smoker's twofold to fourfold increased risk of a myocardial infarction decreases to or near baseline after 2 to 4 years of abstinence. The incidence of lung cancer decreases 80% to 90% in patients abstinent at 15 years. Smoking cessation decreases a patient's risk of pulmonary disease and of oral, esophageal, bladder, cervical, laryngeal, and pancreatic cancer. Children of smokers are at increased risk for respiratory illnesses. Smoking during pregnancy decreases birthweights, increases infant mortality, and leads to reductions in growth and educational achievement. Direct physician advice can produce quit rates of 7% to 10%. If half of US physicians delivered a brief quitting message to their patients who smoke, the national annual cessation rate would double.

Clinical Approach. A minimal-contact approach that can substantially improve cessation rates is the following:

1. Ask patients about smoking at every opportunity.
2. Advise all smokers to stop with a clear, direct message. Personalize the health risks of smoking and the benefits of quitting.
3. Assist the interested smoker by motivating him or her to set a quit date, providing a self-help guide such as "Clearing the Air" available from the National Cancer Institute (1-800-4-CANCER), and prescribing nicotine replacement therapy when appropriate.
4. Arrange follow-up.

To further improve cessation rates:

1. Assess a patient's readiness to quit. Smokers who are not contemplating cessation (precontemplators) benefit from brief motivational counseling and education about the personal health risks of smoking. Those who are contemplating quitting need treatment information and encouragement to set a quit date.
2. Ask about smoking-related symptoms. Smokers who have recently experienced the onset of symptoms or a disease related to smoking have an increased chance of successfully quitting.
3. Discuss a patient's reasons for wanting to quit and employ those reasons to support his or her motivation to stop.
4. Discuss past cessation attempts and portray quitting as a process that

may take several attempts. Patients with a history of multiple failures or who have little confidence in their ability to quit may benefit from referral to a structured smoking cessation program. A list of such programs is available through the American Lung Association.

5. Prescribe nicotine replacement therapy to smokers who are dependent (heavy smokers, those who smoke within 30 minutes of awakening) or those who have failed in past cessation attempts due to withdrawal symptoms (Table 12–1). Patches are generally better tolerated and are probably more efficacious than nicotine polacrilex gum. Heavily dependent patients (cigarette within 5 minutes of awakening) may have a higher rate of success with double-strength (4 mg) gum than with patches.

6. Counsel patients about barriers to quitting, such as withdrawal symptoms (peak 1 to 2 days, last 2 to 4 weeks) and fear of weight gain (averages 5 lb). Briefly introduce self-help materials.

Follow-Up. A visit with a physician or designated staff member is scheduled 1 to 2 weeks after the cessation date. A letter can be sent or a call made reinforcing the patient's decision to stop smoking. The personal health benefits

Table 12–1. NICOTINE REPLACEMENT THERAPY

Administration	Directions for Use	Cost
Nicotine Transdermal System		
Begin with one 21-mg patch every day × 4 weeks (begin with 14 mg every day if cardiovascular disease, weight < 100 lb, or smokes less than ¹/₂ pack/day). Taper to 14 mg every day × 2 weeks then 7 mg every day × 2 weeks. *Note:* No increased benefit has been shown with treatment longer than 8 weeks.	Do not smoke and use patch. Apply a new patch every day to different, nonhairy, dry, intact skin on upper body or upper outer arm; may bathe and exercise during use. 14%–17% experience erythema; 2%–6% discontinue because of skin reactions.	$90–$120/box of 30
Nicotine Polacrilex Gum		
Chew one piece every 1–2 hours; max 30/24 hours (2 mg) or 20/24 hours of double-strength (4 mg) gum. Decrease by one or more pieces every 4–7 days. Stop after reaching 1–2/day.	Do not smoke and chew gum. Chew slowly until a peppery taste develops (approximately 15 chews), place gum between cheek and gum until taste is almost gone. Repeat until nicotine is gone (about 30 minutes), placing gum in a different part of cheek each time. Do not eat or drink for 15 minutes before or while chewing. Chewing too fast increases side effects such as gastrointestinal symptoms, oral ulcers.	$30–$40/box of 96

of quitting can be reemphasized. Those who have not stopped smoking should be praised for any steps taken toward quitting, be helped in identifying quitting obstacles, and be encouraged to set a new quit date. Precontemplators need personalized messages about smoking risks based on symptoms and their medical and family history.

Cross-Reference: Periodic Health Assessment (Chapter 8).

REFERENCES

1. Fiore MC, Smith SS, Jorenby DE, Baker TB. The effectiveness of the nicotine patch for smoking cessation. JAMA 1994;271:1941–1947.

   Meta-analysis of 17 studies of transdermal nicotine shows that abstinence rates at 6 months were 22% with patches versus 9% with placebo. Intensive behavioral therapy showed a reliable but modest impact on cessation rates.

2. Frank E. Benefits of stopping smoking. West J Med 1993;159:83–87.

   The health benefits of smoking cessation are summarized with a patient education handout.

3. Orleans CT, Slade J. Nicotine Addiction: Principles and Management. New York, Oxford University Press, 1993.

   This detailed source of information about tobacco use contains an excellent summary of minimal contact smoking cessation strategies for medical settings.

4. Prochaska JO, Goldstein MG. Process of smoking cessation. Clin Chest Med 1991;12:727–735.

   Research on a stages-of-change model of smoking cessation is summarized. Guidelines are provided for improving cessation rates in the stages they have identified (precontemplation, contemplation, preparation, action, and maintenance).

5. Silagy C, Mant D, Fowler G, Lodge M. Meta-analysis on efficacy of nicotine replacement therapies in smoking cessation. Lancet 1994;343:139–142.

   An analysis of 53 trials found that nicotine replacement increased the odds ratio (OR) of abstinence to 1.71 compared with control interventions. The OR for transdermal nicotine was 2.07 compared with 1.61 for gum (P = .05).

13 Travel Medicine

Problem

ELAINE C. JONG

Epidemiology. International travel has become an increasingly common activity among many sectors of the US civilian population over the past decade. The growth in international travel has been fostered by multinational businesses, collaborative educational and research projects, affordable airfares for tourists, and continued American participation in global relief efforts.

Rationale. In general, travel medicine focuses on the needs of persons going from relatively sanitary, developed areas of the world to areas where conditions of hygiene and sanitation may be relatively less advanced. Preventive health measures to promote the health of the traveler during and after the trip are recommended after a risk assessment of the proposed itinerary. Common ailments associated with disruption of normal sleep/wake cycles, dietary intake, climatic adaptations, and social milieu are also considered. Environmental hazards and personal safety issues are often reviewed.

Clinical Approach. The travel medicine recommendations for a given traveler are based on an assessment of the health risks associated with the proposed itinerary:

I. Geographic destination
   A. Urban or rural travel
   B. Tropical, cold, or temperate climate
II. Purpose of trip
   A. Single or multiple destination(s)
   B. Tourism, short-term business, field work, adventure travel
   C. High-altitude or scuba diving activities
III. Style of travel
   A. Western-style hotel
   B. Local housing
   C. Camping
IV. Anticipated contact with local inhabitants
V. Underlying health status of traveler
VI. Access to health care during travel

Knowledge of updated information on epidemics, environmental hazards, and endemic health problems at one's destination can be obtained from several sources. The Centers for Disease Control and Prevention (CDC) provides authoritative updated information on worldwide epidemiologic conditions with regard to communicable diseases and vaccine requirements (Fax Information Service [404] 332-4565). The CDC travel information Web page is http://www.cdc.gov/travel/travel.html. The US Department of State Citizens Emergency Center is a resource for updated information on political and safety conditions that might impact overseas travelers. The sources listed at the end of this chapter can serve as starting points for the identification of specific health considerations related to geographic location and travel conditions. In general, tropical or extreme climates, trips lasting longer than 1 month with multiple destinations, and remote adventure travel are associated with greater health risks.

The four main preventive health activities in travel medicine are

1. Immunizations for vaccine-preventable diseases
2. Chemoprophylaxis against certain infections (e.g., malaria)
3. Protocols and medications for self-treatment of certain common travel ailments (e.g., traveler's diarrhea)
4. Behavior modification (e.g., use of mosquito nets and insect repellents, use of sunscreens, compliance with malaria chemoprophylaxis, selection of safe food and water, avoidance of high-risk sexual encounters, selection

of safe modes of transportation, avoiding swimming in lakes and rivers in areas of schistosomiasis).

Vaccines for International Travel. Of the routine immunizations, special attention should be given to tetanus, diphtheria, polio, measles, and varicella immune status in persons planning international travel. The recommendations for influenza and pneumococcal vaccines are the same for international travelers and the general population (see Chapter 11, Adult Immunizations).

The vaccines traditionally regulated by the World Health Organization (WHO) are smallpox, cholera, and yellow fever vaccines. At present, the WHO endorses only a yellow fever vaccine requirement for international travelers. The yellow fever vaccine must be received at an official yellow fever vaccine center (designated by state public health departments in the United States) and must be documented on an official WHO international certificate of vaccination. Yellow fever–endemic zones generally include equatorial Africa and Latin America. However, the CDC information sources should be consulted for up-to-date country-by-country recommendations.

The WHO requirement for cholera vaccine has been dropped despite the increased global spread of cholera because the older parenteral cholera vaccine had poor protective efficacy. Two new oral cholera vaccines, an attenuated live vaccine and an inactivated vaccine, show increased efficacy. As these improved cholera vaccines become commercially available worldwide, the WHO may develop a new cholera vaccine policy.

Clinical judgment must be used in the selection of all the other vaccines that are not required but can be appropriately recommended to travelers. Travel in areas of poor hygiene and sanitation prompt consideration of vaccine-preventable diseases transmitted by the oral-fecal route: poliomyelitis, hepatitis A, typhoid fever, and cholera. Work or recreational activities, anticipated living conditions, and lifestyle choices might suggest the need for immunization against hepatitis B, rabies, meningococcal meningitis, and Japanese encephalitis, as well as tuberculosis skin tests before and after travel. The use of bacille Calmette-Guérin (BCG) vaccine in adults to prevent tuberculosis is not recommended.

Data are limited on the risk of communicable diseases among international travelers. However, hepatitis A appears to be the most common vaccine-preventable disease, with an estimated attack rate of 3 per 1000 travelers per month among tourist travelers and an attack rate of as high as 20 per 1000 per month among travelers who went off the normal tourist routes. Immune globulin has been commonly given to provide travelers with short-term protection (3–5 months depending on dose) against hepatitis A infection. However, limited availability of immune globulin for this purpose in the United States and the licensure of two new hepatitis A vaccines that are highly efficacious in eliciting long-lasting immune protection will probably result in increased use of vaccine for hepatitis A prevention. Table 13–1 presents primary immunization schedules, booster intervals, and contraindications for travel vaccines.

Malaria Chemoprophylaxis. Malaria is a blood-borne protozoan infection spread from person to person by female anopheline mosquitoes. A map of areas where malaria transmission occurs is shown in Figure 13–1. Updated country-by-country and regional information may be obtained from the CDC

Table 13–1. SCHEDULES FOR COMMONLY USED TRAVEL IMMUNIZATIONS

Vaccine	Primary Series	Booster Interval
Cholera, parenteral	Two doses 1 week or more apart (0.5 mL SC or IM); (pediatric dose: 0.3 mL for 5–10 y old; 0.2 mL for 6 mo–4 y old)	Six months (see text)
Hepatitis A (Havrix) (1440 EL.U./mL, adult; 720 EL.U./mL, pediatric) (USA)	1.0 mL IM into the deltoid muscle (adult dose: > 18 y old; pediatric dose: 2–17 y old)	Booster dose at 6–12 mo predicted to confer immune protection for 10 y or more
Hepatitis A (VAQTA) (50 U/mL, adult; 25 U/mL, pediatric)	1.0 mL into the deltoid muscle (adult dose: > 18 y old; pediatric dose: 2–17 y old)	Booster dose given at 6 to 18 mo will give long-lasting protection for years
Hepatitis B (Engerix B) (standard schedule)	Three doses at 0, 1, and 6 mo given IM in the deltoid area* (20 μg/mL dose > 10 y old; 10 μg/0.5 mL dose for birth to 10 y old)	Need for booster not determined; predict long-lasting protection for years after completion of primary series
Hepatitis B (Engerix B) (accelerated schedule)†	Three IM doses at 0, 30, and 60 d (age-appropriate doses; see above)	A fourth dose is recommended at 12 mo
Hepatitis B (Recombivax HB) (standard schedule)	Three doses at 0, 1, and 6 mo given IM in the deltoid area* (2.5μg/0.5 mL 1–10 y old; 5 μg/0.5 mL 11–19 y old; 10 μg/1.0 mL > 20 y old; 40 μg/1.0 mL only for adult predialysis/dialysis patients)	Need for booster not determined; predict long-lasting protection for years after completion of primary series; booster dose or revaccination may be considered for anti-HBs < 10 MIU/mL 1 to 2 mo after the third dose
Immune globulin (Human) (Hepatitis A protection)	One dose IM in the gluteus muscle (2 mL dose for 3 mo protection; 5 mL divided dose for 5 mo; pediatric dose: 0.02 mL/kg for 3-mo trip, 0.06 mL/kg for 5-mo trip)	Boost at 3- to 5-mo intervals depending on the initial dose received
Japanese encephalitis	Three doses given 1 week apart (1 mL SC ≥ 3 y old; 0.5 mL SC < 3 y old)	Booster dose 1 at 12–18 mo, then additional doses at 4-y intervals for continued risk of exposure
Meningococcus (A/C/Y/W-127)	1 dose SC‡	None (variable immunogenic response in children < 4 y; reimmunization recommended after 2–3 y for children in this group who continue to be at high risk)
Plague	First dose (1 mL IM); second dose (0.2 mL IM) 4 wk later; dose 3 (0.2 mL IM) 3–6 mo after dose 2	Boost if the risk of exposure persists: give the first two booster doses (0.1–0.2 mL) 6 mo apart; then give one booster dose at 1- to 2-y intervals as needed
Rabies, human diploid cell vaccine (HDCV)	Three doses given 1 week apart (0.1 mL ID) on days 0, 7, and 21 or 28	Boost after 2 y or test serum for antibody level; must not use chloroquine for malaria prophylaxis until 3 wk after completion of third ID dose of vaccine

Table continued on following page

Table 13-1. SCHEDULES FOR COMMONLY USED TRAVEL IMMUNIZATIONS
Continued

Vaccine	Primary Series	Booster Interval
Rabies, human diploid cell vaccine (HDCV) or rabies vaccine absorbed (RVA)	Three doses (1 mL IM in the deltoid area) on days 0, 7, and 28	Boost after 2 y or test serum for protective antibody level
Typhoid VI, capsular polysaccharide, injectable (Typhim VI)	One dose (0.5 mL IM) for ≥ 2 y old	Boost after 2 y for continued risk of exposure (booster interval is 3 y in Canada)
Typhoid, oral (Vivotif)§	One capsule PO every 2 days for four doses (≥ 6 y old)	5 years
Yellow fever§	One dose (0.5 mL SC; pediatric dose: 0.5 mL SC for ≥ 9 mo old)	10 years

SC, subcutaneously; IM, intramuscularly; ID, intradermally; PO, orally.
*Anterolateral thigh region may be used in neonates and small infants.
†Accelerated schedule approved for Engerix B only.
‡See manufacturer's package insert for recommendations on dosage.
§May be contraindicated in patients with any of the following conditions: pregnancy, leukemia, lymphoma, generalized malignancy, immunosuppression due to human immunodeficiency virus infection or treatment with corticosteroids, alkylating drugs, antimetabolites, or radiation therapy.
Adapted from Jong EC, Sharp B. Immunizations for the international traveler. In Bia F, ed. The Travel Medicine Advisor. Atlanta, American Health Consultants, 1996; 2.1–2.16.

(see References). Malaria is a global problem of immense proportion, with 280 million cases per year (according to 1990 WHO statistics) among persons living in endemic areas and in visitors to those areas. Over the past two decades, the emergence of chloroquine-resistant *Plasmodium falciparum* (CRPF) malaria has required the use of increasingly toxic and expensive drugs to prevent and treat disease.

Weekly doses of chloroquine phosphate (500 mg) (adult dose) are recommended for malaria chemoprophylaxis in areas where malaria strains are still chloroquine sensitive, and 250-mg weekly doses of mefloquine (Lariam) (adult dose) are recommended in CRPF areas. Prophylaxis should be started 1 week before travel, continued weekly during travel, and continued for 4 weeks after travel. Daily doses of doxycycline (100 mg) (adult dose) beginning on the day of departure and taken continuously during travel in malaria-endemic areas and for 4 weeks after leaving those areas is the CDC recommendation for adults going to CRPF areas in whom mefloquine is contraindicated.

Vivid dreams, dizziness, and gastrointestinal upset are fairly common side effects associated with mefloquine. Mefloquine is contraindicated in early pregnancy and in persons with a diagnosis of cardiac conduction abnormality, seizure disorder, or depression. Alternative medications should be considered for travelers going to CRPF malaria–endemic areas who are intolerant to both mefloquine and doxycycline. A discussion of the indications, advantages, and disadvantages of these nonstandard CRPF prophylaxis regimens is beyond the scope of this chapter, but further information may be obtained by consulting a tropical medicine specialist or the references at the end of this chapter.

Continuing emergence of drug resistance among malaria strains worldwide means that no malaria chemoprophylaxis regimen can be considered 100%

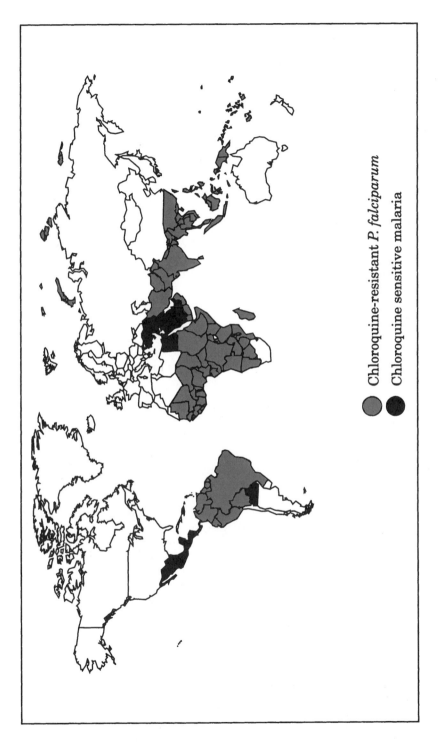

Figure 13–1. Distribution of malaria and chloroquine-resistant *Plasmodium falciparum*, 1996. (From Centers for Disease Control: Health Information for International Travel, 1996–97, HHS Publication No. [CDC] 97-8280, 1997. DHHS, Atlanta, GA, 1997.)

Chloroquine-resistant *P. falciparum*

Chloroquine sensitive malaria

effective. Malaria infection must be considered in the differential diagnosis of a traveler with fever who has returned from the tropics, regardless of a history of having taken on a regular basis antimalarial medications that were appropriately prescribed for a given geographic region.

The use of diethyltoluamide(DEET)-containing insect repellents on exposed areas of skin and sleeping under permethrin-impregnated bed nets are highly recommended to tropical travelers to decrease exposure to mosquitoes that transmit malaria and also to decrease the risk of other vector-borne diseases, such as dengue fever, filariasis, leishmaniasis, various arbovirus infections, Lyme disease, and trypanosomiasis.

Traveler's Diarrhea. Travelers should be advised to follow commonsense guidelines in the safe selection of food and water at destinations where hygiene, sanitation, and food storage are a problem:

- Select thoroughly cooked foods served piping hot.
- Avoid buffet dishes that have been sitting for hours at ambient temperatures.
- Avoid salads containing leafy green and other raw vegetables.
- Avoid salads, casseroles, and desserts with creamy binders or toppings.
- Avoid raw or lightly steamed shellfish and other undercooked seafood.

Travelers going to destinations where tap water is unsafe to drink should be advised to carry water purification tablets for chemical disinfection of the water or a portable water filter for use when there is limited access to safe fluids, such as canned or bottled carbonated beverages or beverages made with boiled water (e.g., coffee, tea, bouillon). Despite good intentions, however, diarrheal illness among travelers is fairly common in developing areas of the world.

Based on clinical field trials in Mexico, the use of prophylactic bismuth subsalicylate (Pepto-Bismol) in doses of 2 tablets orally four times a day for periods of up to 2 weeks of travel has been recommended by some travel health advisors, in addition to the food and water precautions. The use of daily doses of antibiotics for prophylaxis of traveler's diarrhea has been shown to be effective, but concerns about potential adverse side effects and long-term safety of these regimens have made this a controversial practice. Some travel consultants prescribe prophylactic antibiotics for special categories of short-term travelers, such as competitive athletes, political delegates, corporate executives, and honeymooners.

Oral rehydration is the key to preventing dehydration and prostration from illnesses characterized by copious watery diarrhea. Oral rehydration formulas based on the WHO recommendations for fluid and electrolyte replacement are available commercially in convenient foil packets, each of which is formulated to be reconstituted in 1 L of purified water. The formula is given in most travel medicine references and can be made up by individual pharmacies. Approximate replacement of fluid volumes lost through watery diarrhea by drinking oral rehydration solutions is the treatment of choice for cholera and other forms of watery diarrhea. If standard oral rehydration fluids are not available, commercial sports drinks, dilute fruit juices, flavored seltzers, and weak bouillon can supplement purified drinking water.

Symptomatic treatment for frequent stools and intestinal cramping using the over-the-counter antiperistaltic agent loperamide is considered generally safe except when severe abdominal pain, fever, and bloody diarrhea are present. The recommended adult regimen is two 2-mg tablets by mouth for the initial dose, followed by one tablet after each loose stool, up to a maximum dose of 8 tablets in 24 hours. If severe systemic symptoms and signs are present, professional medical evaluation is the optimal course. Travelers who are unable to access medical care may consider empirical self-treatment with antibiotics.

Empirical self-treatment with therapeutic regimens of antibiotics in the quinolone class (ciprofloxacin, ofloxacin, norfloxacin) in combination with loperamide treatment has been reported to effect a clinical cure of traveler's diarrhea within 24 hours after initiation of treatment. The trimethoprim-sulfamethoxazole combination was commonly used for empirical treatment of traveler's diarrhea in the past, but this combination has become less useful in areas of Asia, Latin America, and Africa where antibiotic resistance has emerged among the common bacteria associated with traveler's diarrhea.

Parasitic pathogens and drug-resistant bacteria need to be considered when a travel-acquired diarrheal illness lasts longer than a week or is unresponsive to empirical antibiotic treatment. A thorough evaluation by a knowledgeable clinician is recommended.

Medical consultation is also recommended when severe abdominal pain, fever, and bloody diarrhea are present.

Travel Medicine Kit. The primary care clinician should also discuss the contents of a travel medicine kit, which serves as the "medicine cabinet" away from home. Basic first-aid supplies such as bandages, antibiotic topical ointment, moleskin (for blisters), and a thermometer should be included, even for tourists. Remedies for nasal congestion, headaches, musculoskeletal pain, constipation, indigestion, and allergies should be considered. Adequate supplies of medications taken on a regular basis, as well as copies of current prescriptions, should be included in hand-carried (not checked) luggage. Special needs of travelers might include medications for jet lag, high altitude, and fungal infections. Female travelers need to remember sanitary supplies, and sexually active travelers should include high-quality latex condoms (because the quality of condoms purchased abroad may vary). Adventure travelers will need to consider advanced first-aid items (e.g., splints, sutures, bandages, analgesia for serious injuries) as well as sunscreen and insect repellents.

Summary. Primary care providers can provide useful information and direction to their patients who travel. Because of the complexity of health risks, there should be good coordination of the approach to meeting basic health needs while providing for travel-specific health risks associated with the planned itinerary. Patients with underlying acute or chronic health conditions may benefit by referral to a travel medicine specialist.

Cross-References: Adult Immunizations (Chapter 11), Diarrhea (Chapter 91).

REFERENCES

1. Bia F, ed. The Travel Medicine Advisor. Atlanta, American Health Consultants, 1996.
   This is an excellent general resource.

2. Centers for Disease Control and Prevention: Health Information for International Travel 1996–97. Atlanta, US Department of Health and Human Services, Public Health Service, 1997.

This is an excellent general resource.

3. Ericsson CD, DuPont HL. Traveler's diarrhea: Approaches to prevention and treatment. Clin Infect Dis 1993;16:616–626.

The authors present an overview and useful treatment guidelines.

4. Jong EC, McMullen R, eds. The Travel and Tropical Medicine Manual, 2nd ed. Philadelphia, WB Saunders, 1995.

This is an excellent general resource.

5. Steffen R, Rickenbach M, Wilhelm U, et al. Health problems after travel to developing countries. J Infect Dis 1987;156:84–91.

This is an excellent general resource.

6. US Department of State Citizens Emergency Center, Washington, DC. Telephone (202) 647-5225; (202) 634-3600: after-hours emergencies.

This is an excellent general resource.

SECTION III
Constitutional Symptoms

••

14 Chronic Nonspecific Pain Syndrome

Problem

JODIE K. HASELKORN and DIANA D. CARDENAS

Epidemiology. The perception of pain is highly personal and is dependent on the stimulus, the individual, and the individual's environment. Therefore, an identical painful stimulus can be perceived differently by different individuals and by a single individual at different times. Suffering and pain behaviors often accompany pain perception and tend to reinforce the pain experience.

Because so many factors contribute to pain, the definition of chronic nonspecific pain syndrome is elusive. Persons with chronic nonspecific pain syndrome cannot be characterized by the severity or location of their pain; instead, this name is used to describe a wide range of pain intensity at numerous locations. The pain can occur in any region of the body but most frequently involves the low back, neck, head, abdomen, and soft tissue. One accepted definition of chronic nonspecific pain syndrome is continuing perception of pain after healing or cessation of inflammation should have occurred or suffering and pain behavior that is out of proportion to the residual impairment. Although the normal time of healing varies with the individual and the clinical condition, pain persisting 3 months beyond the time expected for healing can be used as a benchmark.

In addition to this extended pain perception, people with chronic nonspecific pain syndrome tend to exhibit accompanying behaviors such as depression, chronic stress, medication dependence, and frequent visits to a variety of health care providers. Therefore, chronic nonspecific pain syndrome differs from simple chronic pain associated with long-term diseases, such as cancer or arthritis, although some of the individuals with these conditions may also exhibit features of chronic nonspecific pain syndrome.

A risk factor for developing chronic nonspecific pain syndrome is inadequate treatment of an acute injury. Prevention may be enhanced by accurate diagnosis and a thorough explanation of the nature of the acute problem, avoiding associating the pain with a condition not usually associated with pain (e.g., lumbar degenerative disks), avoiding attributing an increase in symptoms to disease progression, providing an estimated recovery date, specifying activity and medications at specifically prescribed doses and frequencies, and providing prompt follow-up.

Other potential risk factors for chronic nonspecific pain syndrome are dissatisfaction with employment and/or employer, disability income that equals or exceeds employment income, pending litigation, substance abuse, and family problems.

Because chronic nonspecific pain syndrome is difficult to define, its epidemiology has not been fully described. The precise prevalence of chronic pain is not known, although roughly one third of the US population report having had chronic pain at some time in their lives, with one half of this group having experienced short-term, long-term, or permanent disability. The cost of this problem is estimated at $79 billion, including 400 million lost days of work and $49 billion in direct health care costs.

Etiology and Syndromes and Signs. Whereas acute pain serves the purpose of warning patients about potential harm or promotes rest and healing after injury, the pain perception in chronic nonspecific pain syndrome serves no useful purpose. In the case of chronic nonspecific pain syndrome, the hurt does not signify impending bodily harm, nor does increased rest serve to promote healing. The suffering behaviors that accompany chronic pain syndrome are learned, goal-directed, and frequently reinforced by family, friends, and the medical and vocational systems.

Unlike acute pain, which is characterized by a heightened sympathetic response, people with chronic nonspecific pain syndrome do not present with hypertension, tachycardia, diaphoresis, and dilated pupils. Instead, symptoms include a depressed affect, sleep disturbance, decreased pain tolerance, disturbed appetite, activity limitation, and substance abuse. Additional clues to the recognition of chronic nonspecific pain syndrome include absence of recovery beyond predicted recovery date, nonphysiologic physical examination findings, poor compliance with follow-up, frequent medical visits to multiple providers, medication-seeking behaviors, and a history of lost medications. These individuals may believe that there is no help or hope and exhibit illness behaviors without a predictable end.

Clinical Approach. Chronic nonspecific pain syndrome can usually be diagnosed with confidence if the risk factors just cited are present and either (1) a source of chronic pain is not identified after a thorough workup or (2) a source is identified but the individual's suffering behaviors are well out of proportion to those usually seen. Intervention should begin promptly.

Once a workup has been completed, there is little to be gained by additional diagnostic efforts, which may, in fact, be detrimental by reinforcing an individual's pain perception and suffering behavior. Instead, all prior diagnostic studies and diagnoses should be reviewed with the individual. The physician should inquire about the individual's beliefs about his or her condition and how readily he or she will accept alternative explanations. The patterns of coping with pain that the individual has observed should be explored. The physician should communicate that (1) he or she understands all that the person has gone through and that the person hurts and is not malingering; (2) the individual's capacity to heal is intact, the original problem has healed, and the person's perceptions of the problem are out of proportion to tissue damage; (3) the physician is confident of the diagnosis and that nothing will be gained by additional diagnostic procedures or treatments used in the management of acute conditions; (4) the individual's pain perception is a "false signal" giving inappropriate information to limit activity; and (5) this is a common problem that can be successfully managed.

The diagnostic goals are to determine the degree of medication use, psychosocial dysfunction, deconditioning, leisure dysfunction, and vocational problems. The clinician should obtain a full inventory of all medications, including prescriptions, over-the-counter remedies, ethanol, and street drugs. The individual should describe both the negative environmental factors that serve to maintain his or her suffering behaviors and the positive factors that can be relied on for support during treatment. A Minnesota Multiphasic Personality Inventory may be useful to help determine the presence of depression and other personal characteristics that may help in treatment (see Chapter 193, Psychological Assessment). Consultation with a psychologist may be helpful.

After establishing the individual's trust and desire to improve, it may be useful to draw up a therapeutic contract specifying the problems, goals, and desired actions. The family and employer may also need to be involved. If goals cannot be reached, all parties should agree to referral to a specialist.

Management. The traditional biomedical model is not useful in the management of chronic nonspecific pain. Instead, the provider must use the biopsychosocial approach. The overall goal in the management of chronic nonspecific pain syndrome is to restore physical and psychological *function*—not necessarily to eliminate pain. Specific treatment goals are to reduce reliance on the medical care system, enhance psychological well-being and coping skills, restore sleep and nutrition, and enhance physical activity, leisure skills, and possibly attendance and performance at work.

Controversy continues about prescription of opioids or sedative/hypnotics in selected individuals with chronic nonspecific pain syndrome. There is, however, general agreement that very few individuals should be treated with these medications, either on a scheduled long-term or on an as-needed basis. Scheduled long-term use of opioids or sedatives impairs the psychological and physical goals of treatment. As-needed use tends to reinforce suffering behaviors.

Many individuals with chronic pain have already been taking opioids and sedative/hypnotics for long periods of time and at high doses. In these cases, it is advisable to begin detoxification using a long-acting opioid, such as methadone, at a total daily dose equal to 120% of the short-acting opioid that they have been taking (Table 14–1). Because the analgesic effect of methadone lasts for 6 hours, the daily dose must be split into four doses over the course of the day. Detoxification from longer-acting sedative/hypnotics (e.g., diazepam) may be accomplished with phenobarbital, but successful detoxification of the shorter-acting benzodiazepines (e.g., alprazolam or lorazepam) is difficult with phenobarbital and may require an "in-between" dose of a short-acting sedative/hypnotic that is withdrawn over time (Table 14–2). Analgesia must be optimized with scheduled anti-inflammatory medications, acetaminophen, and hydroxyzine. Medications may be given in tablet form, although a blind liquid

Table 14–1. EQUIVALENCE AND CONVERSION OF OPIOID MEDICATIONS

Medication	Brand Name	Equivalent Dose (mg) to 10 mg IV Morphine	
		Oral (mg)	IV/IM (mg)
Opioid Agonists			
Morphine	Various	30–60	10
Codeine	Various	200	130
Diacetylmorphine (heroin)			3.0
Fentanyl*	Sublimaze, Duragesic		0.1–0.2
Hydromorphone	Dilaudid	7.5	1.5
Levorphanol	Levo-Dromoran	4	2
Meperidine	Demerol	300	75–100
Methadone	Dolophine, various	10–20	8–10
Oxycodone	Roxidocone	30	10–15
Oxymorphone†	Numorphan	–	1
Propoxyphene HCl‡	Darvon	130	
Propoxyphene napsylate	Darvon-N	200	
Mixed Agonists			
Buprenorphine	Buprenex		0.3
Butorphanol§	Stadol		2–3
Dezocine	Dalgan		10–15
Nalbuphine	Nubain		10
Pentazocine	Talwin	150–200	30–60
Other			
Tramadol	Ultram	120–200	

*Fentanyl also available as transdermal patch, 100 μg/h, which is equivalent to 0.1 to 0.2 mg IM.

†Oxymorphone also available as suppositories of 5 or 10 mg, which are equivalent to approximately 1 mg IM.

‡For replacement of propoxyphene HCL, maximum dose of methadone is 40 mg/24 h.

§Butorphanol also available as Stadol NS; one puff = 1 mg but systemic absorption is variable according to age and gender.

taper using a cherry syrup or an antacid as a vehicle for dissolved medication plus a masking agent, such as a liquid vitamin, may be more effective. Medications should be given only on a fixed time schedule, not as needed, to reduce suffering behaviors. The methadone and phenobarbital may be tapered 10% to 20% per week. Individuals should be counseled that it is essential to taper the medications to achieve other goals and that the taper can be done without escalating symptoms. Alternatively, cognitive-behavioral strategies may also be used instead of the operant strategies presented earlier.

Detoxification may be easier in an inpatient setting where access to other medications and providers can be controlled and symptoms of withdrawal monitored. Nevertheless, an individual can be detoxified on an outpatient basis with close follow-up and with one provider managing all medications. Toxicology screens in either setting may be useful. Withdrawal should be planned around medical and social stressors. When possible, significant others should be involved in the program, and everyone involved should be educated about preventing relapse. If substance abuse of ethanol or street drugs is a problem, this should be managed first (see Chapter 10, Alcohol Problems).

Although detoxification may be critical to achieving the management

**Table 14–2. EQUIVALENCE AND CONVERSIONS OF
SEDATIVE/HYPNOTIC MEDICATIONS**

Medication	Brand Name	Equivalent Dose (mg) to 30 mg Oral Phenobarbital
Benzodiazepines		
Aprazolam	Xanax	1
Chlordiazepoxide	Librium	20–25
Clonazepam	Klonopin	1–4
Clorazepate	Tranxene	15
Diazepam	Valium	10
Flurazepam	Dalmane	15–30
Halazapam	Paxipam	40
Lorazepam	Ativan	2
Oxazepam	Serax	30
Barbiturates		
Amobarbital	Amytal, various	100
Butabarbital	Butisol	100
Butalbital	Fiorinal	100
Pentobarbital	Nembutal	100
Phenobarbital	Various	30
Secobarbital	Seconal	100
Other		
Chloral hydrate	Noctec	500–1000
Ethyl alcohol (100 proof)		90 mL
Meprobamate	Miltown	400

goals, it must be done in conjunction with an overall plan that includes management of psychological dysfunction, sleep disturbance, family dysfunction, exercise, leisure dysfunction, and return to work. Treatment of depression may require medical management and psychological counseling. The use of tricyclic antidepressants is helpful if there is concomitant sleep disturbance, whereas a serotonin-reuptake inhibitor is helpful if activity limitations outweigh sleep disturbance (see Chapter 189, Management of Depression). Family counseling may also be necessary to remedy environment reinforcers of suffering behaviors.

Just as medications must be prescribed specifically in terms of dose and frequency with a taper, exercise must be prescribed with the goal of restoring physical function. Most people will have rested to the point of loss of flexibility, strength, and aerobic fitness. A properly prescribed, graded exercise program can counter these effects of disuse and enhance overall function. The program is developed by establishing "baseline" activities that meet important functional goals, including sitting, standing, walking, climbing stairs, carrying a load, and performing an aerobic activity. The baseline is determined by individual report and observation. The initial quotas are set at a level below the observed or reported baseline, for instance, 20% lower than the level tolerated. The prescription specifies the number of repetitions for each activity per day and the number of days per week. The individual is instructed to exercise to quota, not tolerance, whether he or she feels like it or not. Individuals are counseled that some increased discomfort in the initial aspect of the program is expected. The quotas are increased 10% to 20% per week. A log of success reinforces continued exercise.

Each individual should identify leisure goals that are not associated with ethanol, street drugs, or pain-dependent behavior and develop a plan to enhance leisure time. A log reviewed by the provider will reinforce appropriate leisure activities.

For many individuals return to work is feasible. Whereas the assignment of temporary disability for acute pain may be appropriate, assignment of permanent disability solely because of chronic nonspecific pain is inappropriate. There is no direct link between chronic nonspecific pain and permanent disability. Consultation with a vocational counselor and a provider experienced with the assessment of disability may be beneficial (see Chapter 5, Determining Disability: The Primary Care Physician's Role).

Patients with chronic pain syndrome can be difficult to treat. If the primary care provider cannot facilitate the patient's recovery, the patient can be referred to a program specializing in chronic pain. There are 180 centers accredited by the Commission on Accreditation of Rehabilitation Facilities, including 55 inpatient programs and 125 outpatient programs that offer multidisciplinary treatment.

Cross-References: Effective Communication in the Ambulatory Care Setting (Chapter 2), Diagnosis and Management of Drug Abuse (Chapter 9), Alcohol Problems (Chapter 10), Assessment of Physical Activity (Chapter 72), Abdominal Pain (Chapter 94), Low Back Pain (Chapter 107), Fibromyalgia (Chapter 121), Myofascial Pain Syndromes (Chapter 122), Physical Therapy Care of Outpatients (Chapter 125), Pelvic Pain in Women (Chapter 160), Insomnia (Chapter 187), Management of Depression (Chapter 189), Psychological Assessment (Chapter 193).

REFERENCES

1. International Association for the Study of Pain (Merskey H, ed). Classification of chronic pain: Description of chronic pain syndromes and definitions of pain states. Pain 1986;24(suppl 3):S1.

   This supplement discusses the multidisciplinary efforts to further understand chronic pain.

2. Bonica, JJ. General consideration of chronic pain. In Bonica JJ, ed. Pain. Philadelphia, Lea & Febiger, 1990:180–196.

   This chapter provides a useful overview by a pioneer in the field who edits this two-volume text that covers all aspects of chronic pain.

3. Butler SH, Murphy TM. Use and abuse of drugs in chronic non-cancerous pain states. In Loeser JD, Eagen KJ, eds. Managing the Chronic Pain Patient: Theory and Practice at the University of Washington Multidisciplinary Pain Center. New York, Raven Press, 1989:1162–1168.

   This text presents one center's approach to the management of chronic pain.

4. Cardenas DD, Eagan KJ. Management of chronic pain. In Kottke FJ, Stillwell GK, Lehmann IF, eds. Krusen's Handbook of Physical Medicine and Rehabilitation, 4th ed. Philadelphia, WB Saunders, 1990:1162–1168.

   This chapter in a comprehensive physical medicine and rehabilitation text describes another approach to management of chronic pain.

5. Fordyce WE, ed. Back Pain in the Workplace: Management of Disability in Nonspecific Conditions. Seattle, IASP Press, 1995.

   The management of this often frustrating occupational problem is reviewed.

15 Obesity

Problem

DEBORAH L. GREENBERG

Epidemiology. Obesity, defined as an excess in body fat, is a common chronic condition encountered in primary care practice and one of the most resistant to treatment. The terminology used in discussions of obesity is not uniform, and direct measurement of body fat is difficult. Thus, many studies of prevalence and adverse health outcomes of obesity have used total body weight or body mass index (BMI = weight in kilograms divided by the square of height in meters). These accessible measures correlate well with total body fat. Overweight or mild obesity is defined as 20% to 40% over ideal body weight (BMI of 27.8–31.1 in men and 27.3–32.3 in women). Severely overweight or moderately obese refers to 40% to 100% above ideal weight (BMI of 31.2–39.0 in men and 32.4–39.0 in women). Clinically severe or morbid obesity represents a total weight greater than 100% ideal (BMI above 39.0).

The Second National Health and Nutrition Examination Survey estimated that 34 million American adults (24% of men; 27% of women) were overweight in 1980 and more than 3 million were morbidly obese. The prevalence of overweight has increased over the past several decades despite social and cultural pressures to be thin. Point prevalence and weight trends differ based on sex, ethnic background, socioeconomic status, and age.

Overweight and obese men and women have a higher overall mortality as well as an increased relative risk of death from cardiovascular disease and cancer for their age. Morbidity due to hypertension, dyslipidemia, insulin resistance, diabetes, hepatic steatosis, gallbladder disease, pulmonary dysfunction, sleep apnea, and osteoarthritis is also increased. In addition to overall weight and fat, body fat distribution is also associated with poor health outcomes. Increased intra-abdominal fat (waist-to-hip ratio greater than 0.95 in men and 0.85 in women), independent of overall weight, is associated with an elevated risk for cardiovascular disease and diabetes.

Etiology. Obesity is a heterogeneous disorder reflecting genetic, physiologic, cultural, socioeconomic, and psychologic influences on food intake, perception of food intake, energy expenditure, and fat distribution. In all cases, energy intake exceeds energy expenditure. Secondary obesity accounts for less than 1% of cases. In adults, the clinician should consider medications, hypothyroidism, Cushing's syndrome, and hypothalamic lesions. Common medications associated with weight gain include β-blockers, central sympatholytics (e.g., clonidine), glucocorticosteroids, oral contraceptives, tricyclic antidepressants, sulfonylureas, and insulin. Genetic disorders causing obesity are clinically evident in childhood.

Clinical Approach. Discussions of excess weight can provoke anxiety and frustration in both the patient and the health care provider. An understanding and respectful approach toward obesity is important for the overall psychologic and physical health of the individual patient. The history should focus on the pattern of weight gain, characterization of previous weight loss attempts (e.g., type of program, duration, outcome), motivation to lose weight (e.g., appearance, avoidance of health problems, current health problems, general fitness), weight loss goals, and knowledge about health and diet. The clinician should review all medications, screen for symptoms of neuroendocrine disorders, assess cardiac risk factors and co-morbid conditions (e.g., diabetes, hypertension, hyperlipidemia, sleep apnea), and determine the current level of physical activity. The physical examination, including calculation of BMI, should include a search for underlying disease and complications of obesity and an assessment of the patient's mobility. Laboratory examination will depend on the individual patient but should include a lipid profile, a random glucose test, and determination of levels of hepatic enzymes.

Management. Obesity is a chronic disease. Both the patient and clinician must adopt a long-term approach to therapy. Patients should be motivated to improve their health rather than achieve a specific weight. They must be willing to make lifelong changes in their diet and activity behaviors. Modest weight reduction (5%–10%) can be clinically significant, especially in obese diabetic or hypertensive patients, and can improve the quality of life. Physicians should help patients individualize therapeutic modalities and goals.

Treatment consists of two phases: weight reduction and weight maintenance. Initial attempts at active weight reduction utilize moderate calorie restriction (800–1500 kcal/d). These low-calorie diets usually consist of 15% calories from protein, less than 30% calories from fat, and the rest from carbohydrates. Typical weight loss is 0.5 kg/wk. Very low calorie diets, reserved for moderately to morbidly obese individuals, are modified fasts that enable rapid weight loss while preserving lean body mass and safety. Although intake is restricted to 800 kcal/d or less, protein and recommended daily vitamins, minerals, electrolytes, and fatty acids are maintained. Typical programs consist of four phases: introduction, modified fast, refeeding, and maintenance. These physician-supervised diets generally last 12 to 16 weeks and result in an average weight loss of 1.5 to 2.0 kg/wk. Although very low calorie diets produce superior short-term weight loss compared with low-calorie diets, neither diet alone has been successful in achieving permanent weight loss. Almost all patients return to their original weight within 5 years.

The addition of behavior modification, exercise, and nutritional education to diet therapy has resulted in sustained weight reduction in some patients. Behavior modification uses problem solving to identify and reduce inappropriate eating and exercise habits. Patients keep daily records of food intake, physical activity, and difficulties they encounter. They meet individually with a therapist or in peer groups. Ongoing behavioral treatment is important for relapse prevention and reinforcement of healthy habits.

Exercise enhances overall health and is an essential component of any weight reduction plan. In overweight individuals, exercise alone has not proven effective in initial weight loss. However, exercise is effective in weight maintenance and results in improvement in the waist-to-hip ratio. An exercise program should begin at the patient's current level of activity and increase slowly over time. The duration, intensity, and frequency should be specified. (See Chapter 72, Assessment of Physical Activity.)

Nutritional education emphasizes lifelong dietary changes (e.g., healthy food choices, decreased dietary fat). These changes are important for weight maintenance and have other potential health benefits (e.g., decreased serum lipids, decreased incidence of certain cancers). Some patients experience modest weight loss (i.e., 3 kg) through low-fat diets alone.

Physicians should consider drug therapy for patients who are morbidly obese or have significant co-morbid conditions and cannot lose or maintain their weight with nonpharmacologic interventions. Early compounds used in the treatment of obesity, amphetamines and amphetamine-like drugs, are rarely used owing to their central nervous system stimulation and addictive potential. Over the past several decades, new medications designed to suppress appetite, decrease energy absorption (e.g., lipase inhibitors), or increase energy expenditure (e.g., selective β-adrenergic agonists) have been developed for use in obesity. Appetite suppressants have been the most extensively studied and are the only drugs approved in the United States for weight loss (Table 15–1). Appetite suppressants are more effective than placebo in short-term trials. In the few studies that have looked at long-term (> 6 months) efficacy, most patients regained weight despite continued therapy. A subset of patients continued to lose weight or maintained their weight loss for the duration of the studies (up to 190 months). In general, patients had only mild side effects and no physical addiction. Common side effects of these drugs are similar and include hypertension, tachycardia, insomnia, drowsiness, asthenia, anxiety, nausea, and diarrhea. Of note, fenfluramine has been associated with depression when withdrawn abruptly, and several cases of pulmonary hypertension and valvular heart disease have been reported with the serotonergic agents.

Drug therapy is an option in carefully selected patients in conjunction with other treatment modalities discussed earlier. Therapy is initiated with a noradrenergic or serotonergic medication. If the patient fails to lose weight after several weeks or develops side effects, a drug from a different class or a low-dose combination can be substituted. If the patient responds with minimal side effects, the medication is continued until the patient begins to regain weight.

Table 15–1. APPETITE-SUPPRESSING DRUGS

Drug Class	Drug	Dosage	Cost ($ per month)*
Noradrenergic agents	Diethylpropion†	75 mg qd	47.62
	Mazindol†	1 mg qd	30.55
	Phentermine†	30 mg qd	2.66
Serotonergic agents	Fenfluramine†	20–40 mg tid	27.93–55.85
	Floxetine	20–60 mg qd	64.75–194.24
	Dexfenfluramine	15 mg bid	67.45
Combination	Phentermine and fenfluramine†	15 mg qd and 20 mg tid	29.66

*Average wholesale price, 1995 *Drug Topics Red Book.*
†DEA schedule IV.

Surgical treatment is an option for patients with clinically severe obesity who have failed nonsurgical treatment. Surgeons currently perform gastric bypass or vertical banded gastroplasty. These procedures result in significant perioperative and long-term complications. Gastric bypass results in greater weight loss but has a higher risk for nutritional deficiencies. The clinician should carefully review the benefits and risks for each individual patient before recommending surgery.

Follow-Up. Goals of a successful weight loss program include a decrease in BMI, a decrease in the complications of obesity, long-term weight maintenance, and an improved quality of life. Patients require close observation during periods of rapid weight loss to correct electrolyte abnormalities and provide motivation and support. Obesity, like other chronic diseases, requires regular physician visits for continued education and relapse prevention that are as important as the initial weight loss.

Cross-References: Sleep Apnea Syndromes (Chapter 64), Assessment of Physical Activity (Chapter 72), Essential Hypertension (Chapter 85), Diabetes Mellitus (Chapter 154).

REFERENCES

1. Goldstein DJ, Potvin JH. Long-term weight loss: The effect of pharmacological agents. Am J Clin Nutr 1994;60:647–657.

   Long-term (> 6 months) trials of pharmacologic therapy for weight loss and weight maintenance are reviewed.

2. Kumanyika SK. Special issues regarding obesity in minority populations. Ann Intern Med 1993;119:650–654.

   The increased incidence of obesity and obesity-related conditions in ethnic minorities is discussed along with barriers to prevention and treatment.

3. Manson JE, Willett WC, Stampfer MJ, et al. Body weight and mortality among women. N Engl J Med 1995;333:677–685.

   The association between body mass index and both overall mortality and cause-specific mortality is prospectively examined in the Nurses' Health Study cohort.

4. National Institutes of Health Consensus Development Conference Panel. Gastrointestinal surgery for severe obesity. Ann Intern Med 1991;155:956–961.

   The rationale for surgical procedures is reviewed and also included is a discussion of perioperative and long-term complications and areas for future research.

5. National Task Force on the Prevention and Treatment of Obesity. Very low-calorie diets. JAMA 1993;270:967–974.

   This article includes an overview of published studies on the safety and efficacy of very low-calorie diets.

16 Fever

Problem

BENJAMIN A. LIPSKY

Epidemiology. Most studies of fever have focused either on so-called fever of unknown origin (FUO) or on fever occurring in hospitalized populations. Unlike previously, the workup of FUO is now routinely accomplished in the outpatient setting. Outpatient studies of febrile patients have mainly been conducted in emergency departments, where about 5% of patients (range, 4% to 21% in published studies) are febrile (usually defined as having an oral temperature $\geq$ 37.8°C [100°F] or a rectal temperature of $\geq$ 38.3°C [101°F]).

Etiology. Infections are the cause of fever in most ambulatory patients. Acute febrile illnesses of less than 2 weeks' duration are common, usually uncomplicated, resolve spontaneously, and do not require a specific diagnosis. Bacterial infections and other more serious disorders require diagnostic evaluation and therapy. A prolonged unexplained fever can be classified as classic FUO if it lasts over 3 weeks and defies diagnosis after three outpatient visits or 3 days of hospitalization. In immunocompetent hosts, fever is far more likely to be due to a common disease than to a rare one. Immunocompromised hosts (e.g., those who are neutropenic or infected with human immunodeficiency virus) usually have an infectious cause for their fever. Patients with spinal cord injuries above the T6 level have impaired thermoregulation, but measurements of temperature should be used in a similar manner as in other patients.

The most frequent infectious causes of fever are viral syndromes, pharyngitis, urinary tract infections, cellulitis, pneumonia, and gastrointestinal infections (e.g., bacterial diarrhea, diverticulitis, hepatobiliary infections). Noninfectious causes of fever include malignancies, inflammatory disorders (connective tissue or granulomatous diseases), drug reactions, thromboembolic or neurologic events, hematomas, and alcoholic hepatitis. The relative prevalence of these causes is highly dependent on the age of the population studied and the practice setting. Fevers caused by neoplasms generally last several weeks, do not abate after antimicrobial therapy, and respond promptly to anti-inflammatory agents such as naproxen. In one small study the sensitivity of the "naproxen test" was 0.93 and the specificity was 1.0. Viral syndromes and upper respiratory tract infections cause fever infrequently in adults older than age 60 (< 5%) but commonly in those younger than age 60 (about 40%). Forty percent of febrile outpatients older than age 60 have an identifiable focal or systemic (i.e., bacteremic) bacterial infection. Older outpatients presenting with fever are more likely to have a life-threatening illness (e.g., pneumonia, biliary tract infection, diverticulitis) and to require hospitalization.

The initial evaluation identifies a localized source of the fever in 50% to 80% of patients, although the diagnosis is subsequently revised in 15% of patients. Occult bacterial infection is found in about one third of adult outpatients whose fever was initially unexplained. In parenteral drug users, fever is most often caused by pneumonia (about one third of cases) and endocarditis (about one sixth of cases); less frequent causes include pyrogen reactions, skin and soft tissue infections, and pyelonephritis. Febrile drug users with bacteremia, embolization, or other cardiac disorders should have an echocardiogram. Endocarditis is more likely in those who inject cocaine, have a history of cardiac disorders or weight loss, have a cardiac murmur or petechiae, have injected drugs in the past 5 days, or have previously had endocarditis.

Clinical Approach. The clinician should inquire about localizing symptoms and, when appropriate, about recent or remote travel, exposure to domestic or wild animals, unusual occupations or avocations, prescription and illicit drug use, risk factors for the acquired immunodeficiency syndrome, sexual history, unusual dietary exposures, and contact with sick individuals. The examination should focus on the skin and mucous membranes, lymph nodes, ocular fundi, heart and lung sounds, and palpation of the abdomen. Neither the fever's pattern nor its height is diagnostically reliable, although higher temperatures are more common in bacterial infections, especially in the elderly. Most patients maintain a diurnal temperature variation, especially if they have an infection. Dissociation of the body temperature and the pulse rate (Faget's sign) is of little diagnostic value. Fever lasting more than 2 weeks is unusual in common viral syndromes and most pyogenic infections and suggests subacute or chronic infections (e.g., tuberculosis, endocarditis) or noninfectious disorders.

Two studies have validated an index designed to predict occult bacterial infection in adult outpatients presenting with fever. The independent risk factors were age 50 years or older; diabetes mellitus; white blood cell count of 15,000/mm³ or more; neutrophil band count greater than or equal to 1500/mm³; and erythrocyte sedimentation rate of 30 mm/h or more. Patients who lack all of these features rarely need empirical antibiotic therapy or hospitalization. Among febrile adult outpatients, bacteremia is present in 10% to 15% of patients in whom blood cultures are done. In one study, however, less than 1% of those who were not hospitalized were bacteremic. Blood cultures should usually be done only in patients who are to be hospitalized or in whom subacute bacterial endocarditis is suspected. Because urinary and lower respiratory tract infections account for about half of bacterial infections, urinalysis and chest radiography are often helpful. Other diagnostic tests are indicated only when signs or symptoms suggest a localized infection and in some elderly or cognitively impaired patients.

Management. Hospitalization should be considered for febrile outpatients who are vulnerable hosts (e.g., the elderly, immunocompromised, or those with a serious underlying disease), who appear toxic (e.g., exhibit rigors, hypotension, prostration, extreme pyrexia, central nervous system dysfunction, or cardiopulmonary compromise), or in drug-using or chronically ill patients who have no obvious localizing findings. Studies have shown that febrile neutropenic patients with malignancies who were deemed at a low risk (i.e., relatively stable, with none of the toxic conditions mentioned, with no evidence of deep-organ infections, and with a supportive home environment) can be treated expectantly on an outpatient basis. The predictive index discussed earlier may also help determine who should be hospitalized. Antibiotics are usually indicated only when a bacterial infection is suspected. Empirical antibiotic administration to a patient with fever of uncertain cause usually does more harm than good. If a therapeutic trial is elected for a patient with a prolonged febrile illness, the antibiotic chosen should have as narrow a spectrum as possible. In outpatients with minor febrile illnesses, temperature elevation is only a small determinant of morbidity, and antipyretic therapy provides minimal symptomatic improvement. Except in patients with temperatures above 40°C (104°F) or those with severe cardiac or catabolic diseases, antipyretic therapy is unnecessary, potentially deleterious, and diagnostically confusing.

Follow-Up. Most patients with fever caused by conditions other than a viral respiratory syndrome should be seen (or contacted by telephone) for follow-up in about 3 days. Fifteen percent to 30% of febrile patients initially sent home from an emergency department subsequently require hospitalization.

REFERENCES

1. Eisenberg JM, Rose JD, Weinstein AJ. Routine blood cultures from febrile outpatients: Use in detecting bacteremia. JAMA 1976;236:2863–2865.

   Blood cultures were done in 37% of febrile emergency department patients; bacteremia was present in 10% of those who were hospitalized but only 1 of 124 patients not admitted.

2. Keating HJ, Klimek JJ, Levine DS, Kiernan FJ. Effect of aging on the clinical significance of fever in ambulatory adult patients. J Am Geriatr Soc 1984;32:282–287.

   In a retrospective analysis of adults seen in an emergency department, 93% of febrile patients older than 60 had an illness requiring hospitalization and 32% of them had a focal or systemic bacterial infection.

3. Leibovici L, Cohen O, Wysenbeek AJ. Occult bacterial infection in adults with unexplained fever: Validation of a diagnostic index. Arch Intern Med 1990;150:1270–1272.

   The index developed by Mellors, when prospectively applied within 12 hours of hospitalization to 113 adults with fever without an obvious source, accurately identified patients for whom hospitalization was unnecessary.

4. Mellors JW, Horwitz RI, Harvey MR, Horwitz SM. A simple index to identify occult bacterial infection in adults with acute unexplained fever. Arch Intern Med 1987;147:666–671.

   Of 880 acutely febrile patients presenting to the medicine section of an emergency department, 85% had localizing symptoms or signs. In the remaining 15% of patients, five features were found to be significant independent predictors of occult bacterial infection (see text).

5. Wasserman M, Levinstein M, Keller E, Lee S, Yoshikawa TT. Utility of fever, white blood cells, and differential count in predicting bacterial infections in the elderly. J Am Geriatr Soc 1989;37:537–543.

   In 221 patients age 70 years or older who were seen in an emergency department, temperature greater than or equal to 37.5°C, leukocytosis ($\geq$ 14,500/mm³), and bandemia ($>$ 6%) were each associated with the presence of a bacterial infection.

17 Unintentional Weight Loss

Problem

ERNIE-PAUL BARRETTE

Epidemiology. The exact incidence of involuntary weight loss is not known. In a single outpatient study surveying seven family practice centers over 2 years and including approximately 10,000 patients older than 63 years of age, 45 patients had unexplained weight loss. When weight loss is the presenting complaint, a clinically significant disease is suspected. The consequences of weight loss can be severe. In the Framingham study, a loss of 10% body mass index (body weight in kilograms divided by height in meters squared) correlated with increased mortality.

Etiology. Many diseases cause weight loss from decreased intake, increased losses, or excessive demand. Extensive evaluations yield a physical diagnosis in approximately 65% of patients with unexplained weight loss, whereas 25% remain undiagnosed even after extended follow-up (Table 17–1). Nonmedical causes should also be considered, especially in the elderly. These include poor dentition, loss of taste and smell, and social dysfunction (e.g., inability to cook, lack of funds or transportation).

Cancer is the most common medical cause of weight loss (16%–36% of patients with unexplained weight loss). Anorexia is usually present. Any cancer

Table 17–1. CAUSES OF INVOLUNTARY WEIGHT LOSS

	Number of Patients with Diagnosis (%)		
Causes	Thompson and Morris Outpatient Study	Marton et al. VA Study	Rabinovitz et al. Inpatient Study
Unknown cause	11 (24)	24 (26)	36 (23)
Cancer	7 (16)	18 (19)	56 (36)
Psychiatric disorders	8 (18)	8 (9)	13 (8)
Gastrointestinal disorders	5 (11)	13 (14)	26 (17)
Hyperthyroidism	4 (9)	1	3 (2)
Cardiovascular	—	8 (9)	—
Drug induced	4 (9)	2	—
Alcoholism	—	7 (8)	—
Pulmonary	—	5 (5)	—
Infectious disorders	1 (2)	3 (3)	6 (4)
Diabetes	—	3 (3)	3 (2)
Other diseases	5	4	11
Total	45	91	154

Percentages add up to more than 100 because several patients had more than one diagnosis.

may result in weight loss, but it is frequently seen in tumors of the gastrointestinal tract, particularly in the pancreas. In a Department of Veterans Affairs study, 18% of patients with involuntary weight loss were found to have cancer, and half of these cases involved the lung. Leukemia and lymphoma, especially Hodgkin's disease, may present as constitutional symptoms and loss of weight.

Gastrointestinal causes are frequent (11%–17%). Esophageal diseases cause dysphagia and odynophagia, resulting in decreased intake. Ulcer disease, hepatitis, motility disorders, and malabsorption may all cause significant weight loss. Cardiac cachexia seen in advanced congestive heart failure or severe advanced obstructive lung disease results in a wasted state. Alcoholism often results in malnutrition.

Endocrinologic disorders causing weight loss are more likely to be seen in the ambulatory setting. Hyperthyroidism and diabetes mellitus may present as increased intake and weight loss. Apathetic hyperthyroidism in the elderly may lack the typical symptoms of thyrotoxicosis.

Much like tuberculosis a century ago (hence the name *consumption*), acquired immunodeficiency syndrome (AIDS) has become the predominant chronic infection that causes much wasting and weight loss. In Africa, unremitting wasting is the most common presentation and has been called "slim disease." Patients with human immunodeficiency virus (HIV) infection lose weight because of opportunistic infections, chronic diarrhea, adverse drug reactions, or psychosocial factors. Recovery from repeated infections is incomplete, and long-term weight loss occurs. HIV wasting syndrome (weight loss of > 10% of baseline body weight with diarrhea, chronic weakness, or fevers in the absence of concurrent illness) is an AIDS-defining illness.

Among outpatients, psychiatric illnesses, most commonly depression, are frequent causes (18%) of involuntary weight loss. In the elderly, depression may coexist with dementia, and weight loss may be the only clue to this treatable condition. More common among younger patients are eating disorders such as anorexia nervosa and bulimia. Adverse effects from medications may also cause unexplained weight loss in outpatients. These untoward reactions include nausea, vomiting, dyspepsia, diarrhea, and anorexia. Nonsteroidal anti-inflammatory drugs are among the most frequently prescribed and often result in gastrointestinal problems. Both tricyclic antidepressants and the selective serotonin reuptake inhibitor antidepressants (e.g., fluoxetine and sertraline) are known to cause weight loss.

Clinical Approach. Weight loss of 5% or more of a patient's body weight over 6 months should be evaluated. A patient's perception of weight loss may not be accurate. Review of older records, information from family members, a change in clothing size, and recall of exact weights support the claim. Because weight loss is usually a late symptom in patients with a clinically important disease, the initial history and physical examination will often suggest a diagnosis. A careful review of symptoms and risk factors for malignancies, endocrine disorders, tuberculosis, and HIV infection is necessary. Complete physical examination, including fecal occult blood testing and pelvic examination, should be performed. Nutritional evaluation by a dietitian often discloses the mechanism of weight loss. Laboratory testing includes a complete blood cell count, urinalysis, and determination of electrolytes, blood urea nitrogen, creatinine, glucose, calcium, liver function (aspartate transaminase, alanine transaminase, bilirubin, alkaline phosphatase, lactate dehydrogenase), albumin, total protein, thyroid-stimulating hormone, and sedimentation rate; HIV testing should be done if risk factors are present. Chest radiographs will identify malignancies, potential infections, and pulmonary diseases. Specialized testing is reserved for further evaluation of associated symptoms, such as upper gastrointestinal radiographs to evaluate dysphagia or epigastric pain. Routine computed tomography, ultrasonography, or endoscopy has not been shown to be helpful in the absence of symptoms other than weight loss. Remembering that 25% of patients with unexplained weight loss never receive a diagnosis, it is appropriate after the previous evaluation to observe the patient closely if no cause is found.

Cross-References: Obesity (Chapter 15), Anorexia (Chapter 18), Screening for Depression (Chapter 185), Management of Depression (Chapter 189), HIV Infection: Office Evaluation (Chapter 204).

REFERENCES

1. Marton KI, Sox HC, Krupp JR. Involuntary weight loss: Diagnostic and prognostic significance. Ann Intern Med 1981;95:568–574.

   In a prospective evaluation of 91 patients with documented weight loss at a Veterans Administration Medical Center, almost half of the patients who claimed to have lost weight actually had not lost any weight. Even with extended follow-up, no cause was found in 26%.

2. Rabinovitz M, Pitlik SD, Leifer M, Garty M, Rosenfeld JB. Unintentional weight loss: A retrospective analysis of 154 cases. Arch Intern Med 1986;146:186–187.

   A retrospective chart review of persons with documented weight loss admitted to a tertiary hospital in Israel found a significant number of malignancies and gastrointestinal disorders.

3. Summerbell CD, Perrett JP, Gazzard BG. Causes of weight loss in human immunodeficiency virus infection. Int J STD AIDS 1993;4:234–236.

   In an HIV outpatient clinic, 30% of the patients had weight loss. The majority of cases were due to opportunistic infections, psychosocial factors, or adverse drug reactions. In the remaining cases the patients had symptoms suggestive of an unconfirmed infection or oral lesions that interfered with eating.

4. Thompson MP, Morris LK. Unexplained weight loss in the ambulatory elderly. J Am Geriatr Soc 1991;39:497–500.

   A computer search of the records of seven family practice centers identified 45 patients with documented weight loss among the approximately 10,000 geriatric members. In this outpatient study, depression, hyperthyroidism, and adverse drug reaction were more frequently seen compared with inpatient studies.

18 Anorexia

Problem

DEBORAH L. GREENBERG and STEVEN R. McGEE

Epidemiology. Anorexia, a loss of appetite or desire to eat, may be a prominent symptom in many acute and chronic diseases and in otherwise healthy elderly patients. Anorexia affects 15% to 40% of cancer patients at the time of their presentation and as many as 80% with advanced disease. Point prevalence rates in the elderly approach 20%. Anorexia is distinct from early satiety (i.e., appetite is initially normal but promptly disappears after ingestion of small amounts of food) and sitophobia (i.e., eating provokes unpleasant symptoms such as abdominal angina, dumping, or odynophagia).

Etiology. Although the pathophysiology of anorexia in humans is not clearly understood, animal studies provide some insight. Stimulation of the lateral hypothalamus produces hunger and anabolic responses (increased gastric acid secretion, increased hepatic glycogen synthesis, and increased fat and protein synthesis), whereas stimulation of the ventromedial nucleus causes anorexia and catabolic responses. Specific regulators of appetite within the central nervous system include opioid peptides (which promote feeding) and serotonin, corticotropin-releasing factor, and dopamine (all of which decrease the desire to eat). Many peripheral hormones (e.g., insulin, cholecystokinin, estradiol, bombesin) provide feedback to the hypothalamus and inhibit feeding.

Although speculative, depression and dementia may cause anorexia by altering these central neurotransmitters. The anorexia of normal aging may reflect a decreased opioid feeding drive and an increased appetite suppression by cholecystokinin. Naloxone (an opioid antagonist) and fenfluramine (a serotonin agonist) produce anorexia, whereas cyproheptadine (a serotonin antagonist) causes increased appetite and weight gain. Digoxin and many antihypertensive, antidepressant, and anti-inflammatory medications diminish appetite, particularly in older patients.

Anorexia accompanies most catabolic states, including cancer, chronic infections (e.g., tuberculosis, human immunodeficiency virus infection), and advanced cardiac, pulmonary, and renal disease. Proposed mediators of anorexia in tumor and infection include cytokines such as tumor necrosis factor, interleukins, and interferon gamma.

Other factors that may cause anorexia include (1) abnormal taste and smell—the aging process, multiple medications (e.g., captopril, antibiotics, and carbamazepine), and nutritional deficiencies (e.g., zinc) alter these senses (see Chapter 52, Abnormal Taste and Smell); (2) learned food aversions—cancer patients subconsciously associate unpleasant experiences, such as chemotherapy, with food ingested during that experience; and (3) anorexia nervosa—this disorder may present for the first time in older patients.

Table 18–1. APPETITE-PROMOTING MEDICATIONS

Medications	Dose	Cost ($ per month)*
Cyroheptadine	8 mg tid	8.82, tablets; 25.31, suspension
Dexamethasone	4–8 mg qd	6.30–12.60, tablets
Megestrol acetate	400–800 mg qd	129.75–259.50, suspension
Metoclopramide	10 mg ac and qhs	10.38, tablets; 44.64, suspension
Dronabinol (Marinol)	2.5 mg bid	161.11, tablets

*Average wholesale price, 1995 *Drug Topics Red Book.*

Clinical Approach. The history should focus on the onset of symptoms, associated weight loss, severity of underlying disease (e.g., cardiac, pulmonary, renal), and risk factors for cancer (e.g., smoking) or infection (e.g., human immunodeficiency virus risk factors, tuberculosis exposure). Even in patients with known cancer or the acquired immunodeficiency syndrome (AIDS), the physician should search for a responsible medication, inquire into the possibility of depression, and investigate the patient's ability to prepare, taste, smell, and chew food. After a complete history, physical examination, and routine laboratory tests, the diagnostic search should not go beyond that recommended for involuntary weight loss (see Chapter 17, Unintentional Weight Loss).

Management. The clinician should identify and treat any reversible physical or psychiatric conditions and should discontinue any suspect medication. Therapy for depressed patients with anorexia can be difficult because many newer antidepressants (e.g., fluoxetine, paroxetine, sertraline) depress appetite. Control of the patient's pain, nausea, or constipation may improve appetite. Because not all patients with anorexia benefit from intervention and weight gain (especially those with advanced cancer, AIDS, or other terminal illnesses), the clinician should focus on improving the patient's quality of life. The clinician should limit unpalatable dietary restrictions and increase the patient's socialization during meals. Flavor enhancers may benefit those patients with decreased taste and smell.

Medications that may promote appetite include metoclopramide, dexamethasone, megestrol acetate, tetrahydrocannabinol (dronabinol), and the serotonin antagonist cyproheptadine. Metoclopramide is especially effective in patients with nausea or evidence of gastrointestinal dysmotility. Although cyproheptadine and dexamethasone increase appetite, treated patients may not gain weight and may experience significant side effects. In patients with cachexia from cancer or AIDS, the progesterone derivative megestrol acetate has been shown in short-term, randomized, placebo-controlled studies to stimulate appetite, weight gain, and sense of well-being. Megestrol acetate is available in a liquid formulation, although the cost may be prohibitive (Table 18–1).

Cross-References: Unintentional Weight Loss (Chapter 17), Abnormal Taste and Smell (Chapter 52), Screening for Depression (Chapter 185), End-of-Life Care for Patients with Cancer (Chapter 209).

REFERENCES

1. Beal JE, Olson R, Laubenstein L, et al. Dronabinol as a treatment for anorexia associated with weight loss in patients with AIDS. J Pain Symptom Manage 1995;10(2):89–97.

In this short term, placebo-controlled trial (< 6 weeks), patients taking dronabinol twice daily reported increased appetite and mood and maintained their weight with few side effects.

2. Haller DG. Weight gain in patients with AIDS-related cachexia: Is bigger better? Ann Intern Med 1994;121:462–463.

This editorial reviews the two randomized trials of megestrol acetate in AIDS-related cachexia found in this issue.

3. Kardinal CG, Loprinzi CL, Schaid DJ, et al. A controlled trial of cyproheptadine in cancer patients with anorexia and/or cachexia. Cancer 1990;65:2657–2662.

Patients' appetite improved with cyproheptadine, but they continued to lose weight and reported significant sedation and dizziness.

4. Morley JE, Silver AJ. Review: Anorexia in the elderly. Neurobiol Aging 1988;9:9–16.

This overview of the pathophysiology of anorexia in the elderly includes several articles that deal with anorexia.

5. Nelson KA, Walsh D, Sheehan FA. The cancer anorexia-cachexia syndrome. J Clin Oncol 1994;12:213–225.

A detailed review is presented of the biochemical and metabolic changes, clinical features, and available treatments in the cancer anorexia-cachexia syndrome.

19 Dyspnea

Problem

KATHLEEN JOBE

Although there is no universally accepted definition of dyspnea, it is commonly thought of as a subjective sensation of discomfort associated with difficult or labored breathing. It is a common complaint; in one study, dyspnea accounted for 15% of inpatient admissions to the general medicine service.

Etiology. The sensation of dyspnea is complex and mediated by numerous receptors in the lungs, vasculature, and central nervous system (CNS). Contributing to the sensation of dyspnea are mechanoreceptors in the lungs, muscles, and airway; chemoreceptors in the carotid bodies, aortic bodies, and medulla; and vascular receptors and efferent CNS signals.

Although the differential diagnosis of dyspnea is extensive, four diagnoses account for 70% of patients with dyspnea: asthma, chronic obstructive pulmonary disease (COPD), interstitial lung disease, and cardiomyopathy. In one study of 100 consecutive patients with chronic dyspnea evaluated in a pulmonary clinic, 75% had respiratory disorders. The rest had cardiovascular diseases, gastroesophageal reflux, deconditioning, or psychogenic dyspnea.

The presence of positional dyspnea may suggest an underlying cause. Trepopnea, which is dyspnea in one lateral position but not the other, suggests unilateral lung disease, pleural effusion, mediastinal or proximal endobronchial tumors, and cardiomegaly. Orthopnea, which is recumbent dyspnea, suggests left ventricular dysfunction or pulmonary disease such as COPD. Paroxysmal nocturnal dyspnea, in which the patient awakens short of breath after sound sleep, is specific for cardiomyopathy and elevated left atrial pressure. Platypnea, which is dyspnea in the upright position that is relieved by lying down, is associated with intracardiac shunts and with shunts of the pulmonary vasculature or parenchyma.

Clinical Approach. Although many patients have difficulty characterizing the sensation of breathlessness, a careful clinical assessment can be diagnostic. In one study of 146 inpatients with dyspnea, the initial history-based diagnosis was correct in 74% of cases. History and physical examination findings were most useful in excluding common diagnoses, that is, they had high negative predictive value. A negative smoking history ruled out COPD (100% negative predictive value), but only 20% of smokers had COPD. A previous diagnosis of asthma or wheezing had a positive predictive value for asthma of less than 50%. The overall accuracy of the clinical assessment based on the findings of history, physical examination, and chest radiograph was correct in 66% of cases but was correct in only 33% for less common causes of dyspnea.

Several instruments are available for quantifying the degree of dyspnea the patient is experiencing. A combination of the Baseline Dyspnea Index (BDI) and Transition Dyspnea Index (TDI) and the dyspnea component of the Chronic Respiratory Questionnaire (CRQ) provide a more comprehensive measurement of dyspnea. The BDI and TDI consider task, effort, and function; and the dyspnea component of the CRQ considers the five most common activities that cause exertional dyspnea for a given patient. These instruments have been found valid and reliable. They provide a baseline for evaluation of future therapy and provide the physician with information regarding the impact of the patient's symptoms on their activities of daily living.

A careful stepwise approach to the complaint of dyspnea will yield a diagnosis in virtually all cases. The history should be comprehensive, including occupational and environmental exposures, a review of current medications, past medical and surgical history, and prior trauma. A detailed physical examination may help differentiate cardiac from pulmonary disease. The most useful studies include chest radiography and pulmonary function studies. Hemoglobin level, thyroid function studies, and an electrocardiogram should be done early in the evaluation of dyspnea. Provocative testing with methacholine for reactive airway or interstitial disease is useful in patients whose pulmonary function tests are unrevealing. Oximetry during exercise may be useful in patients with normal oximetry at baseline. Cardiopulmonary exercise testing is indicated for patients whose symptoms are out of proportion to objective findings. It defines the relative contributions of cardiac and pulmonary components of the patient's dyspnea and is useful for evaluation of psychogenic dyspnea and deconditioning.

Management. With the exception of asthma, which may improve with treatment in the emergency department, acute dyspnea is generally evaluated and managed during urgent admission to the inpatient medicine service. Chronic dyspnea is usually managed in the outpatient clinic.

The goal of treatment is to relieve the underlying disorder responsible for the patient's dyspnea. However, many patients including those with COPD and interstitial lung disease may not have relief of dyspnea even with specific therapy. There are several types of symptomatic therapies that may be helpful. Home oxygen therapy reduces dyspnea and hypoxic symptoms (confusion, headache, sleeplessness) and improves survival in patients with severe chronic hypoxemia ($PO_2 < 55$ mm Hg). Oxygen may be of value in relieving dyspnea in some patients with only mild hypoxia who do not meet criteria for supplemental oxygen based on mortality data. In some patients, pulmonary training may be useful. Inspiratory muscle training strengthens the pulmonary muscles and may improve dyspnea. Pursed-lip breathing reduces the amount of airway collapse and improves dyspnea. Theophylline may be of value in patients with COPD by decreasing central neural drive and the perceived respiratory effort. Opiates, benzodiazepines, and phenothiazines have been shown to relieve dyspnea, but owing to problems with addiction and mental status changes these agents are generally avoided. They may be used in low doses in carefully monitored treatment regimens.

Cross-References: Asthma and Chronic Obstructive Pulmonary Disease (Chapter 68), Pulmonary Function Testing (Chapter 69), Congestive Heart Failure (Chapter 79), Generalized Anxiety (Chapter 186), Hyperventilation Syndrome (Chapter 194), Dyspnea in Patients with Cancer (Chapter 208).

REFERENCES

1. Gillespie DL, Staats BA. Unexplained dyspnea. Mayo Clin Proc 1994;69:657–663.

    This case report illustrates a stepwise approach to the evaluation of dyspnea and the value of cardiopulmonary exercise testing in cases where initial testing is nondiagnostic.

2. Mahler DA, Horowitz MB. Clinical evaluation of exertional dyspnea. Clin Chest Med 1994;2:259–269.

    The causes and the evaluation of exertional dyspnea are reviewed with discussion of the appropriate use of various diagnostic tests.

3. Manning HL, Schwartzstein RM. Pathophysiology of dyspnea. N Engl J Med 1995;333:1547–1554.

    The current understanding of mechanisms of dyspnea is reviewed.

4. Pratter MR, Curley FJ, Dubois J, Irwin RS. Cause and evaluation of chronic dyspnea in a pulmonary disease clinic. Arch Intern Med 1989;149:2277–2282.

    Prospective evaluation was done of 89 consecutive patients referred to a pulmonary subspecialty clinic with chronic dyspnea (mean duration of dyspnea, 2.9 years). The diagnosis was made in 100%.

5. Schmitt BP, Kushner MS, Wiener SL. The diagnostic usefulness of the history of the patient with dyspnea. J Gen Intern Med 1986;1:386–393.

    Of 146 consecutive hospital admissions for dyspnea, the initial diagnosis (obtained by a 5- to 15-minute history) was correlated with the final diagnosis in 74% of cases.

20 Dizziness

Problem

STEVEN R. McGEE

Epidemiology. General practitioners evaluate two thirds of all patients with dizziness, which is the fifth most common complaint among patients older than age 65. Dizziness is more common in women and the elderly. One-year prevalence rates approach 20% in those older than age 60.

Etiology. Among patients with dizziness who consult general practitioners, three diagnostic groups account for more than 75% of the final diagnoses: peripheral vestibular disorders, psychiatric disorders, and multiple sensory deficits (Table 20–1). *Benign positional vertigo* produces short (less than 1 minute) episodes of vertigo brought on by head movements; over 50% have had previous ear trauma or infection. Neurologic examination, other than the Hallpike-Dix test, is normal. *Vestibular neuronitis*, also called acute vestibulopathy or acute labyrinthitis, causes acute temporary vertigo, nausea, and vomiting. Most patients are young and have experienced a recent viral illness. *Ménière's syndrome* causes vertigo that lasts hours and, in contrast to other vestibular disorders, is associated with cochlear symptoms (neurosensory hearing loss, tinnitus, and ear fullness). *Central vestibular disorders* (brain stem and cerebellar ischemia) occur in elderly patients with known cerebrovascular disease and produce acute dizziness associated with diplopia, dysarthria, headache, altered mental status, or cerebellar, motor, or sensory abnormalities. *Multiple sensory deficits* describes combinations of poor vision, neuropathy, orthopedic deformity, or mild vestibular deficits, which progressively diminish the patient's orientation to the environment. Most patients are elderly, often diabetic, and experience no dizziness

Table 20–1. ETIOLOGY OF DIZZINESS

Etiology of Dizziness	% of Cases
Peripheral vestibular disorders	38–43
Benign positional vertigo	12–16
Vestibular neuronitis	3–9
Ménière's disease	3–4
Other	14–20
Psychiatric disorders	16–24
Multiple sensory deficits	13–17
Central vestibular disorders	7–10
Cardiovascular disorders*	4–6
Unknown	8–9

*Hypotension (e.g., vasovagal, orthostatic, arrhythmia-induced).
Adapted from McGee SR. Dizzy patients: Diagnosis and treatment. West J Med 1995; 162:37–42. Reprinted by permission of *The Western Journal of Medicine.*

at rest but vague unsteadiness during walking and turning. Patients with *psychiatric disorders* lack the key diagnostic features of the disorders just described and instead meet the diagnostic criteria for a psychiatric condition (most often depression or somatization) and experience dizziness often provoked by hyperventilation.

Other causes of dizziness include cardiovascular disorders (e.g., carotid sinus hypersensitivity; see Chapter 75, Syncope), various toxins (welder's fumes, carbon monoxide, hydrocarbon solvents), and medications (quinine, alcohol, and antihypertensive, anticonvulsant, antidepressant, or cardiovascular medications).

Clinical Approach. The most useful diagnostic test, in both primary care and sophisticated referral centers, proves to be a careful history, which provides the diagnosis in over 70% of cases. The physician should review the patient's own description of dizziness, its duration, what brings it on, the patient's medications, and any symptoms of neurologic or cardiac disease. Categories of dizziness include (1) vertigo, a sensation of movement (twirling, rolling, tilting) in the head, which implies vestibular disease (peripheral or rarely central); (2) sensation of impending fainting or loss of consciousness, which implies hypotension; and (3) unsteadiness, *not* in the head, which implies cerebellar or proprioceptive disorders. Unfortunately, the symptoms of 40% of patients, some with multiple sensory deficits or psychiatric disorders, are too vague or diverse to classify neatly.

The physical examination carefully reviews the ears, heart, and nervous system (proprioception, cranial nerves, and cerebellum). Nystagmus is normal if present only on extreme lateral gaze. Rotary nystagmus suggests peripheral or central vestibular disease, and pure horizontal or vertical nystagmus implies a central cause. In all patients, the clinician should perform tests intended to provoke the patient's dizziness, including (1) postural blood pressure determinations; (2) hyperventilation (30/min for 3 minutes); (3) Hallpike-Dix (Nylen-Bárány) maneuver; and (4) sudden turns when walking (if dizziness appears during this test, relief by touching the examiner's finger suggests multiple sensory deficits). The Hallpike-Dix maneuver evaluates patients with dizziness provoked by head movements; with the patient seated, the examiner turns the patient's head to one side and directs the patient to lie down, hyperextending the head over the edge of the table (because most elderly patients tolerate hyperextension poorly, many clinicians allow the patient's head to land squarely on the table). If vertigo appears after a pause of 2 to 20 seconds (latency), then dies away after seconds (adaptation) and is less prominent during immediate repeat testing (fatigability), the patient has common *benign* (peripheral) positional vertigo. The rare patient with central positional vertigo, due to brain stem or cerebellar causes, experiences milder vertigo without latency, adaptation, or fatigability during this test.

Measuring the blood cell count and electrolyte levels is appropriate if the patient has orthostatic hypotension (to address the possibilities of gastrointestinal bleeding, prerenal azotemia, or diabetes). Patients with associated hearing loss or tinnitus should be promptly referred for audiometry to screen for Ménière's disease. Other laboratory tests are rarely useful. Bithermal calorics and electronystagmography, although frequently abnormal, merely support diagnoses obvious from the history and physical examination.

Table 20–2. ANTIVERTIGO MEDICATIONS

Drug	Dose	Cost ($ per 3 Days)
Antihistamine		
Dimenhydrinate* (Dramamine)	50 mg PO q6h, prn	3.12
Meclizine* (Antivert)	25 mg PO q6h, prn	.60

*Available over-the-counter. 1996 *Drug Topics Red Book.*
Prices for generic where available.

Management. Some cardiovascular disorders, such as carotid sinus hypersensitivity, require specific therapy. Postural hypotension improves with wearing of support hose and reduction of responsible medications. Multiple sensory deficits are partially offset by correct eyeglass prescriptions, use of night-lights at home, and a referral to a physical therapist for a cane or other appropriate ambulatory aids.

Patients with acute or chronic vertigo benefit from specific rehabilitative exercises: seated at home, the patient lies down quickly to one side to provoke vertigo repeatedly until it disappears. Antihistamine medications may also help (Table 20–2), although evidence from human trials is meager and most recommendations derive from animal studies, human caloric responses, and military motion sickness experiments. Benzodiazepines are recommended for severe sustained vertigo (e.g., vestibular neuronitis) but are ineffective in controlled trials of episodic positional vertigo. Because medications may retard the central nervous system's adaptation to vertigo and prolong recovery, they should not be used for long periods. In a single randomized trial of 26 patients with Ménière's syndrome, treatment with hydrochlorothiazide reduced vertigo and hearing loss but not the tinnitus.

Follow-Up. Vestibular neuronitis resolves after 10 to 14 days; benign positional vertigo disappears after weeks or months or, infrequently, years. Predictors of persistent dizziness include a psychiatric cause, idiopathic vertigo, daily dizziness, and dizziness aggravated by walking. Dizzy patients rarely require hospitalization or referral and do not have increased risk of death or institutionalization. If vertigo is disabling and unresponsive to treatment, a neurology or otolaryngology referral is indicated.

Cross-References: Tinnitus (Chapter 51), Syncope (Chapter 75), Cerebrovascular Disease (Chapter 146), Somatization (Chapter 188), Panic Disorder (Chapter 191), Hyperventilation Syndrome (Chapter 194).

REFERENCES

1. Baloh RW, Sloane PD, Honrubia V. Quantitative vestibular function testing in elderly patients with dizziness. Ear Nose Throat J 1989;68:935–939.

   Electronystagmograms, abnormal in 65% of patients, contributed little to assessment from history and physical examination. The test added new information in only 4 of 75 patients, all with unsuspected bilateral vestibular disease.

2. Brandt T, Daroff RB. Physical therapy for benign paroxysmal positional vertigo. Arch Otolaryngol 1980;106:484–485.

Exercises are described that produced relief in 66 of 67 patients with benign positional vertigo, usually within 7 to 10 days.

3. Fisher CM. Vertigo in cerebrovascular disease. Arch Otolaryngol 1967;85:529–534.

   In this study, 77% of patients with basilar vertebral ischemia experienced dizziness: in 75%, dizziness and other neurologic symptoms (e.g., diplopia) occur together; in 25%, dizziness is the sole initial symptom, although other revealing neurologic symptoms appear within 6 weeks.

4. Kroenke K, Lucas C, Rosenberg ML, Scherokman B, Herbers JE. One-year outcome for patients with a chief complaint of dizziness. J Gen Intern Med 1994;9:684–689.

   Results of a 1-year follow-up on a classic cohort of 100 patients with chronic dizziness are presented. The dizziness resolved or improved in most patients, and none developed a serious illness. A point-system classified a patient's prognosis accurately.

5. McGee SR. Dizzy patients: Diagnosis and treatment. West J Med 1995;162:37–42.

   A comprehensive overview of recent literature is provided including historical insights.

● ●

21 Fatigue

Problem

STEVEN R. McGEE and MARGUERITE J. McNEELY

Epidemiology. In the primary care setting, fatigue is one of the most common chief complaints, with a point prevalence of 24% and an annual incidence of 3% to 7%. Fatigue is more common in women than in men.

Etiology. Evaluation of fatigue identifies a physical cause in 20% to 40% of affected patients, a psychiatric cause in 50% to 65%, and no cause in 10% to 30%. The leading physical causes are infections (especially viral diseases), metabolic disorders (thyroid disease, hypokalemia), and medications (sedatives, diuretics, β-blockers, antihistamines, psychotropic medications). Although fatigue may persist long after infections with Epstein-Barr virus (EBV) and influenza viruses have resolved, the exact role of the virus is unclear, because some studies suggest that those with prolonged recovery were prone to depression before their infection. The most common psychiatric disorders are depression, anxiety, and somatization disorder. The evaluation of fatigue present for less than 4 weeks yields a physical diagnosis in 70% of cases, whereas fatigue exceeding 4 months leads to a psychiatric diagnosis in 76%.

Only 5% of patients with chronic fatigue satisfy the criteria of the chronic fatigue syndrome, a disorder characterized by fatigue persisting longer than 6 months, the absence of known physical causes of fatigue, and the presence of sore throat, lymphadenopathy, myalgia, headache, and sleep disturbance, among other associated symptoms. Early studies attempted to link this syndrome to chronic EBV infection, but subsequent work has demonstrated that abnormal EBV serology is very nonspecific and no such association exists for most, if any, patients.

In one study, 70% of patients with chronic fatigue also experienced diffuse musculoskeletal pain, had multiple tender muscle points on examination, and otherwise met the diagnostic criteria for fibromyalgia (see Chapter 121, Fibromyalgia).

Clinical Approach. The physician should carefully distinguish the patient's complaint of fatigue from the exertional dyspnea of cardiopulmonary disease, the muscle weakness of neuromuscular disease (myasthenia gravis, multiple sclerosis, polymyositis), and the daytime hypersomnolence of sleep apnea (usually associated with morning headache and night-time snoring and apnea). The finding of weakness or fever on physical examination requires a different diagnostic approach (see Chapter 16, Fever, and Chapter 137, Muscular Weakness).

If the cause of fatigue is not obvious after the initial history and physical examination, recommended laboratory testing includes a complete blood cell count, electrolytes, glucose, calcium, phosphorus, blood urea nitrogen, creatinine, thyroid-stimulating hormone, liver function tests, total protein, albumin, globulin, urinalysis, and erythrocyte sedimentation rate. Such routine testing, however, provides clues to the diagnosis of chronic fatigue in only 5% of patients. Other tests, including EBV serology, are appropriate only when directed by suggestive signs and symptoms. No specific electromyography, muscle biopsy, or muscle enzyme defects have ever been identified in patients with fatigue.

The physician should address with all patients the possibility of excessive life stresses, substance abuse, risk factors for human immunodeficiency virus infection, and symptoms of depression and anxiety. Even in patients with physical disease, depression or anxiety may contribute significantly to fatigue.

Management. Double-blind, placebo-controlled, randomized trials have shown that acyclovir or combined liver extract–folate–vitamin B_{12} injections are no better than placebo in the chronic fatigue syndrome and that the placebo effect is powerful in these patients. Amantadine has a meager benefit for the disabling fatigue of multiple sclerosis, but its use for fatigue remains restricted to this group of patients.

Specific therapy may benefit patients with known physical or psychiatric disease. For patients with fatigue of unknown cause, a logical approach includes the following:

1. Consider withdrawal of medications suspected as a cause.
2. Prescribe moderate, not excessive, exercise (see Chapter 72, Assessment of Physical Activity).
3. Reduce stresses in the patient's life.
4. Consider empirical antidepressant medications.

This approach is untested, but a similar disorder, fibromyalgia, does improve with very low doses of tricyclic medications. Nonsedating antidepressants are probably best, unless insomnia is a significant problem.

Follow-Up. Patients with fatigue are not at increased risk of hospitalization or death but do have a significantly greater number of clinic visits than nonfatigued patients. Most patients remain employed. Chronic fatigue tends to wax and wane over years and may remit; some 30% to 50% of affected patients show improvement at 1-year follow-up.

Cross-References: Assessment of Physical Activity (Chapter 72), Fibromyalgia (Chapter 121), Common Thyroid Disorders (Chapter 153), Screening for Depression (Chapter 185), Generalized Anxiety (Chapter 186), Somatization (Chapter 188).

REFERENCES

1. Epstein KR. The chronically fatigued patient. Med Clin North Am 1995;79:315–327.

   This is a nice overall review.

2. Fukuda K, Strauss SE, Hickie I, Sharp MC, Dobbins JG, Komaroff A, and the International Chronic Fatigue Syndrome Study Group. The chronic fatigue syndrome: A comprehensive approach to its definition and study. Ann Intern Med 1994;121:953–959.

   A revision of the 1988 working definition for chronic fatigue syndrome is proposed and clinical evaluation including inability to confirm diagnosis with laboratory tests such as EBV titers is discussed.

3. Kroenke K, Wood DR, Mangelsdorff AD, Meier NJ, Powell JB. Chronic fatigue in primary care: Prevalence, patient characteristics, and outcome. JAMA 1988;260:929–934.

   A prospective analysis of 102 patients with chronic fatigue (>1 month) was done. Laboratory testing was unhelpful in diagnosis, and most fatigued patients had high depression or anxiety ratings.

4. Morrison JD. Fatigue as a presenting complaint in family practice. J Fam Pract 1980;10:795–801.

   The longer the fatigue, the more likely is a psychiatric diagnosis.

5. Swartz MN. The chronic fatigue syndrome: One entity or many? N Engl J Med 1988;319:1726–1728.

   This is an outstanding historical review.

Disorders of the Skin

22 Principles of Dermatologic Diagnosis and Therapy

Diagnosis

JAN V. HIRSCHMANN

DIAGNOSIS

The ability to diagnose dermatologic disorders depends heavily on visual recognition of patterns of skin abnormalities, a skill that requires considerable knowledge and experience. A systematic approach to the history and the physical examination is necessary for an accurate appraisal of cutaneous problems. The clinician should inquire about the duration and evolution of the disorder, including any relationship to season, ambient temperature, occupation, travel, animal exposure, hobbies, other illnesses, drug use (including illicit drugs and over-the-counter medications), and similar skin diseases in family or other contacts. Especially important is information about previous or current treatment, not only because it may indicate the efficacy of such therapy but also because certain treatments alter the appearance of the skin lesions. For example, topical corticosteroids often significantly diminish the erythema and scaling of a superficial fungal infection, making it more difficult to identify. Sometimes, treatment will replace one disease with another. For example, topical neomycin erroneously given for a mild, self-limited eruption may result in a contact dermatitis to that antibiotic. This, then, is the problem that the clinician sees, rather than the initial rash, which has resolved spontaneously. The symptoms of dermatologic disease to elicit are mainly pruritus, pain, or paresthesias in the skin; but because some skin lesions may be manifestations of a systemic disease, it may be important to inquire about other problems, such as weight loss, fever, and arthralgias.

The clinician should scrupulously examine the entire skin surface (including the scalp, nails, axillae, and anogenital area), the conjunctivae, and the oral cavity. The examiner should use the dermatologic terminology of macule, papule, nodule, and so on to characterize the abnormalities seen. Other important elements to note are the color, palpable features (e.g., consistency, temperature, tenderness), and shape (e.g., round, oval, annular) of the individual lesions. If several lesions are present, the clinician should identify their arrangement (grouped or widespread) and distribution (e.g., symmetric, sun-exposed areas, extensor surfaces). Many dermatologic diseases have such typical patterns of skin involvement that the location of lesions is one of the most important characteristics in identifying them. Sometimes, the use of a hand lens will reveal information not appreciated by the naked eye.

Lesions are frequently altered or destroyed by scratching, leaving nonspecific excoriations as the only finding. Similarly, certain topical therapies may so change the appearance of a skin disorder that it is unrecognizable. In these circumstances, other features, such as the distribution of the eruption, may suggest the proper diagnosis, but finding undisturbed ("primary") lesions is most helpful.

TOPICAL THERAPY

Wet Dressings. Wet dressings are often useful for acute conditions in which erythema, vesicles, crusting, pruritus, and oozing are present. They cool through evaporation, reducing itching and causing vasoconstriction of the dilated vessels found in acute inflammation. Because of capillary action, moistened crust and superficial dead skin adhere to the dressing, the removal of which provides gentle débridement. Tap water alone may suffice, but aluminum acetate (Burow's) solution, one packet or tablet dissolved in 2 cups of cool or lukewarm water, is more drying and has mild antimicrobial activity. Items found in most households, such as washcloths, towels, or sheets, are excellent dressings when applied loosely in two to three layers (wet, but not dripping) to the affected area and changed every 5 minutes for a period of about 20 minutes three to five times a day. Longer use may cause skin maceration. Wet dressings are rarely necessary for more than 24 to 48 hours.

Moisturizers. Certain preparations help the epidermis retain the moisture necessary to keep the skin's surface smooth and soft. They are especially useful in patients with xerosis (dry skin), which is a common problem in the elderly, and in those with atopic eczema.

Moisturizers may be occlusive or humectants. The occlusive types create a partially permeable barrier that helps the skin retain its moisture. They are creams or ointments that contain emulsions of oil in water or water in oil. When the amount of oil exceeds that of water by a certain amount, the formulation changes from a pourable cream to a semisolid ointment. Oil-in-water emulsions that are useful moisturizers include hydrophilic ointment (e.g., generic, Cetaphil Lotion, Keri Lotion, Lubriderm Cream, Nivea Cream). Water-in-oil emulsions that rehydrate the skin include cold creams and lanolin preparations (e.g., Eucerin). Oil-in-water emulsions are less greasy and more easily removed, but water-in-oil emulsions provide better lubrication and occlusion. Water-absorbent ointment bases contain no water but will absorb water and become water-in-oil emulsions. Examples are hydrophilic petrolatum and anhydrous lanolin (e.g., Aquaphor). All these occlusive moisturizers are nonprescription drugs.

Humectants, when absorbed, help the skin to retain its moisture. Examples include urea lotion 10% (e.g., Nutraplus, Carmol 10) or cream 20% (Carmol

20) and lactic acid (Lac-Hydrin). These preparations are especially useful with dry, scaly conditions such as atopic dermatitis.

Patients with dry skin should use one of these moisturizing agents several times a day, particularly after washing the hands or bathing, when they should be applied to damp but not dripping skin. They will help the water present on the skin surface to penetrate into the epidermis rather than evaporate. When moisturizers are put over dry skin, little water is added, but they will help protect the epidermis from further loss.

Topical Corticosteroids. In general, creams and lotions, which are more drying than ointments, are appropriate for acute or subacute inflammatory disorders characterized by oozing, erythema, crusting, and vesiculation. Ointments are superior with chronic, dry, scaling, and lichenified conditions and are better absorbed than creams. Because creams and lotions blend into the skin readily and do not have the greasy feel of ointments, they are often more acceptable to patients. Lotions are especially useful in hairy areas, where creams and ointments are difficult to apply.

The absorption of topical corticosteroids markedly varies according to the site on the skin, being much greater where it is thin, such as on the face and scrotum. It is also increased severalfold with well-hydrated skin. Therefore, when possible, patients should moisten the area to be treated by bathing or brief soaking before applying the medication. Some disorders that respond poorly to conventional topical corticosteroid therapy may improve when a cream preparation is covered with occlusive dressings. An ointment is not ordinarily used under occlusion because it is more likely to produce folliculitis and maceration. The patient should apply the cream to moist skin and cover the area for a minimum of 6 hours (overnight use is usually most convenient) with a plastic wrap such as Saran Wrap for large areas, plastic gloves for hands, plastic bags for the hands or feet, and a bathing cap for the scalp. The edges should be sealed with tape, elastic bandages, or items of clothing such as underwear or panty hose, depending on the area being treated.

Topical corticosteroids, of which there are many types, vary considerably in potency. It is useful to learn one or two in each group. In general, therapy should begin with a medium-strength formulation in mild to moderately severe conditions, reserving the most potent formulations for severe or refractory disorders. In chronic dermatoses, after the condition has responded to a potent preparation, a lower-strength corticosteroid is often appropriate for maintenance therapy. Chronic use of the strong corticosteroids, especially when applied under occlusion, may cause atrophy, telangiectasia, and striae. The face, axillae, and genital areas are particularly susceptible, and, ordinarily, only low-potency preparations are indicated for long-term treatment in these areas.

The following list includes a few of the available topical corticosteroids according to their potency. Trade names are included to help identify the products, but those preparations available as generic prescriptions are marked by an asterisk (*). In each category, the medications are listed in approximate descending order of strength, although frequently the difference, if any, is slight.

Very High Potency
Clobetasol propionate cream, ointment, solution 0.05% (Temovate)
*Betamethasone dipropionate cream, ointment 0.05% (Diprolene)

High Potency
Betamethasone dipropionate cream, ointment 0.05% (Diprosone) (different vehicle than Diprolene)
Fluocinonide *cream, ointment, lotion 0.05% (Lidex)
Halcinonide cream 0.1% (Halog)
*Betamethasone valerate ointment 0.1% (Valisone)

Intermediate Potency
*Fluocinolone acetonide cream 0.2%, ointment 0.025% (Synalar)
*Triamcinolone acetonide ointment 0.1% (Aristocort, Kenalog)
*Betamethasone valerate cream, lotion 0.1% (Valisone)
*Triamcinolone acetonide cream 0.025% (Aristocort)

Low Potency
Desonide cream 0.05% (Tridesilon)
*Hydrocortisone cream, ointment, lotion 1.0%, 2.5%

Frequency and Amount of Application. With topical corticosteroids, twice-daily application nearly always suffices; more frequent use is rarely more effective. With some disorders, particularly for maintenance therapy of chronic conditions, a single treatment a day is adequate. Patients should apply the medication in a thin layer to the skin; thick applications are wasteful, because only the material directly touching the skin exerts any therapeutic benefit. It takes about 30 g of topical medication to cover the entire body for one application, with the following approximate amounts (the monthly amount when the medication is used twice daily is given in parentheses):

Head, both hands, buttocks (each area): 2 g (120 g)
Neck, genitals, feet (each area): 1 g (60 g)
Both arms: 4 g (240 g)
Trunk: 8 g (480 g)
Both legs: 10 g (600 g)

REFERENCES

1. Arndt KA: Manual of Dermatologic Therapeutics: With Essentials of Diagnosis, 5th ed. Boston, Little, Brown & Co, 1995.

   This book is a superb, concise, and very practical summary of the management of common dermatologic disorders.

2. Sams WM, Lynch PJ, eds: Principles and Practice of Dermatology, 2nd ed. New York, Churchill Livingstone, 1995.

   An excellent medium-sized textbook, it is appropriate for primary care clinicians. Numerous, first-rate clinical color photographs are included.

23 Pruritus

Symptom

JAN V. HIRSCHMANN

Epidemiology. Although pruritus is the most common symptom in dermatologic diseases, its prevalence in the general population is unknown.

Etiology. Often, skin lesions that clarify the cause of itching are present. Common skin diseases typically associated with pruritus are xerosis (dry skin), scabies, pediculosis, urticaria, atopic or contact dermatitis, insect bites, fiberglass dermatitis, and fungal infections. When no skin lesions are present except excoriations, the cause may be a systemic disorder, primarily uremia; cholestasis from drugs, primary biliary cirrhosis, or extrahepatic biliary obstruction; lymphomas (especially Hodgkin's disease); polycythemia vera; and, perhaps, thyroid disease. Of patients with itching but no diagnostic skin lesions, about 15% will have an associated systemic disease at initial evaluation; lymphoma will emerge as a cause on follow-up in a very small number. About 65% of patients in whom no cause is found will continue to have pruritus for years.

Clinical Approach. History should include information about the nature and duration of the itching, the precipitating factors, occupation and hobbies, previous therapy, medications taken, similar symptoms in close contacts, systemic symptoms such as weight loss, and travel. With Hodgkin's disease the pruritus is frequently burning in quality and typically occurs on the legs. The itching of polycythemia vera is often "prickling" and tends to develop when the patient abruptly cools off after emerging from a warm bath or shower. The itching of scabies is particularly intense at night. Xerosis is especially likely in an older patient, particularly after frequent bathing or during the winter months when indoor heating reduces the ambient humidity.

The physical examination should include a thorough examination of the entire cutaneous surface, including the genitalia. Burrows of scabies tend to occur in the interdigital webs, volar wrists, axillae, umbilicus, and genital areas. Xerosis is indicated by dryness of the skin, fine platelike scaling, and delicate fissuring with erythema. Stroking the back firmly with the blunt end of a pen and examining the area for a wheal 2 to 3 minutes later will reveal dermographism, an accentuated wheal and flare, which can cause itching (see Chapter 34, Urticaria). The examination should also include palpation for abdominal masses, hepatosplenomegaly, and lymph node enlargement in those with no obvious cause of the itching.

If no primary skin lesions are present, the cause of pruritus is inapparent, and the patient has failed to respond to a 2-week trial of treatment for xerosis (see later), a reasonable laboratory evaluation includes a complete blood cell count (to detect polycythemia, iron-deficiency anemia, or a leukemia); evaluation of alkaline phosphatase (to seek evidence of cholestasis); determination of levels of thyroid-stimulating hormone, thyroxine, and triiodothyronine (to detect hypothyroidism or hyperthyroidism); and a chest radiograph (to detect mediastinal lymph node enlargement in lymphomas, metastatic disease, or evidence of primary pulmonary neoplasm). If these are unrevealing, further testing without other evidence of systemic disease is usually unrewarding.

Management. For xerosis, infrequent bathing, use of mild soaps such as Dove or Tone, generous application of emollients such as Aquaphor or Carmol 20 (urea cream 20%), and humidification of dry air in heated environments are useful.

Antihistamines are helpful for some forms of pruritus. They are the drugs of choice for symptomatic dermographism. Hydroxyzine, 25 to 50 mg three times a day, is a reasonable agent that is also sedating, which is a helpful feature for those with nocturnal itching. Doxepin, an antidepressant and a potent antihistamine, is a good alternative, especially for those with chronic symptoms that have led to depression. A topical formulation of 5% doxepin (Zonalon) may be useful for short-term therapy for itching caused by atopic dermatitis, lichen simplex chronicus, or other disorders when applied four times a day. When used on more than 10% of the body surface, drowsiness from systemic absorption may occur.

Pramoxine, a topical anesthetic with low sensitizing potential, may be useful when combined with hydrocortisone cream (Pramosone) in some pruritic disorders, especially lichen simplex chronicus involving the anogenital areas.

Patients with uremic pruritus may benefit from ultraviolet B therapy, parathyroidectomy (in those with secondary hyperparathyroidism), oral activated charcoal, 6 g daily, or oral cholestyramine, 5 g twice daily. Patients with itching from cholestasis may improve with cholestyramine, 4 g one to three times a day; occasionally, ultraviolet B light treatment is helpful.

REFERENCE

1. Bernhard JD, ed. Itch. Mechanisms and Management of Pruritus. New York, McGraw-Hill Book Company, 1994.

   The entire book is devoted to various aspects of itching, including differential diagnosis and management.

24 Corns and Calluses

Problem

JAN V. HIRSCHMANN

Epidemiology. Corns and calluses are common hyperkeratotic lesions of the feet arising from chronic trauma to areas of pressure over bony prominences. The most frequent cause is poorly fitting shoes, but sometimes an abnormal gait or unusual bony architecture of the feet is responsible.

Symptoms and Signs. When symptomatic, corns and calluses cause pain on pressure. Corns are small, well-defined areas of skin thickening with a central hyperlucency that are most common around the fifth toe. Sometimes, they occur as a whitish hyperkeratosis in the toe webs ("soft corns"). Calluses are larger and less well-delineated areas of skin thickening and hardness that usually develop under the first and fifth metatarsal heads.

Clinical Approach. Paring the surface of corns will reveal a central clear area (nucleus) that disappears with deeper cuts, while shaving plantar warts, often confused with corns, will demonstrate black and red specks representing thrombosed capillaries. Furthermore, warts tend to be painful with lateral pressure, whereas corns tend to be painful with vertical pressure. Some patients, particularly the elderly, have hyperkeratotic, fissured areas on the heel that seem to occur from a combination of severely dry skin and pressure. These are not calluses in the usual sense, and they respond best to aggressive hydration of the skin with emollients.

Management. The pain produced by the thickened skin will abate after paring the surface of corns and calluses with a scalpel blade. Patients can often achieve good results by applying a 40% salicylic acid plaster every night, soaking the area in water the following morning, and then abrading the surface with a pumice stone, emery board, or callus file. These lesions return unless the underlying problem, such as ill-fitting footwear, is corrected. For difficult or recurrent lesions, consultation with a podiatrist may be helpful.

25 Warts

Problem

JAN V. HIRSCHMANN

Epidemiology. Warts result from intraepidermal infection with human papillomaviruses. DNA hybridization techniques have identified more than 50 types of these viruses, many associated with different clinical appearances of the warts. They are most common in childhood, with a peak incidence at ages 12 to 16, but occur at all ages. Infection develops by contact with another affected person or by autoinoculation from a site elsewhere on the body; the wart appears 1 to 12 months later, most commonly after 2 to 3 months. They present in areas of frequent pressure, especially on the plantar surfaces. Warts are usually categorized by their location or appearance. A common wart (verruca vulgaris) is a papule with an irregular surface that tends to occur on the hands and fingers, often in the periungual area. A flat wart (verruca plana) is a slightly elevated, flat-topped papule primarily found on the face, neck, forearms, and hands. Plantar warts are flat or elevated, thickened lesions that interrupt the skin lines (unlike calluses); often have black or red dots on the surface, representing thrombosed capillaries; and are usually surrounded by a collar of thickened skin. Filiform warts are small, slender papules, usually present on the neck or face. Anogenital warts (condylomata accuminata) are typically soft, moist, hyperplastic lesions found primarily on the foreskin and head of the penis in men, on the labia in women, and in the anal and urethral openings in both sexes.

Warts may demonstrate the Koebner phenomenon, which is the tendency to appear in areas of trauma. This characteristic explains some configurations of warts, such as their linear arrangement where a previous scratch has occurred.

Clinical Approach. The clinical appearance is usually diagnostic; occasionally, a biopsy is necessary. Because about 65% of warts spontaneously disappear in 2 years, not all require treatment.

Management. The simplest treatment of most warts is cryotherapy with liquid nitrogen applied for 5 to 30 seconds with a cotton applicator or with a spray from a special instrument. The wart and a 1-mm rim of normal surrounding skin should turn white with freezing. Repeating the liquid nitrogen freezing after the area defrosts probably yields greater success than a single treatment. A blister, sometimes hemorrhagic, may form but is unnecessary for effective therapy. Repeated treatment at about 2-week intervals is often necessary for resolution. An alternative approach, especially for warts on the hands or feet, is a salicylic acid–lactic acid paint (e.g., Duofilm) applied daily. This treatment is more effective if the area of the wart is soaked in hot water and gently abraded with an emery board before application of the solution. Improvement usually begins in 1 to 2 weeks, and 70% to 85% of patients are cured by 3 months.

REFERENCE

1. Cobb MW: Human papillomavirus infection. J Am Acad Dermatol 1990;22:547–566.

   A complete review is presented of the cutaneous manifestations of human papillomaviruses, with some excellent color photographs.

· ·

26 Superficial Fungal Infections

Problem

JAN V. HIRSCHMANN

DERMATOPHYTE INFECTIONS

Epidemiology. Dermatophytes, fungi that can invade the hair, skin, and nails of living hosts, belong to the genera *Epidermophyton*, *Microsporum*, and *Trichophyton*. Some species are confined to humans; others live in the soil or on other animals, and humans become infected after contact with these sources. About 10% of adults with apparently normal skin on their feet harbor dermatophytes; an additional 5% to 10% have clinical disease of the feet (tinea pedis) due to these organisms, primarily in the interdigital toe spaces.

Symptoms and Signs. The most common manifestations of tinea pedis are boggy whiteness and fissuring in the toewebs, especially the fourth interspace. A second form is redness and dry scaling of the sole and lower portion of the dorsal foot (moccasin distribution). Sometimes, erythema and vesicles or bullae develop, the roofs of which demonstrate fungi on microscopic examination. Onychomycosis, also called tinea unguium, is dermatophyte infection of the nails and is very common on the toenails. It causes yellow, opaque, thickened nails that may crumble easily and often have extensive hyperkeratosis and debris beneath, with separation of the nail plate from the nail bed (onycholysis). Often, both feet are infected with fungi; and when concomitant hand involvement occurs, inexplicably only one hand is typically affected (two feet, one hand disease).

Dermatophyte infections elsewhere on the skin usually occur as patches of erythema and scaling with raised red borders and central clearing. Tinea cruris involves the upper thighs and pubic area but spares the scrotum in men. On the trunk (tinea corporis) usually only one lesion develops. Infection may also occur on the face (tinea facei) and the scalp (tinea capitis), the latter usually in children.

Clinical Approach. Examination of skin or nail scrapings immersed in 10% to 30% potassium hydroxide (KOH) and gently heated is a very sensitive and specific test but requires experience for reliable interpretation. Positive preparations demonstrate translucent, septate hyphae, often with individual barrel-shaped segments that represent arthrospores. The different genera of dermatophytes are indistinguishable by this test, but scrapings inoculated onto fungal media will grow the organism and allow specific identification. Cultures are usually unnecessary, however, if the KOH preparation is positive, unless the history or epidemiologic setting suggests an unusual organism.

Management. Most cases of tinea pedis, tinea corporis, tinea facei, and tinea cruris respond to topical antifungal agents applied twice a day for about 4 weeks. Available agents, all equally effective against both dermatophytes and *Candida* species, include ciclopirox (Loprox), clotrimazole (Lotrimin, Mycelex), econazole (Spectazole), ketoconazole (Nizoral), miconazole (Micatin, Monistat-Derm), oxiconazole (Oxistat), and sulconazole (Exelderm). Clotrimazole and miconazole are available without prescription.

With extensive disease, involvement of the hands or with scalp infection, oral griseofulvin is the drug of choice. It is a very safe medication; the traditional teaching that it is significantly hepatotoxic or that its use requires monitoring of liver tests is untrue. The usual daily dose is 500 mg of the ultramicrosized form given for 1 to 2 months depending on clinical response. Oral ketoconazole, equally effective but not superior for most cases, is occasionally necessary for those who cannot tolerate or do not respond to griseofulvin. The usual dose is 200 mg/d. Hepatic injury rarely occurs (about 1 in 10,000 persons is affected), usually early in the course of therapy. Another option is oral fluconazole given 150 mg once a week.

Fingernail infection commonly responds to 500 mg of griseofulvin daily for 4 to 12 months. Toenail involvement is much more resistant, especially in the elderly, and many clinicians attempt treatment only in younger patients, giving griseofulvin, 1 g/d for 12 to 18 months. Another option is oral fluconazole, 150 mg once a week. Topical therapy for toenails is not very effective, but surgical removal of the nail with destruction of the nail matrix by phenol to prevent regrowth eliminates the infection and is sometimes indicated for symptomatic disease. For many patients, careful nail trimming and filing with an emery board or nail file, while not curative, relieves any discomfort caused by the dystrophic nail.

Follow-Up. Dermatophyte infection, especially tinea pedis, often recurs, and many patients learn to resume therapy when symptoms or signs reappear. Patients receiving ketoconazole should know the symptoms of hepatotoxicity, stop treatment if they appear, and seek prompt medical attention.

TINEA (PITYRIASIS) VERSICOLOR

Epidemiology. Tinea (pityriasis) versicolor is due to a yeast that is a normal skin organism and resides primarily on the face, neck, and upper trunk. This fungus has several names, *Pityrosporum ovale, P. orbiculare,* or *Malassezia furfur.* In some individuals the oval yeast forms become filamentous and cause the cutaneous lesions of tinea versicolor. This disorder occurs in up to 50% of people in tropical climates, compared with 5% in dry, temperate areas. Systemic corticosteroid therapy, Cushing's disease, compromised cell-mediated immunity, and pregnancy may increase the incidence.

Symptoms and Signs. Most patients are asymptomatic, but mild pruritus occasionally occurs. Many patients complain of the altered pigmentation that the characteristic macular lesions cause. In dark-skinned patients (including whites with suntans) they are often hypopigmented; in those with light complexions they are usually darker than the surrounding skin. The colors of the macules range from white to brown (versicolor). The borders are well delineated, but individual macules often coalesce to form larger patches. Gentle scratching produces a fine scale. The areas most involved are the trunk and neck, although lesions may occur on the abdomen, upper arms, and genital area.

Clinical Approach. KOH preparations of skin scrapings establish the diagnosis by demonstrating abundant yeasts and hyphae ("spaghetti and meatballs"). Parker's blue-black ink will stain them blue, making their identification easier. Culturing this organism, which requires special media, is of no diagnostic value because it is normally present on the skin.

Management. Treatment is usually successful, but relapse is common, unless the agents are continued. Selenium sulfide suspension (Selsun) applied overnight from the chin to the waist and from the shoulders to the wrists and then rinsed off is effective. Re-treatment 1 week later and repeated every few weeks as necessary will usually control this disorder. If this program causes skin irritation, the shampoo may be rinsed off 5 to 15 minutes after application, and the treatment repeated for 3 consecutive days. The use of topical antifungal agents such as clotrimazole is also effective but more expensive. With very extensive involvement or when the patient is unable to apply topical therapy, a single oral dose of 400 mg of ketoconazole is very effective and may be repeated once a month to prevent recurrence. With either topical or systemic treatment, the scaling resolves quickly, but the pigmentary changes may require several weeks to months to disappear.

Follow-Up. Patients can learn to re-treat any relapses, which should respond to the same agent used before, without further visits to the clinician.

CANDIDA INFECTIONS

Epidemiology. *Candida* species are normal inhabitants of the alimentary tract but not the skin. *Candida* infections most commonly seen in ambulatory care are thrush, perlèche, intertriginous candidiasis, and vulvovaginitis (see Chapter 164, Vaginitis). Conditions predisposing to thrush are diabetes, decreased saliva (as in Sjögren's syndrome), recent broad-spectrum antibacterial therapy, or diminished cell-mediated immunity, especially the acquired immunodeficiency syndrome. Perlèche (angular cheilitis) usually occurs in older patients with increased moisture and maceration at the angles of the mouth, especially from poorly fitting dentures or drooling because of neurologic disorders. *Candida* is commonly, but not universally, present in the characteristically red and fissured lesions. Intertriginous candidiasis usually occurs in the skin folds of obese people.

Symptoms and Signs. Thrush consists of whitish plaques, usually resting on an erythematous base, affecting the tongue, buccal mucosa, gums, or palate. They may be asymptomatic or cause soreness of the mouth. Perlèche causes soreness of the angles of the mouth, where moisture, erythema, and fissuring are present. Intertriginous candidiasis occurs in any body fold, especially beneath pendulous breasts, between folds of fat on the abdomen, or in the groin. Erythema, moisture, and whitish debris are present, often with an irregular peeling edge and pustules or reddish papules outside these borders (satellite lesions).

Clinical Approach. Scraping the oral lesions of thrush with a tongue blade, smearing the material onto a slide, and examining it under a microscope will establish the diagnosis. Gram stains, easier than a KOH preparation for most persons to interpret, disclose large gram-positive yeasts and pseudohyphae characteristic of the organism. Cultures are not indicated because *Candida* species are part of the normal mouth flora. For skin lesions, KOH preparations or Gram stains will reveal the fungi. If these are positive, cultures are usually unnecessary.

Management. For thrush, nystatin, 4 to 6 mL (400,000 to 600,000 units), swished four times a day around in the mouth for several minutes and then swallowed, is very effective when given for 1 to 2 weeks. Clotrimazole troches (10 mg) dissolved slowly in the mouth and swallowed five times a day also work. Occasionally, with very severe or refractory disease, oral ketoconazole, 200 mg daily, or fluconazole, 50 to 100 mg/d for 2 weeks, is required. Perlèche usually responds to topical antifungal creams effective against *Candida* species such as clotrimazole given twice daily. Correction of predisposing factors, such as poorly fitting dentures, is important to prevent recurrences. Intertriginous candidiasis can be treated with topical creams as well. Weight loss for obese patients, keeping the area dry, and wearing loose-fitting clothing are helpful measures. Some patients with intertriginous inflammation do not have a fungal infection. They usually respond to topical corticosteroids—1% hydrocortisone in the groin or axilla, and more potent agents, such as triamcinolone 0.1%, in other areas.

REFERENCES

1. Crislip MA, Edwards JE: Candidiasis. Infect Dis Clin North Am 1989;3:103–133.

   A thorough review is presented of both superficial and deep infections due to Candida *species.*

2. Gupta AK, Sauder DN, Shear NH: Antifungal agents: An overview: I and II. J Am Acad Dermatol 1994;30:677–698, 911–933.

   Both topical and systemic agents are discussed.

27 Scabies and Lice

Problem

JAN V. HIRSCHMANN

SCABIES

Epidemiology. *Sarcoptes scabiei* var. *hominis* is an obligate human parasite that usually cannot survive for more than a few days off the human skin. Close physical contact, especially sexual intercourse, allows transmission of the mites from person to person. Family outbreaks are common.

Symptoms and Signs. In previously uninfected patients symptoms begin 4 to 6 weeks after infestation. Generalized pruritus, characteristically worse at night, is the most prominent symptom. Burrows—short, wavy lines, especially likely to occur between fingers, on the penis, or on the flexor areas of the wrist—are usually the earliest lesions but may not develop or may disappear after vigorous scratching. Other common sites are the nipples, umbilicus, buttocks, or axillae. The head is usually spared, but it may be involved, particularly in children, elderly persons, or bedridden patients. Frequently, the major or only lesions are excoriations and erythematous papules. Occasionally, vesicles, bullae, or nodules occur. Pustules develop in areas of secondary infection, which is especially likely to occur in hot, humid climates.

Clinical Approach. Definitive diagnosis depends on finding mites or their eggs or feces on skin samples, best obtained by applying a drop of mineral oil over burrows or papules and scraping with a scalpel blade. This material, placed on a slide, is examined under low power on a microscope. Because the number of mites on the skin of an infested person is small, frequently no definitive findings are present, and the clinical diagnosis depends on the patient's response to empirical (antiscabetic) therapy.

Management. Lindane 1% (Kwell) remains very effective therapy in the United States when given as a lotion to cover the body from head to the soles of the feet, left on for 8 to 12 hours, and then washed off. If new lesions develop, a second treatment 10 days later is necessary. Permethrin 5% cream (Elimite) applied in the same manner as lindane is an effective, but not superior, alternative in the United States. Close contacts should receive simultaneous therapy, but special treatment of clothing is probably unnecessary.

Follow-Up. Pruritus often persists for 2 to 4 weeks and is not an indication for re-treatment. For this symptom, antihistamines such as hydroxyzine, 25 mg three times a day, or topical corticosteroids may be useful. For intolerable itching a short course of systemic corticosteroids (e.g., 40 mg of prednisone for 5 to 7 days, then tapered off over the following week) provides relief.

All of the material in Chapter 27 is in the public domain, with the exception of any borrowed figures and tables.

LICE

Epidemiology. Body lice reside mostly in clothing, where they lay eggs and from which they emerge, mostly at night, to feed on the host's blood. Therefore, they usually infest those with poor personal hygiene, who do not wash or change clothes frequently. Head lice live in the scalp, attached to hair, on which they lay their eggs. They infest mostly children. They are probably transmitted from person to person by close head contact or the sharing of hats, combs, and brushes. Pubic lice live mostly in the hairs of the pubic area but can also reside in the beard, eyelashes, scalp, or axillae. Close body contact, commonly sexual activity, transmits the lice; fomites such as bed clothing or towels may occasionally be responsible, but pubic lice survive for only about 12 hours off the host.

Symptoms and Signs. The most common symptom in all forms of infestation is pruritus. Occasionally, patients may notice the lice on their bodies or have the sense of movement on their skin as the lice migrate. Excoriations are frequent; some patients get secondary skin infections with purulent lesions, tender lymph nodes, fever, and malaise ("feeling lousy"). With head lice the scalp usually reveals excoriations and crusts, often with enlarged posterior cervical lymph nodes. With pubic lice, some patients have asymptomatic *maculae ceruleae* ("sky-blue spots") 0.5 to 1 cm in diameter in the area of infestation, probably representing alteration of the host's blood pigments by the louse's saliva.

Clinical Approach. The diagnosis of infestation depends on detecting the lice or their eggs ("nits"), which are brown or white and, with pubic or head lice, are cemented to the hairs. In the scalp they may resemble dandruff but are not easily movable along the hair shaft. Microscopic examination of a plucked hair with an attached nit that is covered by a drop of oil will reveal the egg and developing embryo. Because neither lice nor nits are usually present on the skin with body lice infestation, the diagnosis typically rests on finding them in the patient's clothing, usually along the seams.

Management. Lindane is effective for all lice. For head lice, lindane shampoo left on for 10 minutes or the lotion left on overnight and then rinsed off is effective. An alternative therapy is permethrin creme rinse (Nix) left on for 10 minutes, then washed off. Removing all nits with a comb or tweezer ("nitpicking") should follow these treatments. All household contacts should receive simultaneous treatment. For pubic lice, lindane lotion left on for 12 hours and then washed off is effective. All sex partners should also be treated. Permethrin creme rinse is equally efficacious.

Because body lice live on clothing, the patient's skin does not usually require treatment, but if lice or nits are present, lindane lotion left on for 12 hours and then rinsed off is appropriate. The patient's clothes should be laundered with hot water or dry-cleaned.

Follow-Up. Reexamination of patients about 1 week after treatment of head and pubic lice determines the efficacy of therapy. If viable nits or live lice are present, re-treatment is necessary.

REFERENCE

1. Elgart ML: Scabies. Pediculosis. Dermatol Clin North Am 1990;8:219–228, 253–263.
   Both entities are well reviewed.

28 Eczema

Problem

JAN V. HIRSCHMANN

Eczema (or dermatitis) is a pattern of skin inflammation with clinical features of erythema, itching, scaling, lichenification, papules, and vesicles in varying combinations. Several distinctive forms exist, but some cases defy simple classification. The types commonly seen are atopic eczema, asteatotic eczema, nummular (coinlike) eczema, pompholyx (hand and foot eczema), prurigo nodularis, lichen simplex chronicus, venous eczema (stasis dermatitis), and contact dermatitis. The overall prevalence of all forms of eczema is about 18 per 1000 in the United States.

ATOPIC ECZEMA

Epidemiology. The prevalence of atopic eczema in the United States is about 7 per 1000. It typically begins in childhood, usually before 5 years of age, and commonly subsides by adulthood, although in some patients it recurs after years of quiescence. Only occasionally does the disease begin after age 30.

Symptoms and Signs. In adults the usual lesions are dry, lichenified, and hyperpigmented patches in flexor areas of the elbows, knees, wrists, neck, and ankles and around the eyes. With exacerbations, erythematous papules and vesicles may develop, sometimes diffusely over the body. Itching is the major symptom.

Clinical Approach. The clinician should seek and eliminate factors that exacerbate the disease, such as extremes of temperature, sweating, irritating clothing (especially silk and wool), and harsh soaps. Although atopic patients have a lower incidence of contact dermatitis than the general population, unexplained worsening, particularly in well-delimited areas of topical therapy, should suggest the possibility of sensitivity to the agent being applied.

Management. Because dry skin is a major component of atopic eczema, a most important element of treatment is adequate cutaneous hydration. Immediately after bathing or washing their hands, patients should pat the skin, not rub it, with a towel and apply emollients such as Aquaphor or Eucerin to the damp but not dripping skin. In addition, they should use these agents several times a day to keep the skin moist. Potent topical corticosteroids such as betamethasone valerate 0.1% two to three times a day are the mainstay of treatment and should be prescribed as ointments because creams are more drying. For stubborn lesions topical corticosteroid creams under occlusion, usually most convenient at night, may be helpful. Systemic corticosteroids given in short courses are sometimes necessary for severe, widespread exacerbations, but chronic use is rarely appropriate. *Staphylococcus aureus* is very commonly present on eczematous skin in all phases of the disease, but when its presence indicates infection rather than colonization is often unclear. Certainly, treatment is appropriate for pustules or cellulitis; many dermatologists, however, prescribe systemic antistaphylococcal agents such as dicloxacillin or erythromycin, 250 to 500 mg four times a day, for widespread exudative lesions as well. The evidence for this practice is weak.

Follow-Up. During exacerbations clinicians should see patients frequently until the problem subsides. Sometimes, hospitalization is necessary for adequate therapy, and often a brief stay results in remarkable, rapid improvement.

ASTEATOTIC ECZEMA (ECZEMA CRAQUELÉ)

Epidemiology. Asteatotic eczema occurs primarily in the elderly and seems to arise from decreased skin lipids. The drying effect of indoor heating during winter, frequent bathing, and diuretic therapy for edema are common initiating or exacerbating factors.

Symptoms and Signs. The lesions may be asymptomatic or pruritic. They occur primarily on the anterior legs as areas of dryness, scaling, and a fine fissuring of the skin resembling the cracks seen in porcelain china. Erythema may be diffuse in the involved area or most prominent along the edges of the fissures, from which clear fluid may exude. Asteatotic eczema may also involve the backs of the hands and fingertips, where dryness, cracking, and a shrunken appearance are common.

Management. Emollients such as Aquaphor, Eucerin, or 20% urea cream provide the necessary hydration. Topical corticosteroids such as triamcinolone ointment 0.1% twice daily are also helpful. Patients should use bland soaps containing cold cream such as Dove or Tone and avoid excessive bathing.

NUMMULAR ECZEMA

Epidemiology. Nummular eczema has a prevalence in the United States of about 2 per 1000, primarily in adults over age 50, especially men.

Symptoms and Signs. The lesions may be asymptomatic or pruritic. They are rounded (nummular), erythematous plaques, sometimes with central clearing, that contain vesicles, exudation, and crusting or are dry and scaling. Although they may be single, sparse, or widespread, the lesions are discrete, with normal intervening skin. They most commonly appear on the back and legs but can also involve the hands and arms.

Management. Emollients may be helpful for dry skin, but the major treatment is a potent corticosteroid ointment such as betamethasone valerate 0.1%. Lesions often respond slowly, and higher-potency preparations such as clobetasol propionate (Temovate) may be necessary. New lesions form unpredictably. Often, patients have periods of disease activity for weeks to months, and then the disorder subsides, sometimes to relapse later. In other patients, mild disease may become extensive without any clear explanation, although low humidity, especially during the winter months, and exposure to irritating substances on the skin may sometimes be provocative factors.

POMPHOLYX (DYSHIDROTIC ECZEMA)

Epidemiology. The prevalence of this eczema is about 2 per 1000 in the United States with most cases beginning before age 40.

Symptoms and Signs. Pompholyx usually involves the hands alone; sometimes both hands and feet are affected; occasionally, it is confined to the feet. The main symptom is itching; the major sign is the presence of tiny deep-seated vesicles that look like tapioca pudding and occur symmetrically on the palms, soles, and borders of the fingers. The vesicles may coalesce to form bullae. Sometimes, the main finding is dryness, cracking, and scaling of the palms, soles, and digits.

Clinical Approach. Especially when unilateral, particularly on the foot, a potassium hydroxide examination of the roofs of vesicles or scrapings from a scaly area is necessary to exclude a dermatophyte infection. A careful history should help ensure that contact dermatitis (e.g., from an unprescribed topical preparation) is not the cause of or an exacerbating factor in the eczema.

Management. For acute weeping lesions, wet dressings of aluminum acetate (Burow's) solution over the affected area three to four times a day may be soothing. Potent topical corticosteroids are usually necessary to control the inflammation, and oral antihistamines such as hydroxyzine may be useful for the pruritus. Occasionally, a short course of oral corticosteroids is appropriate for severe disease. Patients should avoid irritating substances, such as detergents, polishes, and cleansing agents. With prolonged exposure to water, which removes skin lipids, they should wear rubber or, preferably, vinyl gloves with cotton liners beneath. For dry work and gardening, leather or heavy fabric gloves are advisable, and patients should wear warm gloves during cold, dry weather, which worsens the eczema. They should use little soap when hand washing. Because rings often exacerbate dermatitis by trapping irritating substances beneath them, patients should remove them during housework and before hand washing and should clean them frequently on the inside.

PRURIGO NODULARIS

Epidemiology. Prurigo nodularis (nodular prurigo or "picker's nodules") is most common in middle age, especially in women.

Symptoms and Signs. Intense pruritus is the major complaint, and a tendency to scratch is overwhelming. Early lesions are papules, but they become firm, reddish or purple 1- to 3-cm nodules, with an excoriated surface. They occur primarily on the arms and back but not in the interscapular area, where the patient cannot readily reach. On regression, hyperpigmented or hypopigmented scars may remain.

Management. Treatment can be very difficult. Oral antihistamines, such as hydroxyzine, 25 mg three times a day, may diminish the pruritus. Potent corticosteroids in ointments such as betamethasone valerate 0.1% or in tape form (Cordran) may help, but intralesional corticosteroid injection may be the most effective therapy for many. Some patients benefit from ultraviolet light treatments or liquid nitrogen cryotherapy.

LICHEN SIMPLEX CHRONICUS (NEURODERMATITIS)

Epidemiology. This disorder may occur at any age but is most common between 30 and 50 years of age. It is more frequent in women than in men.

Symptoms and Signs. Lichen simplex chronicus occurs from repeated scratching or rubbing of the skin. The most common sites are the back or sides of the neck, ankle, lateral aspect of the lower leg, upper thighs, and anogenital region. The affected areas are markedly pruritic and demonstrate lichenification and erythema or, sometimes, hyperpigmentation.

Clinical Approach. Other entities to consider include contact dermatitis and psoriasis.

Management. A potent corticosteroid ointment such as betamethasone valerate 0.1% used twice daily or the daily application of Cordran tape usually suffices, but intralesional injection of corticosteroids may be indicated in refractory cases. Hydrocortisone 1% to 2.5% alone or with the topical anesthetic pramoxine (Pramasone) is usually effective in anogenital areas where stronger corticosteroids are not indicated for chronic therapy. Topical doxepin (Zonalon) may be useful for short periods to relieve intolerable pruritus.

VENOUS ECZEMA (STASIS DERMATITIS)

Epidemiology. Venous eczema is a complication of venous insufficiency of the legs, a disorder most common in the elderly, especially women.

Symptoms and Signs. Venous eczema may be asymptomatic or cause pruritus or burning discomfort. It may also be the site of entry for streptococci that cause cellulitis. It almost always occurs around the malleoli, especially the medial ones, but it may extend up the leg. It consists of erythematous scaling, often with exudation, crusts, and superficial ulcerations. Signs of venous hypertension are present, including varicosities, hemosiderin pigmentation, edema, venous ulcers, and dilated venules.

Management. Burow's (aluminum acetate) wet dressings 20 minutes three to four times a day are useful for acute weeping dermatitis. Topical corticosteroid creams, such as triamcinolone 0.1% twice daily, will usually relieve the eczema. Treatment of the venous hypertension with leg elevation and elastic support stockings is crucial to control the edema and prevent future exacerbations.

CONTACT DERMATITIS

Epidemiology. Contact dermatitis, which may occur from irritating substances or because of allergy to a material, is frequent, especially on the hands and in certain occupations. Contact allergy may develop to topical medications, the most common agents being neomycin, lanolin, and topical anesthetics such as benzocaine.

Symptoms and Signs. The eruption may occur several days after first exposure to the agent; in those sensitized by previous contact, it usually appears 12 to 48 hours after exposure. Pruritus is the main complaint. Acute lesions show vesicles, oozing, erythema, and crusting. Chronic lesions are scaly, lichenified, and fissured. Sometimes, the diagnosis is obvious by history, but physical findings suggesting a contact cause are straight borders or lines, or a configuration conforming to some object touching the skin, such as a band around the wrist from an allergy to a component of a watchband. Failure of another skin disorder to improve despite apparently adequate topical therapy should suggest the possibility of contact allergy to an element of the treatment.

Clinical Approach. After resolution of the dermatitis, skin testing to confirm the diagnosis and the identity of the contact allergen may be indicated.

Management. Removal of the responsible agent is obviously crucial. The dermatitis should respond to topical corticosteroids.

REFERENCES

1. Champion RH, Burton JL, Ebling FJG, eds. Textbook of Dermatology. Oxford, Blackwell, 1992:537–715.

   Superb clinical discussions of the various eczemas are included in the best dermatology textbook in English.

2. Epstein E: Hand dermatitis: Practical management and current concepts. J Am Acad Dermatol 1984;10:395–424.

   This is a very practical guide to the management of hand dermatitis with good instructions for patients.

· ·

29 Seborrheic Dermatitis

Problem

JAN V. HIRSCHMANN

Epidemiology. Seborrheic dermatitis, a chronic disorder probably caused by overgrowth of a normal skin yeast, *Pityrosporum orbiculare*, is rare before puberty and usually begins in adults between 18 and 40 years of age. It is more common in males and is especially frequent in patients with Parkinson's disease and in those with the acquired immunodeficiency syndrome (AIDS), in whom it is often very severe.

Symptoms and Signs. Seborrheic dermatitis occurs predominantly on the scalp, face, and upper trunk. These areas have abundant sebaceous glands; the sebum that they produce contains the lipids necessary for *P. orbiculare* to grow. Erythema and scaling, often of a "greasy" nature, are the most common findings. In the scalp the scaling is usually diffuse, often with patches of redness and thick, sometimes weeping crusts. Common areas of facial involvement are the forehead, the eyebrows, the skin around the nasal alae, the external auditory canal, and the postauricular region. In those with mustaches or beards, yellowish white scales may adhere to the hairs, and the skin surrounding the follicles is often red. Blepharitis, inflammation of the eyelid margins, commonly occurs. On the trunk, yellowish brown or red patches of scaling may occur on the presternal or interscapular regions. Seborrheic dermatitis may also involve the axillary, submammary, or groin areas, typically as patches of bright, moist erythema with mild scaling.

Management. For scalp involvement, selenium sulfide shampoo applied for 5 to 10 minutes before rinsing is usually effective when used daily or less often as necessary. Alternative shampoos include those containing zinc pyrithione (e.g., Head and Shoulders), salicylic acid-sulfur (e.g., Ionil), or tar (e.g., Ionil T, Zetar). Topical corticosteroid lotions (e.g., fluocinolone) used twice daily are helpful for those with substantial inflammation or a poor response to a shampoo alone. Removal of thick crusts often requires nighttime application of keratolytic medications such as Baker's P&S (phenol and saline), covering the scalp with a shower cap overnight, and shampooing in the morning.

Seborrheic dermatitis elsewhere usually responds to topical corticosteroids—hydrocortisone 1% on the face and groin and more potent agents (e.g., triamcinolone 0.025%), if necessary, on the trunk. Patients with recalcitrant disease, especially those with AIDS, may require topical ketoconazole twice a day (instead of, or in addition to, corticosteroids) or even oral ketoconazole (200 mg/d) to achieve control. For most immunocompetent hosts, topical corticosteroids seem slightly better and much less expensive than topical ketoconazole, although refractory disease sometimes requires combined topical treatment with both agents.

Involvement of the eyelid margins usually subsides with hot compresses, débridement with a cotton-tipped applicator stick and baby shampoo, or use of 10% sodium sulfacetamide ophthalmic ointment (Sodium Sulamyd) two to four times a day.

Follow-Up. Seborrheic dermatitis is a chronic disease that usually relapses quickly when treatment ends. Most patients learn to manage their disease, resuming therapy when the symptoms and signs recur, and require infrequent return visits for this problem. Chronic use of hydrocortisone on the face and elsewhere is safe, as are potent corticosteroids on the scalp.

Cross-References: Redness of the Eye (Chapter 37), Otitis Media and Externa (Chapter 56), HIV Infection: Disease Prevention and Antiretroviral Therapy (Chapter 203), HIV Infection: Office Evaluation (Chapter 204), HIV Infection: Evaluation of Common Symptoms (Chapter 205).

REFERENCES

1. Bergbrant IM, Faergemann J: The role of *Pityrosporum ovale* in seborrheic dermatitis. Semin Dermatol 1990;9:262–268.

   This article presents a thorough review of the microbiology of this organism and the evidence of its role in seborrheic dermatitis.

2. Stratigos JD, Antoniou C, Katsambas A, et al: Ketoconazole 2% cream versus hydrocortisone 1% cream in the treatment of seborrheic dermatitis. J Am Acad Dermatol 1988;19:850–853.

   This double-blind trial showed that hydrocortisone had a better result than ketoconazole (clinical response 94% vs. 81%).

. . . .

30 Herpes Zoster

Problem

JAN V. HIRSCHMANN

Epidemiology. Ten percent to 20% of all people have herpes zoster during their lifetime. The incidence increases with age from less than 50 per 100,000 person-years for those younger than 15 years old to more than 400 per 100,000 person-years for people older than age 74. The average age of patients with herpes zoster is about 45. The presence of cancer modestly increases the risk, whereas immunocompromising conditions such as Hodgkin's disease, acquired immunodeficiency syndrome (AIDS), or organ transplantation are associated with incidences as high as 10% to 30% per year. A second attack occurs in about 5% of patients, although the risk of recurrence is higher in immunocompromised patients.

Symptoms and Signs. A prodrome of burning, tingling, pain, and hyperesthesia in a dermatome is frequent and may last for a few days (occasionally as long as a week or more) before skin lesions appear. These begin as erythematous papules that transform into vesicles, with contents that are originally clear but later turn yellow and turbid or, occasionally, bloody. Darkening of the roofs is frequent, and the skin may become black, representing focal gangrene. The vesicles usually evolve over 4 to 7 days before crusts appear. The crusts fall off several days later, leaving scars in many patients.

Herpes zoster occurs in the thoracic dermatomes in 60% of patients and involves the cranial nerves in about 15%, usually the trigeminal nerve in one of its three subsegments—ophthalmic, maxillary, or mandibular. About 20% of patients with herpes zoster of the trigeminal nerve have eye involvement; most of these (85%) have Hutchinson's sign (the presence of lesions on the tip of the nose). The cervical dermatomes are affected in 10%, the lumbar dermatomes in 10%, and the sacral dermatomes in 5%. Immunocompetent patients often have scattered lesions distant from the original dermatome. Only the presence of numerous extradermatomal lesions (at least 25) qualifies as clinically significant dissemination, which is virtually confined to severely immunocompromised patients. In these patients, evidence of cutaneous dissemination begins 6 to 10 days after the original lesions appear; involvement of visceral organs such as lung, liver, or brain occurs in only about 10% of untreated immunocompromised patients with disseminated disease.

Postherpetic neuralgia, generally defined as pain lasting more than 1 month, occurs in 10% to 60% of patients overall, is more frequent in older patients, especially those older than 60 years of age, and may be more common in immunocompromised patients. The distribution of the dermatomes involved reflects that of herpes zoster in general, except that postherpetic neuralgia is uncommon in the lumbar area.

Clinical Approach. The appearance of papules, vesicles, and pustules in a dermatomal distribution is virtually pathognomonic of herpes zoster. Viral cultures and immunofluorescent or electron microscopic techniques can confirm the diagnosis but are rarely necessary. In confusing cases a simple diagnostic test is the Tzanck smear, in which material is scraped from the base of vesicles, pustules, or erosions; placed on a slide; and treated with Wright's stain. A positive test—the presence of characteristic nuclear changes, including enlargement and multinucleation—is present in 91% of patients with varicella or zoster but does not distinguish these lesions from those of herpes simplex.

Because herpes zoster may be an early complication of AIDS, patients with risk factors for this disease should undergo testing for human immunodeficiency virus antibody. Herpes zoster is rarely a sign of occult malignancy; without other clinical evidence, further tests are unnecessary.

Patients with herpes zoster are contagious to people who have not had varicella in the past. By age 20, about 90% of the population is immune. During the first trimester of pregnancy, varicella causes congenital abnormalities in about 10% of fetuses. This infection is especially risky close to the time of delivery (with onset of disease from 5 days before to 2 days after), when infant mortality is 20% to 30%. Patients with herpes zoster should carefully avoid contact with pregnant women and immunocompromised patients who have not had varicella; in them, the disease can be severe.

Management. Herpes zoster ordinarily requires no topical therapy, although wet dressings may be useful for exudative lesions. Painful disease may require narcotics. In most immunocompetent patients acyclovir has little clinical benefit and does not decrease the frequency of postherpetic neuralgia. In patients with ophthalmic involvement, however, oral acyclovir reduces the incidence and severity of the most common eye complications if begun within 7 days of the appearance of skin lesions. For those with normal renal function the recommended oral dose is 800 mg five times a day for 10 days; the same regimen is appropriate for immunocompromised patients with herpes zoster at any cutaneous site. Those with severe disease may require hospitalization and intravenous acyclovir.

For patients with postherpetic neuralgia—either a steady or lancinating pain in the dermatome lasting for more than 1 month—the most effective treatment is amitriptyline beginning at 25 mg at bedtime, increasing the dose by 25 mg every 2 to 5 days until pain subsides or side effects preclude further use. Seventy-five milligrams (range: 25–137.5 mg) was the median daily dose necessary in one study to provide good to excellent pain relief, a goal achieved in about two thirds of patients. A nonsedating tricyclic antidepressant such as desipramine is also effective. Topical capsaicin (Zostrix) applied three times a day furnishes some benefit in about 80% of patients, but often the effect is only modest.

Cross-References: Redness of the Eye (Chapter 37), HIV Infection: Disease Prevention and Antiretroviral Therapy (Chapter 203), HIV Infection: Office Evaluation (Chapter 204), HIV Infection: Evaluation of Common Symptoms (Chapter 205).

REFERENCES

1. Hirschmann JV. Herpes zoster. Semin Neurol 1992;12:322–328.
   This is a thorough review, with special emphasis on the neurologic complications.

2. Rowbotham MC: Postherpetic neuralgia. Semin Neurol 1994;14:247–254.
   The author presents a sensible, detailed assessment of the published information.

• •

31 Acne

Problem

JAN V. HIRSCHMANN

Epidemiology. Acne is virtually universal during adolescence, with peak incidences at age 14 to 17 in girls and 16 to 19 in boys. Occasionally, especially in girls, acne begins before other features of puberty appear. In about 85% of patients acne is mild; in 15% it is more troublesome. Usually, acne disappears in the late teens or early 20s, but in a few persons, especially women, it continues until age 40 or beyond. Occasionally, acne begins in the early 20s or later. The distribution and severity of acne tend to be similar in family members, suggesting a hereditary component in this disease. Acne frequently worsens just before or during menstruation, but diet seems unimportant. Moderate exposure to sunlight is usually beneficial; excessive sweating in tropical climates, however, may worsen the disease.

Symptoms and Signs. The face is nearly always involved, and patients usually have lesions on the chest and back as well. Most have several types of cutaneous abnormalities in varying combinations: noninflammatory—open comedones (blackheads), closed comedones (whiteheads)—and inflammatory lesions—

papules, pustules, nodules, and, less commonly, cysts. Scarring is frequent in severe disease, causing hypertrophic lesions, depressed areas (icepick scars), or small regions of increased or decreased pigmentation, especially in persons with dark skin.

Clinical Approach. The diagnosis of acne is evident on physical examination. Clinicians should inquire about medications that can precipitate or exacerbate acne, such as androgenic hormones, anabolic steroids, topical or systemic corticosteroids, phenobarbital, isoniazid, lithium, and cyclosporine. Cosmetics, oily hair products, and occupational exposure to cutting oils (e.g., in machinists) can also cause or worsen the disease.

Management. Medications used to treat acne alter one or more of the four major etiologic factors in acne: (1) increased sebum production, resulting from the effects of endogenous androgenic hormones; (2) hypercornification of the follicular orifice, causing duct obstruction; (3) colonization of the pilosebaceous duct with *Propionibacterium acnes*; and (4) inflammation, perhaps to microbial products of *P. acnes*. Most patients with mild acne respond to topical agents. Benzoyl peroxide, which decreases the population of *P. acnes* and diminishes the inflammatory response to it, is used twice daily, or less frequently, to produce mild erythema and dryness. Topical antibiotics, either clindamycin or erythromycin, which also reduce the numbers of *P. acnes*, are effective in about 70% of patients. Tretinoin (Retin-A) decreases ductal hypercornification and possibly colonization with *P. acnes*; when applied overnight it is very useful, especially in those with predominantly comedonal acne. These topical agents may be given alone or in tretinoin—combination at night, benzoyl peroxide or topical antibiotics in the morning—but not applied at the same time. These medications require at least 3 months of use to attain their optimal effect, although improvement is usually evident by 2 to 3 weeks.

For moderate or severe involvement, oral tetracycline, 500 mg twice daily, is effective and well tolerated. Patients should use it for at least 6 months to achieve its maximum benefit. Long-term administration (several years) appears safe and effective. For those unable to tolerate tetracycline, erythromycin, 500 mg twice daily, or trimethoprim-sulfamethoxazole, one double-strength tablet daily or twice daily, is an acceptable alternative. Patients who fail to respond to these measures or who have very severe acne should consult a dermatologist, who might consider estrogens or prednisone in females or isotretinoin, a very potent medication with dramatic effects on acne, in both sexes. Local measures that are sometimes helpful are gentle removal of blackheads and whiteheads by a comedone extractor and drainage, intralesional corticosteroids, or cryotherapy for cysts.

Follow-Up. During early therapy, monthly review may be wise to monitor improvement, reassure patients, and offer encouragement. Later, follow-up every 3 to 4 months usually suffices.

REFERENCES

1. Cunliffe WJ: Acne. Chicago, Year Book Medical Publishers, 1989.
   Superb color photographs are included in this thorough and practical book on acne.
2. Kaminer MS, Gilchrest BA: The many faces of acne. J Am Acad Dermatol 1995;32:S6–S14.
   This is a succinct review of the subtypes of acne and other disorders that resemble it.

32 Psoriasis

Problem

JAN V. HIRSCHMANN

Epidemiology. Psoriasis occurs in about 1.5% of American adults of both sexes. Onset is typically in the 20s and somewhat earlier in women than in men. A family history is common.

Symptoms and Signs. The most common form consists of well-defined plaques of white to silver scale of varying thickness, adherent to an erythematous base. They tend to occur in one or more of the following areas: the lower back, including the gluteal cleft; the scalp; the extensor surfaces of the elbows and knees; and the genital area. Where scale is removed, bleeding points may occur (Auspitz' sign). The appearance of lesions 1 to 2 weeks after trauma to a previously uninvolved area (Koebner's phenomenon) is common; paradoxically, many note that injury to an area of psoriasis may result in improvement. The lesions may cause no symptoms, but itching, soreness, or pain are common. Many patients seek treatment for the cosmetic appearance of the skin.

Nail changes occur in 25% to 50% of patients, especially those over age 40, and include pitting, separation of the nail from the nail bed (onycholysis), subungual hyperkeratosis, splinter hemorrhages, areas of salmon-pink discoloration under the nail, and opaque yellowing. The palms and soles may have thick hyperkeratosis and pustules.

Some patients develop widespread small, scaling papules called guttate (droplike) psoriasis; another uncommon form is erythrodermic psoriasis, with confluent erythema and fine scaling involving nearly the entire skin surface.

About 10% of patients with psoriasis develop arthritis. This may be (1) predominantly a sacroiliitis or spondylitis; (2) a symmetric polyarthritis resembling rheumatoid arthritis and mostly affecting the hands; (3) arthritis mutilans, a form associated with osteolysis of the phalanges; (4) distal interphalangeal joint involvement; and (5) asymmetric oligoarthritis affecting the distal or proximal interphalangeal joints, often with swelling of a single digit.

Management. Emollients hydrate and soften the hyperkeratotic, scaly surface when applied twice a day, and they may help relieve itching, redness, and soreness. For mild plaque psoriasis, topical corticosteroids may control the disease. Hydrocortisone 1% or 2.5% is recommended for the face, genitals, and axillae; more potent agents such as triamcinolone ointment 0.025% to 0.1% or even stronger preparations are appropriate for other areas. Treatment once a day may be as effective and produce fewer side effects than twice-daily therapy. Patients often become resistant to corticosteroids despite an initial response. Coal tar formulations such as Estar gel may be used daily or twice daily, combined or alternated with corticosteroids.

An excellent, simple alternative treatment of chronic plaque psoriasis is anthralin (dithranol) in a cream base (Drithocreme). Available in strengths of 0.1%, 0.25%, 0.5%, and 1.0%, it can be applied to affected skin for 20 to 30 minutes a day and then washed off. Beginning with 0.1% or 0.25%, the strength can be increased every few days to weeks if the response is slow or absent. This preparation often induces remissions for several weeks to months. Its main side effects are a burning sensation (which suggests too potent a concentration or too lengthy an application) and staining of the skin purplish brown. This discoloration, which is not a reason for discontinuing the medication, fades quickly when the treatment ends, which should occur when the plaques have disappeared. The anthralin can then be resumed at the earliest signs of recurrence. For patients who do not respond or cannot tolerate the above topical treatments, a very expensive option is the twice-daily application of calcipotriene (Dovonex), but many have found this vitamin D derivative disappointing.

Scalp psoriasis is often difficult to manage. A tar shampoo such as Zetar or T-gel is frequently effective for mild involvement. For more severe or inflammatory disease the twice-daily addition of a corticosteroid lotion or solution such as fluocinolone (Synalar) or betamethasone valerate (Valisone) is recommended. The most potent topical corticosteroid currently available, clobetasol propionate 0.05% scalp application (Temovate), used twice daily for several weeks, is effective for severe disease. Whether long-term use of clobetasol causes adverse effects such as cutaneous atrophy is unknown, and some experts recommend intermittent use (e.g., rest periods of at least 1 week between 2-week treatment courses). Chronic use of the lower-potency corticosteroids on the scalp, however, seems safe. Overnight treatment with Baker's P&S (phenol and saline) applied to a wet scalp and covered by a shower cap will help loosen very thick scale, and the patient can then shampoo with a tar preparation, followed by application of a corticosteroid solution when the scalp is still wet to increase absorption. An alternative is to use anthralin (Dritho-Scalp) overnight, followed by a tar shampoo. This preparation can cause a brownish discoloration of those with blonde, gray, or white hair.

Nail psoriasis is generally unresponsive to topical therapy. Application of a corticosteroid ointment (e.g., betamethasone valerate) to affected skin around the nail may help a little. Usually, keeping the nails trimmed and removing the subungual debris represent the most that can be achieved.

When patients have widespread disease or fail to respond to the simple measures outlined above, they should see a dermatologist, who can offer more complicated therapy such as ultraviolet light treatment or systemic agents such as methotrexate.

Cross-Reference: General Approach to Arthritic Symptoms (Chapter 106).

REFERENCES

1. Buxton PK: Psoriasis. BMJ 1987;295:904–906.
   The author presents a succinct summary of diagnosis and treatment.

2. Going SM: Treatment of psoriasis. BMJ 1987;295:984–986.
   Brief overviews, with a distinctive British flavor, come from a series of simple, but rewarding articles on skin diseases entitled ABC of Dermatology, *later published in book form.*

3. Greaves MW, Weinstein GD: Treatment of psoriasis. N Engl J Med 1994;332:581–588.
   This is a good summary of the pathophysiology and current treatments.

33 Malignant Melanoma

Problem

JAN V. HIRSCHMANN

Among the primary skin cancers that primary care clinicians are likely to see—basal cell carcinomas, squamous cell carcinomas, and malignant melanomas—only melanomas cause significant mortality. Whether widespread screening of asymptomatic people for this disorder is worthwhile remains uncertain. When clinicians encounter pigmented lesions because of patients' concerns or during routine examinations, however, they should know about the epidemiologic and clinical features that help distinguish lesions that deserve further dermatologic evaluation from those that are not worrisome.

Epidemiology. In the United States the incidence of malignant melanoma is currently increasing at a more rapid rate than any other cancer. The annual incidence is about 12 per 100,000 people but is higher in the Southwest. The available evidence strongly implicates sunlight as an important etiologic factor, especially infrequent, brief, and intense exposures leading to sunburns in youth rather than regular, protracted exposure. Darkly pigmented persons have a much lower risk than fair-skinned ones; for example, among blacks in the United States the incidence is about 0.8 per 100,000. In the white population, significant risk factors, reflecting the importance of skin melanin as a protective factor, are red or blonde hair, blue eyes, a tendency to freckle, and an inability to tan. A past history of melanoma increases the risk of developing another melanoma ninefold, and a family history increases the risk eightfold.

Symptoms and Signs. Some melanomas cause itching, bleeding, crusting, or inflammation, but most patients have no symptoms except, perhaps, a concern about a lesion's identity, enlargement, or changed appearance. Nearly all melanomas are pigmented. Features that help distinguish these cancers from other pigmented lesions are summarized by the mnemonic ABCD: A = asymmetry in shape (one half unlike the other); B = border is irregular (edges scalloped); C = color is a haphazard variety of hues (blue, red, white, gray in a brown to black lesion); D = diameter is large (greater than 6 mm). Another scheme to suggest which pigmented lesions are worrisome is a 7-point checklist:

Major Features
1. Change in size
2. Change in shape
3. Change in color

Minor Features
4. Size 7 mm or more in diameter
5. Inflammation
6. Crusting or bleeding
7. Altered sensation, usually itch

All of the material in Chapter 33 is in the public domain, with the exception of any borrowed figures and tables.

The authors of this list suggest referral to a dermatologist when patients have any major feature; the concurrent presence of any minor feature increases the likelihood that melanoma is present.

Four basic types of melanomas occur: superficial spreading (60% to 80% of melanomas in the United States), nodular (10% to 20%), acral lentiginous (5%), and lentigo maligna (5%). Superficial spreading melanoma tends to occur on the legs of females and the backs of males. About 50% of patients report a preexisting, apparently benign lesion at the site. These tumors have a lengthy radial growth phase (lateral extension of the cancer) that may last from months to years before vertical growth (invasion into deeper structures) occurs and clinically detectable nodules form. In nodular melanoma the vertical growth phase is present when the lesion is first clinically apparent. It is a raised pigmented nodule with normal surrounding skin. Acral lentiginous melanomas involve the palms, soles, or subungual areas, often initially as a pigmented macule that later becomes nodular. This is the most frequent form of melanoma in blacks. Lentigo maligna melanoma occurs mostly on the face in elderly persons. It begins as a slowly growing area of macular pigmentation, typically on the temple or cheek, sometimes with central regression. At this stage it is called lentigo maligna and is a melanoma in situ with malignant-appearing cells that have not invaded from the epidermis into the dermis. When such penetration occurs, with papule formation, the lesion is called lentigo maligna melanoma.

Clinical Approach. Clinicians should inspect and palpate the areas around suspicious lesions to detect "satellite" metastases and the regional lymph nodes for lymphatic involvement. A careful search of the remaining skin surface for other intracutaneous metastases and palpation of the liver and spleen complete the preliminary assessment before referring the patient to a dermatologist for further evaluation. Routine laboratory or radiographic studies are not warranted at this stage in the absence of suggestive symptoms or signs.

Management. Although primary care clinicians generally do not manage patients with malignant melanoma, they should know about some important issues. The melanoma staging system identifies three stages: I, localized disease; II, regional lymph node involvement; and III, distant metastases. Overall 5-year survival rates for these are about 90%, 60%, and 0%, respectively. For stage I lesions the most important prognostic feature is the depth of tumor, measured in millimeters from the granular layer of the epidermis to the deepest penetration into the dermis or subcutaneous tissue. The 5-year survival according to the thickness of the tumor is less than 0.76 mm, 96% to 99%; 0.76 to 1.5 mm, 87% to 94%; 1.51 to 4.0 mm, 66% to 77%; and more than 4.0 mm, less than 50%. Factors other than tumor depth that suggest a poor prognosis include lesions on the head, neck, trunk, hands, and feet; age older than 50; male sex; and ulceration of the lesion.

Excisional biopsy is the treatment of choice. For thin melanomas (< 1 mm), a 1-cm margin is adequate; for thicker lesions, margins of 1 to 3 cm are appropriate. Elective regional dissection of clinically normal lymph nodes is controversial, but regional lymph node dissection is clearly indicated for patients with histologically involved nodes (stage II).

Follow-Up. A common practice is evaluation monthly for 3 months, every 3 months for up to 2 years, every 6 months for up to 5 years, and annually thereafter. Lengthy follow-up is necessary because about 2.5% of patients will have their first recurrence more than 10 years after removal of a malignant melanoma, most commonly at the original site or in its draining lymph node area. Furthermore, about 5% of patients will develop a second primary melanoma. Accordingly, at each visit the clinician should examine the excision site, the regional lymph nodes, and the remainder of the skin surface.

REFERENCES

1. Healsmith MF, Bourke JF, Osborne JE, Graham-Brown RAC: An evaluation of the revised seven-point checklist for the early diagnosis of cutaneous malignant melanoma. Br J Dermatol 1994;130:48–50.

   An attempt to evaluate screening criteria for malignant melanoma suggests that the seven-point list is quite sensitive and perhaps better than the ABCD system.

2. Koh HK: Cutaneous melanoma. N Engl J Med 1991;325:171–182.

   This succinct overview has 16 color photographs.

3. MacKie RM: Skin Cancer. Chicago, Year Book Medical Publishers, 1989.

   Included in this excellent book are discussions of both benign and malignant skin tumors. Superb color illustrations are included of both clinical and histologic examples.

■ ■

34 Urticaria

Problem

JAN V. HIRSCHMANN

Epidemiology. Urticaria occurs once or more in the lifetime of about 20% of the population. Most attacks are acute, short-lived, and frequently provoked by identifiable causes, such as medications or food (e.g., nuts, seafood, eggs). In chronic urticaria, defined as lasting more than 6 weeks, a cause usually remains undiscovered. Some forms of urticaria, called physical urticaria, are due to physical stimuli, usually easily discernible by history, including cold (cold urticaria), exercise or heat (cholinergic urticaria), or sunlight (solar urticaria). Dermographism, an exaggerated wheal and flare response to stroking the skin, is present in 4% to 5% of the population, but only a minority of these people develop symptoms.

Symptoms and Signs. Urticaria usually occurs as raised, erythematous, pruritic plaques with sharply defined borders and often whitish centers. Individual lesions typically last up to 12 hours, although new ones may continue to appear. Those remaining unchanged for more than 24 hours (especially if associated with arthralgias and accompanied by scaling, purpura, or pigmentation on resolution) should suggest the diagnosis of urticarial vasculitis, a disorder with different diagnostic and therapeutic implications. Lesions of the physical urticarias usually disappear within 30 minutes of the provoking stimuli, and one form, cholinergic urticaria, has a distinctive morphology—tiny (1 to 3 mm) papular wheals with surrounding erythema. Patients with symptomatic dermographism (most commonly, young adults) typically have attacks of itching and subsequent wheals from scratching that may be provoked by heat or pressure from various sources such as tight clothing, sitting, or working with tools.

Clinical Approach. A detailed history searching for such provocative factors as food or drug intake and physical stimuli is the most important investigation. If an etiology is discovered, it is usually by history. In chronic urticaria, no cause is apparent in 90% of cases, and laboratory tests are rarely rewarding. Stroking the back firmly with the blunt end of a pen and examining the area 1 to 3 minutes later for an accentuated wheal and flare reaction will confirm the diagnosis of dermographism in patients with a suggestive history. The wheal is 2 mm or more in diameter, and erythema of 5 to 10 mm in width spreads out from it. The wheal reaches its maximum size in 6 to 7 minutes and then fades within 10 to 15 minutes.

Management. Antihistamines are the mainstay of treatment. Hydroxyzine, 25 mg three to six times a day, is an excellent agent. When drowsiness is a significant complication, a nonsedating antihistamine such as terfenadine, 60 mg twice daily, is a useful substitute. Doxepin beginning in doses of 10 mg three times a day is another effective alternative. At these low doses dryness of the mouth and sedation may not occur; at higher doses these side effects, although common, often diminish with time. With refractory cases, particularly for patients with symptomatic dermographism, the addition of an H_2 blocker such as cimetidine, 300 mg four times a day, or ranitidine, 150 mg twice daily, may be helpful. Patients with chronic urticaria should avoid aspirin, nonsteroidal anti-inflammatory agents, and angiotensin-converting enzyme inhibitors, all of which may provoke or worsen attacks.

Follow-Up. Acute urticaria usually resolves by 1 to 2 weeks and, by definition, abates within 6 weeks. Chronic urticaria usually subsides over several months, but, occasionally, the condition is much more protracted.

REFERENCES

1. Casale TB, Sampson HA, Hanifin J, et al: Guide to physical urticarias. J Allergy Clin Immunol 1988;82:758–763.
   The authors present an excellent, brief summary.
2. Greaves MW: Chronic urticaria. N Engl J Med 1995;332:1767–1772.
   This article is a thoughtful and practical discussion of the topic.

Disorders of the Eye

· ·

35 Screening for Glaucoma

Screening

HOWARD BARNEBEY

Epidemiology. *Glaucoma* can be defined as a progressive anterior optic neuropathy that frequently develops in patients with elevated eye pressure. This definition emphasizes the optic nerve and its appearance and does not emphasize intraocular pressure (IOP). Most studies screening for glaucoma have used elevated IOP to identify persons at risk for the development of glaucoma. In fact, IOP is elevated in 2% to 4% of the population (IOP > 21 mm Hg).

Screening for glaucoma traditionally depended on IOP measurement. Unfortunately, IOP as a sole predictor of glaucoma lacks both sensitivity (50%–70%) and specificity (30%), thus limiting its usefulness as a sole screening strategy.

In addition, the IOP normally fluctuates throughout the day. Even in patients with suspected glaucoma who have known elevations in IOP, there is a one in five chance that IOP will be normal on a single reading. Screening sensitivity is dramatically improved by ophthalmoscopic evaluation of the optic disc, which focuses on the finding of a large cup-disc ratio (i.e., ≥ 0.6), vertical elongation of the cup, or loss of rim inferiorly or superiorly.

Rationale for Screening. Early diagnosis and treatment can prevent or minimize progressive optic nerve atrophy and visual loss. Because the disease is relatively common, with a presymptomatic stage, and there are benefits from treatment, it is a suitable condition for screening programs.

Unfortunately, no single test has adequate predictive power to identify all patients with glaucoma. One approach, however, which combines tonometry (IOP measurement) with optic disc evaluation (ophthalmoscopy), will detect the most affected persons. Most studies have suggested that screening for glaucoma be directed toward high-risk populations, including the elderly (> 50 years old), blacks, diabetics, "high myopes," and those with a family history of glaucoma.

Action. Once high-risk individuals have been identified and screened, referral to an ophthalmologist is required.

Cross-Reference: Glaucoma (Chapter 40).

REFERENCES

1. Sommer A, Tielsch JM, Katz J, Quigley HA, Gottsch JD, Javitt JC, Martone JF, Royall RM, Witt KA, Ezrine S. Racial differences in the cause-specific prevalence of blindness in east Baltimore. N Engl J Med 1991;325:1412–1417.

   Primary open-angle glaucoma accounted for 19% of all blindness among blacks; it was six times as frequent among blacks as whites and began 10 years earlier.

2. Tielsch JM, Sommer A, Katz J, Royall RM, Quigley HA, Javitt J. Racial variations in the prevalence of primary open-angle glaucoma: The Baltimore Eye Survey. JAMA 1991;266:369–374.

   The prevalence of primary open-angle glaucoma among blacks ranged from about 1% in 40- to 49-year olds to 11% of those 80 or older; prevalence among blacks was four to five times higher than among whites.

· ·

36 Visual Impairment

Screening

KENNETH E. HAMRICK

Epidemiology. Of the 95.2 million people 40 years of age and older in the United States, an estimated 2.3 million are visually impaired (i.e., Snellen acuity between 20/40 and 20/200). An additional 900,000 are legally blind (i.e., best corrected acuity 20/200 [and worse] or usable field of vision less than 20 degrees). The prevalence of both visual impairment and legal blindness increases with age and is higher among blacks, although the racial difference narrows with advancing age.

The four main causes of vision loss in this age group are macular degeneration, cataracts, diabetic retinopathy, and glaucoma. More than 13 million persons in the United States have some degree of macular degeneration, a damaged central retina, whereas 1.2 million suffer the more advanced vision-threatening stages. Presently, 12.9 million people age 40 and older have cataracts or lens opacities, with the incidence increasing with age. Nearly half of the 14 million Americans with diabetes have diabetic retinopathy, with 700,000 having serious retinal disease. The duration of diabetes is the main risk factor for retinopathy, with nearly all patients with disease type I and 60% of patients with disease type II having signs of diabetic retinopathy 20 years after the onset of diabetes. Glaucoma, optic nerve damage, and subsequent visual field loss usually associated with increased intraocular pressure affect between 2 and 3 million Americans age 40 and older.

Rationale. Between 40% and 50% of blindness is thought to be preventable or treatable with possible restoration of sight, delay of visual deterioration, or maintenance of current visual acuity. More than half of persons could enhance their functional vision with proper correction of refractive error. When diagnosed early, about 20% of cases of exudative macular degeneration are amenable to laser treatment that may prevent further visual loss. Rehabilitative services and training with low-vision devices may allow patients with severe vision loss to more fully utilize their remaining sight.

Treatment for cataracts with extraction and, in most cases, implantation of an intraocular lens is the most common surgical procedure performed in the elderly. Visual improvement is expected in about 95% of cases.

The Diabetic Retinopathy Study and the Early Treatment Diabetic Retinopathy Study have shown a 50% reduction in vision loss with recommended laser intervention protocols for patients with proliferative diabetic retinopathy (PDR) and patients with clinically significant macular edema (CSME). Stereoscopic photography performed and interpreted by skilled personnel is more accurate than standard ophthalmoscopy in screening for diabetic retinopathy. Under ideal conditions dilated ophthalmoscopy has been found to be about 80% sensitive for detecting PDR and CSME; specificity for detecting PDR is 99%, and for detecting CSME it is 79%. Undilated photography may be as accurate as standard ophthalmoscopy, whereas undilated ophthalmoscopy is least accurate, especially when performed by general medical personnel. Effective screening for glaucoma may require a complete ophthalmic evaluation. The Baltimore Eye Survey demonstrated that half of Americans older than age 40 in an urban population who have glaucoma are not aware that they have it. Glaucomatous optic nerve damage and abnormal visual fields often progress without symptoms; no single screening test has been found to be effective in predicting glaucoma. Known risk factors for glaucoma are race (black more commonly than white), age, positive family history, myopia, microvascular disease, ocular trauma, and chronic corticosteroid medication.

Strategy. Visual acuity testing can effectively screen for refractive error and cataracts but is ineffective in screening for earlier stages of macular degeneration, diabetic retinopathy, or glaucoma. Snellen acuity less than 20/40 in either eye should initiate a referral unless the decreased vision is established and stabilized. Factors from the history that should prompt earlier referral include a family history of eye disease (e.g., glaucoma), history of serious eye injury (e.g., blunt trauma to the globe), advanced age (e.g., cataract and macular degeneration), and black (glaucoma) or white race (macular degeneration).

Systemic diseases associated with increased risk for eye disease require close investigation. Patients with type I diabetes should be screened using dilated ophthalmoscopy annually, beginning 5 years after onset of diabetes. Because of the timing of the onset of type II diabetes, annual screening should be started soon after the diagnosis is established. When screening is performed using retinal photography and the initial screen in a patient with type II diabetes is negative, some authorities recommend that repeat screening need not be performed for another 4 years. This strategy presumes reliable patient follow-up and does not address detection of ocular problems that are not detected by retinal photography.

Action. Patients with unexplained visual impairment or with risk factors for serious eye disease should be referred to an ophthalmologist or optometrist. Appropriate intervention is indicated for cataracts, glaucoma, diabetic retinopathy, and macular degeneration to prevent, delay, or reverse visual loss. After confirming functional impairment due to visual loss, rehabilitative and social services should be arranged.

Cross-References: Screening for Glaucoma (Chapter 35), Glaucoma (Chapter 40), Cataracts (Chapter 41), Diabetic Retinopathy (Chapter 44).

REFERENCES

1. DeSylvia DA. Low vision and aging. Optom Vis Sic 1990;67:319–322.
   Functional losses, visual needs, low vision solutions, and rehabilitation suggestions for the visually impaired are described.

2. Prevent Blindness America. Vision Problems in the U.S. Schaumberg, IL, Prevent Blindness America, 1994.
   A compilation of state-by-state information on the scope of eye disease and vision loss is presented.

3. Singer DE, Nathan DM, Fogel HA, Schachat AP. Screening for diabetic retinopathy. Ann Intern Med 1992;116:660–671.
   Appropriate patients, methods, and timing for screening for diabetic retinopathy are determined.

4. Strahlman E, Ford D, Whelton P, Sommer A. Vision screening in a primary care setting: A missed opportunity? Arch Intern Med 1990;150:2159–2164.
   Effective screening for serious eye disease in an internal medicine setting is described.

5. Tielsch JM, Sommer A, Witt K, Katz J, Royal RM. Blindness and visual impairment in an American urban population: The Baltimore Eye Survey. Arch Ophthalmol 1990;108:286–290.
   The prevalence of blindness and visual impairment and their epidemiologic significance are delineated.

37 Redness of the Eye

Symptom

JOYCE E. WIPF and STEPHAN D. FIHN

Epidemiology and Etiology. After changes in visual acuity, redness of the eye is the most common ocular problem encountered by primary care providers. Redness of the eye is nonspecific. Causes can be separated into disorders related to the globe, disorders of the surrounding soft tissue and supporting structures, and trauma (Table 37–1).

Disorders affecting the eye itself include conjunctivitis, keratitis, scleritis/episcleritis, uveitis, keratoconjunctivitis sicca, and acute angle-closure glaucoma. Conjunctivitis is the most frequent cause of a red eye and is usually a result of viral infection, bacterial infection, or allergy (see Chapter 43, Conjunctivitis). Keratitis may result from wearing contact lenses for long periods of time or

Table 37–1. DIFFERENTIAL DIAGNOSIS OF A RED EYE

Ocular Problem	Vision	Pain, Photophobia	Pupils	Intraocular Pressure	Discharge/ Smear	Conjunctival Injection	Cornea	Referral	Comments
Conjunctivitis									
Bacterial	Normal	Minimal to absent	Normal	Normal	Purulent/ neutrophilic	Diffuse	Normal	No, unless unresponsive to treatment	Eyes stick together
Viral	Normal	Minimal to absent	Normal	Normal	Watery/ lymphocytic	Diffuse/follicular infiltrates	Normal	No	Associated upper respiratory tract infection; preauricular lymph node enlargement
Allergic	Normal	Minimal to absent	Normal	Normal	Stringy/ eosinophilic	Minimal	Normal	No	Associated atopy, itching, puffy eyes
Keratitis									
Infectious	Diminished, depends on extent and area of corneal involvement	Yes, less prominent in herpes and zoster	Usually normal	Normal	Possibly mild	Diffuse	Opacified ulcer, hypopyon, dendritic ulcer	Yes	
Abrasions	Usually mild blurring	Yes, sharp foreign body sensation	Normal	Normal	Tearing	Diffuse	Epithelial defects	Yes	
Iritis	Mild to moderate blurring	Yes	Miotic	Normal	No	Circumcorneal	Hazy, keratic precipitates	Yes	May have associated systemic disease
Glaucoma	Marked blurring	Yes, acute onset	Mid-dilated and fixed	Increased	No	Diffuse with circumcorneal prominence	Hazy with decreased light reflex	Yes	May complain of nausea and vomiting, headaches, colored halos

Adapted from Bauman R, Fihn SD. The red eye. Med Rounds 1989;2:267–278.

from corneal exposure related to paralysis of cranial nerve VII or ectropion. Keratitis can also be caused by primary or recurrent herpes simplex virus (HSV) infection, by varicella-zoster virus infection, or, less commonly, by other viruses, such as measles, mumps, rubella, or Epstein-Barr virus.

Episcleritis is an inflammation of the episclera, the thin vascular layer covering the sclera. The cause is uncertain but may be allergic. Scleritis is a more severe problem associated with systemic inflammatory disease such as rheumatoid arthritis, polyarteritis nodosa, systemic lupus, and Wegener's granulomatosis.

Inflammation of the uveal tract (iris, ciliary body, and choroid) may be anterior (iritis, iridocyclitis), posterior (choroiditis, chorioretinitis), or diffuse. Although 50% of cases are associated with rheumatologic disease, many cases of anterior uveitis are idiopathic. Uveitis occurs in 25% to 40% of patients with ankylosing spondylitis, 20% to 30% of those with Reiter's syndrome, and 20% to 25% of those with sarcoidosis. Acute iridocyclitis is common in young women with sarcoidosis, especially those with erythema nodosum. Chronic iridocyclitis occurs more commonly in elderly patients. Rarely, uveitis results from an infection (e.g., toxoplasmosis, histoplasmosis, candidiasis, tuberculosis, cytomegalovirus [CMV] infection, HSV infection, or syphilis); the posterior uveal tract is most commonly involved. CMV retinitis is an important cause of visual loss in patients with acquired immunodeficiency syndrome (AIDS); early symptoms include visual floaters.

Keratoconjunctivitis sicca (dry eyes) occurs in 16% of persons older than age 80 and in patients with connective tissue diseases (see Chapter 38, Dry Eyes and Excessive Tearing).

Acute angle-closure glaucoma may be precipitated by pupillary dilation from entering a dark room or by the use of mydriatics or anticholinergics and can rapidly lead to blindness (see Chapter 40, Glaucoma).

Redness of the eye may also be due to inflammation of the sebaceous glands in the tarsal plate (meibomian glands) or the glands along the margin of the eyelid (glands of Zeis or Moll). A *hordeolum* is a localized abscess usually caused by staphylococci. When the glands of Zeis or Moll are involved, it is called an external hordeolum or, more commonly, a stye. When the meibomian glands are involved, a larger abscess, called an internal hordeolum, occurs. Blepharitis is a common inflammatory condition of the eyelid margins caused by infection (usually staphylococci) or by seborrhea.

Cellulitis may also redden the structures around the eye. Orbital cellulitis results from direct spread from the sinuses, trauma, or conjunctivitis and must be distinguished from preseptal cellulitis.

Subconjunctival hemorrhage is a common, benign cause of a red eye that can be disconcerting to patients. Patients with thrombocytopenia can present with subconjunctival hemorrhage. Petechiae on the distal extremities are a clue to the diagnosis.

Clinical Approach. The presence of ocular pain or impaired visual acuity suggests a serious disorder (e.g., keratitis, iritis, or acute angle-closure glaucoma). Conjunctivitis typically causes burning and itching, whereas iritis and glaucoma cause a deep throbbing pain. Corneal injury is accompanied by a sharp foreign body sensation. The details of any ocular trauma should be obtained as well as information on the use of contact lenses or ophthalmic preparations. The presence of an underlying systemic disease such as rheumatoid arthritis or sarcoidosis may point to specific ocular disorders.

Visual acuity should be documented using a Snellen chart and corrective lenses, if available, or a pinhole card. Examination of the eye should begin with inspection of the globe and the periorbital structures and elicitation of pupillary reflexes. Although anisocoria can be a normal variant, the pupils should be round and equal unless there is a history of surgery or trauma. Most corneal opacities are obvious, but epithelial defects may require fluorescein staining for identification. Measurement of intraocular pressure helps to diagnose glaucoma but should be avoided if there is a purulent discharge or the possibility of globe perforation.

In *viral conjunctivitis* the discharge is watery, and conjunctival hyperemia is accompanied by follicular infiltrates (focal lymphoid hyperplasia) on the tarsal conjunctiva (creating a mild foreign body sensation and tearing). Conjunctival hyperemia tends to be most prominent at the fornices and decreases toward the limbus. Signs of an upper respiratory tract infection and preauricular adenopathy may be present. Everting the lids is important in making the diagnosis, because the tarsal conjunctiva is not typically involved in bacterial conjunctivitis. *Allergic conjunctivitis* commonly occurs in atopic patients or those exposed to allergens such as animal dander or eye preparations such as contact lens solutions. Patients complain of itching and tearing that is often bilateral. The discharge is typically watery to mucoid with a stringy consistency. Chemosis and swollen eyelids may be prominent. Conjunctival hyperemia tends to be mild compared with viral or bacterial conjunctivitis. The discharge of *bacterial conjunctivitis* is copious and purulent, and patients complain of adherent eyelids on awakening. Blepharitis may coexist, especially with a staphylococcal infection. The presence of pain, visual changes, pupillary abnormalities, or a ciliary flush (circumcorneal vessel dilation) suggests a diagnosis other than conjunctivitis.

Keratitis commonly produces visual impairment and pain made worse by lid movement, except when caused by HSV or zoster, which produces corneal hypoesthesia and less pain and tearing. Pupils are normal unless there is an associated uveitis, in which case they may be miotic. Penlight examination reveals a hazy appearance of the cornea with loss of the normal corneal light reflex. Visualization of epithelial disruption is enhanced by touching a sterile fluorescein-impregnated strip to the wet conjunctiva in the lower fornices and having the patient blink. Bacterial infection may cause a hypopyon (collection of inflammatory cells in the anterior chamber) or centrally located ulcers. Herpes keratitis is usually unilateral with associated conjunctivitis and cutaneous vesicles. Corneal ulcerations are rare, although recurrent herpes may produce dendritic (branching) ulcers that are enhanced by staining with fluorescein. Eye involvement should be suspected in facial zoster, because about 50% of patients with zoster of cranial nerve V_1 will have associated keratitis. The presence of lesions on the tip of the nose (Hutchinson's sign) is helpful. The absence of nasal involvement does not rule out keratitis.

Patients with *episcleritis* typically present with a unilateral red eye and excessive tearing, photophobia, and mild ocular discomfort. Visual acuity and pupillary examination are normal. Unlike conjunctivitis, episcleritis does not involve the palpebral conjunctiva. In *scleritis*, there is moderate to severe pain, excessive tearing, photophobia, and violaceous discoloration of the sclera. Visual acuity may be reduced if there is associated corneal or retinal involvement.

Patients with *keratoconjunctivitis sicca* often complain of a gritty sensation in the eye as well as burning, redness, mild pain and itching, and a mucoid discharge. Many patients note a paradoxic increase in tearing. The eye may appear grossly normal but is often red with a stringy mucoid discharge.

Unlike chronic open-angle glaucoma, which is usually asymptomatic, *acute angle-closure glaucoma* causes severe eye pain, headache, nausea and vomiting, and impaired vision. Patients may note colored halos around lights owing to the corneal edema. The conjunctiva is injected, with prominent perilimbal vessels (ciliary flush), producing a violet hue. The pupils are characteristically mid-dilated and minimally reactive and appear hazy. Intraocular pressure is elevated, usually greater than 40 mm Hg (normal, 12–20 mm Hg). The depth of the anterior chamber can be estimated by shining a penlight from the temporal side of the head, parallel to the plane of the iris. If two thirds or more of the nasal iris is in shadow, the anterior chamber is probably shallow and the angle narrowed.

An *internal hordeolum* is characterized by localized swelling, erythema, and pain. *Blepharitis* commonly manifests as crusting, scaling, erythema, and swelling of the eyelid.

Periorbital cellulitis, better termed *preseptal cellulitis,* involves the eyelid and surrounding skin. It is prevented from extending to the globe by the fibrous orbital septum. The globe itself is usually not red unless there is associated conjunctivitis. Patients with *orbital cellulitis* are often systemically ill and have erythema and chemosis of the lids and globe, as well as pain on eye movement that may be restricted from the swelling.

Trauma to the eye is usually apparent from the history and examination.

Management. Mild conjunctivitis and blepharitis can usually be managed by the primary care provider (see Chapter 43, Conjunctivitis), as can keratoconjunctivitis sicca (see Chapter 38, Dry Eyes and Excessive Tearing). Any patient with ocular pain, visual disturbance, or pupillary abnormalities should be examined as soon as possible by an ophthalmologist.

Measures to *avoid* in managing a red eye are giving topical anesthetics or corticosteroids to patients for use at home, using nonsterile ophthalmic preparations, dilating pupils before assessing anterior chamber depth, and performing ocular manipulation if perforation is suspected.

Follow-Up. Patients with conjunctivitis who have not improved within 48 hours should be reexamined.

Cross-References: Eye Pain (Chapter 39), Glaucoma (Chapter 40), Foreign Bodies and Corneal Abrasions (Chapter 42), Conjunctivitis (Chapter 43).

REFERENCES

1. Albert DM, Jakobiec FA. Principles and Practice of Ophthalmology. Philadelphia, WB Saunders, 1994.
   This is a practical reference guide.

2. Bauman R, Fihn SD. The red eye. Med Rounds 1989;2:267–278.

   This article proves a thorough and practical review for the primary care provider.

3. Buehler PO, Schein OD, Stamler JF, Verdier DD, Katz J. The increased risk of ulcerative keratitis among disposable soft contact lens users. Arch Ophthalmol 1992;110:1555–1558.

   The hazards of wearing contact lens, particularly extended-wear lenses, are described. This controlled study found a relative risk of 14.2 of ulcerative keratitis in disposable extended-wear lenses compared with daily-wear soft lenses.

4. Kanski JJ. The Eye in Systemic Disease. London, Butterworths, 1986.

   This atlas of eye involvement in various systemic conditions includes illustrations and a review of other physical findings.

5. Spalton DJ, Hitchings RA, Hunter PA. Atlas of Clinical Ophthalmology. Philadelphia, JB Lippincott, 1984.

   This is an excellent atlas.

■ ■

38 Dry Eyes and Excessive Tearing

Symptom

THOMAS D. LINDQUIST

Epidemiology and Etiology. Keratoconjunctivitis sicca, or aqueous-deficient dry eye, is an often-overlooked condition that affects 20% to 25% of patients visiting eye clinics. The incidence is greatest between 40 and 60 years of age, with a 6:1 female-male predominance.

Keratoconjunctivitis sicca most commonly is caused by lymphocytic infiltration and fibrosis of the lacrimal gland but may, on occasion, be associated with sarcoidosis, rheumatoid arthritis, or other connective tissue disease.

Symptoms and Signs. The symptoms are typically worse on awakening and include burning, grittiness, or foreign body sensation; discharge in the inner canthus or lower cul-de-sac; redness of the eye; blurred vision; and difficulty opening the eyelids. Paradoxically, patients frequently describe excessive tearing due to a relative response to drying of the cornea.

Signs include sticky, ropy discharge; dilated bulbar conjunctival vessels (particularly within the interpalpebral fissure); filaments; punctate epithelial defects; and keratinization. Filaments are discrete strands of mucus intertwined with desquamated cells and cellular debris that dangle from an attachment to the corneal epithelium.

Clinical Approach. Drying causes a loss of the smooth refractive surface of the tear film and an irregular light reflex. Epithelial abnormalities are best elucidated by rose bengal or fluorescein staining of the epithelium. Drying, keratinization, filaments, and mucous plaques are readily seen with rose bengal. Frank epithelial defects stain brilliantly with fluorescein.

Tear production can be measured by Schirmer tests, in which a Whatman No. 41 filter paper, 5 mm in width, is placed for 5 minutes at the junction of the lateral and middle thirds of the lower lid. The inferior conjunctival cul-de-sac must be dried gently with a cotton-tipped applicator stick before testing. The length of the wet portion of the filter paper is measured after 5 minutes. Less than 5 mm of wetting is always suggestive of significant tear dysfunction. A normal test result in the unanesthetized eye is 15 mm or more of wetting; with topical anesthesia it is 10 mm or more of wetting.

Although a tearing eye may be a nuisance to the patient, it never causes permanent visual loss, whereas absence of tears may lead to keratinization of the corneal and conjunctival epithelium. Epiphora is a condition in which drainage of tears through the lacrimal system is faulty, with the result that tears overflow onto the cheek. This condition should be evaluated by an ophthalmologist.

Management. A tear substitute should be prescribed, but many preparations contain preservatives (e.g., thimerosal and benzalkonium chloride) that cause hypersensitivity reactions when used frequently. Nonpreserved tear preparations are now commercially available in varying viscosities (Refresh, HypoTears PF, Celluvisc, Occucoat, Tears Naturale Free). Application of a nonpreserved tear substitute ointment at bedtime is highly recommended. Patients who continue to have symptoms and signs despite frequent supplemental lubrication should be referred to an ophthalmologist for punctal occlusion. This may be performed by punctal cautery using local anesthetic, or a permanent silicone plug that may be removed if necessary at a later date may be placed in the punctum. Severe tear deficiency may even require lateral tarsorrhaphy to decrease the exposed surface area and retard evaporation.

Follow-Up. Patients with severe dry eyes should be followed by an ophthalmologist at 4- to 6-month intervals because they are at greater risk for persistent epithelial defects, infectious ulcers, and stromal melting.

REFERENCES

1. Baum JL. Systemic disease associated with tear deficiencies. Int Ophthalmol Clin 1973;13:157–184.

   A thorough review is presented of systemic diseases associated with tear deficiency.

2. Holly FJ, Lemp MA. Tear physiology and dry eyes. Surv Ophthalmol 1977;22:69–87.

   The dry eye syndromes can be divided as follows: aqueous tear deficiency, mucin deficiency, lipid abnormalities, lid surfacing abnormalities, and epitheliopathies.

3. van Bijsterveld OP. Diagnostic tests in the sicca syndrome. Arch Ophthalmol 1969;82:10–14.

   The role of rose bengal 1% is emphasized in the diagnosis of dry-eye conditions.

39 Eye Pain

Symptom

JAMES C. ORCUTT

Etiology. Pain in or around the eye occurs in one of four patterns: ocular pain, pain with eye movement, orbital pain, and referred pain.

Ocular pain is generally accompanied by additional ocular symptoms, such as foreign body sensation, decreased visual acuity, pupillary abnormalities, redness of the eye, or visual halos. Common causes are corneal abrasion (see Chapter 42, Foreign Bodies and Corneal Abrasions), acute angle-closure glaucoma (see Chapter 40, Glaucoma), and iritis (see Chapter 37, Redness of the Eye). Ocular pain may stimulate the vagal reflex, producing nausea and vomiting. Chronic open-angle glaucoma is rarely painful.

Pain with eye movements can be due to optic neuritis, sinusitis, or idiopathic inflammation of the extraocular muscles (pseudotumor). Except in cases of pseudotumor, the pain is usually mild. Associated diplopia suggests pseudotumor, whereas associated impairment in vision with a noninflamed eye suggests optic neuritis.

Orbital pain is usually severe, constant, boring, localized behind the eye, and associated with proptosis. Primary orbital inflammation (pseudotumor), orbital hemorrhage, and orbital cellulitis are common causes. Because orbital malignancies are occasionally painful, the presence of pain does not help differentiate malignancies from other cause of orbital pain. Fleeting, shooting, sharp, stabbing pains lasting 1 to 5 seconds and unaccompanied by eye signs or symptoms are generally unassociated with a pathologic process.

Referred pain is the most common cause of ocular pain. The pain is generally diffusely related to the eyes, brow, and forehead or, in rare cases, is dermatomal. A common cause of diffuse referred pain is one of the common headaches (see Chapter 138, Headache); in such cases the eye examination is normal. Pain referred in a dermatomal pattern may be caused by nasopharyngeal carcinomas, intracranial aneurysms, cavernous sinus tumors, or herpes zoster infections. Dermatomal referred pain may be accompanied by other signs of cranial nerve involvement such as diplopia, numbness, or ptosis.

Clinical Approach. An eye examination including visual acuity, pupil evaluation, extraocular movements, external examination, cranial nerve examination, fluorescein staining, intraocular pressure, and funduscopy is required. The absence of specific findings would be most compatible with a diagnosis of referred pain. Additional diagnostic tests depend on the type of eye pain: for example, patients with pain on eye movement and normal results of an eye examination should be evaluated for sinusitis (see Chapter 57, Sinusitis); patients with referred pain and no ocular findings should be further evaluated for the causes of headache.

Management. Various chapters in this section review the management of redness of the eye, conjunctivitis, blepharitis, foreign bodies, and corneal abrasion. Patients describing fleeting pain who have normal results of an eye examination should be reassured. In general, all patients with ocular pain, painful eye movements (unless due to sinusitis), orbital pain, or abnormal findings on an eye examination should be referred to an ophthalmologist.

Follow-Up. If the results of the initial examination are unremarkable, a follow-up appointment should be scheduled for 2 to 4 weeks to monitor for any new ocular findings.

Cross-References: Redness of the Eye (Chapter 37), Foreign Bodies and Corneal Abrasions (Chapter 42), Conjunctivitis (Chapter 43), Sinusitis (Chapter 57), Headache (Chapter 138).

REFERENCES

1. Hitchings RA. The symptoms of ocular pain. Trans Ophthalmol Soc UK 1980;100:257–259.
   This article discusses pathophysiology of eye pain and is part of a four-article symposium on eye pain.

2. Kalina RE, Orcutt JC. Ocular and periocular pain. In Bonica JJ, ed. The Management of Pain in Clinical Practice, 2nd ed, vol 1. Philadelphia, Lea & Febiger, 1990:759–768.
   This is an up-to-date review of diagnosis and management.

40 Glaucoma

Problem

HOWARD BARNEBEY

Epidemiology. One percent to 2% of the US population will develop glaucoma. The prevalence is increased among the elderly, myopic (near-sighted) persons, blacks, diabetics, and persons with hypertension.

Symptoms and Signs. Open-angle glaucoma is asymptomatic until quite late in the disease, when complaints of visual loss may occur. *Angle-closure glaucoma* is less common than open-angle glaucoma but often is symptomatic, causing blurred vision, eye pain, headache, and even nausea and vomiting. Clinical examination reveals a red eye, corneal edema, and a mid-dilated pupil. The intraocular pressure (IOP) is often quite high (> 45 mm Hg).

Management. Once open-angle glaucoma is detected, treatment to lower the IOP includes medications (Table 40–1), laser treatment, and surgery.

Angle-closure glaucoma is a true emergency and requires the immediate

Table 40–1. MEDICAL MANAGEMENT OF GLAUCOMA

Medication	Mechanism	Side Effects	Cost ($ per Month)
β-Blockers	Decrease aqueous secretion	Ocular: punctate keratitis, corneal anesthesia	
Timolol (Timoptic)		Other: bronchospasm, congestive heart failure, arrhythmias, mood changes, impotence	11.96
Levobunolol (Betagan)			10.84
Betaxolol (Betoptic)			14.06
Mitipranolol (OptiPranolol)			10.79
Carteolol (Ocupress)			
Miotics	Improve aqueous outflow	Ocular: constrict pupil, dim vision, decreased night vision, retinal tear/detachment	
Pilocarpine			4.00 (15 mL)
Pilocarpine (Ocusert)		Other: headache, nausea, diarrhea, sweating, bronchospasm	3.83 (7 d)
Carbachol (Isopto Carbachol)			12.50 (15 mL)
Pilocarpine gel (Pilopine)			18.13 (5 g)
Adrenergic agonists	Improve aqueous outflow	Ocular: local erythemia, allergy	
Dipivefrin (Propine)			11.48
Epinephrine			9.23
Selective agonists	Decrease production	Ocular: local allergy, contact dermatitis	
Apraclonidine (Iopidine)		Systemic: hypotension malaise, fatigue	33.75
Brimonidine			43.55
Carbonic anhydrase inhibitors	Decrease production	Ocular: blurred vision	
Topical:			
Dorzolamide (Trusopt)		Systemic: dry mouth, bitter taste, malaise, fatigue, confusion, renal calculin metabolic acidosis, blood dyscrasias	21.78 (5 mL)
Systemic:			
Acetazolamide (Diamox)			22.80
Methazolamide (Neptazane)			53.60
Dichlorphenamide (Daranide)			29.40
Prostaglandin analog	Increase uveal-scleral outflow	Ocular: conjunctival erythemia, iris color change	
Latanoprost (Xalatan)			37.81

*Average wholesale price, 1996 *Drug Topics Red Book.*

lowering of IOP with medications, followed by laser iridectomy. Once an iridectomy has been performed and the attack broken, the glaucoma can be considered "cured."

Follow-Up. Often, multiple visits are required to properly titrate medical therapy for each individual patient. Once stable, the patient needs to be monitored two to four times a year. Particular attention should be directed to any side effects from medication, which may not be apparent during the initial part of the treatment.

Cross-References: Screening for Glaucoma (Chapter 35), Visual Impairment (Chapter 36), Redness of the Eye (Chapter 37), Eye Pain (Chapter 39).

REFERENCES

1. Becker B. Shaffer's Diagnosis and Therapy of the Glaucomas. St. Louis, CV Mosby, 1989.
2. Shields MB, Ritch R, eds. The Glaucomas. St. Louis, CV Mosby, 1989.

   These are two excellent textbooks.

41 Cataracts

Problem

THOMAS D. LINDQUIST

Epidemiology. A cataract is an opacity of the natural lens of the eye. The most common cause of cataract formation is related to the normal aging process, and some degree of clouding of the lens can be expected in persons older than age 70. Other causes of cataract formation may be (1) congenital, from hereditary, infectious, or inflammatory causes; (2) traumatic; (3) metabolic, as in diabetes mellitus; (4) toxic, as in corticosteroid use; or (5) secondary to ocular inflammation or intraocular disease.

Symptoms and Signs. The principal symptom of an acquired cataract is a gradual decrease in vision unassociated with pain or inflammation. Monocular diplopia, photophobia, and the complaint of glare are other symptoms. Signs of a cataract are best seen with the slit lamp biomicroscope after pupillary dilation; however, direct ophthalmoscopy does allow estimation of the degree of media opacity. The principal types of lens opacities are nuclear, cortical, and subcapsular. A nuclear cataract is a yellow or brunescent opacity of the lens nucleus; a cortical cataract frequently forms radial opacities in a spokelike pattern, whereas a posterior subcapsular cataract appears as a granular opacity just anterior to the posterior capsule itself. Posterior subcapsular cataract is the most visually disabling for its density and size, because it anatomically approximates the nodal point of the eye and also frequently involves the visual axis early. A mature cataract is white, does not allow visualization of the ocular fundus, and causes reversible blindness in the affected eye.

Clinical Approach. Patients should be asked about their continued ability to read, drive, and perform other daily activities. An acquired cataract warrants surgical extraction only when it significantly interferes with the patient's visual needs.

A hypermature cataract may leak lens protein through an intact capsule, resulting in a secondary glaucoma in which macrophages distended with lens material obstruct the trabecular meshwork. Prompt cataract extraction is indicated.

Management. Acquired cataracts are usually removed by extracapsular extraction or phacoemulsification, leaving the posterior capsule intact. A posterior chamber intraocular lens is preferred for optical correction of aphakia in adults without proliferative diabetic retinopathy or chronic uveitis. Severe complications of this surgery include endophthalmitis and expulsive choroidal hemorrhage, but they occur in less than 0.1% of patients.

Follow-Up. After cataract surgery, patients are treated with topical antibiotics until the surface reepithelializes and with topical corticosteroids until intraocular inflammation resolves. The wound is secure by 6 weeks postoperatively, at which time patients may resume normal activities.

Cross-Reference: Visual Impairment (Chapter 36).

REFERENCES

1. Jaffe NS. Cataract Surgery and Its Complications, 4th ed. St. Louis, CV Mosby, 1984.

   Preoperative workup, surgical technique, and complications of cataract surgery are described.

2. Lane SS, Kopietz LA, Lindquist TD, Leavenworth N. Treatment of phacolytic glaucoma with extracapsular cataract extraction. Ophthalmology 1988;95:749–753.

   Phacolytic glaucoma may be treated by extracapsular cataract extraction with implantation of a posterior chamber intraocular lens.

3. Lindquist TD, Lindstrom RL, eds. Ophthalmic Surgery, 3rd ed. Chicago, Year Book Medical Publishers, 1994.

   Extracapsular cataract and phacoemulsification techniques, intraocular lens insertion, and epikeratoplasty technique are illustrated and described.

42 Foreign Bodies and Corneal Abrasions

Problem

THOMAS D. LINDQUIST

Epidemiology. Each year, over 1 million persons sustain eye injuries; over 90% of these are preventable. Corneal abrasions are frequently caused by branches, fingernails, paper cuts, or contact lenses. Foreign bodies on the surface of the cornea account for about 25% of all eye injuries. Most intraocular foreign bodies are caused by small particles penetrating the cornea or sclera; the majority of such particles come from the striking of metal on metal.

Symptoms and Signs. Symptoms of a corneal foreign body may vary from minimal discomfort to severe pain. The patient may sense a foreign body and usually inaccurately localizes it to the outer portion of the upper eyelid. Corneal abrasions are associated with intense pain, photophobia, ciliary injection, and tearing. A corneal abrasion may be visualized readily by instillation of a sterile 2% fluorescein solution that stains the denuded epithelium. A corneal foreign body may be seen by careful inspection, preferably aided by magnification with a loupe or direct ophthalmoscope when a slit lamp is unavailable.

Clinical Approach. Corneal foreign bodies should be removed entirely to allow reepithelialization and to minimize pain. An attempt should be made to remove a corneal foreign body by irrigation before removing it with a spud or the tip of a needle (see Chapter 45, Foreign Body Removal).

The conjunctiva and cornea should be examined carefully for a possible penetrating injury from an intraocular foreign body. A small conjunctival hemorrhage or a suspicious corneal lesion requires slit lamp examination and indirect ophthalmoscopy of the fundus by an ophthalmologist. Radiography or computed tomography of the orbit is indicated in suspected cases of penetrating injuries to rule out intraocular foreign bodies. Retained iron foreign bodies slowly oxidize within the eye to form an irreversible ferrous compound that results in gradual loss of vision (siderosis). Retention of copper particles (chalicosis) is much more rapidly injurious to the eye, but the tissue reaction is reversible if the copper particle is removed. Retention of an intraocular foreign body must be ruled out in any patient who develops uveitis after an eye injury.

Management. Treatment of a corneal abrasion with or without prior foreign body removal should include the use of topical antibiotic solution. Tobramycin, a fluoroquinolone, or trimethoprim–polymyxin-B solutions provide broad antibacterial coverage. A cycloplegic such as cyclopentolate (Cyclogyl) 1% or homatropine 5% may be instilled for patient comfort if there is ciliary injection or photophobia. Topical atropine 1% may have a duration as long as 2 weeks and therefore should not be used acutely. A pressure dressing may be applied to immobilize the eyelids but should not be used if it causes discomfort. Patching does not increase the rate of reepithelialization.

Follow-Up. Because any foreign body may introduce microorganisms, the eyes should be examined daily until the epithelium resurfaces.

Cross-References: Eye Pain (Chapter 39), Foreign Body Removal (Chapter 45).

REFERENCES

1. De Juan E Jr, Sternberg P Jr, Michels RG. Penetrating ocular injuries. Ophthalmology 1983;90:1318–1322.

    Initial acuity after injury is correlated closely with the final visual outcome.

2. Lobes LA Jr, Grand MG, Reece J, Penkrot RJ. Computerized axial tomography in the detection of intraocular foreign bodies. Ophthalmology 1981;88:26–29.

    Computed tomography is particularly useful in evaluating multiple foreign bodies and foreign bodies adjacent to the ocular wall and, in some cases, in distinguishing metallic from nonmetallic foreign bodies.

3. Schein OD, Hibberd PL, Shingleton BJ, Kunzweiler T, Franbach DA, Seddon JM, Fontan NL, Vinger PF. The spectrum and burden of ocular injury. Ophthalmology 1988;95:300–305.

    Only 10% of injured individuals were wearing protective eyewear; many injuries could be prevented.

- -

43 Conjunctivitis

Problem

THOMAS D. LINDQUIST

Epidemiology and Etiology. Conjunctivitis is the most common eye disease worldwide. It is characterized by inflammation with cellular infiltration and exudation. The cause may be bacterial, viral, allergic, toxic, mechanical, or parasitic.

Symptoms and Signs. The onset of conjunctivitis is usually insidious. Patients complain of foreign body sensation, itching, and burning. Discomfort from infectious causes is most severe on awakening: the eyelids are swollen and the eyelashes are matted. The conjunctiva is diffusely injected, in contrast to the perilimbal flush more characteristic of iritis or uveitis or the sectorial injection seen with episcleritis or scleritis.

Clinical Approach. *Bacterial conjunctivitis* is accompanied by an acute purulent or mucopurulent discharge. Both *Streptococcus pneumoniae* and *Haemophilus aegyptius* can occur in epidemics and may be associated with small petechial subconjunctival hemorrhages. Most cases of bacterial conjunctivitis are self-limited, with the exception of those caused by *Neisseria* species.

Viral conjunctivitis is accompanied by a follicular response except in infants younger than 6 to 8 weeks old, who have an immature immune system. The conjunctival follicle is a smooth elevation of the conjunctiva, representing a lymphocytic response with an active germinal center. Whereas follicles represent a specific response, the conjunctival papillary response is a nonspecific conjunctival sign that can result from any type of inflammation. Papillae are characterized by a central fibrovascular core with the vessel breaking into a fine spokelike pattern on reaching the surface. In viral conjunctivitis a preauricular node is usually palpable and may be quite prominent and tender. The infection usually begins in one eye and often spreads to involve the other eye, although the first eye is always more severely affected. Adenovirus is the most common cause of acute conjunctivitis and is associated with copious tearing, minimal mucopurulent discharge, swollen lids, and significant injection. Epidemic keratoconjunctivitis, caused by adenovirus types 8 and 19, is associated with keratitis in 80% of cases, leading to severe photophobia and foreign body sensation. Small granular subepithelial corneal opacities may develop that may be visually significant and persist for months to years after resolution of the conjunctivitis. Because epidemic keratoconjunctivitis is spread with ease through fomites, affected health care personnel should restrict direct contact with patients for 2 weeks.

Primary herpesvirus conjunctivitis may be associated with vesicles on the eyelids and may progress to involve the cornea. Because most people have antibodies to herpesvirus type 1 by 15 years of age, herpetic blepharoconjunctivitis in adults usually represents recurrent disease.

Adult inclusion conjunctivitis (caused by *Chlamydia trachomatis*) results from sexually transmitted disease and is generally spread to the eyes from the genital area. It is frequently unilateral and associated with large follicles, foreign body sensation, and conjunctival injection. A conjunctival scraping should be sent for immunofluorescence and culture to establish the diagnosis.

Lyme disease may be associated with follicular conjunctivitis and keratitis.

Allergic conjunctivitis is characterized by bilaterality, recurrences, and marked itching. A papillary conjunctival response is seen, with only a mild mucoid discharge. Conjunctival scrapings frequently reveal eosinophils. Soft contact lens wearers may develop giant papillary conjunctivitis that is most prominent on the upper tarsal plate.

Management. Mild bacterial conjunctivitis generally resolves within 1 to 3 days when treated with broad-spectrum topical antibiotics such as sulfacetamide 10% or trimethoprim–polymyxin-B, which may be given four times a day for 5 to 7 days or until the conjunctivitis resolves. Bacterial conjunctivitis with copious purulent discharge or corneal ulceration should be cultured and Gram and Giemsa stains performed; referral to an ophthalmologist is recommended. Topical corticosteroids should be avoided in infectious conjunctivitis.

Adenovirus conjunctivitis is usually self-limited. Cool compresses bring relief; prophylactic topical antibiotic solution may be given but is unnecessary. Patients with herpetic conjunctivitis should be referred to an ophthalmologist and treated with topical trifluridine (Viroptic) or vidarabine (Vira-A). Inclusion conjunctivitis requires systemic treatment with tetracycline or doxycycline for 3 weeks in adults.

Acute allergic conjunctivitis may be treated with cool compresses, systemic antihistamines, and topical decongestant-antihistamines. Disodium cromoglycate 4% or lodoxamide 0.1% four times a day may be used for chronic allergic conditions.

Cross-References: Redness of the Eye (Chapter 37), Sexually Transmitted Disease (Chapter 176).

REFERENCES

1. O'Day DM, Guyer B, Hierholzer JC. Clinical and laboratory evaluation of epidemic keratoconjunctivitis due to adenovirus types 8 and 19. Am J Ophthalmol 1976;81:207–215.

   Considerable variability in disease severity may be seen in patients with epidemic keratoconjunctivitis due to adenovirus types 8 and 19.

2. Rapoza PA, Quinn TC, Terry AC, Gottsch JD, Kiessling LA, Taylor HR. A systematic approach to the diagnosis and treatment of chronic conjunctivitis. Am J Ophthalmol 1990;109:138–142.

   The proper approach to diagnosing chronic conjunctivitis is outlined.

3. Sheppard JD, Kowalski RP, Meyer MP, Amortegui AJ, Slifkin M. Immunodiagnosis of adult chlamydial conjunctivitis. Ophthalmology 1988;95:434–443.

   Direct monoclonal fluorescent antibody and enzyme and immunosorbent assays for chlamydial antigens are available to supplement culture and Giemsa staining.

4. Steere AC, Bartenhagen NH, Craft JE, Hutchinson GJ, Newman JH, Rahn DW, Sigal LH, Spieler PN, Stenn KS, Malawista SE. The early clinical manifestations of Lyme disease. Ann Intern Med 1983;99:76–82.

   Conjunctivitis is the most commonly reported ocular complication of Lyme disease; its incidence was 10% in this series.

. . . .

44 Diabetic Retinopathy

Problem

HOWARD J. KAPLAN and JAMES L. KINYOUN

Epidemiology. Diabetic retinopathy continues to be one of the leading causes of blindness in the United States. Approximately 25% of diabetic patients have retinopathy, with 5% having the sight-threatening proliferative form of diabetic retinopathy. The prevalence of diabetic retinopathy increases as a function of disease duration. Seven years after initial diagnosis, 50% of patients with type I diabetes will have retinopathy. After 17 to 25 years of disease, 90% of patients with type I diabetes will have visible retinopathy. The most severe, sight-threatening form of disease, proliferative retinopathy, is found in 26% of individuals after 26 to 50 years of disease duration.

Pathogenesis. Early microvascular damage results in increased retinal vascular permeability and the loss of the integrity of the blood–retina barrier. Capillary closure leads to retinal ischemia. Studies indicate that retinal ischemia may result in the production of an angiogenic growth factor that promotes retinal neovascularization.

Symptoms and Signs. Diabetic retinopathy has a variable clinical presentation. Patients may have severe vision-threatening proliferative retinopathy with no symptoms or change in visual acuity. The clinically silent nature of diabetic retinopathy cannot be overemphasized. Commonly, a complaint of a minor loss in visual acuity can be an early sign of macular edema. The sudden appearance of floaters may represent new vitreous or preretinal hemorrhages.

Nonproliferative diabetic retinopathy is defined by pathologic changes that stay within the confines of the retina, including the formation of microaneurysm, retinal hemorrhages, and nerve fiber layer infarcts (cotton-wool spots), focal hemorrhages (dot-blot), retinal edema, and hard exudates (serum lipoproteins).

Proliferative diabetic retinopathy is defined by the appearance of retinal neovascularization. New retinal vessels are both fragile and highly permeable. A vicious cycle ensues whereby these vessels leak protein, leading to fibrosis and contraction of the surrounding vitreous gel. This contraction places increased traction on the new vessels, which may in turn bleed, resulting in a vitreous hemorrhage. Further traction may cause a retinal detachment.

The need for stereoscopic viewing of the retina precludes the diagnosis of macular edema with a direct ophthalmoscope. However, the presence of the previous findings, especially hard exudates, is presumptive evidence that macular edema may be present.

New retinal vessels are commonly found on the optic nerve head. Neovascularization may also be found in any area of the retina. Neovascularization has the appearance of very fine tortuous capillaries that are best seen with high magnification. Preretinal or vitreous hemorrhages are also indicative of proliferative diabetic retinopathy.

Clinical Approach. The clinical evaluation should include a clear history of the patient's diabetes, including date at onset and level of metabolic control. The patient should be questioned about changes in visual acuity, increase in floaters, and sudden loss in vision. A dilated retinal examination should be performed using a direct ophthalmoscope, with particular attention to the optic nerve and macula. However, the physician should be cautioned that direct ophthalmoscopy is a poor method for detecting diabetic retinopathy. Any patient with visual complaints or retinal changes should be referred to an ophthalmologist.

The differential diagnosis of diabetic retinopathy includes the following: (1) hypertensive retinopathy, (2) collagen vascular disease, (3) retinal vein occlusion, (4) radiation retinopathy, (5) acquired immunodeficiency syndrome (AIDS) retinopathy, and (6) leukemia.

Management. The Diabetes Control and Complications Trial examined the effect of strict metabolic control on diabetic retinopathy, as determined by levels of glycosylated hemoglobin. The study found that strict metabolic control both significantly delays the onset and decreases the severity of diabetic retinopathy in insulin-dependent diabetic patients.

Patients with historically poor metabolic control whose disease is suddenly brought under tight control are at risk for sudden acceleration of diabetic retinopathy. Similarly, pregnancy can also cause rapid worsening of both nonproliferative and proliferative retinopathy.

Visual loss secondary to diabetic retinopathy is both preventable and treatable. Several important randomized prospective clinical trials have led to the current standard of care for diabetic retinopathy: panretinal laser photocoagulation reduces severe visual loss by 60% in eyes that had proliferative diabetic retinopathy; focal laser photocoagulation can stabilize and prevent vision loss due to clinically significant macular edema. Aspirin has no effect on proliferative or nonproliferative diabetic retinopathy but is not contraindicated for use in other medical conditions by the presence of diabetic retinopathy.

Patients with vision loss secondary to advanced diabetic retinopathy complicated by vitreous hemorrhage and retinal detachment can now have sight restored by modern vitreoretinal surgical techniques. In eyes that have nonclearing vitreous hemorrhage without retinal detachment, vitrectomy resulted in visual improvement in 80% of operated eyes. In addition, vitrectomy also arrests the development of neovascularization and provides stable long-term visual improvement.

Follow-Up. The American Academy of Ophthalmology recommends that all patients with diabetes (diagnosed after age 30 years) have a routine yearly dilated retinal examination by an ophthalmologist; for those patients in whom diabetes mellitus was diagnosed before age 30, yearly dilated retinal examinations are recommended after 5 years of disease duration. Pregnant women with diabetes should have a dilated retinal examination every trimester.

Cross-References: Visual Impairment (Chapter 36), Diabetes Mellitus (Chapter 154).

REFERENCES

1. Aiello L. Diagnosis, management, and treatment of nonproliferative diabetic retinopathy and macular edema. In Albert D, Jakobiec F, eds. The Principles and Practice of Ophthalmology, vol 2. Philadelphia, WB Saunders, 1994:747–759.
   The author provides a good overview illustrated with excellent color photographs.

2. Diabetes Control and Complications Trial Research Group. The effect of intensive treatment of diabetes on the development and progression of long-term complications in insulin-dependent diabetes mellitus. N Engl J Med 1993;329:977–986.
   Tight metabolic control reduced the development of diabetic retinopathy by 76% and slowed progression of retinopathy by 54%.

3. Diabetic Retinopathy Research Group. Photocoagulation treatment of proliferative diabetic retinopathy. Ophthalmology 1981:88:583–600.
   Laser photocoagulation reduced vision loss from proliferative diabetic retinopathy.

4. Early Treatment Diabetic Retinopathy Study Research Group. Early photocoagulation for diabetic retinopathy. Ophthalmology 1991;98(suppl):766–785.
   Laser photocoagulation reduced vision loss from proliferative diabetic retinopathy.

5. Miller J, D'amico D. Proliferative diabetic retinopathy. In Albert D, Jakobiec F, eds. The Principles and Practice of Ophthalmology, vol 2. Philadelphia, WB Saunders, 1994:760–781.
   This is a useful general reference.

45 Foreign Body Removal

Procedure

THOMAS D. LINDQUIST

Rationale. All corneal foreign bodies should be removed entirely to allow reepithelialization, minimize pain, and remove contaminated material.

Methods. Slit lamp examination is the optimal means of assessing the depth of a foreign body. Foreign bodies or corneal abrasions involving only the epithelium do not leave a scar. Scarring results from injuries deep to Bowman's layer. A full-thickness corneal foreign body should be removed by an ophthalmologist because it is likely to result in a shallow or flat anterior chamber unless the perforation site is sutured. Intraocular foreign bodies need to be removed in the operating room using an operating microscope.

An initial attempt should be made to remove a conjunctival or corneal foreign body by irrigation using a syringe and sterile saline solution. If a corneal foreign body cannot be removed by irrigation, it should be removed with a sharp instrument rather than a cotton-tipped applicator stick, which can significantly damage the corneal epithelium. A sterile spud or a 25- or 27-gauge needle on a tuberculin syringe should be used. The instrument should be held tangential to the cornea such that the cornea would not be perforated if the patient lunged forward. The spud is used to gently elevate the foreign body off the cornea. Corneal anesthesia is accomplished by use of topical proparacaine or tetracaine. A slit lamp is best suited because it provides adequate illumination and magnification, but a binocular loupe may be used. Many emergency departments are equipped with slit lamps.

A rust ring may be present if an iron foreign body has been retained for several hours or days. This is best removed by an ophthalmologist with a battery-operated, slow-speed drill with a fairly rounded bur. Rust rings that cannot be removed readily at the first attempt can often be removed easily 24 hours later, after leukocytes have softened the surrounding corneal tissue.

Topical antibiotics should be used until the corneal surface reepithelializes. Topical cycloplegics may be given, depending on patient discomfort. The eye should be examined daily until it has healed to ensure that a corneal ulcer has not developed.

Cross-Reference: Foreign Bodies and Corneal Abrasions (Chapter 42).

46 Ophthalmoscopy

Procedure

CRAIG G. WELLS

Indications. Ophthalmoscopy may be useful during directed examinations in patients with visual symptoms, vascular disorders, and neurologic disease. Ophthalmoscopy by nonophthalmologists is not reliable, and examination should be performed by an ophthalmologist if findings are critical or if a potentially blinding disorder such as diabetic retinopathy is under consideration. Guidelines for screening have been published.

Rationale. Ophthalmoscopy allows direct examination of the inside of the eye.

Methods. Pupillary dilation facilitates examination, improving clarity and field of view.

The pupil is dilated with either tropicamide 0.5% or phenylephrine 2.5% or with both in combination. Tropicamide is an anticholinergic agent that may blur near vision but produces dilation unaffected by the examining light. Phenylephrine does not blur vision but the pupil constricts with bright light, limiting the examination. A single drop is applied in the inferior conjunctival fornix with the patient's gaze directed upward.

After dilation, the patient's eyeglasses are removed. The examiner's right hand and right eye are used to examine the patient's right eye, and the left hand and left eye are used for the patient's left eye. A +6 (black numbers) lens at a distance of about 1 foot is used to examine the ocular media for opacities, which appear black in the red reflex. The patient's eye is then approached closely, and the ophthalmoscope lens power is reduced until the optic disc is visualized. The examiner's middle finger rests on the malar eminence to stabilize the ophthalmoscope. Systematic inspection of the optic disc, retinal vessels, retinal background, and macula is then performed. Peripheral examination is facilitated by having the patient look in the direction the examiner wishes to see and by the examiner's moving his or her head so that the examiner's eye, the patient's pupil, and the part of the fundus in which inspection is desired are all on a straight line.

Opacities in the media may be due to corneal, lens, cataract, or vitreous pathology. Optic disc pallor indicates neuronal death from neurologic or vascular disease. Optic nerve edema obscures vessel borders at the disc margins and may be due to increased cerebrospinal fluid pressure, inflammation, or ischemia. Cupping greater than 50% of the optic nerve head width usually indicates glaucomatous damage. Abnormal neovascular blood vessels are in front of normal retinal vessels and frequently arranged in a spoked wheel pattern. Leakage of serum causes macular edema and waxy, yellow, "hard" exudates.

Complications. Rarely, angle-closure glaucoma is precipitated. Individuals at risk may be detected by shining a penlight parallel to the iris plane (see Chapter 36, Visual Impairment).

Cross-References: Screening for Glaucoma (Chapter 35), Visual Impairment (Chapter 36), Diabetic Retinopathy (Chapter 44), Diabetes Mellitus (Chapter 154).

REFERENCES

1. American Academy of Ophthalmology. Comprehensive Adult Eye Examination: Preferred Practice Pattern. San Francisco, American Academy of Ophthalmology, 1989.
2. American Academy of Ophthalmology. Diabetic Retinopathy: Preferred Practice Pattern. San Francisco, American Academy of Ophthalmology, 1989.

   Two documents from an ophthalmologic society review recommended intervals for screening and follow-up.

3. Sussman EJ, Tsiaras WG, Soper KA: Diagnosis of diabetic eye disease. JAMA 1982;247:3231–3234.

   Nonophthalmologists frequently miss the diagnosis of diabetic retinopathy.

SECTION VI

Disorders of the Ears, Nose, Mouth, and Throat

· ·

47 Detection and Initial Management of Oral Cancer

Screening

NEAL D. FUTRAN and ALLAN D. HILLEL

Epidemiology. Malignant tumors of the oral cavity account for 3% of all new cancers per year and for 1.6% of cancer deaths per year. Over 5000 new cases of oral cancer are reported nationwide each year. Tumors occur twice as often in men as in women. The most common histologic type is squamous cell carcinoma (90%), which is almost always associated with a history of tobacco use (cigarette, cigar, pipe, or chewing tobacco). Excessive use of alcohol potentiates the risk of developing disease. Other histologic types include melanoma and minor salivary gland cancers such as adenoid cystic, mucoepidermoid, and malignant mixed carcinomas.

Rationale. Examination of the oral cavity should be conducted as part of a physical examination of all smokers and tobacco chewers. Teenagers should be included in this risk category because the widespread use of chewing tobacco has increased their incidence of oral cancer. Whereas lesions on the lips are usually easily seen, lesions inside the mouth often remain asymptomatic and undetected until bleeding or pain results from advanced lesions. Dentists discover oral cancers more often than physicians because they usually perform screening examinations before dental treatments and because a frequent presenting symptom of oral cancer is ill-fitting dentures.

The presence of neck adenopathy indicating nodal metastases may be an initial sign of asymptomatic oral cancer and necessitates careful examination of the upper aerodigestive tract.

Strategy. A comprehensive examination of the oral cavity requires a strong light, preferably a headlight that will allow the examiner to use a tongue blade in each hand. One systematic approach includes the following steps:

1. After the tongue blade has been inserted in the open mouth, the patient is instructed to close the mouth halfway, allowing the cheeks to relax for easy examination of the buccal mucosa and the buccal side of the alveolar ridges.
2. The mouth is widely opened to examine the lingual side of the alveolar ridges, the tongue, and the palate.
3. With appropriate positioning of the tongue, the anterior floor of the mouth, the undersurface and sides of the tongue, and the retromolar trigones (corner on each side where the tongue, jaw, and palate meet) are examined.
4. The tongue is depressed to view the anterior tonsillar pillars and the tonsillar fossae (or tonsils, if present).
5. Finally, a gloved finger should carefully palpate the just-mentioned structures for any irregularities.

Squamous cell cancers usually present as ulcerations, although early lesions may appear as leukoplakia or erythroplakia. Tumors of salivary gland origin usually present as submucosal masses without ulceration.

Action. Patients with lesions that do not resolve within 7 to 10 days should be referred to a specialist for further evaluation and biopsy.

Tumors are classified by site (lip, anterior tongue, buccal mucosa, alveolar ridge, hard palate, soft palate, or retromolar trigone) and graded T1 through T4 on the basis of size and invasion of adjacent structures. Treatment options for malignant lesions include surgery with or without adjuvant radiation therapy. Small tumors are often successfully managed by local resection with primary closure or placement of skin grafts. For advanced cases that require resection of large areas of mucosa or bone, reconstructive options include pedicled myocutaneous flaps and free tissue transfer.

Cross-Reference: Periodic Health Assessment (Chapter 8).

REFERENCES

1. Baker SR. Malignant neoplasms of the oral cavity. In Cummings CW, et al, eds. Otolaryngology—Head and Neck Surgery. St. Louis, Mosby–Year Book, 1992.
   Anatomy, description of lesions, and treatment are reviewed.

2. Hillel AD, Fee WE. Malignant tumors of the palate. In English GM, ed. Otolaryngology. Philadelphia, Harper & Row, 1982.
   This detailed account of palatal lesions includes nonsquamous cell malignancies.

3. Sullivan MJ, Urken ML, Glenn MG, Baker SR. Free tissue transfer: Head and neck reconstruction. In Cummings CW, ed. Otolaryngology—Head and Neck Surgery. Update II. St. Louis, CV Mosby, 1990.
   An overview of reconstruction for advanced oral cancers is given.

4. Urken ML. The restoration or preservation of sensation in the oral cavity following ablative surgery. Arch Otolaryngol Head Neck Surg 1995;121:607–612.
   New concepts in reconstruction of the oral cavity are presented.

48 Screening for Hearing Impairment

Screening

CYNTHIA D. MULROW

Epidemiology. Hearing impairment is one of the three most common chronic health problems of elderly Americans. One fourth of individuals older than age 65 report problems with their hearing, and audiologically detectable hearing loss is present in more than one third of individuals older than age 65. Most are affected by presbycusis, the bilateral high-frequency hearing loss that occurs and progresses with advancing age. The etiology of presbycusis is not known, although exposure to occupational and environmental noise is thought to be a factor.

Rationale. Adverse effects on physical, cognitive, emotional, and social function are associated with hearing loss. Many of these effects are reversible with the use of hearing aids. Simple accurate methods for screening hearing exist. One is a hand-held audioscope, which is an otoscope that emits tones of calibrated frequencies and intensities. Reported sensitivities for the audioscope range from 93% to 96%, specificities range from 70% to 90%, and positive likelihood ratios range from 3.1 to 9.4. In the absence of audioscopy, a self-reported screening questionnaire such as the Hearing Handicap Inventory for the Elderly (Fig. 48–1) or a whispered voice test may be used. Reported sensitivities and specificities are in the range of 60% to 80% and 75% to 85%, respectively. Positive likelihood ratios range from 2.0 to 6.7. Tuning fork tests are not recommended.

Strategy. Primary care providers should screen for hearing impairment in elderly persons as part of their annual preventive health care examinations. Portable audioscopy should be considered the screening test of choice. Failure to respond to a 40-dB tone at any one frequency (1000, 2000, or 4000 Hz) in either ear constitutes a fail; in adults younger than 65, failure to hear these frequencies using a 25-dB signal constitutes a fail.

Action. Persons who fail screening examinations should be referred to audiologists for comprehensive audiometric evaluations and possible amplification interventions. Five percent to 10% of such persons may benefit from medical or surgical interventions. Costs for formal audiometry and hearing aids vary depending on the type of aid (i.e., behind-the-ear, in-the-ear, programmable) but range from $500 to $1000.

Question	Yes	No	Sometimes
1. Does a hearing problem cause you to feel embarrassed when you meet new people?			
2. Does a hearing problem cause you to feel frustrated when talking to members of your family?			
3. Do you have difficulty hearing when someone speaks in a whisper?			
4. Do you feel handicapped by a hearing problem?			
5. Does a hearing problem cause you difficulty when visiting friends, relatives, or neighbors?			
6. Does a hearing problem cause you to attend religious services less often than you would like?			
7. Does a hearing problem cause you to have arguments with family members?			
8. Does a hearing problem cause you difficulty when listening to TV or radio?			
9. Do you feel that any difficulty with your hearing limits or hampers your personal or social life?			
10. Does a hearing problem cause you difficulty when in a restaurant with relatives or friends?			

Scoring: No = 0; Sometimes = 2; Yes = 4.

Interpretation of total scores: 0–8 = no handicap; 10–24 = mild to moderate handicap; 26–40 = severe handicap.

Figure 48–1. Hearing Handicap Inventory for the Elderly.

REFERENCES

1. Frank T, Peterson DR. Accuracy of a 40-dB HL audioscope and audiometer screening for adults. Ear Hear 1987;8:180–183.

   The use and accuracy of a portable audioscope is described.

2. Lichtenstein MJ, Bess FH, Logan SA. Validation of screening tools for identifying hearing-impaired elderly in primary care. JAMA 1988;259:2875–2878.

   Screening protocol, including audioscopy, that is useful in the general practice setting is described.

3. McBride WS, Mulrow CD, Aguilar C, Tuley MR. Methods for screening for hearing loss in older adults. J Med Sci 1994;307:40–42.

   Performance and patient preferences for audioscope versus self-report hearing handicap questionnaire are compared.

4. Mulrow CD, Lichtenstein MJ. Screening for hearing impairment in the elderly: Rationale and strategy. J Gen Intern Med 1991;6:249–258.

   Operating characteristics of multiple hearing screening tests are reviewed.

5. US Department of Health and Human Services Public Health Service. Clinician's Handbook of Preventive Services: Put Prevention into Practice. Washington, DC, 1994:187–190.

   Screening recommendations from multiple authorities are reviewed.

49 Hiccough (Singultus)

Symptom

KATHLEEN H. MAKIELSKI

Epidemiology. Hiccoughs are inspiratory sounds made by abrupt glottic closure associated with rhythmic spasms of the accessory respiratory muscles and diaphragm. Hiccoughs occur at any age (including during fetal life) and may last up to 60 years. There is a strong male predominance.

Etiology. Hiccoughs result from a wide variety of conditions affecting a reflex arc that includes the vagus nerve as the afferent limb, brain stem centers, and the phrenic nerve as the efferent limb. Causes may be peripheral (more often left-sided than right-sided) or central. Lesions or postsurgical states of the abdomen, chest, or neck are common peripheral causes, especially when the disease is adjacent to the diaphragm or along the course of the phrenic or vagus nerves. Examples include gastric distention (common), esophagitis, pancreatic carcinoma, peritonitis, subphrenic abscess, myocardial infarction, pneumonia, and aortic aneurysm.

Examples of central causes include central nervous system (CNS) lesions (meningitis, stroke, tumor, trauma, multiple sclerosis), metabolic disorders (diabetes mellitus, gout, uremia, hypokalemia, hypocalcemia, hyponatremia), drugs (alcohol, general anesthetics, barbiturates, diazepam, midazolam, α-methyldopa, dexamethasone, methylprednisolone), and psychogenic disorders (more common in women).

A foreign body in the ear canal may also produce hiccoughs by stimulating the auricular branch of the vagus nerve.

Clinical Approach. Persistent hiccoughs (lasting more than 48 hours) suggest a serious underlying disease and require evaluation. The patient interview and physical examination should focus on the CNS, ears, throat, esophagus, chest, and abdomen, with a careful review of alcohol intake and medications. Diagnostic tests include chest radiography, electrocardiography, complete blood cell count, electrolyte and blood glucose determinations, and liver and renal function tests.

Management. There is no single most effective treatment, and few controlled trials exist. One reasonable approach is to start with mechanical stimulation of the pharynx or esophagus, which attempts to interrupt the reflex arc. Any of the following may be tried:

1. Have the patient swallow a tablespoon of granulated sugar.
2. Pass a catheter into the patient's nasopharynx.
3. Massage the soft palate or apply traction to the tongue.
4. Pass a nasogastric tube.

If these steps are ineffective and the diagnostic evaluation fails to reveal a treatable disorder, specific pharmacologic treatment may benefit the patient, probably by acting on the CNS hiccough center. Treatment is largely empirical. Successes have been reported with anesthetics, anticonvulsants, calcium channel blockers, dopamine antagonists, γ-aminobutyric acid agonists, hypnotics, muscle relaxants, narcotics, sedatives, tranquilizers, and tricyclic antidepressants. Response to treatment may require hours or days. Reasonable initial choices are chlorpromazine (50 mg given intravenously, then 25–50 mg given orally every 6 hours) or metoclopramide (10 mg orally every 4 hours for 10 days).

Hypnosis, acupuncture, and digital rectal massage are also reported to be effective, but no controlled data exist.

Severe cases refractory to all pharmacologic options should be referred to an anesthesiologist for anesthetic infiltration of the left phrenic nerve. If hiccoughs recur after anesthetic blocks, a phrenic nerve crush (usually on the left side, rarely bilaterally) may be effective but should be considered only if the anesthetic block produced at least transient relief without adversely affecting pulmonary function.

Complications of severe, protracted hiccoughs include vomiting, dehydration, weight loss, fatigue, surgical wound dehiscence, and death.

REFERENCES

1. Jones JS, et al. Persistent hiccups as an unusual manifestation of hyponatremia. J Emerg Med 1987;5:283–287.

    The authors provide a concise review, with an emphasis on the etiology and a description of the hiccough reflex.

2. Lewis JH. Hiccups: Causes and cures. J Clin Gastroenterol 1985;7:539–552.

    This is a detailed review that includes specific treatment regimens.

3. Nathan MD, et al. Intractable hiccups. Laryngoscope 1980;90:1612–1618.

    This article provides an overview of the etiology and treatment of hiccoughs.

• •

50 Hoarseness

Symptom

HEIDI POWELL

Epidemiology and Etiology. Normal vocal sound is produced by the coordinated movements of the abdominal, chest wall, and laryngeal muscles. Hoarseness, a coarse, scratchy vocalization, occurs when the vocal cords vibrate abnormally. It can be caused by local disorders of the larynx, lesions affecting the innervation of the larynx, or regional or systemic illnesses.

The most common local disorders are vocal abuse or misuse and upper respiratory tract viral infections. Vocal cord paralysis, usually unilateral and more common on the left side, can be caused by any lesion affecting the vagus nerve or its upper two branches, the superior and recurrent laryngeal nerves. Table 50–1 lists the causes of hoarseness.

Clinical Approach. The history should emphasize duration of symptoms, medications, substance abuse, and general health. In addition, a complete head and neck examination is necessary. Acute or intermittent hoarseness, most often benign, is usually caused by voice abuse or upper respiratory tract infections. Chronic hoarseness is more worrisome. Symptoms and signs of malignancy include neck mass, otalgia, stridor, weight loss, dysphagia, hemoptysis, cough, and odynophagia. Other causes of persistent hoarseness include gastroesophageal reflux disease (nocturnal cough, acid taste in mouth, heartburn, halitosis, sore throat, throat clearing), hypothyroidism (fatigue, weight gain), vocal use pattern (public speaking, singing, shouting), previous neck surgery or intubation, allergies (rhinorrhea, cough), substance abuse (alcohol, smoking), rheumatoid arthritis (cricothyroid arthritis), neurologic disorders, pulmonary diseases, and systemic illnesses.

Management. Most cases of hoarseness seen by the primary care physician are self-limited (viral infection) and respond to initial treatment. Patients with acute or intermittent hoarseness can be treated with voice rest (avoid complete voice abstinence), hydration, and discontinuation of offending agents (smoking, medications). Hydration and humidification of the home and workplace are especially important in the elderly. Gastroesophageal reflux disease can be treated with lifestyle measures (raise head of bed to 30 degrees, avoid eating 3 to 4 hours before sleeping, avoid caffeine) and antacids or H_2 blockers. If symptoms persist for more than 2 weeks, indirect laryngoscopy can be done by the indirect mirror method in the primary care physician's office. With this technique one can assess vocal fold abduction and adduction symmetry and evaluate for inflammation or mass lesions. If hoarseness has been present for more than 4 weeks, the patient should be referred to an ear, nose, and throat specialist for evaluation and flexible fiberoptic nasolaryngoscopy or fiberoptic strobovideolaryngoscopy. Direct laryngoscopy requiring general anesthesia is usually not required. If a patient is found to have unilateral vocal cord paralysis, a chest radiograph to evaluate for a possible lung mass is appropriate. If this is negative, magnetic resonance imaging or computed tomography of the neck/chest/skull base should be done. Panendoscopy is indicated if the results of the previous tests are normal.

Hoarseness secondary to systemic illnesses generally responds to treatment of the underlying illness. Patients with structural lesions may require surgical excision or laser treatment but also benefit from voice rehabilitation with a skilled speech pathologist. There is a high cure rate for laryngeal cancers detected early, and often the voice can be restored. Patients with unilateral vocal cord paralysis and vocal muscle atrophy may benefit from techniques that improve glottic closure (Teflon injection, vocal fold augmentation with a silicone block, surgery), in addition to speech therapy.

Cross-References: Smoking Cessation (Chapter 12), Dysphagia and Heartburn (Chapter 96).

Table 50–1. CAUSES OF HOARSENESS

Local Disorders of the Larynx	Vocal Cord Paralysis	Regional Diseases and Systemic Illnesses	Muscular Weakness or Discordance
Benign lesions: polyps, nodules, cysts, calluses, papillomas, laryngeal webs, leukoplakia (precancerous), contact granulomas	Neoplasms: lung, esophagus, thyroid, jugular foramen, glomus, deep lobe parotid, schwannomas, paragangliomas	Endocrine abnormalities: hypothyroidism, acromegaly, hypoparathyroidism, hypogonadism, increased progesterone states such as pregnancy and oral contraceptives	Pulmonary diseases: chronic obstructive pulmonary disease, bronchiectasis, lung cancer, pneumonia
Neoplasms: squamous cell carcinoma, chondrosarcoma	Head/neck/chest trauma and surgery	Collagen vascular diseases: rheumatoid arthritis, systemic lupus erythematosus, Wegener's granulomatosis, scleroderma, polyarteritis nodosa	Neurologic diseases: amyotrophic lateral sclerosis, Guillain-Barré syndrome, Parkinson's disease, Alzheimer's disease, myoclonus
Throat irritants: smoke, atmospheric chemicals/particles repetitive throat clearing, coughing	Neuromuscular disorders: myasthenia gravis, multiple sclerosis	Infections: bacterial, viral, fungal, chronic granulomatous	Spastic dysphonia
Gastroesophageal reflux	Neuropathies: heavy metals, endocrine abnormalities	Cystic fibrosis	
Postnasal drip: sinusitis, allergic rhinitis	Brain stem strokes	Amyloidosis	
Recurrent tonsillitis	Arnold-Chiari malformations		
Drugs/medications: alcohol, nicotine, major tranquilizers, diuretics, tricyclic antidepressants, steroid inhalers, theophylline	Thoracic aorta aneurysm		
Trauma and surgery: hematoma, laryngeal fractures, intubation complications, and thyroid/parathyroid surgery	Cardiomegaly		

REFERENCES

1. Lancer JM, et al. Vocal cord nodules: A review. Clin Otolaryngol 1988;13:43–51.

   The histology, clinical appearance, symptoms, incidence, and causes of vocal cord nodules are detailed.

2. Maragos NE. Hoarseness. Prim Care 1990;17:347–363.

   The anatomy, pathophysiology, etiology, and management of hoarseness are reviewed.

3. Sataloff RT, et al. Gastroesophageal reflux laryngitis. Ear Nose Throat J 1993;72:113–114.

   The signs, symptoms, confirmatory tests, and treatment of gastroesophageal reflux laryngitis are provided in this article.

4. Terris DJ, et al. Contemporary evaluation of unilateral vocal paralysis. Otolaryngol Head Neck Surg 1992;107:84–90.

   The evaluation of 181 patients diagnosed with unilateral vocal paralysis is discussed and a cost-effective algorithm regarding diagnostic tests to determine the etiology is provided.

51 Tinnitus

Symptom

KATHLEEN C. Y. SIE

Epidemiology. Tinnitus refers to the perception of sound in the absence of an appropriate acoustic stimulus. Although estimates of the prevalence of tinnitus are misleading, the National Center for Health Statistics survey (1968) showed that 32% of adults in the United States have complained of tinnitus at one time or another; 6.4% of these persons described their symptoms as severe or debilitating. The prevalence of tinnitus increases with age until 70 years, most commonly affecting persons between 40 and 70 years old. Men and women are equally affected. Tinnitus can be described as objective (i.e., appreciable by the patient and the examiner) or subjective (i.e., appreciable by only the patient).

Etiology. Objective tinnitus is unusual and suggests either a vascular or a mechanical cause. Vascular causes of tinnitus include arteriovenous malformation, high jugular bulb, arterial bruit, or aberrant large vessels in the middle ear. Arterial causes of tinnitus are generally associated with a pulsatile quality. Venous causes may be associated with a low-pitched hum. Mechanical causes of tinnitus include patulous eustachian tube, palatal myoclonus, or stapedial muscle myoclonus. Tinnitus related to myoclonus may have a clicking quality.

The most common type of tinnitus is continuous, high-pitched, nonpulsatile, and subjective. This type of tinnitus is usually bilateral and associated with sensorineural hearing loss due to noise exposure, presbycusis, or other causes. The cause of this tinnitus is generally thought to be related to spontaneous neural activity unrelated to an acoustic stimulus. This "head noise" tends to be most bothersome in a quiet setting, when the patient is trying to rest or relax. Other common causes of tinnitus are middle and external ear pathologic processes, such as middle ear effusions, negative middle ear pressure, tympanic membrane perforation, and cerumen impaction. Inner ear disorders such as Meniere's disease (fluctuating hearing loss, aural fullness, and vertigo), ototoxicity (Table 51–1), and neurosyphilis can also cause tinnitus. Drug-related tinnitus is generally dose related, reversible after cessation of the offending agent, and not always associated with hearing loss. For example, tinnitus associated with aspirin ingestion usually occurs with doses of greater than 4 g/d and usually resolves within 2 to 3 days after discontinuing the aspirin.

Tinnitus may also be a manifestation of cerebellopontine angle (CPA) lesions. In these cases the tinnitus is usually unilateral and may be continuous or pulsatile. Associated signs and symptoms are asymmetric hearing loss, vertigo, and facial numbness. The most common CPA tumor is the acoustic neuroma, a benign neoplasm originating from Schwann cells surrounding the vestibular division of the auditory nerve. Up to 90% of patients with acoustic neuromas complain of tinnitus. Other CPA tumors include meningiomas, cholesterol granulomas, primary cholesteatoma, and metastases.

Other, less common causes of tinnitus include temporomandibular joint syndrome, hypothyroidism, hyperthyroidism, hyperlipidemia (particularly when associated with hearing loss and vertigo), and head trauma. Cardiovascular disease may also be associated with tinnitus. Psychological factors, such as stress and depression, are known to exacerbate the perceived severity of tinnitus.

Clinical Approach. Tinnitus is characterized by its quality (ringing, humming, roaring, pulsatile), pitch (high, low), fluctuation, location (unilateral, bilateral) and relationship to activity (chewing, Valsalva's maneuver, breathing, and pulse), as well as its impact on the patient's life. Important related symptoms are hearing loss, aural fullness, vertigo, and dysequilibrium. The patient should also be asked about past noise exposure, infections (particularly meningitis), head injury, and medications, especially over-the-counter preparations containing aspirin.

The clinician should perform a head and neck examination including pneumatic otoscopy, auscultation of the carotid arteries, and assessment of cranial nerve and cerebellar function. Blood pressure should be measured. All patients who complain of tinnitus should have an audiogram with speech discrimination testing. Unilateral tinnitus, audiometric findings of asymmetric sensorineural hearing loss, or disproportionately poor speech discrimination suggests the possibility of a retrocochlear lesion such as an acoustic neuroma. These patients should be referred to an otolaryngologist. Further testing may include auditory brain stem responses. Fine-cut computed tomography of the

Table 51–1. SUBSTANCES THAT CAUSE OR EXACERBATE TINNITUS

Aspirin	Alcohol
Heavy metals	Caffeine
Oral contraceptives	Cocaine
Quinine	Marijuana
Aminoglycoside antibiotics	Tobacco
Heterocyclic antidepressants	

internal auditory canal with contrast medium enhancement or magnetic resonance imaging with gadolinium enhancement is required to demonstrate lesions of the internal auditory canal. Magnetic resonance imaging is the most sensitive test for detection of acoustic neuromas.

If the clinician sees a middle ear mass or palpates a neck mass suggesting a glomus tumor, computed tomography or angiography may be required. These patients should also be referred to an otolaryngologist.

The evaluation of tinnitus can be performed on an outpatient basis, unless the patient demonstrates signs of increased intracranial pressure.

Management. Management of the patient with tinnitus should include identification and treatment of an underlying pathologic process, identification of associated problems (e.g., hearing loss), assessment of symptom severity, and symptom suppression. Treatment options include treatment of underlying medical disorders, surgical treatment of mass lesions, masking, biofeedback, stress management, and reassurance.

Underlying medical disorders, including hypertension and depression, should be treated appropriately. Also, any medications that cause or exacerbate tinnitus should be adjusted or discontinued, if possible. Special attention should be given to over-the-counter medications that may contain aspirin or nonsteroidal anti-inflammatory medications.

Mass lesions, such as acoustic neuromas and glomus tumors, generally require excision, although poor surgical candidates may sometimes be treated with radiation therapy. Otitis media or cerumen impaction should be treated (see Chapter 56, Otitis Media and Externa, and Chapter 58, Cerumen Removal), and ototoxic medications should be discontinued if possible.

Masking may be accomplished with masking devices, hearing aids, or home devices such as a radio tuned between stations to provide white noise.

Many other means, including anticonvulsants, lidocaine, and electrical stimulation, have been studied for their potential benefit in the management of patients with tinnitus. None is clinically useful. Alprazolam seems to be the most promising agent, although its mechanism of action may be in treating underlying depression when present.

If there is not an identifiable treatable cause of the tinnitus, the patient should be reassured that the tinnitus is benign.

Follow-Up. Patients complaining of tinnitus with symmetric sensorineural hearing loss or normal hearing and no treatable cause should have audiograms every 1 to 2 years to detect progression of hearing loss or development of retrocochlear signs. Patients with unilateral tinnitus, asymmetric hearing loss, pulsatile tinnitus, or vestibular symptoms should be referred to an otolaryngologist for further evaluation. Patients with asymmetric sensorineural hearing loss in whom acoustic neuroma has been ruled out should be observed every 6 to 12 months. Progression of asymmetric sensorineural hearing loss should prompt reassessment to rule out a retrocochlear process.

REFERENCES

1. Hazell JW. Tinnitus: II: Surgical management of conditions associated with tinnitus and somatosounds. J Otolaryngol 1990;19:6–10.

This article discusses surgical options for some of the more unusual causes of tinnitus (e.g., palatal myoclonus, stapedial myoclonus).

2. Hazell JW. Tinnitus: III: The practical management of sensorineural tinnitus. J Otolaryngol 1990;19:11–18.

   This article provides a comprehensive discussion of management strategies, including a decision algorithm used in a large tinnitus clinic.

3. McFadden D. Tinnitus: Facts, Theories, and Treatment. Washington, DC, National Academy Press, 1982.

   The author provides an overview of the incidence of tinnitus, review of etiologies, and treatment.

4. Schleuning AJ. Management of the patient with tinnitus. Med Clin North Am 1991;75:1225–1237.

   The author provides a review of etiologies and management of tinnitus.

- -

52 Abnormal Taste and Smell

Symptom

JOHN B. STIMSON

Epidemiology. It is estimated that more than 2 million Americans suffer from disorders of taste and smell.

Etiology. Taste is mediated by specialized taste buds, served by cranial nerves VII, IX, and X, which are spread over the tongue, soft palate, pharynx, larynx, epiglottis, uvula, and upper one third of the esophagus. There are four types of receptors, responding to salty, sweet, bitter, and sour substances. Nuances of taste are provided by olfaction, which appears to have unlimited capacity for recognition of distinct odors. As a result, the symptom of diminished or absent taste most commonly results from loss of smell (anosmia) rather than loss of taste (ageusia). Olfactory receptors are confined to a 1-cm^2 area at the top of the nasal cavities, and afferent impulses are transmitted by cranial nerve I through the cribriform plate of the ethmoid bone. Because the olfactory system is spatially confined, local problems, such as tumors, airflow obstruction, trauma, or mucosal disruption, are much more likely to cause anosmia than ageusia. Conditions affecting taste are more often systemic (e.g., drug effect, uremia, hepatitis) and more commonly produce distorted taste (dysgeusia) than absence of taste.

Table 52–1 is a list of causes of abnormal taste or smell organized by the anatomic level of the defect. In recent series of patients evaluated for anosmia, 25% to 34% had nasal and sinus inflammatory conditions (allergic rhinitis, sinusitis, or polyps), 14% to 30% of cases followed a viral infection, and 10%

Table 52–1. CAUSES OF ABNORMAL TASTE AND SMELL

Level of Defect	Smell Disorders	Taste Disorders
Substance delivery	Nasal obstruction Nasal polyps Mucosal edema (rhinitis) Sinusitis Adenoid hypertrophy Airflow diversion Laryngectomy Tracheostomy	
Mucosa	Dryness Sjögren's syndrome Smoking Destruction Viral infections Leprosy Ozena Caustic exposure (e.g., ammonia)	Sjögren's syndrome Smoking Radiation therapy Dysautonomia Viral infections Thermal burn
Receptor abnormality	Absence Kallmann's syndrome (hypogonadotropic hypogonadism with anosmia)	
Peripheral nerve	Head injury Craniotomy Postsubarachnoid hemorrhage Meningitis Tumor	Bell's palsy (unilateral) Chorda tympani nerve injury (tumor, dental anesthetic injection) (unilateral)
Central nervous system	Meningioma or other tumor Parkinson's disease Multiple sclerosis	
Systemic	Vitamin B_{12} deficiency Myxedema Depression	Drugs* Hepatitis Uremia Malignancy Pregnancy Myxedema Addison's disease Deficiencies of zinc or niacin

*Some common examples are griseofulvin, amitriptyline, antithyroid drugs, chlorambucil, cholestyramine, penicillamine, procarbazine, vincristine, vinblastine, angiotensin-converting enzyme inhibitors, and propafenone.

to 19% of cases followed head injury. Similar data for disorders of taste do not exist.

Clinical Approach. Inquiry should focus on recent upper respiratory tract infections, rhinitis or sinusitis, medications, and symptoms of systemic conditions such as uremia, hepatitis, pregnancy, hypothyroidism, and depression. A history of head injury or other central nervous system disease (Parkinson's disease, multiple sclerosis, subarachnoid hemorrhage) is important in the evaluation of anosmia. Fluctuating anosmia strongly suggests nasal or sinus inflammatory disease. A taste disorder associated with anorexia should bring malignancy to mind.

The nasal examination should evaluate airway patency and look for evidence for infection and the presence of allergic discoloration (pallor), polyps, and moisture. Oral examination should include assessment for adequate salivation, poor dentition, glossitis, or purulent postnasal drainage. If uncertainty exists about the presence of polyps or sinusitis, endoscopic nasal examination or computed tomography (CT) of the sinuses may be indicated. Although less expensive than CT, traditional radiography of the sinuses is insensitive. Physical examination may provide clues to systemic conditions such as liver disease, endocrine disorders, or malignancies.

Testing of taste or smell in a symptomatic patient is probably of little value in a primary care setting unless confusion exists between ageusia and anosmia or there is suspicion of malingering. Smell is tested by presenting aromatic substances and odorless controls (water) in a patient-blinded fashion and testing one nostril at a time. Pungent or irritating substances such as ammonia or oil of wintergreen can be misleading because they stimulate trigeminal nerve endings and are primarily used to detect malingerers. Taste testing is probably unnecessary.

Selected laboratory tests to exclude pregnancy, vitamin B_{12} deficiency, hypothyroidism, and liver or kidney dysfunction are appropriate when clinically indicated.

Management. Cases of recent onset and no evident cause may resolve spontaneously, and it is often sensible to defer a detailed evaluation for 1 to 2 months. Allergic rhinitis and sinusitis frequently coexist and often respond to a combination of antibiotics, intranasal corticosteroids, and a short course of oral corticosteroids, although results are sometimes temporary. Nasal polyps or obstructing adenoids can be removed surgically. Vitamin B_{12} deficiency and hypothyroidism are easily treatable. If diagnosis of an untreatable cause of taste or smell dysfunction, such as anosmia after head injury, is established, further costly workup should be avoided and patient concerns should be addressed. Potentially offending medications, such as angiotensin-converting enzyme inhibitors, should be stopped on a trial basis. Smokers are advised to stop smoking before extensive evaluation. Conditions due to mucosal dryness (Sjögren's syndrome, radiation effects, dysautonomia) do not respond to moisturizing agents, but patients with Sjögren's syndrome may respond to specific therapy for their disorder. Lastly, zinc-deficient patients frequently are ageusic, but this condition is rare, and the widespread use of zinc supplements in the treatment of idiopathic ageusia has not been beneficial.

Patients with permanent anosmia have lost the warning function of olfaction. They should be advised to install smoke detectors in their homes, to avoid natural gas appliances, and to date all groceries to prevent consumption of spoiled foods.

Cross-References: Smoking Cessation (Chapter 12), Anorexia (Chapter 18), Sinusitis (Chapter 57).

REFERENCES

1. Davidson TM, Jalowayski A, Murphy L, Jacobs RD. Evaluation and treatment of smell dysfunction. West J Med 1987;146:434–438.
   This series comes from a smell disorder clinic.

2. Henkin RI, Schecter PJ, Friedewald WT, Demets DL, Raff M. A double blind study of the effects of zinc sulfate on taste and smell dysfunction. Am J Med Sci 1976;272:285–299.

   No significant benefit occurred with zinc supplements.

3. Henkin RI, Talal N, Larson AL, Mattern CFT. Abnormalities of taste and smell in Sjögren's syndrome. Ann Intern Med 1972;76:375–383.

   No benefit was derived from moisturizing agents, but corticosteroids or irradiation helped if increased salivary flow resulted.

4. Mott AE, Leopold DA. Disorders in taste and smell. Med Clin North Am 1991;75:1321–1353.

   This is an excellent current overview.

5. Scott AE. Clinical characteristics of taste and smell disorders. Ear Nose Throat J 1989;68:297–315.

   A general review summarizes practical experience in a taste and smell dysfunction clinic.

53 Dental Disease

Problem

MARK M. SCHUBERT

Epidemiology and Etiology. The two most common dental diseases are decay and periodontal disease. Untreated disease may lead to loss of the involved teeth or, especially in immunocompromised patients, extension of infection into surrounding bone and soft tissue. Additionally, patients with valvular heart disease and dental infections are at risk for bacterial endocarditis. The most important dental infections are dental caries, which may spread to the dental pulp (causing severe pain) or farther into periapical tissues, and acute periodontal abscesses.

The oral microflora is extremely complex and consists of at least 35 to 40 species of aerobic and anaerobic bacteria and fungal organisms. The predominant organisms depend on whether the problem is an orofacial odontogenic infection (polymicrobial, with obligate anaerobes comprising 65% of isolates), dental caries (gram-positive facultative anaerobes or microaerophilic cocci), pulpal infection (anaerobes), or periodontal infections (anaerobic gram-negative rods and motile forms, including spirochetes).

Signs and Symptoms

DENTAL CARIES. Decay is initially asymptomatic and appears as a darkly stained cavitation of the tooth surface. Decay can also proceed adjacent to existing restorations and under crowns. The involved tooth structure is soft or leathery when examined with a dental explorer. As decay deepens and approaches the pulp, the tooth becomes sensitive to hot and cold as well as sweet foods (which rapidly increase bacterial acid production). When bacteria invade the pulp, constant severe pain occurs. Stimulated pain that lasts for a few seconds is generally referred to as "reversible pulpitis," indicating that decay removal and placement of dental restoration will allow healing of pulpal tissues. However, stimulated pain that lasts longer than 30 to 60 seconds indicates more severe pulpal disease that generally will require root canal therapy or extraction to cure. Although patients can initially localize pain to the involved tooth, this becomes more difficult as disease progresses. Periapical infection makes the tooth sensitive to percussion. Radiographically, carious tooth structure and periapical infections appear as radiolucent changes, although radiolucent dental filling materials and normal anatomic structures can have a similar radiographic appearance.

GINGIVITIS AND PERIODONTITIS. These low-grade localized infections are usually asymptomatic but can cause symptoms of gingival pain and tooth sensitivity to hot and cold and sweets. Gingivitis refers to infection of the gingiva, whereas periodontitis denotes infection that results in the loss of supporting bone and ligaments for the teeth. The first sign of gingivitis is gingival bleeding, usually associated with localized erythema and edema. Although erythema and edema may be absent with periodontitis, probing of the involved periodontal pocket causes bleeding or, in severe cases, reveals pus. Progressive periodontitis deepens the periodontal pockets (normal, 2 to 3 mm), increases bone loss, loosens the involved teeth, and increases the risk of an acute periodontal abscess. Gingivitis and periodontitis can be the source of bacteremia and cause endocarditis or fevers of unknown origin.

OROFACIAL ODONTOGENIC INFECTIONS. Acute odontogenic infections produce localized and painful soft tissue swelling (sometimes with cellulitis or fluctuance) with associated fever, local lymphadenitis, leukocytosis, and an increased erythrocyte sedimentation rate. Accumulated pus from periapical infections usually perforates bone and drains into the mouth but may track along tissue planes and spread to deeper facial spaces, most commonly the sublingual, submandibular, pterygomandibular, and buccal spaces and less commonly the temporal, masseteric, parotid, lateral pharyngeal, and retropharyngeal spaces. Deep space infections that spread into pharyngeal spaces can cause significant trismus and compromise the airway and thus constitute a medical emergency requiring immediate treatment. Periodontal abscesses may also cause deep space infections.

Clinical Approach. The diagnosis of dental caries and periodontal disease depends on the patient's symptoms, clinical examination (caries detection, periodontal probing, percussion, and palpation), tests to determine pulp vitality (e.g., cold and hot testing and electrical stimulation of teeth), and radiographic examination. Pulp vitality tests determine the pain responsiveness of pulpal tissue, a measure of tooth vitality.

A number of nondental conditions may produce facial pain and mimic odontologic pathology. Maxillary sinusitis can cause toothache symptoms in upper posterior teeth. Myofascial pain arising in the muscles of mastication, especially the masseter muscles, can cause pain referred to dental structures. Angina pectoris may be referred to the jaw, most commonly the mandible, but maxillary pain has also been reported. Other conditions to be considered are trigeminal neuralgia and atypical orofacial pain. Local and metastatic tumors may produce radiolucencies that are confused with a pathologic dental process.

Management. The prevention of dental infectious diseases depends on consistent removal of dental plaque from teeth and gingival tissue. The treatment of established odontogenic infections requires instrumentation or surgical techniques, including decay removal, root canal therapy, tooth extraction, periodontal curettage, or, in the case of acute abscesses, incision and drainage. In addition to tooth brushing and flossing to remove plaque, topical antimicrobial rinses (e.g., tetracycline, chlorhexidine, povidone-iodine) can be beneficial.

Most of the microorganisms implicated in orofacial infections, including anaerobes, are susceptible to penicillin. Because of its excellent absorption and high serum levels, amoxicillin is especially effective. Erythromycin has similar antimicrobial activity and is used in patients allergic to penicillin. When β-lactamase–producing anaerobes are suspected (e.g., serious orofacial odontogenic infections), metronidazole is an excellent alternative.

Antibiotic prophylaxis (see Chapter 222, Preoperative Infectious Disease Problems) is necessary before invasive dental procedures are undertaken in patients at risk for bacterial endocarditis or with intravascular dialysis catheters in place. Similar recommendations for patients with prosthetic implants, especially joint implants, have not been clearly established.

Patients who are at particular risk for medical complications from dental disease and who would benefit from referral to an oral surgeon or a specialist include patients at risk for bacterial endocarditis, patients with indwelling venous access lines for dialysis, immunocompromised patients (e.g., human immunodeficiency virus–infected patients, patients scheduled to receive cancer chemotherapy or high-dose systemic corticosteroids, organ transplant recipients), and patients who are to receive radiation therapy to the jaws and oral cavity.

Cross-References: Sinusitis (Chapter 57), Myofascial Pain Syndromes (Chapter 122), Preoperative Infectious Disease Problems (Chapter 222).

REFERENCES

1. Dajani AS, Bisno AL, Chung KJ, et al. Prevention of bacterial endocarditis: Recommendations by the American Heart Association by the Committee on Rheumatic Fever, Endocarditis, and Kawasaki Disease. JAMA 1990;264:2919–2922.

    The most recent recommendations are presented.

2. Kureishi A, Chow AW. The tender tooth: Dentoalveolar, pericoronal, and periodontal infections. Infect Dis Clin North Am 1988;2:163–182.

    Clinical and pathologic features of dental caries, pulpitis, periapical abscess, pericoronitis, and periodontal infections are discussed.

3. Moenning JE, Nelson CL, Kohler RB. The microbiology and chemotherapy of odontogenic infections. J Oral Maxillofac Surg 1989;47:976–985.

    The rationale for the use of recommended antibiotics is reviewed.

4. Odell PF. Infections of the fascial spaces of the neck. J Otolaryngol 1990;19:201–205.

    Anatomy, microbiology, and treatment of these life-threatening infections are reviewed.

54 Pharyngitis

Problem

ROBERT M. CENTOR

Epidemiology and Etiology. Pharyngitis leads to more than 16 million office visits each year, accounting for 2.5% of all visits to primary care physicians. In adult patients with sore throat, pharyngeal cultures are positive for group A β-hemolytic streptococci in about 10% of cases seen in an office practice setting and in about 25% of cases seen in an emergency (or urgent) care setting.

Other probable causes include *Arcanobacterium haemolyticum* (formerly *Corynebacterium haemolyticum*), non–group A streptococci (especially group C), a variety of viral infections, *Chlamydia trachomatis* (or perhaps *C. pneumoniae*, the Taiwan acute respiratory [TWAR] agent), *Mycoplasma pneumoniae*, and *Neisseria gonorrhoeae*.

Symptoms and Signs. The most common symptoms are difficulty swallowing, fever, cough, and coryza. Patients who have severe pain on swallowing or fever are more likely to have a group A β-hemolytic streptococcal infection, whereas both cough and coryza occur more often with viral infections. On examination, findings of pharyngeal exudates or redness, fever, and swollen anterior cervical nodes all support the diagnosis of streptococcal pharyngitis.

Clinical Approach. Four clinical variables (absence of cough, history of fever, exudates, and swollen, tender anterior cervical nodes) help one estimate the probability of streptococcal pharyngitis (Table 54–1). This initial screening test allows the clinician to select a group of patients who need no further evaluation, that is, patients with a very low probability of having the infection. Many

Table 54–1. ESTIMATING THE PROBABILITY OF GROUP A STREPTOCOCCAL PHARYNGITIS

Strep Score*	Prevalence	
	10%†	*20%‡*
0	1%	3%
1	4%	8%
2	9%	18%
3	21%	38%
4	43%	62%

*Points for strep score come from four clinical variables (one point each): lack of a cough; presence of tonsillar exudates; presence of swollen, tender anterior cervical nodes; recent history of fever.

†Most office practices.

‡Most emergency departments.

physicians prescribe antibiotics for high-probability patients ($\geq$ 38% probability of streptococcal pharyngitis) without performing any diagnostic tests.

Rapid antigen tests have a sensitivity of 80% and a specificity of 98% for streptococcal pharyngitis. The clinician should be confident when treating patients with positive test results. In those with negative test results, however, a throat culture may be beneficial (to detect the 20% of patients with streptococcal pharyngitis who have negative tests). This strategy, while having a higher cost, greatly decreases the probability of missing the diagnosis and decreases the possibility of rheumatic fever.

Management. Penicillin is the drug of choice for suspected streptococcal pharyngitis (either a single intramuscular injection of penicillin G benzathine, 1.2 million units, or a full 10-day course of penicillin V potassium, 125 to 250 mg orally four times a day or 250 to 500 mg orally twice a day). For patients allergic to penicillin, erythromycin is the drug of choice.

At the current time no other common cause of sore throats requires treatment. Some clinicians use erythromycin to treat patients with pharyngitis, reasoning that it has activity against other causes of pharyngitis such as *Chlamydia* species and *Mycoplasma*. No data support or refute this practice.

Patients often receive symptomatic benefit from a variety of over-the-counter minor-pain and cold-relief preparations.

Follow-Up. Follow-up of patients with sore throats is generally unnecessary. Most patients' symptoms are self-limited. If symptoms persist, the clinician may consider retesting for group A β-hemolytic streptococci and, if noncompliance is suspected, treating the patient with parenteral penicillin. Alternatively, a penicillinase-resistant antibiotic may be used to cover β-lactamase-producing organisms.

Because asymptomatic carriers require no treatment, routinely performing cultures on specimens from patients after resolution of symptoms is unnecessary.

Cross-Reference: Upper Respiratory Infection (Chapter 66).

REFERENCES

1. Belsey RE, Hale DC, Marcy SM. Rapid office tests: How useful? Patient Care 1990;24:103–125.

   The available rapid antigen tests are listed, with data on the majority of streptococcal pharyngitis test kits currently on the market.

2. Centor RM, Meier FA, Dalton HP. Throat cultures and rapid tests for diagnosis of group A streptococcal pharyngitis in adults. In Sox HC Jr, ed. Common Diagnostic Tests: Use and Interpretation, 2nd ed. Philadelphia, American College of Physicians, 1990:253.

   This comprehensive review is revised from the 1986 Annals of Internal Medicine *article by the same authors.*

3. Kaplan EL, Johnson DR. Eradication of group A streptococci from the upper respiratory tract by amoxicillin with clavulanate after oral penicillin V treatment failure. J Pediatr 1988;113:400–403.

   The management of "treatment failure" is discussed.

4. Meier FA, Centor RM, Graham L, Dalton HP. Clinical and microbiological evidence for endemic pharyngitis among adults due to group C streptococci. Arch Intern Med 1990;150:825–829.

   Evidence is presented for group C streptococci as a cause of pharyngitis.

55 Epistaxis

Problem

MICHAEL G. GLENN

Epidemiology. Nosebleeds are common and affect more than half of us at some time in our lives, but it is estimated that fewer than 1 in 10 persons ever seek medical attention for epistaxis. Severe or refractory nasal hemorrhage in the absence of major trauma is even more rare. Nosebleeds are considerably more common in dry and cold climates.

Etiology. Dryness and crusting of the anterior septum is the major cause of minor nosebleeds. This area is richly vascularized by way of an interconnecting vascular network (Kiesselbach's plexus). Minor trauma or removal of crusts can lead to brisk, but usually easily controlled, bleeding. Hypertension is usually associated with posterior arterial bleeding sites. Coagulopathies, especially platelet disorders, and use of aspirin or nonsteroidal anti-inflammatory drugs (NSAIDs) may be associated with recurrent or refractory bleeding episodes. Atrophic mucosae from chronic use of corticosteroid sprays has become a frequent cause of minor bleeding. More than half of sinonasal tumors present as recurring, unilateral epistaxis as a primary symptom.

Clinical Approach. The primary goal is to stop active bleeding. Secondarily, one needs to determine the cause and the source of bleeding to prevent further episodes. It is important to inquire about any history of trauma, prior nosebleeds, or bruising and bleeding elsewhere. Medication history should elicit any use of aspirin, NSAIDs, or nasal sprays. A family history of bleeding may be important.

On physical examination the first priority is to determine if there is active bleeding. The posterior pharynx should be inspected to rule out posterior drainage of blood if there is no bleeding from the nostrils. The nasal cavity should be examined carefully to look for clots or dried blood and to exclude tumors, polyps, or significant septal deviation. Vital signs should be checked, with measurement of orthostatic changes if there has been significant or lengthy bleeding. Routine laboratory studies are not needed for a patient with isolated minor epistaxis. Hematocrit should be measured in patients with heavy or recurrent bleeding, and platelet counts and coagulation studies should be checked if bleeding is frequent or difficult to control.

Management

NO ACTIVE BLEEDING. Humidification, especially the use of nasal saline sprays, will often prevent further bleeding. If a visible vessel or discrete old bleeding site can be identified, silver nitrate cautery may be beneficial. Control of hypertension and cessation of aspirin, NSAIDs, or nasal corticosteroid sprays may be useful as well.

ACTIVE BLEEDING. Direct, sustained pressure on both nasal alae against the septum is the best way to stop most bleeding. It should be maintained firmly, with the head elevated to minimize venous pressure, for 10 to 15 minutes. Suction removal of clot and decongestant spray may also help control bleeding. If bleeding is not controlled with these measures, an anterior pack should be placed. Compressed sponge packs (Merocel) are easy to insert and relatively comfortable for patients. Antibiotic ointment coating of the sponge facilitates insertion and reduces bacterial colonization. Gauze or intranasal balloon devices are appropriate alternatives. Packing should be left for 3 days. The use of antistaphylococcal antibiotics has not been proven to prevent toxic shock syndrome when packing is in place and is not routinely necessary.

Bleeding not controlled with an anterior pack may require otolaryngologic consultation. Alternatives at that point include (1) placement of a posterior pack (one that fills the nasopharynx as well as the entire nasal cavity), (2) angiographic embolization, (3) surgical vessel ligation, and (4) direct surgical cautery with use of endoscopic instrumentation. The latter approach is becoming more common and may be most cost-effective and least uncomfortable for patients. Nosebleeds in thrombocytopenic or factor-deficient individuals can be exceedingly difficult to control and typically require otolaryngologic consultation.

Follow-Up. Hypertensive patients should be observed to ensure adequacy of their blood pressure control. Patients with recurrent, especially unilateral, nosebleeds should be evaluated by an otolaryngologist to exclude occult tumors, sinus infections, or septal deformities.

Cross-References: Sinusitis (Chapter 57), Essential Hypertension (Chapter 85), Bleeding (Chapter 195).

REFERENCES

1. Jackson KR, Jackson RT. Factors associated with active refractory epistaxis. Arch Otolaryngol Head Neck Surg 1988:114:862–865.

   This article provides useful diagrams and guidelines for when to refer a patient.

2. Josephson GD, Godley FA, Stierna P. Practical management of epistaxis. Med Clin North Am 1991;75:1311–1320.

   The authors give a good general review.

3. Shaw CB, Wax MK, Wetmore SJ. Epistaxis: A comparison of treatment. Otolaryngol Head Neck Surg 1993;109:60–65.

   This study compares the costs of medical versus surgical management.

56 Otitis Media and Externa

Problem

ANDREW F. INGLIS, JR.

OTITIS MEDIA

Epidemiology and Etiology. Acute otitis media is an acute bacterial middle ear infection with a mucopurulent effusion. The usual causative organisms are *Streptococcus pneumoniae, Haemophilus influenzae, Streptococcus pyogenes,* and *Moraxella catarrhalis.* Acute otitis media is extremely common in children but relatively rare in adults. Otitis media with effusion refers to a middle ear effusion that is usually sterile and persists behind an intact tympanic membrane for several weeks to months. Chronic otitis media is an active or smoldering infection, present for weeks to years, associated with a foul-smelling otorrhea that drains through a tympanic membrane perforation. It is usually associated with some combination of enteric gram-negative rods, *Staphylococcus aureus,* or anaerobes. Chronic otitis media may be caused or accompanied by an epithelial cyst (cholesteatoma), which if left untreated will expand to fill the middle ear and mastoid, injuring associated structures such as the ossicular chain, facial nerve, dural sinuses, or brain. All forms of otitis media are more common in patients with a predilection for eustachian tube dysfunction; risk factors include Native American or Southeast Asian race, cleft palate (repaired or not), nasopharyngeal carcinoma, ciliary dysmotility syndromes, and immunocompromise.

Symptoms and Signs. Patients with acute otitis media initially experience symptoms of an upper respiratory tract infection (rhinorrhea, sore throat, cough) associated with a growing ear pressure sensation. This is followed by fever, severe otalgia, hearing loss, and sometimes vertigo or unsteady gait. The tympanic membrane is usually bulging with dilated blood vessels on a cream or yellow background. Pneumatic otoscopy reveals reduced tympanic membrane mobility. The tympanic membrane may spontaneously rupture, with profuse otorrhea and rapid reduction of otalgia. Otitis media with effusion usually follows acute otitis media and causes a sensation of aural pressure and hearing loss. The tympanic membrane is usually thickened, slightly retracted, opaque, and hypomobile. If the diagnosis is in doubt, a tympanogram should be obtained. In chronic otitis media the examination reveals thick, foul otorrhea that becomes copious during exacerbations, draining through a perforated tympanic membrane or tympanostomy tube. Granulation tissue from the middle ear may obscure the perforation or cholesteatoma.

Clinical Approach. The initial approach in suspected acute otitis media and otitis media with effusion is empirical antibiotic administration; no further tests are necessary. In immunocompromised patients, however, the potential pathogens are too diverse to allow accurate prediction of infecting organisms, and middle ear culture by tympanocentesis should precede antibiotic treatment. In chronic otitis media, a hearing screening evaluation or formal audiogram should precede therapy. The therapeutic goals in these patients are to sterilize the middle ear and mastoid cavity, either medically or surgically, to exclude cholesteatoma, and ideally to restore the integrity of the tympanic membrane.

Management. The symptoms of acute otitis media usually respond to a 10-day course of amoxicillin or trimethoprim-sulfamethoxazole (Table 56–1). Medical management of otitis media with effusion is problematic, because antibiotics are only infrequently beneficial. A trial of antibiotics can be considered; and in selected cases, a 1-week trial of prednisone with a 3-week trial of amoxicillin plus clavulanate is appropriate.

In chronic otitis media, the ear should be gently cleaned with miniature cotton swabs or a No. 6 French nasotracheal suction catheter set on low suction. Appropriate antibiotics include both topical preparations (e.g., an ophthalmologic gentamicin drop) and an antistaphylococcal oral agent such as cephalexin. Patients in whom this regimen fails should have drainage cultured

Table 56–1. OTITIS MEDIA AND OTITIS EXTERNA: SUGGESTED TREATMENT

Drug	Dose and Duration for Adults	Cost ($)*
Acute Otitis Media		
Amoxicillin	500 mg tid × 10 d	8.50
Trimethoprim-sulfamethoxazole	1 double-strength tablet bid × 10 d	23.50
Amoxicillin-clavulanate	875 mg bid × 10 d	62.10
Cefuroxime axetil	250 mg bid × 10 d	49.00
Cefixime	400 mg qd × 10 d	78.00
Otitis Media with Effusion†		
Trimethoprim-sulfamethoxazole	1 double-strength tablet bid × 10 d	23.50
or		
Amoxicillin-clavulanate	500 mg bid × 10 d	50.00
plus		
prednisone	1 mg/kg × 7 d	1.36‡
Chronic Otitis Media		
Systemic		
Cephalexin	250 mg qid × 14 d	57.68
Amoxicillin-clavulanate	500 mg bid × 14 d	63.84
Ciprofloxacin	500 mg bid × 14 d	71.40
Ototopical§		
Polymyxin B sulfate–neomycin sulfate–hydrocortisone suspension	4 drops tid × 5–10 d	3.75 for 10 mL
Gentamicin ophthalmic solution	Same as above	3.75 for 5 mL
Tobramycin ophthalmic solution	Same as above	12.75 for 5 mL

*Average wholesale price, *1995 Drug Topics Red Book,* for duration listed unless otherwise noted.

†Efficacy of antibiotic/corticosteroid combination established in children; trials in adults lacking.

‡Cost for 50 mg/d × 7 days.

§The potential for ototoxicity exists with prolonged use; patients should be instructed to stop administering drops when otorrhea resolves.

and may require an antipseudomonal agent such as ciprofloxacin. Patients should use ototopical antibiotics only as long as the otorrhea persists, because of the theoretic risk of ototoxicity.

Follow-Up. Patients with acute otitis media should be instructed to call back if otalgia and fever do not improve within 2 to 3 days; many patients subsequently note a response to broader-spectrum antibiotics such as amoxicillin-clavulanate, cefixime, or cefuroxime. The physician should examine all patients again in 2 to 4 weeks to ensure that the middle ear effusion has resolved. Patients with otitis media with effusion should be seen monthly. If the effusion does not clear in 2 to 3 months despite antibiotic therapy, the patient should be referred to an otolaryngologist for consideration of tympanostomy tube placement and exclusion of nasopharyngeal carcinoma. Patients with chronic otitis media should return in 1 month, and sooner if there is otalgia. Patients who do not respond, who have persistent tympanic perforations, or who have membrane abnormalities suggestive of a cholesteatoma should be referred to an otolaryngologist.

OTITIS EXTERNA

Epidemiology and Etiology. Otitis externa usually refers to a bacterial infection of the external auditory canal. Predisposing factors include humid climate and trauma; collapse or stenosis of the external auditory canal; or overly vigorous cleaning of naturally bactericidal cerumen. Conditions that mimic bacterial otitis externa include eczema of the external auditory canal and fungal, herpetic, and necrotizing (malignant) otitis externa. Malignant otitis externa is a life-threatening pseudomonal infection that occurs in diabetic or immunocompromised hosts; it is marked by granulation tissue in the external auditory canal and periostitis of the skull base and often presents with cranial nerve palsies.

Symptoms and Signs. Pruritus typically precedes mild to excruciating otalgia in bacterial otitis externa. Manipulation of the pinna is painful. There is a scant amount of discharge and debris. Edema is usually present and may occlude the canal and produce a hearing loss.

Clinical Approach. The diagnosis is based on the combined findings of severe otalgia, auricular tenderness, swelling and erythema of the skin in the canal, and scant, cheesy discharge. Denudation of the skin of the canal or adjacent meatus with little edema suggests an atopic or eczematous process. If the pinna itself is inflamed or swollen, the diagnosis is most likely perichondritis, cellulitis, or erysipelas; otologic consultation is indicated. Microscopic examination of ear canal scrapings may reveal hyphal elements in fungal otitis externa. Vesicular lesions suggest herpetic otitis externa. The history should carefully identify diabetic or immunocompromised patients and consider the possibility of necrotizing (malignant) otitis externa. If granulation tissue (which appears as fleshy, friable, polypoid tissue) is present in the canal, blood glucose levels should be screened.

Copious otorrhea with a slightly macerated or erythematous canal suggests chronic otitis media through a tympanic membrane perforation.

Management. Simple pruritus of the external auditory canal responds to topical hydrocortisone cream, applied with a swab three times daily as needed. In bacterial otitis externa, a narcotic-containing pain medicine, including oxycodone or meperidine, may be necessary. Mild cases are treated with a homemade preparation of 50% isopropyl alcohol (for a drying agent) and 50% vinegar (to create a hostile pH for *Pseudomonas*) applied three times daily for 1 to 2 weeks. In more severe cases, an aminoglycoside-containing ophthalmologic drop should be substituted. Formulations containing neomycin may cause severe dermatitis, which confuses the clinical picture.

If edema of the external auditory canal skin does not completely occlude the lumen, the canal should be gently cleaned with a miniature cotton-tipped applicator stick or a soft No. 6 French nasotracheal suction catheter set on low suction. An ear wick (e.g., a Pope Oto-wick) should be inserted when swelling obstructs the canal lumen.

Vesicles should be cultured for viruses since herpes otitis may benefit from oral acyclovir. Fungal infections can be treated with topical amphotericin B lotion.

Necrotizing (malignant) otitis externa requires prolonged (6 weeks or more) courses of parenteral antipseudomonal antibiotics or ciprofloxacin. An otologic consultation should be obtained whenever this disorder is suspected.

Follow-Up. Mild cases of bacterial otitis externa that respond to topical therapy do not require follow-up. In more severe cases, ear wicks should be replaced daily and the external auditory canal cleaned until the swelling goes down enough to allow ototopical drops to penetrate. These infections resolve only very slowly, and adequate analgesia is important.

Cross References: Eczema (Chapter 28), Herpes Zoster (Chapter 30), Upper Respiratory Infection (Chapter 66).

REFERENCES

1. Klein JO: Otitis media. Clin Infect Dis 1994;19:823–833.

   The author has compiled an outstanding review of the current thinking on the pediatric aspects of otitis media.

2. Pelton SI, Klein JO: The draining ear, otitis media and externa. Infect Dis Clin North Am 1988;2:117–129.

   A detailed review of these similarly presenting diseases is provided.

3. Rosenfeld RM: What to expect from medical treatment of otitis media. Pediatr Infect Dis J 1995;14:731–737.

   Recent meta-analyses pertaining to acute otitis media, recurrent acute otitis media, and otitis media with effusion are summarized, making this a "must-read" review, especially for those dealing with pediatric patients.

4. Rubin J, Yu VL: Malignant external otitis: Insights into pathogenesis, clinical manifestations, diagnosis, and therapy. Am J Med 1988;85:391–398.

   This is a good clinical guide for this very difficult disease.

57 Sinusitis

Problem

JOHN W. WILLIAMS, JR.

Epidemiology. Inflammation, with or without bacterial infection, of the paranasal sinuses leads to an estimated 6% of office visits to primary care physicians annually. Sinusitis usually follows ostial obstruction that is caused by mucosal edema or inflammation (allergens and air pollutants, viral upper respiratory tract infection, overuse of topical decongestants) or anatomic obstruction (deviated nasal septum, nasopharyngeal intubation, nasal polyps, and tumors). Patients with immunodeficiency and mucociliary dysfunction syndromes are predisposed to sinusitis. The maxillary sinuses are the most frequently involved in adults with acute sinusitis. The frontal and ethmoid sinuses are infected less frequently but carry a greater risk of serious complications; isolated sphenoid sinusitis is rare and constitutes a medical emergency because of potential cavernous sinus thrombosis or central nervous system infection.

The microbial causes of infectious sinusitis vary with the duration of symptoms. In adults with acute sinusitis (symptoms up to 3 weeks) the most common pathogens are *Streptococcus pneumoniae* (35%) and *Haemophilus influenzae* (35%). β-Lactamase–producing strains of *H. influenzae* and *Moraxella catarrhalis* are amoxicillin resistant but are not prevalent in acute sinusitis. The microbiology is not well defined for subacute sinusitis; but for chronic sinusitis (symptoms greater than 3 months), anaerobic organisms are much more common (> 50%) and infections are more likely to be polymicrobial. Fungal infections, uncommon in otherwise healthy patients, occur most frequently in patients with granulocytopenia or diabetes mellitus.

Symptoms and Signs. Acute sinusitis should be suspected when a patient has a prolonged (> 7 to 10 days) or unusually severe "cold." Usually the patient is afebrile or has a low-grade fever and does not appear very ill. Mucopurulent nasal discharge, cough, and pain in the upper teeth are characteristic symptoms and signs. Facial pain that increases when bending over or that is unilateral and failure to improve with over-the-counter decongestants or antihistamines increase the likelihood of sinusitis. Ethmoid sinusitis may be associated with orbital symptoms (e.g., edema of the eyelid, chemosis), whereas headache is frequently the most prominent symptom of sphenoid sinusitis.

Inspection of the nasal mucosa and transillumination of the sinuses are useful diagnostic maneuvers. A limited examination of the nasal mucosa can be performed using a nasal speculum mounted on a hand-held otoscope. The nasal mucosa should be examined for erythema or pallor, edema, character of nasal secretions, and polyps. Purulent secretions, particularly when coming from the middle meatus, suggest bacterial sinusitis. Facial tenderness elicited by palpation does not distinguish between acute sinusitis and other causes of nasal symptoms.

Transillumination must be performed in a completely darkened, windowless room (the examiner must close the door, turn off the lights, and allow time to adapt to darkness). The maxillary sinuses are transilluminated by placing a Welch Allyn–Finnoff transilluminator or Mini Mag-Lite over the infraorbital rim and judging light transmission through the hard palate. Normal light transmission through both maxillary sinuses makes sinusitis much less likely. Decreased or no light transmission on either side makes sinusitis more likely, but false-positive results may be caused by intrasinus polyps or a hypoplastic sinus. The frontal sinuses can be transilluminated by placing a light against the floor of the frontal sinus at the superomedial edge of the orbit. A glow should be transmitted through the anterior wall of the sinus. When interpreting this test, the clinician should remember that in approximately 5% of persons, one or both frontal sinuses have not developed and for many persons the frontal sinuses develop asymmetrically.

A predictive rule, developed in a primary care population, uses maxillary toothache, colored rhinorrhea, a history of poor response to over-the-counter nasal decongestants or antihistamines, abnormal transillumination, and mucopurulent or purulent discharge on nasal inspection. When none of the key symptoms and signs were present, the probability of sinusitis was less than 10%; when all were present, the probability of sinusitis exceeded 90%.

Clinical Approach. Diagnostic testing is recommended when considerable uncertainty exists after the clinical examination or the patient fails an initial course of therapy. Compared with sinus aspiration and culture, conventional radiographs are approximately 80% to 90% sensitive and 75% specific for maxillary sinusitis. A single Waters view is relatively inexpensive, visualizes well the maxillary and frontal sinuses, and correlates highly with the standard four-view sinus series. However, conventional radiographs visualize the ethmoid sinuses poorly. Sinus computed tomography images the ethmoid sinuses well, is a more sensitive test for sinusitis (90%–100%), but may have poor specificity (60%, therefore many false-positive results). It is used most appropriately for the evaluation of chronic sinusitis or for evaluating complications of sinusitis such as orbital abscess or cavernous sinus thrombosis. Magnetic resonance imaging is the most sensitive test for cavernous sinus thrombosis, is useful for differentiating soft tissue tumors from inflammation, and may be useful for distinguishing bacterial from fungal sinusitis.

Cultures of nasal secretions are not useful because they do not correlate with cultures from sinus antral aspirates. Although sinus aspiration and culture is the research "gold standard" for establishing sinusitis, it is recommended clinically when sinus drainage is essential and for guiding antibiotic therapy in patients with complicated or refractory sinusitis. Flexible rhinopharyngoscopy allows detailed inspection of the nasal cavity and posterior nasopharynx. Otolaryngologists frequently use this technique to establish the diagnosis of chronic sinusitis and to inspect for anatomic abnormalities that may predispose to recurrent sinusitis.

Management. Treatment is aimed at improving drainage of the sinuses and eradicating pathogens. Because randomized controlled trials have shown similar efficacy for many antibiotics, selection is based on cost, ease of dosing, and side effect profiles. At least 80% of patients with community-acquired acute sinusitis (symptoms ≤ 3 weeks) will respond to 10 to 14 days of trimethoprim-sulfamethoxazole, 160/800 mg twice daily, or amoxicillin, 500 mg three times a day. One study found that 3 days of therapy was as efficacious as 10 days, suggesting that 3-day therapy may be appropriate for selected patients with uncomplicated sinusitis. In communities with a high prevalence of amoxicillin-resistant *H. influenzae* or *M. catarrhalis* infection, broader-spectrum antibiotics such as amoxicillin-clavulanate, cefaclor, cefuroxime axetil, clarithromycin, or azithromycin are recommended. Patients with protracted symptoms may benefit from a 2- to 3-week course of antibiotics.

Topical or systemic decongestants promote sinus drainage and may be used safely in patients with mild to moderate hypertension. However, prolonged use of topical decongestants (> 5 days) may cause rebound vasodilation and rhinitis medicamentosa. For adults, one can prescribe oxymetazoline nasal spray 0.05%, 2 sprays twice daily for 3 to 5 days; pseudoephedrine sustained release, 120 mg twice daily; or phenylpropanolamine sustained release, 75 mg twice daily.

Although antibiotics and decongestants are the mainstay of therapy, a number of ancillary treatments may be beneficial.

1. Mucolytics (guaifenesin, potassium iodide) may thin secretions, and ciliatory activators (acetylcysteine) may promote sinus drainage. Evidence from one clinical trial suggests that guaifenesin, 30 mL four times a day, speeds recovery.
2. Nasal corticosteroids have a limited role in acute bacterial sinusitis but may be useful for selected patients with underlying allergic rhinitis. Nasal corticosteroids inhibit inflammatory responses without inducing adrenal suppression at usual doses and act to decrease edema of the ostiomeatal complex.
3. Steam inhalation or nasal saline may liquefy secretions, decrease crusting, and facilitate sinus drainage.
4. Antihistamines may thicken nasal secretions and therefore they are not recommended for the initial treatment of acute sinusitis. For patients with underlying allergic rhinitis, the nonsedating antihistamines are less likely to thicken secretions and may be useful ancillary treatment when topical corticosteroids have failed.

Follow-Up. Most patients feel substantially improved or cured after an average of 5 days of appropriate therapy, and consequently no specific follow-up is needed. However, patients who do not improve or who develop recurrent disease need further evaluation and treatment. If not already done, sinus radiographs should be performed to confirm the diagnosis. Once confirmed, a longer course of a broad-spectrum antibiotic effective against β-lactamase–producing organisms should be prescribed. Consultation with an otolaryngologist is appropriate for patients who appear toxic, are immunocompromised, or have complications. Serious complications of sinusitis occur rarely but include osteomyelitis, orbital abscess that can progress to blindness, or intracranial disease (meningoencephalitis, brain abscess, or cavernous sinus thrombosis). In patients with sinusitis that is refractory to medical management or that recurs three or more times per year, further evaluation by an otolaryngologist is indicated. This evaluation should include a search for anatomic factors that may predispose to sinusitis.

Cross-References: Upper Respiratory Infection (Chapter 66), Headache (Chapter 138).

REFERENCES

1. Kroenke K, Omori DM, Simmons JO, Wood DR, Meier NJ. The safety of phenylpropanolamine in patients with stable hypertension. Ann Intern Med 1989;111:1043–1044.

   A crossover trial of phenylpropanolamine (25 mg every 4 hours) in patients with systemic blood pressure less than 160 mm Hg and diastolic blood pressure less than 100 mm Hg on or off medication for hypertension showed short-term safety of this drug in patients with controlled hypertension.

2. Mabry RL. Therapeutic agents in the medical management of sinusitis. Otolaryngol Clin North Am 1993;26:561–570.

   The author provides a good general discussion of therapeutic agents used to manage sinusitis.

3. Roithmann R, Shankar L, Hawke M, Kassel E, Noyek AM. CT imaging in the diagnosis and treatment of sinus disease: A partnership between the radiologist and the otolaryngologist. J Otolaryngol 1993;22:253–260.

   The indications for CT scanning in sinusitis are discussed along with its role in the evaluation of chronic sinusitis.

4. Williams JW Jr, Holleman DR Jr, Samsa GP, Simel DL. Randomized controlled trial of 3 vs. 10 days of trimethoprim/sulfamethoxazole for acute maxillary sinusitis. JAMA 1995;273:1015–1021.

   Eighty patients were randomized to trimethoprim-sulfamethoxazole for 3 versus 10 days plus nasal sprays for 3 days. At 2-week follow-up clinical symptoms and radiograph scores improved equally (77% of the 3-day subjects and 76% of the 10-day subjects rated symptoms as cured or much improved). Symptomatic relapse and recurrence were similar between groups.

5. Williams JW Jr, Simel DL. Does this patient have sinusitis? Diagnosing acute sinusitis by history and physical examination. JAMA 1993;270:1242–1246.

   A critical review is presented of the clinical diagnosis for sinusitis in the primary care setting.

58 Cerumen Removal

Procedure

STEVEN R. McGEE

Indications and Contraindications. Common indications for removal of cerumen, or ear wax, include conductive hearing loss and the sensation of ear fullness. Hearing loss may appear suddenly, especially after swimming or showering (the epithelial component of cerumen absorbs water, swells, and occludes the canal). Tinnitus, vertigo, or intractable cough also may resolve after cerumen removal. Indications in asymptomatic patients include preparation for audiologic evaluation or tympanic membrane examination. Otitis externa, prior tympanic membrane perforation, or previous ear surgery are contraindications to ear syringing.

Rationale. Cerumen is a normal product of apocrine and sebaceous glands located in the outer one third of the external ear canal. Simple mendelian genetics determines a person's cerumen type; the dry type of cerumen, common in Asians and Native Americans, is recessive to the wet sticky type, common in whites and blacks. Cerumen inhibits the growth of bacteria and fungi in vitro; patients with inadequate cerumen, such as those with seborrheic dermatitis, may experience repeated external ear infections. Normal migration of the underlying epithelium from the tympanic membrane toward the outer canal continuously clears cerumen from the canal. Movements of the mandibular condyle during chewing also promote the exit of cerumen. Despite these self-cleansing mechanisms, cerumen sometimes becomes impacted. Predisposing factors include older age, narrow external ear canals, and the prolonged or repeated use of cotton-tipped applicator sticks, stethoscope earpieces, or hearing aid molds. Impacted cerumen may contain hair and, because of associated desquamated epithelium, may appear to have a membranous lining.

Methods. Three different techniques clear cerumen impaction: use of instruments, ear syringing, or suction. The physician may use dull ring curets to tease the edges of the cerumen away from the canal wall. The cerumen block may then be removed with the curet or tiny forceps. Because the canal is extremely sensitive and susceptible to bleeding, the use of instruments requires direct visualization and great care. During ear syringing, the physician pulls the auricle up and back and directs a stream of body-temperature tap water against the posterior-superior canal wall. Small gaps in the cerumen blockage at this location frequently allow the flow of water to pass behind the cerumen and push it out from the inside. A basin held under the ear collects the returning stream. If the cerumen is hard and does not clear easily, the patient should use a ceruminolytic (Table 58–1) for 3 days before repeat attempts at syringing. If the second attempt fails, the patient should be referred to a specialist, who may use suctioning tools to clean the canal.

Controlled clinical trials demonstrate that olive oil, used to soften ear wax for over 100 years, is as effective as proprietary ceruminolytics. Other specialists recommend a light mineral oil, such as baby oil. Most ear drops are applied twice a day (the exception is Cerumenex, which the manufacturer recommends be given only as a single dose). The patient retains each dose for 15 minutes, either by keeping the head tilted or by plugging the ear with cotton. A

Table 58–1. CERUMEN-SOFTENING AGENTS

Chemical	Product Name	OTC/Rx*	Cost†
Mixed glycerides of oleic acid	Olive oil	OTC	$ 2.83/250 ml
Trolamine polypeptide oleate-condensate	Cerumenex	Rx	$29.61/12 ml
Carbamide peroxide	Debrox drops	OTC	$ 4.58/15 ml
	Murine ear drops	OTC	$ 4.52/15 ml

*Over-the-counter (OTC) or prescription (Rx) drug.
†Average wholesale price.

ceruminolytic's ability to dissolve wax in vitro correlates poorly with its clinical efficacy.

Cross-References: Dizziness (Chapter 20), Screening for Hearing Impairment (Chapter 48), Tinnitus (Chapter 51), Cough and Sputum (Chapter 63).

REFERENCES

1. Carne S. Ear syringing. BMJ 1980;280:374–376.

   This article is a thorough illustrated guide to ear syringing.

2. Fraser JG. The efficacy of wax solvents: In vitro studies and a clinical trial. J Laryngol Otol 1970;84:1055–1064.

   A randomized double-blind controlled trial of ceruminolytics was done in elderly patients with bilateral cerumen impaction: olive oil was as effective as any other available medication.

3. Hanger HC, Mulley GP. Cerumen: Its fascination and clinical importance: A review. J R Soc Med 1992;85:346–349.

   A comprehensive review of pathophysiology, genetics, and management is presented.

SECTION VII
Respiratory Disorders

· ·

59 Screening for Occupational and Environmental Lung Disease

Screening

GRIFFITH M. BLACKMON

Epidemiology. Occupational and environmental exposures commonly cause or exacerbate respiratory illness. Workplace exposures may cause as many as 15% of adult-onset asthma cases and contribute to a similar proportion of lung cancer cases. Irritant bronchitis, occupational asthma, bronchogenic carcinoma, asbestosis, silicosis, and coal workers' pneumoconiosis are the most common occupational lung diseases in the United States. Asbestos-related lung disease remains an important clinical problem because of the characteristic 20- to 30-year lag between exposure and disease onset. Nineteen million US workers had significant asbestos exposure between 1940 and 1979, and approximately 2 million US workers (primarily in the construction industry) have ongoing, albeit lower, exposure. The incidence of work-related exacerbation of preexisting respiratory conditions (e.g., asthma, chronic obstructive pulmonary disease, rhinosinusitis) is unknown but likely a major contributor to occupational morbidity. Complaints of chest tightness and mucous membrane irritation, prominent features of sick-building syndrome, have increased over the past decade and may affect 20% of office workers.

The latency, or lag time, between exposure and disease is often helpful in the diagnosis of occupational lung disease. Patients may present within hours of exposure as with metal fume fever—a flulike syndrome after inhalation of welding fumes—or after several days with irritant bronchitis after exposure to irritant gases or dust. Occupational asthma may develop within 2 weeks but more often occurs after months or, occasionally, several years of exposure. The pneumoconioses generally present more than a decade after first exposure, although silicosis may develop within 1 year. Asbestos-related disease is variable; pulmonary fibrosis (asbestosis), pleural plaques, and malignancy almost always exhibit at least a 20-year latency, whereas benign asbestos effusions may occur within a few years of exposure.

Rationale. Identification of potential exposures, early diagnosis of disease, and prompt intervention to reduce exposure are crucial to limiting impairment and mortality. Patients may be unaware of workplace hazards or unfamiliar with safety precautions. Occupational asthma may resolve if the offending agent is withdrawn quickly but usually persists or worsens in patients with long-term or continuing exposure. Respiratory symptoms associated with sick-building syndrome generally resolve when sources of indoor pollutants are reduced (e.g., tobacco smoke, photocopying, microorganisms) and the proportion of fresh versus recirculated air within the office is increased. Even a delayed diagnosis directs subsequent therapy and often provides for additional insurance coverage or compensation for the patient through workers' compensation programs.

Occupational lung diseases are distinguished from their nonoccupational counterparts primarily by a compatible exposure history. Thus, a complete and concise work history is the best screening tool available to the clinician. Although many experts advocate annual or biannual screening of patients with asbestosis or a history of significant exposure, routine chest radiography, even in cohorts at high risk for lung cancer, does not improve survival. Conversely, the fortuitous finding of interstitial lung disease on a chest radiograph should prompt a search for occupational exposures to dusts, hard metals, and fibers. Occasionally, pathognomonic changes are encountered on the chest radiograph. Symmetric focal calcified or noncalcified pleural thickening (pleural plaques) along the lateral chest wall or diaphragms strongly suggests asbestos exposure. "Eggshell" calcification of hilar lymph nodes is classically associated with silicosis.

Pulmonary function testing (spirometry, lung volumes, and diffusing capacity) is a sensitive but nonspecific adjunct when occupational lung disease is suspected clinically.

Strategy. Primary care providers should be alert to the possibility of occupational and environmental lung disease and consider the diagnosis early in the course of any respiratory illness.

A temporal relationship between work and illness should be sought. Diagnosis of pneumoconiosis requires that a plausible latency between first exposure and disease be established. A patient with occupational asthma may present with symptoms during the workday or the following evening depending on whether the antigen elicits an immediate or delayed response. Nonspecific irritant symptoms such as rhinitis and conjunctivitis usually occur within a few hours of entering the workplace and improve rapidly with cessation of exposure. Transient improvement over weekends or vacations and reports of similar symptoms in coworkers strongly suggest an occupational link.

Offending agents should be identified as directed by the initial diagnostic impression (e.g., asthma, interstitial fibrosis, bronchitis). Careful attention to the entire work history is mandatory and often yields surprising dividends. A detailed chronology of all jobs held and description of the current or primary lifetime occupation may identify unsuspected exposures. Nonoccupational exposures such as amiodarone- or bleomycin-induced pulmonary fibrosis and recreational exposures must be sought and excluded. Preliminary information that can be obtained from material safety data sheets includes outlines of the chemical properties, adverse health effects, and recommended safety precautions for all compounds used in a workplace. Employers are legally bound to provide workers or their physicians with these documents. In the healthy patient a work review enforces primary prevention. Potentially hazardous exposures and unsafe work practices may be identified and remedied through appropriate management, union, or government channels.

Diagnostic testing should exclude nonoccupational disease. For example, collagen vascular disease should be excluded in cases of pulmonary fibrosis. Occupational asthma can be confirmed with self-measured peak expiratory flow (three efforts, six times daily over 2 weeks at work and 2 weeks off work) but requires exceptional patient compliance. A 20% decrement in flow after exposure is diagnostic.

Action. Once a diagnosis of occupational disease is made the patient must be informed of the prognosis, the health risks of continuing exposures, and the right to apply for workers' compensation. With the patient's permission, the physician may contact the employer regarding whether the patient may return to work and to prescribe specific restrictions. Beyond this, confidentiality should be strictly preserved. The employer should be contacted immediately if ongoing exposures pose an acute risk to other workers. Requirements for reporting occupational diseases should be obtained from the local health department.

The primary goal of therapy is to eliminate or reduce the causal exposure. Improving ventilation, substituting safer materials, and establishing rotating job assignments are preferable and more effective than simply providing the worker with a "gas mask" or protective respirator. Often a combined approach is required. The effective use of respirators requires continuing education and quality-control programs. Exposure should be eliminated in most cases of occupational asthma; job reassignment or retraining may be necessary. Medical therapy for occupational lung disease is identical to treatment of the nonoccupational counterpart. Inhaled corticosteroids and bronchodilators are the cornerstones of asthma therapy. Smoking cessation is strongly encouraged, and pneumococcal and influenza vaccines are indicated in patients with chronic pulmonary disease.

It is often appropriate to refer patients with known or suspected occupational disease to an occupational medicine specialist. Their training and familiarity with workers' compensation and legal issues allows a coordinated effort with the employer, industrial hygienists, local agencies, and Occupational Safety and Health Administration to return the patient to good health and a safe work environment.

Cross-References: Determining Disability: The Primary Care Physician's Role (Chapter 5), Periodic Health Assessment (Chapter 8), Adult Immunizations (Chapter 11), Dyspnea (Chapter 19), Asthma and Chronic Obstructive Pulmonary Disease (Chapter 68), Pulmonary Function Testing (Chapter 69).

REFERENCES

1. Bascom R. Occupational and environmental respiratory diseases: A medicolegal primer for physicians. Occup Med 1992;7:331–345.
   The author provides a practical introduction to the legal aspects of occupational lung disease.

2. Chan-Yeung M, Malo JL. Aetiological agents in occupational asthma. Eur Respir J 1994;7:346–371.

This excellent review includes an annotated list of known occupational sensitizers.

3. Cullen MR, Cherniack MG, Rosenstock L. Occupational medicine. N Engl J Med 1990;322:594–601, 675–683.

A comprehensive review of occupational medicine is presented.

4. Goldman RH, Peters JM. The occupational and environmental health history. JAMA 1981;264:2831–2836.

This well-written clinically oriented review includes specific recommendations.

5. Mossman BT, Gee JBL. Asbestos-related diseases. N Engl J Med 1989;320:1721–1730.

This is an extensive review, but many clinicians believe the authors understated the risks of asbestos exposure.

· ·

60 Tuberculosis Screening

Screening

JOYCE E. WIPF

Epidemiology. After a steady decline during the previous 30 years, the incidence of tuberculosis in the United States rose dramatically between 1986 and 1992 and has decreased steadily since 1992, with approximately 19,000 cases reported in 1996. However, the number and percentage of tuberculosis cases in foreign-born persons is increasing. Reasons for the recent decline in the overall number of cases include improved laboratory tests for prompter diagnosis, expanded use of preventive therapy in human immunodeficiency virus (HIV)–infected and other high-risk groups, and increased funding for tuberculosis surveillance and control. High-risk groups include individuals with HIV infection, injection drug users, alcoholics, the homeless, immigrant minority groups, and confined populations such as those in nursing homes and prisons. The only acceptable screening method is the tuberculin skin test (PPD, purified protein derivative), a test that detects delayed or cell-mediated immunity to tuberculosis infection. An estimated 10 million Americans are infected (defined as asymptomatic tuberculin skin test–positive). Eighty percent of active tuberculosis cases result from reactivation of latent infection in tuberculin reactors.

Rationale. The goals of screening are to identify infected individuals at high risk of developing active disease and to eventually eradicate tuberculosis by preventive treatment with isoniazid. Active tuberculosis ultimately develops in about 10% of infected persons; actual probabilities vary between 5% over 5 years for recent (within 2 years) converters and 0.1% per year for other reactors without additional risk factors. The risk of tuberculosis in a tuberculin-positive person with HIV infection may be as high as 8% per year. One year of isoniazid therapy is over 90% effective in preventing activation of tuberculosis, although studies of chemoprophylaxis efficacy in HIV-infected or immunocompromised patients are limited.

Strategy. The standard test is 5 tuberculin units of intermediate strength, administered intradermally with controls, and read at 48 to 72 hours. A positive test is defined as an induration greater than or equal to 5 mm in an HIV-infected person, a close contact of a patient with tuberculosis, or a patient with a chest radiograph suggestive of tuberculosis. A reaction of an induration greater than or equal to 10 mm in diameter at the site is positive in persons with any other risk factors. A skin test performed on a person without a defined risk factor for tuberculosis is positive if it produces an induration greater than or equal to 15 mm. Positive results for control antigens are defined as induration greater than or equal to 10 mm for *Candida* and *Trichophyton* and erythema greater than or equal to 5 mm for mumps.

Waning immunity or loss of immunologic recall years after exposure may cause a false-negative PPD. Therefore, elderly persons who are negative on initial testing require a second test within 2 weeks because many will show a "booster" reaction. False-positive tuberculin reactions are usually 5 to 10 mm in diameter and due to mycobacteria other than *Mycobacterium tuberculosis*. False-negative reactions are typically due to anergy and are confirmed by negative control tests. They occur in 15% of patients with proven active pulmonary tuberculosis and in up to 50% of those with miliary tuberculosis.

The Centers for Disease Control and Prevention and the American Thoracic Society recommend tuberculin testing in the following groups:

1. Persons suspected of having active tuberculosis
2. Close contacts of persons with known or suspected tuberculosis
3. HIV-infected individuals
4. Alcoholics or injection drug users
5. Residents of long-term-care facilities and prisons
6. High-risk racial minorities (blacks, Asians, Hispanics, Native Americans)
7. Newly arrived immigrants, foreign workers
8. Health care employees
9. Persons with chronic medical conditions that may put them at increased risk (data limited for most): silicosis, previous gastrectomy, end-stage renal disease, diabetes mellitus, immunosuppressive therapy or diseases, glucocorticoid therapy, myeloproliferative malignancies, and malnutrition

Action. PPD test and control results should be recorded in the patient's medical record. Periodic retesting is recommended only for nonreactors at high risk such as household contacts. Tuberculin reactors require evaluation for active tuberculosis. Six to 12 months of isoniazid, 300 mg/d, is recommended for the following asymptomatic tuberculin-reactive patients:

1. Household members and other close contacts of persons with tuberculosis (≥ 5-mm reaction)
2. Persons with HIV infection (≥ 5-mm reaction)—12 months of therapy recommended. (Injection drug users with HIV infection and cutaneous

anergy should be considered for prophylaxis because their risk of active tuberculosis appears similar to that of untreated HIV-positive tuberculin reactors.)

3. Newly infected persons (recent converters, within 2 years)
4. Persons with an abnormal chest radiograph in whom active tuberculosis has been excluded
5. Persons with associated medical conditions such as silicosis, diabetes mellitus, hematologic malignancies, end-stage renal disease, or malnutrition or those receiving chronic corticosteroid or other immunosuppressive therapy
6. All other tuberculin reactors younger than age 35

These recommendations for chemoprophylaxis are debated, particularly in healthy young adults and patients with chronic diseases, in whom data on the risk of developing active tuberculosis are limited. Patients who have probable exposure to multidrug-resistant tuberculosis should be considered for prophylaxis with ethambutol and pyrazinamide; for these cases an expert in tuberculosis should be consulted. Compliance and abstinence from alcohol are important during isoniazid therapy. Twice-weekly directly observed therapy should be considered for high-risk patients with questionable compliance.

Adverse reactions to isoniazid include rash, nausea, malaise, fever, chills, arthralgias, and peripheral neuropathy. Because the risk of isoniazid-associated hepatitis increases with age older than 35 or because patients of any age with a history of alcohol use should receive baseline liver function tests, a monthly review of symptoms and periodic liver function tests are required. If liver enzyme levels become elevated three to five times the normal value or the patient becomes symptomatic, isoniazid should be discontinued. Patients at increased risk of isoniazid-associated neuropathy due to diabetes mellitus, end-stage renal disease, history of alcohol abuse, malnutrition, pregnancy, or seizure disorder should be given 50 mg pyridoxine daily.

Cross-References: Periodic Health Assessment (Chapter 8), Fever (Chapter 16), HIV Infection: Disease Prevention and Antiretroviral Therapy (Chapter 203), HIV Infection: Office Evaluation (Chapter 204), HIV Infection: Evaluation of Common Symptoms (Chapter 205).

REFERENCES

1. American Thoracic Society. Guidelines for treatment and prevention of tuberculosis. Am J Respir Crit Care Med 1994;149:1359–1374.

   The latest statement recommendations for screening high-risk groups are presented including therapy for tuberculosis-infected persons without active disease.

2. Centers for Disease Control. Tuberculosis morbidity—United States, 1995. MMWR 1996;45:365–370.

   This issue reports statistics on changing epidemiology of tuberculosis.

3. Markowitz N, Hansen NI, Hopewell PC, et al. Incidence of tuberculosis in the United States among HIV-infected persons. Ann Intern Med 1997;126:123–132.

   In this prospective cohort study of HIV-positive patients without AIDS, 31 of 1130 developed tuberculosis (0.7 cases per 100 person-years). Tuberculosis occurred more frequently in patients with CD4 counts < 200/mm³, in tuberculin converters, and in patients living in the eastern United States.

4. Rose DN, Schechter CB, Silver AL. The age threshold for isoniazid chemoprophylaxis: A decision analysis for low risk tuberculin reactors. JAMA 1986;256:2709–2713.

Decision analysis concludes that prophylaxis is beneficial for tuberculin reactors of all ages, even low-risk individuals. Issues in the debate on chemoprophylaxis are reviewed.

5. Wipf JE, Lipsky BA. Tuberculosis screening and chemoprophylaxis: An update for clinicians. Med Rounds 1988;1:188–196.

This detailed review of the tuberculin test, mechanics of testing, and data on high-risk populations includes recommendations for testing and chemoprophylaxis with isoniazid and outlines the controversial aspects of chemoprophylaxis.

61 Pleuritic Chest Pain

Symptom

JOSHUA BENDITT

Epidemiology. Pleuritic chest pain that is related to inflammation or irritation of the parietal pleura results from a wide variety of disorders. Little data are available regarding the frequency of the disorder.

Etiology. Pleuritic chest pain is caused by inflammatory, neoplastic, and other processes that irritate the surface of the parietal pleura that covers the inner aspect of the rib cage and the diaphragm. The visceral pleura has no pain receptors. Disorders in the lung parenchyma that give rise to pleuritic pain do so because of irritation or inflammation of the parietal pleura that is in close contact with the lung.

The term *pleuritic chest pain* has been incorrectly applied to any pain that varies with the respiratory cycle (respirophasic chest pain). The most common cause of respirophasic pain is musculoskeletal injury that occurs when the injured muscle, bone, or joint is moved during the respiratory cycle. Pleuritic chest pain is sharp, usually abrupt in onset, unilateral, and worse with deep inspiration, cough, or sneeze. Musculoskeletal pain is frequently less severe and sharp and is associated with tenderness over the involved area. Musculoskeletal pain is also worsened by movement of the arm and shoulder, unlike pain arising from the pleura.

Conditions that cause pleuritic chest pain include infections such as empyema, pneumonia, tuberculosis, lung abscess, and pleurodynia. Pleurodynia is a disorder caused by viral infection of the pleura by coxsackievirus B or, rarely, coxsackievirus A and echoviruses. It occurs most frequently in the summer and fall in younger patients. Systemic diseases such as rheumatoid arthritis and systemic lupus erythematosus are associated with both pleural effusions and pleuritic chest pain, as is asbestos exposure. Pneumothorax either spontaneous or secondary to trauma, emphysema, sarcoidosis, eosinophilic granuloma, endometriosis, and lymphangioleiomyomatosis are associated with pleuritic pain. Tumors that invade the pleura and result in respirophasic pain include bronchogenic carcinoma, mesothelioma, and metastatic cancers (most frequently from breast and colon). Pulmonary embolism is associated with pleuritic chest pain, particularly when infarction of the lung that extends to the parietal pleura occurs. Pericarditis and postmyocardial injury syndrome that occur 2 to 3 weeks after an acute myocardial infarction can result in pleuritic chest pain. Abdominal processes such as subdiaphragmatic abscess can also cause pleuritic chest pain.

Clinical Approach. The initial clinical evaluation should focus on history and associated symptoms indicating a disorder requiring immediate attention and hospitalization, such as pulmonary emboli, empyema, or pneumothorax. Other causes can frequently be evaluated in the outpatient setting. Pulmonary embolism is suggested by associated dyspnea, hemoptysis, leg swelling, and a history of appropriate risk factors. A history of pneumonia or loss of consciousness, high fever, and systemic symptoms suggests empyema. Pneumothorax is associated with chest trauma, emphysema, and the other diagnoses noted above. Symptoms of arthritis and polyserositis indicating a collagen vascular disease should be sought. In the patient with systemic symptoms such as weight loss and fatigue, tuberculosis, lung cancer, and empyema are possible diagnoses.

Findings on physical examination that should be sought include pleural friction rub and findings consistent with pleural effusions as well as physical findings associated with the underlying cause of the effusion. Evaluation should include a chest radiograph that may immediately reveal the cause of the pain, for example pneumonia, pleural effusion, pneumothorax, or lung cancer. In pulmonary embolism the chest radiograph is usually normal, although focal decrease in pulmonary blood flow, pleural effusion, or an infiltrate representing pulmonary infarction may be seen. An electrocardiogram may show a pattern consistent with pulmonary embolism such as right-axis deviation or an S1 Q3 T3 pattern, evidence of pericarditis or recent myocardial infarction in the postmyocardial injury syndrome. Other laboratory investigations including a complete blood cell count and electrolyte levels including blood urea nitrogen and creatinine should be obtained. An antinuclear antibody level and a rheumatoid factor are helpful in patients in whom a connective tissue disease is suspected.

If pulmonary embolism is suspected, a ventilation-perfusion scan should be obtained, followed by bilateral lower extremity Doppler examination if the diagnosis is not established by the scan alone. If evaluation of the lower extremities is negative and pulmonary embolism is still suspected, a pulmonary arteriogram should be ordered.

Management. Management depends entirely on the underlying diagnosis responsible for the pain. Infections such as pneumonia and tuberculosis will need appropriate antibiotic therapy. Empyema will need to be treated additionally with chest tube drainage. Pneumothoraces of greater than 15% to 20% of the volume of the hemithorax also require chest tube drainage. Pulmonary embolism is treated with intravenous heparin, followed by oral anticoagulation. The pain of pulmonary embolus frequently responds within hours after heparin therapy. Pleurodynia may respond to nonsteroidal anti-inflammatory medications. Pleuritic chest pain associated with collagen vascular disease may be particularly difficult to treat. Non-narcotic pain medications are the initial therapy in these conditions also. Occasionally, intercostal nerve blocks with injections of an anesthetic agent such as lidocaine are helpful.

Follow-Up. Follow-up is tailored to the specific cause of the pleuritic chest pain.

Cross-References: Pleural Effusion (Chapter 65), Thoracentesis (Chapter 70), Recurrent Chest Pain (Chapter 74), Painful and Swollen Calf (Chapter 130).

REFERENCES

1. Branch WT, McNeil BJ. Analysis of the differential diagnosis and assessment of pleuritic chest pain in young adults. Am J Med 1983;75:671–679.

   This articles suggests methods to differentiate the more common causes of pleuritic chest pain in young adults emphasizing physical examination and chest radiographic findings in differentiating the etiology.

2. Donat WE. Chest pain: Cardiac and noncardiac causes. Clin Chest Med 1987;8:241–252.

   This excellent review of chest pain in general focuses on pathophysiologic mechanisms.

3. Hull RD, et al. A noninvasive strategy for the treatment of patients with suspected pulmonary embolism. Arch Intern Med 1994;154:289–297.

   A method is presented for diagnosing pulmonary embolism that relies predominantly on the ventilation-perfusion scan and noninvasive evaluation of the lower extremities. Pulmonary arteriogram is reserved for those cases in which noninvasive evaluation is equivocal, thus sparing patients invasive and costly procedures.

4. Light RW. Pleural Diseases. Baltimore, Williams & Wilkins, 1995.

   An excellent, up-to-date and brief review of all aspects of pleural disease is presented with an emphasis on the clinical approach to the patient.

62 Hemoptysis

Symptom

JOSHUA BENDITT

Epidemiology. Hemoptysis as a presenting clinical symptom is less common since the advent of effective antibiotic chemotherapy for tuberculosis and pneumonia. In the United States, tuberculosis and bronchiectasis, previously the most common causes of hemoptysis, have been replaced by bronchitis and lung cancer. On a worldwide basis the most common cause of hemoptysis is the parasite *Paragonimus westermani*.

Etiology. *Hemoptysis* is defined as blood that is coughed up from the lower respiratory tract—the tracheobronchial tree and the lung parenchyma. Hemoptysis may be scant, with only slight blood streaking of the sputum, or "massive," defined as the expectoration of more than 200 mL/24 h. Blood arising from the gastrointestinal tract (hematemesis) or the nasopharynx can be confused with blood from the lower respiratory tract. History, physical examination, and laboratory findings can help to differentiate these causes.

There are many diagnoses associated with hemoptysis (Table 62–1). All of these conditions lead to bleeding by one of two pathophysiologic mechanisms: (1) disruption of the integrity of the vascular wall in pulmonary blood vessels or (2) inhibition of the blood clotting system.

Clinical Approach. The initial consideration in approaching the patient with hemoptysis is to decide whether the patient is at immediate risk of massive hemoptysis, which can lead to exsanguination or respiratory embarrassment and death. Defining which patients are at risk for this complication is difficult. Most authors agree that patients who present with hemoptysis of 50 mL or more should be admitted to the hospital. Once this is established, the focus shifts to localizing the source of bleeding. Nasopharyngeal and gastrointestinal bleeding sources should be excluded. Blood originating from the gastrointestinal tract tends to be dark red or brown, has a low pH, and may contain food particles, whereas blood from the respiratory tract is usually bright red and alkaline. Nasopharyngeal bleeding can often be identified by physical examination.

Associated symptoms may suggest a specific diagnosis. Cough, fever, and purulent sputum suggest infection such as bronchitis, bronchiectasis, or pneumonia. Fetid sputum is associated with lung abscess. Pleuritic chest pain is associated with pulmonary emboli, lung abscess, and fungal cavities contiguous with the parietal pleura. A history of blunt trauma to the chest suggests lung contusion or a bronchial tear. A careful medication history should focus on drugs that may interfere with blood clotting, such as warfarin and aspirin.

The physical examination may provide crucial clues to the diagnosis. The

Table 62–1. CAUSES OF HEMOPTYSIS

Type	Frequent Causes	Infrequent Causes
Inflammatory	Bronchitis Bronchiectasis	Wegener's granulomatosis Goodpasture's syndrome
Infectious	Bronchitis Bronchiectasis Pneumonia Lung abscess Tuberculosis Paragonimiasis (worldwide)	Cystic fibrosis Fungal infection Broncholithiasis
Vascular	Pulmonary embolus	Bleeding disorders Osler-Weber-Rendu syndrome Arteriovenous malformation Mitral stenosis Chest trauma
Neoplastic	Lung cancer	Bronchial adenoma Metastatic cancer

finding of a pleural friction rub is associated with pulmonary emboli, pneumonia, and lung contusion. Clubbing suggests bronchiectasis or cancer, and a localized wheeze suggests an endobronchial lesion such as lung cancer or a benign tumor. A diastolic heart murmur may be found in mitral stenosis, and a continuous murmur is heard over the lung fields in a patient with intrapulmonary arteriovenous malformation. Telangiectases are seen in hereditary hemorrhagic telangiectasia (Osler-Weber-Rendu syndrome). A careful ear, nose, and throat examination should be performed in all patients, particularly those with a smoking history, because head and neck cancer may present as blood-streaked sputum.

The chest radiograph is invaluable in assessing the patient with hemoptysis. Cavitation and scarring in one or both upper lobes suggest tuberculosis. Bronchiectasis is associated with ring shadows and parallel "tram track" markings, both representing thickened bronchial walls. Consolidation and pleural effusion may be found with pneumonia or pulmonary embolus. A rounded opacity within a cavity suggests a fungus ball within a preexisting cavity. An enlarged left atrium, enlarged pulmonary arteries, and ossified densities at the lung bases are seen in patients with mitral stenosis. A mass lesion may signify lung cancer. Diffuse patchy infiltrates suggest alveolar hemorrhage associated with processes such as Goodpasture's syndrome or Wegener's granulomatosis.

Chest computed tomography has not been shown to add significant information to the workup of the patient with hemoptysis and a normal chest radiograph. A complete blood cell count, coagulation studies, and blood urea nitrogen and creatinine levels should be obtained.

Management. Hospitalization is recommended for those patients suspected to be at risk for massive hemoptysis: those with an initial hemorrhage of more than 50 mL or evidence of bronchiectasis, lung abscess, or a tuberculous cavity on chest radiography. Antitussive therapy, antibiotics to treat concurrent bacterial infection, and light sedation of the patient are useful initial measures in reducing bleeding. Chest physical therapy should be avoided because it may increase bleeding. Thoracic surgical consultation should be sought.

When the suspected risk of massive bleeding is low, the workup may be performed in the outpatient setting. After careful history, physical examination, and laboratory evaluation most patients will need referral to a pulmonologist for bronchoscopy. Bronchoscopy identifies the bleeding site in many cases and provides material for cytology and microbiology studies. Most outpatient episodes of hemoptysis are associated with bronchitis and respond to appropriate oral antibiotics. However, a significant number may be due to more serious but potentially treatable causes such as lung cancer and tuberculosis. In most cases, tuberculosis is identified by chest radiographic findings, skin testing, and acid-fast stained and cultured sputum samples. Treatment is with appropriate multidrug therapy. In the situation of suspected lung cancer, early and aggressive evaluation, including sputum cytologic study and bronchoscopy, is necessary. Risk factors for lung cancer diagnosed at bronchoscopy are (1) age 40 or older, (2) coughing blood for more than 1 week, (3) a smoking history, and (4) an abnormality on chest radiography. In the younger, nonsmoking patient with a clear chest radiograph in whom hemoptysis is of limited duration and associated with respiratory infection, bronchoscopy is not warranted. In older patients in whom the chest radiograph is clear and the bronchoscopy is negative, the likelihood of lung cancer is very low. These patients should have a careful ear, nose, and throat evaluation by an otolaryngologist to exclude head and neck cancer.

Follow-Up. Follow-up depends on the cause of hemoptysis and ranges from follow-up visits only if additional symptoms occur in the young, nonsmoking patient with bronchitis, to frequent outpatient follow-up in the patient with tuberculosis or bronchiectasis in whom adjustment of antibiotic therapy and assessment of treatment effect are critical.

Cross-References: Tuberculosis Screening (Chapter 60), Cough and Sputum (Chapter 63), Lower Respiratory Infection (Chapter 67), Bleeding (Chapter 195).

REFERENCES

1. Cahill BC, Ingbar DH. Massive hemoptysis: Assessment and management. Clin Chest Med 1994;15:147–167.
   The authors present an excellent review of this subject.

2. Johnston H, Reisz G. Changing spectrum of hemoptysis: Underlying causes in 148 patients undergoing diagnostic flexible fiberoptic bronchoscopy. Arch Intern Med 1989;149:1666–1668.
   This article documents the decreasing incidence of tuberculosis and its sequelae.

3. Weaver LJ, Solliday N, Cugell DW. Selection of patients with hemoptysis for fiberoptic bronchoscopy. Chest 1979;76:7–10.
   A study was done of 110 patients with hemoptysis to identify what clinical characteristics are associated with the finding of malignancy on bronchoscopy. Three factors emerged: (1) age older than 40 years, (2) any abnormality on chest radiography, and (3) hemoptysis of greater than 1 week's duration.

63 Cough and Sputum

Symptom

SHAWN J. SKERRETT

Epidemiology. Cough is a normal reflex that becomes symptomatic when unusually frequent or productive. In the 1985 National Ambulatory Medical Care Survey, cough was the sixth most common reason for consulting a physician and the second most common symptom, accounting for 2.5% of office visits. A chronic cough afflicts most smokers of more than a pack of cigarettes per day and 8% to 22% of nonsmokers.

Etiology. Involuntary coughing most often results from the stimulation of cough receptors in the larynx, trachea, or major bronchi; but it may follow irritation of the nose and paranasal sinuses, the external auditory canal, the pharynx, the diaphragm, the pleura, the pericardium, the esophagus, or the stomach.

Acute cough is accompanied by symptoms of respiratory tract infection in over 85% of cases. Chronic cough, variably defined as lasting at least 3 to 8 weeks, is often related to cigarette smoking. Among patients with chronic cough referred to pulmonologists, the most common causes are postnasal drip (30%–50%), asthma (25%–35%), gastroesophageal reflux (10%–20%), recent respiratory tract infection (10%–15%), and chronic bronchitis (5%–12%). Pertussis or chlamydial respiratory infection may cause a protracted cough lasting several weeks. Other causes include exposure to dust or noxious gases, interstitial lung disease, bronchiectasis, neoplasm (primary or metastatic), recurrent aspiration, hair or cerumen in the external ear, congestive heart failure, drugs (particularly angiotensin-converting enzyme inhibitors and β-blockers), and psychiatric disorders. Up to 25% of cases of chronic cough have more than one cause, and in 1% to 12% of cases no cause can be identified.

Clinical Approach. The history and physical examination usually suggest the diagnosis. The history should focus on smoking habits, environmental exposures, medications, the duration and character of the cough, and associated symptoms of respiratory, gastrointestinal, neurologic, and heart disease. The examination should be directed at the ears, nose, throat, neck, chest, and heart.

Postnasal drip from allergic rhinitis, perennial nonallergic rhinitis, or sinusitis is suggested by a cough productive of scant mucoid or mucopurulent sputum, worse in the morning, often associated with a sensation of secretions draining down the posterior pharynx and a need to frequently clear the throat. Nasal discharge and symptoms of sinus congestion (facial pain, headache) also occur, and examination of the nose and pharynx may reveal mucoid or mucopurulent secretions and a "cobblestone" appearance of the mucosa due to prominent submucosal lymphoid follicles. An asthmatic cough may be productive or nonproductive and is typically paroxysmal, precipitated by exertion or specific environmental exposures (e.g., cold air, perfume, smoke, pollen, dander). Although usually accompanied by dyspnea and wheezing, cough may be the sole manifestation of asthma. Most patients with gastroesophageal reflux admit to heartburn, a sour taste in the mouth, or morning hoarseness, but cough may be the only symptom. Although the cough in this setting is often nocturnal or postprandial, the absence of this pattern does not exclude reflux. A persistent cough after a viral respiratory tract infection may have features of postnasal drip or asthma; bronchial hyperreactivity may persist for up to 7 weeks after infection. Chronic bronchitis is defined by a productive cough on most days for at least 3 months of 2 or more consecutive years. Daily or recurrent production of purulent sputum is suggestive of bronchiectasis. Lung cancer may present as a new or changing cough, but additional symptoms, such as hemoptysis, chest pain, dyspnea, and weight loss, are elicited in more than 80% of cases. A dry cough precipitated by deep inhalation and associated with dyspnea on exertion is suggestive of interstitial lung disease. Patients with left ventricular failure and mitral stenosis may present with cough that is worse with exertion or supine posture. A history of neurologic, oropharyngeal, or esophageal disease or of coughing while eating should prompt consideration of recurrent aspiration.

When history and physical examination do not provide a diagnosis or grounds for a therapeutic trial, further evaluation should include a chest radiograph and spirometry. A deep nasopharyngeal culture using special swabs and culture media is required to diagnose pertussis. Methacholine challenge testing is necessary to diagnose most cases of cough-variant asthma, but bronchial provocation studies should be delayed for 8 weeks after a respiratory tract infection. Esophageal reflux may be demonstrated by barium swallow or endoscopic evidence of esophagitis, but 24-hour esophageal pH monitoring is the most sensitive method. Laryngoscopy may reveal evidence of chronic laryngeal irritation, consistent with postnasal drip or recurrent aspiration. If empirical therapy is ineffective in patients with chronic postnasal drip, sinus radiographs or limited computed tomography scans should be ordered to exclude sinusitis. Computed tomography of the chest is the preferred means of demonstrating bronchiectasis. Fiberoptic bronchoscopy and cardiac studies may be indicated in selected cases.

Management. The treatment of cough should be directed at a specific diagnosis, such as asthma, gastroesophageal reflux, chronic bronchitis, or sinusitis. Oral bronchodilators should be considered for the treatment of asthma if inhaled agents provoke coughing. Postnasal drip in the absence of infection is best treated with a long-acting oral decongestant–antihistamine combination, adding nasal corticosteroids (e.g., beclomethasone, 1 or 2 puffs in each nostril two to four times a day), if necessary. Specific treatment is effective in 87% to 98% of patients with chronic cough.

Antitussive agents should be used with caution, because cough serves to protect the airway and expel secretions. Syrups, lozenges, and topical anesthetics may be helpful in the setting of dry or irritated pharyngeal mucosa. Among the centrally active antitussives (Table 63–1), opiates are the most effective, and dextromethorphan is a useful nonprescription agent.

Mucolytics and expectorants are of uncertain value in the management of chronic productive cough, with the exception of aerosolized DNase, which reduces sputum viscosity, dyspnea, and airflow obstruction in patients with cystic fibrosis. The other agents listed in Table 63–1 have been shown to produce subjective improvement in at least one controlled trial, but the benefits are slight and inconsistently demonstrated. Postural drainage and chest physical therapy can be helpful in some patients with copious sputum or impaired airway clearance.

Table 63–1. NONSPECIFIC TREATMENT OF COUGH

Class/Agent	Dose	Daily Cost ($)*
Central Antitussives		
Codeine	15–60 mg qid	0.92
Propoxyphene	65 mg qid	0.28
Dextromethorphan†	15–30 mg qid	0.51
Diphenhydramine†	12.5–25 mg qid	0.12
Mucolytics/Expectorants		
Recombinant human DNase	2.5 mg by aerosol bid	64.80
N-Acetylcysteine	3–5 mL of 20% solution by aerosol tid–qid	8.39
Guaifenesin†	400 mg qid	0.58

*Average wholesale cost, lower daily dose listed, 1995 *Drug Topics Red Book*.
†Over-the-counter medications.

Cross-References: Sinusitis (Chapter 57), Screening for Occupational and Environmental Lung Disease (Chapter 59), Lower Respiratory Infection (Chapter 67), Asthma and Chronic Obstructive Pulmonary Disease (Chapter 68), Dysphagia and Heartburn (Chapter 96).

REFERENCES

1. Irwin RS, Curley FJ: The treatment of cough: A comprehensive review. Chest 1991;99:1477–1484.

   A thorough compendium by two investigators in the field is presented.

2. Irwin RS, Curley FJ, French CL. Chronic cough: The spectrum and frequency of causes, key components of the diagnostic evaluation, and outcome of specific therapy. Am Rev Respir Dis 1990;141:640–647.

   A specific diagnosis was made in 101 of 102 patients, and directed treatment was successful in 98%.

3. Israili ZH, Hall D: Cough and angioneurotic edema associated with angiotensin-converting enzyme inhibitor therapy: A review of the literature and pathophysiology. Ann Intern Med 1992;117:234–242.

   Cough afflicts up to 39% of patients taking these agents, occurs more commonly in women than in men, and usually resolves within 4 days of discontinuing therapy.

4. Patrick H, Patrick F: Chronic cough. Med Clin North Am 1995;79:361–372.

   This article is a recent review.

5. Pratter MR, Bartter T, Akers S, DuBois J. An algorithmic approach to chronic cough. Ann Intern Med 1993;119:977–983.

   A stepwise approach to empirical treatment and selected diagnostic testing was effective in 43 of 45 patients.

6. Nennig ME, Shinefield HR, Edwards KM, Black SB, Fireman BH. Prevalence and incidence of adult pertussis in an urban population. JAMA 1996;275:1672–1674.

   In a large health maintenance organization, the prevalence of adult pertussis was 12.4% of persons over age 18 presenting with cough for 2 weeks or longer. The annual incidence was estimated at 176 cases/100,000 population—higher than the incidence in the prevaccine era.

■ ■

64 Sleep Apnea Syndromes

Problem

HUGH F. HUIZENGA

Epidemiology. Sleep apnea syndromes are characterized by recurrent cessation of airflow during sleep sufficient to cause frequent awakening, fragmented sleep, and subsequent excessive daytime sleepiness. Sleep apnea is classified as obstructive, central, or mixed. Obstructive sleep apnea is the most common form (> 80%) and is caused by upper airway collapse during inspiration, resulting in airway obstruction. Patients with central sleep apnea (10%) have impaired respiratory drive, usually secondary to neurologic disorders or congestive heart failure. The remainder of patients (5%–10%) have mixed central and obstructive sleep apnea.

Obstructive sleep apnea affects an estimated 2% to 4% of the middle-aged population (ages 30 to 60) with a male-to-female ratio of 2:1. Sleep apnea is a significant public health problem, costing an estimated $20 billion annually in lost productivity. Individuals with sleep apnea have a two- to fourfold increased risk of automobile accidents.

Signs and Symptoms. The most common features in sleep apnea syndromes are snoring (up to 90%) and daytime hypersomnolence (50%). Morning headache (5%–10%), restless sleep, impotence, and nocturnal angina may also be reported. Nocturnal gasping or witnessed apneic events may be reported by the bed partner. The most helpful physical sign is obesity (70%). Hypertension is more common in individuals with a sleep apnea syndrome; and in more severe cases of sleep apnea syndrome, patients may develop signs and symptoms of right-sided heart failure, biventricular failure, and polycythemia.

Clinical Approach. Sleep apnea should be considered in any individual who presents complaining of daytime hypersomnolence, witnessed sleep disturbances, or unexplained pulmonary hypertension and right-sided heart failure. The history should focus on sleep habits, perceived functional impairment, psychiatric symptoms, and use of alcohol, sedatives, or other sleep-altering medications. A bed partner, if present, may also provide useful history. Careful examination of the upper airway may reveal macroglossia, hypertrophied adenoids and tonsils, nasal obstruction, droopy soft palate, or mandibular abnormalities predisposing the patient to upper airway obstruction. Elevated jugular venous pressure may be detected in patients with right-sided heart failure. Findings of left-sided heart failure may suggest central apnea as a cause of sleep-disordered breathing. Thyroid function tests should be obtained to exclude hypothyroidism.

The overall sensitivity of the history and physical examination for detecting sleep apnea is poor. The most important clinical predictors of sleep apnea syndromes are increasing age, male sex, obesity, and a history of snoring. In a study of patients referred to a sleep center with suspected sleep apnea, the subjective impression of the examiner based on history and examination had a diagnostic sensitivity of 52% and a specificity of 70%. Accurate diagnosis of sleep apnea syndromes requires a sleep study with monitoring of respiratory and neurologic parameters. The traditional gold standard for diagnosis has been polysomnography, in which patients are evaluated in a sleep center during an overnight stay with monitoring of electroencephalogram, electromyogram, respiratory airflow, respiratory muscle effort, pulse oximetry, and limb movement. The high cost of these studies ($1000) and their limited availability have led to the use of less elaborate, portable, at-home monitoring systems that generally dispense with the electroencephalographic monitoring but do include measurement of airflow, respiratory muscle effort, pulse oximetry, and limb movement. The sensitivity of these systems approaches 90% for diagnosing obstructive sleep apnea syndromes compared with formal polysomnography. They are considerably less expensive and are a reasonable initial diagnostic step. Formal polysomnography can be reserved for individuals with equivocal portable studies or suspected sleep disorders other than sleep apnea syndromes.

The severity of sleep apnea is determined on the basis of the apnea-hypopnea index, which is expressed as the number of apneic and hypopneic episodes per hour of sleep. Apneic episodes are defined as cessations of airflow lasting 10 seconds or more. Hypopneic episodes are usually defined as reduction in airflow of 50% or more associated with a decrease in oxygen saturation of 4% or more. An apnea-hypopnea index of less than 5/h is considered normal, whereas values of 10 to 30, 30 to 50, and more than 50 are considered mild, moderate, and severe sleep apnea syndromes, respectively.

Management. Once the diagnosis of a sleep apnea syndrome has been confirmed, the mainstay of therapy is nasal continuous positive airway pressure (CPAP), which effectively maintains airway patency in most individuals with obstructive sleep apnea and may be effective in some forms of central sleep apnea. The level of CPAP must be titrated to a level sufficient to prevent airway obstruction. This should be documented by a repeat sleep study. Long-term compliance with CPAP is quite variable (50%–75%) and dependent on patient motivation and perceived benefit. The most common reasons for intolerance of CPAP are rhinorrhea, nasal irritation, claustrophobia, and inconvenience.

For patients with a significant sleep apnea syndrome who are intolerant of CPAP, surgical therapy may be considered. The most common surgical procedure performed for this disorder is uvulopalatopharyngoplasty. This is effective in reducing snoring but leads to resolution of sleep apnea syndrome in only 30%. More extensive surgical procedures including genioglossus or mandibular advancement may be effective in selected patients.

Oral appliances such as tongue-retaining devices or mandibular advancement devices also may be beneficial in selected patients but can aggravate sleep apnea syndromes. Data are conflicting on the benefits of pharmacologic therapy. Protriptyline and fluoxetine may be effective in mild obstructive apnea. Medroxyprogesterone is used in patients with obesity-hypoventilation (pickwickian) syndrome who have impaired respiratory drive.

All patients should be counseled to lose weight, avoid respiratory depressants, and maintain regular sleep habits, including avoiding sleeping in the supine position if possible.

Follow-Up. Individuals should be followed for improvement in their sleep apnea syndrome symptoms. For individuals on CPAP, recurrence of previously resolved symptoms may indicate malfunctioning of the CPAP device, poor compliance, or a need to retitrate the level of CPAP. A follow-up sleep study may be required to determine the continued efficacy of therapy.

Cross-Reference: Asthma and Chronic Obstructive Pulmonary Disease (Chapter 68).

REFERENCES

1. American Thoracic Society. Indications and standards for use of nasal CPAP in sleep apnea syndromes. Am J Respir Crit Care Med 1994;150:1738–1745.

   This is an excellent review of the appropriate use, titration, and monitoring of nasal CPAP.

2. Phillipson EA, Bradley TD, eds. Breathing disorders in sleep. Clin Chest Med 1992;13(3):383–554.

A comprehensive review of pathophysiology, diagnosis, and management of sleep apnea syndromes is provided.

3. Riley RW, et al. Obstructive sleep apnea: Trends in therapy. West J Med 1995;162:143–148.

The author presents a concise review of treatment options for sleep apnea, giving special attention to surgical treatment.

4. Viner S, et al. Are history and physical examination a good screening test for sleep apnea? Ann Intern Med 1991;115:356–359.

The limits of the history and physical examination in screening for sleep apnea are discussed.

■ ■

65 Pleural Effusion

Problem

FEROZA DAROOWALLA and JOSHUA BENDITT

Epidemiology. A pleural effusion is a collection of fluid in the space between the visceral pleura lining the lungs and the parietal pleura covering the diaphragm and the chest wall. Pleural effusions are classified according to their chemical characteristics into transudates and exudates. Exudates are protein-rich fluids that result from an alteration of the pleural surface that allows protein molecules to move from the serum into the pleural space. Transudates are protein-poor effusions that form in the pleural space as a result of excessive capillary hydrostatic pressure or low plasma oncotic pressure.

Pleural effusions have a wide range of causes (Table 65–1). The most common causes of pleural effusions in the United States are congestive heart failure (~500,000 cases/year), pneumonia (~300,000 cases/year), and malignancy (~200,000 cases/year).

Transudative pleural effusions are most often associated with congestive heart failure or cirrhosis. Exudative effusions most commonly result from pneumonia, malignant pleural disease, pulmonary embolism, or gastrointestinal disease.

Symptoms and Signs. Pleural effusions may be asymptomatic or associated with dyspnea and sometimes pleuritic chest pain. Other symptoms associated with this disorder are related to the underlying cause of the effusion. The degree of shortness of breath is related to the size of the effusion and the preexisting function of the lung. Signs on physical examination include decreased chest excursion over the effusion, reduced tactile fremitus, dullness to percussion, and decreased breath sounds.

Clinical Approach. Clinical suspicion or an abnormal chest radiograph should initiate an investigation for a pleural effusion. An upright, lateral chest radiograph with an obscured posterior costophrenic sulcus or posterior diaphragm

Table 65–1. CAUSES OF PLEURAL EFFUSIONS

Transudates	Exudates
Congestive heart failure	Infectious
Cirrhosis	Bacterial pneumonia
Nephrotic syndrome	Tuberculous pleurisy
Peritoneal dialysis	Subphrenic abscess
Hypoalbuminemia	Hepatic abscess
Urinothorax	Drug induced
Atelectasis	Esophageal perforation
Constrictive pericarditis	Malignancy
Trapped lung	Carcinoma, lymphoma
Superior vena cava obstruction	Chylothorax
	Meigs' syndrome
	Pancreatitis
	Connective tissue disease
	Hypothyroidism
	Lymphangioleiomyomatosis
	Benign asbestos pleural effusion

suggests the need to determine the presence of free fluid in the pleural space. This is achieved with bilateral decubitus chest films. Almost all patients with free fluid that forms a layer of more than 10 mm between the inside of the thoracic cavity and the outside of the lung should undergo a diagnostic thoracentesis. Laboratory tests on the initial diagnostic fluid sample should include those for lactate dehydrogenase (LDH), protein, and glucose, with accompanying values for serum, and a Gram stain. The results of these tests aid in classification of the effusion as either a transudate or an exudate. Exudates are characterized by one of the following criteria: (1) LDH pleural fluid/serum ratio more than 0.6, (2) total LDH more than two thirds of the upper value of normal, or (3) protein pleural fluid/serum ratio more than 0.5. When the suspicion for a transudate is very high, the LDH level in fluid and serum can be checked first. If the fluid is in fact a transudate, no further tests need to be ordered, resulting in a more cost-effective approach.

Most transudative effusions result from extrapulmonary causes, and further workup should focus on identifying other organ systems that may be involved. This investigation should include history, physical examination, and routine tests, such as electrocardiography; determination of electrolyte, blood urea nitrogen, and creatinine levels; and screening liver function tests.

Thoracentesis can be deferred in clear-cut cases of congestive heart failure until the cardiac disease is better controlled because this is frequently accompanied by the resolution of the effusion. However, a diagnostic thoracentesis should be performed in cases of congestive heart failure with an effusion that is unilateral, growing, associated with fever or pleuritic chest pain, unequal to the other side, causing symptoms, or not accompanied by clear cardiomegaly. A diagnostic thoracentesis and paracentesis should also be performed in cases of hepatic hydrothorax with associated cirrhosis and ascites to confirm the transudative nature of the effusion and the ascitic fluid.

The differential diagnosis of an exudative effusion is more extensive (see Table 65–1) and may require detailed laboratory investigation. For exudates of unknown cause, cytologic studies and cultures for bacteria (aerobic and anaerobic), mycobacteria, and fungi should be performed. Bloody-appearing effusions should be sent for hematocrit, cell count, cultures, and cytology. In a suspected case of pleural malignancy or in an undiagnosed exudate, repeated thoracenteses can be useful: three separate specimens of fluid will yield positive cytology 90% of the time with such a malignancy. Exudates associated with pneumonia should be checked for pH, glucose, Gram stain, culture and sensitivity, and LDH. Antinuclear antibody and rheumatoid factor levels may be helpful to diagnose effusions associated with collagen vascular disease.

Management. Appropriate treatment of a pleural effusion depends on the underlying etiology. Generally, however, a symptomatic effusion should be drained after diagnostic tests are sent. One thousand milliliters can be safely drained at a time.

Effusions in cases of congestive heart failure can be managed medically with diuretics and afterload reduction. They can be drained if necessary to give symptomatic relief. Effusions associated with liver disease are treated by management of the ascites with diuretics.

A parapneumonic effusion, that is, fluid associated with a pneumonia, is managed with antibiotics (no increase in dose needed) unless the thoracentesis reveals pus (called an empyema), pH is less than 7.1, glucose is less than 40 mg/dL, the Gram stain is positive for microorganisms, or there are loculations (detected by ultrasonography or computed tomography of the chest). These findings imply active infection in the pleural space and represent a complicated parapneumonic effusion or empyema. In this situation, drainage can be achieved by chest tube or by more invasive surgical procedures if the fluid cannot be drained with the chest tube alone.

A hemothorax is defined as pleural fluid with hematocrit greater than or equal to 50% of the serum hematocrit and usually requires a chest tube for drainage. Further invasive investigation should follow if bleeding continues or if the chest tube is ineffective in draining the pleural space secondary to clotting blood.

Tuberculous pleuritis classically presents 3 to 6 months after a primary tuberculous infection as an exudative effusion without evidence of parenchymal involvement on plain radiographs. A delayed-type hypersensitivity reaction is thought to play a role in this presentation, and the mycobacterial burden in this pleural fluid is low. In this presentation, the fluid will reabsorb but can be followed by pleural thickening. Another clinical presentation in the patient with tuberculosis involves effusion associated with reactivation of disease. Pleural fluid in this case is more likely to have a positive acid-fast bacillus smear and culture for mycobacteria. Tuberculous pleuritis is treated as active pulmonary disease with antituberculous medicines. Drainage is not indicated unless the fluid is thick with a large number of organisms on acid-fast smear, making it consistent with a tuberculous empyema.

Follow-Up. Follow-up of a pleural effusion depends on the underlying cause. If an effusion is not tapped on the initial evaluation, radiographs should be obtained within 2 weeks to look for enlargement of the effusion. Enlargement mandates thoracentesis. For recurrent effusions that are symptomatic, invasive procedures such as chemical or mechanical pleurodesis can be attempted to approximate the layers of the pleura and prevent further fluid collection.

Cross-References: Pleuritic Chest Pain (Chapter 61), Pulmonary Function Testing (Chapter 69), Thoracentesis (Chapter 70).

REFERENCES

1. Broaddus VC. Infections in the pleural space: An update on pathogenesis and management. Semin Respir Crit Care Med 1995;16:303–331.

   The author discusses pathogens in empyemas and tuberculous pleuritis in human immunodeficiency virus–positive patients.

2. Hott JW. Malignant pleural effusions. Semin Respir Crit Care Med 1995;16:333–339.

   One third of malignant effusions are secondary to lung carcinoma. Breast cancers and lymphomas are the second and third leading causes of malignant effusions.

3. Light RW. Pleural Diseases. Baltimore, Williams & Wilkins, 1995.

   This is a recent text on pleural diseases including effusions by one of the experts.

4. Sahn SA. Management of complicated parapneumonic effusions. Am Rev Respir Dis 1993; 148:813–817.

   One well-accepted approach to parapneumonic effusions is presented.

5. Sahn SA. The diagnostic value of pleural fluid analysis. Semin Respir Crit Care Med 1995;16:269–278.

   A pleural fluid glucose level between 0 and 30 is associated with rheumatoid pleurisy; if it is between 30 and 59 it is associated with malignancy, tuberculosis, and lupus pleuritis. Many other diagnostic "pearls" are included.

- -

66 Upper Respiratory Infection

Problem

SHAWN J. SKERRETT

Epidemiology. Infections of the upper respiratory tract, including the overlapping clinical syndromes of the common cold, influenza, sinusitis, otitis media, pharyngitis, and laryngitis, are the most common acute illnesses affecting humans. Adults average two to four colds per year, with exposure to children in the home being an important risk factor. Colds occur year-round, with different viruses prominent in each season. Sinusitis and otitis media are infrequent complications of common colds, developing in fewer than 1% of cases in adults. Influenza occurs every winter with overall attack rates of 10% to 20%, higher in epidemic and pandemic years. Lower respiratory tract complications of influenza, including tracheobronchitis and viral or bacterial pneumonia, develop in 10% of all patients, mainly in a high-risk group composed of persons older than age 65, residents of chronic care facilities, and persons with diabetes, immunodeficiencies, hemoglobinopathies, and chronic heart, lung, or kidney disease.

Although most upper respiratory tract infections do not come to medical attention, acute respiratory symptoms are the most common reasons for consulting a physician, accounting for 12% to 14% of outpatient physician contacts. Over 40% of time lost from work and school is due to acute respiratory illnesses.

The common cold is caused by rhinoviruses in 30% to 40% of cases in adults, coronaviruses in 10% to 20%, other respiratory viruses in 10% to 20%, and unidentified agents in 30% to 40%. Laryngitis is viral in origin in over 90% of cases; the most common causes are influenza, rhinovirus, adenovirus, and parainfluenza. The etiologic agents of otitis, pharyngitis, and sinusitis are discussed in other chapters.

Symptoms and Signs. The clinical manifestations of the common cold are familiar to everyone. After a 2- to 5-day incubation period, the prototypical rhinovirus infection begins with a scratchy discomfort in the throat, followed by rhinorrhea (initially watery, then mucopurulent), nasal congestion, sneezing, and cough. Fever is rare and low grade when present. The acute symptoms usually resolve within 7 days, but cough, due to postnasal drip, viral tracheobronchitis, or bronchial hyperreactivity, may persist for several weeks. Symptoms of sinusitis may include facial or dental pain, fever, anosmia, and purulent nasal discharge. Ear pain, drainage from the ear, and hearing loss are common manifestations of otitis media. Influenza may present as symptoms similar to the common cold, but nasal features are typically less prominent, whereas cough and systemic manifestations such as fever, malaise, headache, and myalgias are more severe. Most symptoms of uncomplicated influenza resolve within 7 days, but lassitude and cough may persist for weeks.

Examination of the patient with the common cold reveals erythema and crusting of the nares, erythema and edema of the nasal mucosa, and nasal discharge; mild pharyngeal injection may be seen. The presence of a pharyngeal exudate and tender cervical adenopathy is suggestive of bacterial pharyngitis, mononucleosis, or adenovirus infection; the latter often causes an associated conjunctivitis (pharyngoconjunctival fever). Vesicles on the palate suggest infection with coxsackievirus or herpes simplex virus. A purulent nasal discharge, facial tenderness, and loss of maxillary transillumination are indicative of sinusitis. Otitis media is diagnosed by the presence of fluid in the middle ear, most reliably identified on pneumatic otoscopy by an immobile tympanic membrane.

Clinical Approach. Most patients with upper respiratory infections are self-diagnosed; evaluation is directed at confirming the diagnosis and excluding complications. Allergic and vasomotor rhinitis may mimic the common cold but can be distinguished by the exposure history and chronicity, respectively. Influenza should be differentiated from the common cold on the basis of clinical features. Specific virologic diagnosis of colds and influenza is unnecessary. The clinical approaches to pharyngitis, otitis media, sinusitis, and pneumonia are discussed in separate chapters.

Management. The treatment of the common cold is aimed at relief of symptoms (Table 66–1). Sympathomimetics effectively relieve nasal congestion but do not reduce rhinorrhea. Topical decongestants are at least as effective as oral agents and have fewer side effects, but rebound symptoms may occur if topical decongestants are used for more than 3 or 4 days. Topical parasympatholytics, such as ipratropium bromide, are effective in reducing nasal discharge. The use of antihistamines is controversial, but their anticholinergic effects may help dry unwanted secretions. Acetaminophen and aspirin are helpful for pain and fever. Multiple-combination preparations should be avoided. There is no role for antibacterial antibiotics, and antiviral therapy for the common cold remains elusive. Although topical interferon alfa-2 has shown prophylactic efficacy, its therapeutic activity has been disappointing, and irritation of the nasal mucosa has been a limiting side effect. Vitamin C, zinc, and countless folk remedies are popular but of uncertain value.

Table 66–1. OVER-THE-COUNTER NASAL DECONGESTANTS
(WITH REPRESENTATIVE DRUGS)

Medication	Dose	Cost ($)*
Topical Sympathomimetics		
Phenylephrine 0.5%	2–3 sprays or drops qid	
Dristan		3.84 (15 mL)
Neo-Synephrine		3.52 (15 mL)
Naphazoline 0.05%	2–3 sprays or drops qid	
Privine		3.64 (15 mL)
Oxymetazoline 0.05%	2–3 sprays or drops bid	
Afrin		4.36 (15 mL)
Neo-Synephrine 12 Hour		4.13 (15 mL)
Xylometazoline	2–3 sprays or drops bid	
Otrivin		4.88 (20 mL)
Oral Sympathomimetics		
Pseudoephedrine	60 mg qid or 120 mg bid	
Sudafed		3.94 (24 tablets, 30 mg)
Sympathomimetic/Antihistamine Combinations		
Pseudoephedrine plus	60 mg qid or 120 mg bid	
Brompheniramine	6 mg qid or 12 mg bid	
Bromfed		6.25 (120 mL, 30/2)†
Pseudoephedrine plus	60 mg qid or 120 mg bid	
Chlorpheniramine	4 mg qid or 8 mg bid	
Allerest Tabs		3.98 (24 tablets, 30/2)
Sudafed Plus		4.73 (24 tablets, 60/4)
Phenylpropanolamine plus	25 mg qid or 75 mg bid	
Brompheniramine	4–6 mg qid or 12 mg bid	
Dimetapp Tabs		4.46 (24 tablets, 25/4)
Phenylpropanolamine plus	25 mg qid or 75 mg bid	
Chlorpheniramine	4 mg qid or 8 mg bid	
Contac		4.10 (10 tablets, 75/8)
Coricidin D		4.36 (24 tablets, 12.5/2)‡
Triaminic		5.42 (24 tablets, 25/4)

*Average wholesale price, 1995 *Drug Topics Red Book.*
†Quantity of first medication/quantity of second medication per tablet or 5 mL.
‡Also contains 325 mg acetaminophen.

Vaccination is effective in reducing the incidence and severity of influenza A and B and should be offered to all patients at high risk. Amantadine and rimantadine are active against influenza A and should be considered as supplements to vaccination for prophylaxis in high-risk patients during an outbreak of influenza A. These agents are also effective as therapy for influenza A if they are given within 48 hours of the onset of symptoms; therapeutic use should be considered in high-risk patients. Both drugs are given in doses of 100 mg twice daily for patients younger than 65 years of age and 100 mg daily for older patients. The dose must be reduced for patients with renal dysfunction. Rimantadine appears to have fewer gastrointestinal and central nervous system side effects. Prophylactic antiviral therapy should be continued through the period of exposure, and treatment of established influenza should be given for 3 to 5 days. The treatment of sinusitis, pharyngitis, and otitis is discussed elsewhere.

Follow-Up. Follow-up of the common cold is unnecessary unless patients develop symptoms of otitis or sinusitis. Patients with influenza, particularly the elderly, should be warned about lower respiratory tract symptoms (dyspnea, worsening cough, recurrence of fever) that suggest the development of pneumonia.

Cross-References: Adult Immunizations (Chapter 11), Pharyngitis (Chapter 54), Otitis Media and Externa (Chapter 56), Sinusitis (Chapter 57), Cough and Sputum (Chapter 63), Lower Respiratory Infection (Chapter 67).

REFERENCES

1. Centers for Disease Control and Prevention. Prevention and control of influenza: Recommendations of the advisory committee on immunization practices (ACIP). MMWR 1996;45(RR-5):1–24.
   A concise summary of immunization, chemoprophylaxis, and treatment is provided.

2. Forstall GJ, Macknin ML, Yen-Lieberman BR, Medendrop SV. Effect of inhaling heated vapor on symptoms of the common cold. JAMA 1994;272:1109–1111.
   Chicken soup revisited? The authors present a negative study.

3. Lowenstein SR, Parrino TA. Management of the common cold. Adv Intern Med 1987;32:207–233.
   The authors engagingly present a review of fact and fancy about the common cold.

4. Mossad SB, Macknin ML, Medendorp SW, Mason P. Zinc gluconate lozenges for treating the common cold: a randomized, double-blind, placebo-controlled study. Ann Intern Med 1996;125:81–88.
   The duration of most symptoms was reduced if zinc was started within 24 hours of onset.

5. Smith MBH, Feldman W. Over-the-counter cold medications: A critical review of clinical trials between 1950 and 1991. JAMA 1993;269:2258–2263.
   This article includes a helpful analysis of the literature.

67 Lower Respiratory Infection

Problem

SHAWN J. SKERRETT

Epidemiology and Etiology. Lower respiratory tract infections include tracheo-bronchitis and pneumonia. In the United States there are over 3 million cases of community-acquired pneumonia in adults each year, leading to more than 500,000 hospital admissions. Risk factors for lower respiratory tract infection include chronic airway disease (e.g., chronic bronchitis, bronchiectasis, or bronchogenic carcinoma), an aspiration diathesis (such as alcoholism or a seizure disorder), recent upper respiratory tract infection (especially influenza), advanced age, and immunodeficiency.

Table 67–1 lists the common causes of community-acquired pneumonia in hospitalized patients. *Mycoplasma, Chlamydia,* and viruses often cause relatively mild illnesses that are typically treated in the ambulatory setting and may be underrepresented in the table. Acute tracheobronchitis is most often caused by viruses, followed by *Mycoplasma pneumoniae, Chlamydia pneumoniae,* and *Bordetella pertussis.* Acute exacerbations of chronic bronchitis associated with purulent sputum are commonly due to *Haemophilus influenzae, Streptococcus pneumoniae,* and *Moraxella (Branhamella) catarrhalis.*

Symptoms and Signs. Acute tracheobronchitis presents as cough that is often productive and usually accompanied by concurrent or recent symptoms of upper respiratory tract infection. Examination may reveal rhonchi or wheezes, but there are no signs of pneumonia.

The cardinal symptoms of pneumonia are cough (75% to 90%, productive in 60% to 70%) and fever (60% to 70%). Dyspnea and chills each occur in

Table 67–1. ETIOLOGIC AGENTS OF COMMUNITY-ACQUIRED PNEUMONIA IN HOSPITALIZED ADULTS

Organism	% of Cases
Streptococcus pneumoniae	10–40
Haemophilus influenzae	5–15
Viruses	5–15
Mixed oral flora	3–15
Mycoplasma pneumoniae	2–15
Chlamydia pneumoniae	5–10
Pneumocystis carinii	2–13
Legionella species	2–4
Gram-negative bacilli	1–8
Staphylococcus aureus	1–8
Unknown	30–50

All of the material in Chapter 67 is in the public domain, with the exception of any borrowed figures and tables.

about 50% and chest pain in 30% to 40%. Most patients have fever, often with tachycardia and tachypnea. The chest examination is abnormal in over 90% of patients, revealing crackles, diminished breath sounds, rhonchi, and egobronchophony, in decreasing order of frequency. Elderly patients may present with more subtle signs, such as an isolated alteration in mental status.

Clinical Approach. Routine laboratory tests for suspected pneumonia should include a chest radiograph, complete blood cell count, and, when available, sputum for Gram stain and culture. Although most patients with fever, cough, and an infiltrate on chest radiograph have infection, a similar presentation can result from a variety of noninfectious processes, such as pulmonary embolism, gastric aspiration, malignancy, drug toxicity, hypersensitivity, and vasculitis.

Clues to the microbial etiology of pneumonia may be found in the patient's medical history. Aspiration diatheses and poor dentition predispose to infection with mixed aerobic and anaerobic oral flora. Alcoholism, diabetes mellitus, and chronic renal failure are associated with colonization of the upper respiratory tract with gram-negative bacilli and *Staphylococcus aureus* and an increased risk of pneumonia due to these organisms (although pneumococcus is the most common agent in this group of patients). The lower respiratory tract of patients with chronic obstructive pulmonary disease is often colonized with pneumococcus, *H. influenzae*, or *M. catarrhalis*, predisposing to infection with these agents. Neutropenia or defective neutrophil function predisposes to infection with gram-negative bacilli, *S. aureus*, and *Aspergillus*. Impaired humoral immunity, as may be found in multiple myeloma or chronic lymphocytic leukemia, leads to an increased risk of infection with encapsulated organisms such as pneumococcus and *H. influenzae*. Defective cell-mediated immunity may result from T-cell lymphomas or corticosteroid therapy, for example, and increases the risk of infection with mycobacteria, *Legionella*, fungi, cytomegalovirus, and *Pneumocystis carinii*. Human immunodeficiency virus infection predisposes to a wide variety of respiratory infections, reflecting damage to both humoral and cell-mediated immune responses. Pneumonia in previously healthy young adults is usually caused by *M. pneumoniae*, *C. pneumoniae*, a respiratory virus, pneumococcus, or *H. influenzae*.

The clinician should inquire about exposure to specific infectious agents. Illness in the community may suggest influenza, other viruses, or pertussis. Exposure to sick children raises the possibility of *Mycoplasma* infection. Residence in a dormitory or barracks increases the risk of epidemic infection with *M. pneumoniae*, *C. pneumoniae*, *Neisseria meningitidis*, or adenovirus. Nursing home residents are at risk for outbreaks of influenza, respiratory syncytial virus, and tuberculosis, as well as staphylococcal and gram-negative infection. Prisoners and residents of shelters are at particular risk for tuberculosis and epidemic pneumococcal infections. A travel history may suggest exposure to geographically restricted airborne fungi such as *Histoplasma* (Ohio, Mississippi, and Missouri River valleys), *Blastomyces* (central and southeastern United States), and *Coccidioides* (southwestern United States), or regionally distributed bacteria such as *Pseudomonas pseudomallei* (Southeast Asia) and *Legionella* (often resident in community water towers and hot-water systems of old hotels). Also helpful is an occupational or recreational history of exposure to poultry or birds of the parrot family (psittacosis), domestic livestock such as cattle, sheep, and goats (Q fever, brucellosis, and anthrax), and wild rodents (tularemia, plague, and hantavirus).

The typical acute pneumonia syndrome consisting of an abrupt onset of fever, chills, pleuritic chest pain, and cough productive of purulent sputum suggests infection with pyogenic bacteria such as pneumococcus, *Staphylococcus*, or *H. influenzae*. The atypical pneumonia syndrome, defined by a more insidious onset, nonproductive cough, and prominent extrathoracic symptoms such as headache, myalgias, and diarrhea, is commonly associated with *Mycoplasma*, *Chlamydia*, viruses, and Q fever *(Coxiella burnetii)*. There is substantial overlap between these syndromes, however, and clinical features are not reliable predictors of microbial etiology.

The chest radiograph may reveal evidence of endobronchial obstruction, such as mass lesions, or volume loss. Lobar or segmental consolidation is usually due to a bacterial process, whereas bilateral mixed alveolar–interstitial infiltrates most likely represent viral or *Pneumocystis* infection. Nodular infiltrates suggest fungi, mycobacteria, *Legionella*, or *Nocardia*. Cavitation usually indicates infection with mixed anaerobes, gram-negative bacilli, *S. aureus*, hemolytic streptococci, fungi, or mycobacteria. Pleural effusions are evidence against viral or *Mycoplasma* infection. All parapneumonic effusions producing more than blunting of the costophrenic angle should be tapped to exclude empyema.

A sputum Gram stain with fewer than 10 squamous epithelial cells and more than 25 neutrophils per low-power field and a single predominant organism when examined under high power is very accurate in directing therapy. Unfortunately, a diagnostic Gram stain is available in less than 50% of patients with community-acquired pneumonia. Other rapid diagnostic methods, which detect microbial antigens or nucleic acids in respiratory specimens, are expensive and usually unnecessary in the outpatient setting. In patients with acute purulent bronchitis, microbiologic studies of sputum are necessary only if empirical therapy has failed.

Management. The indications for hospital admission include the following:

1. Features of severe illness, including hypotension (systolic blood pressure < 90 mm Hg), marked tachycardia (heart rate > 140 beats per minute), altered mental status, respiratory distress or hypoxemia (arterial Po_2 < 60 mm Hg or oxygen saturation < 90% by pulse oximetry), multilobar involvement, evidence of a suppurative complication (such as empyema or metastatic infection), or severe hematologic or metabolic abnormalities (such as neutropenia, marked hyponatremia, or new azotemia)
2. A high risk for a complicated course because of immunodeficiency, postobstructive pneumonia, or suspected infection with particularly virulent organisms, such as *S. aureus* and gram-negative bacilli
3. Suspicion of an opportunistic or unusual infection that warrants further diagnostic evaluation under observation

Further, hospital admission should be considered in patients older than 65 years, those with underlying chronic disease that may impair host defenses or pulmonary reserve (e.g., chronic renal insufficiency, diabetes mellitus, congestive heart failure, and chronic obstructive pulmonary disease), and patients whose socioeconomic circumstances interfere with reliable treatment and follow-up.

Table 67–2. ORAL ANTIBIOTICS FOR LOWER RESPIRATORY INFECTION

Antibiotic	Dose	Cost ($)*
Erythromycin	500 mg qid	15.50
Clarithromycin	500 mg bid	62.94
Azithromycin	500 mg then 250 mg qd	36.23
Amoxicillin	500 mg tid	9.00
Amoxicillin/clavulanate	875 mg/125 mg bid	78.00
Cefaclor	500 mg tid	122.10
Cefuroxime axetil	500 mg bid	123.98
Cefprozil	500 mg bid	106.51
Loracarbef	400 mg bid	75.60
Doxycycline	100 mg bid	6.89
Trimethoprim/sulfamethoxazole	160 mg/800 mg bid	4.48

*Average wholesale cost of 10-day supply (5 days for azithromycin), 1995 *Drug Topics Red Book.*

The antibiotic treatment of pneumonia should be based on the sputum Gram stain, whenever possible. Empirical therapy can be directed at the likely etiologic agents according to risk factors and clinical presentation. For healthy adults younger than 60 years of age, a macrolide such as erythromycin, clarithromycin, or azithromycin is usually the drug of choice when sputum is nondiagnostic. For older patients and those with underlying diseases, a second-generation cephalosporin or amoxicillin (with or without clavulanate) is recommended, with macrolides, trimethoprim-sulfamethoxazole, or doxycycline as acceptable alternatives for those with penicillin allergy. Antibiotics are unnecessary in most cases of acute bronchitis, but patients with underlying chronic obstructive pulmonary disease and newly purulent sputum may benefit from treatment with amoxicillin, trimethoprim-sulfamethoxazole, or tetracycline. Dosages and costs are listed in Table 67–2.

Follow-Up. Treatment failures result from an incorrect presumptive etiologic diagnosis, obstruction to bronchial drainage, development of a suppurative complication such as empyema, or noncompliance. Patients should be seen routinely within 1 week and should be advised to return for increasing dyspnea or chest pain, alteration in mental status, or persistent fever after 3 days of treatment. All patients with pneumonia should have a follow-up chest radiograph 6 to 12 weeks after presentation to document complete resolution.

Cross-References: Cough and Sputum (Chapter 63), Pleural Effusion (Chapter 65), Upper Respiratory Infection (Chapter 66), Asthma and Chronic Obstructive Pulmonary Disease (Chapter 68), HIV Infection: Disease Prevention and Antiretroviral Therapy (Chapter 203).

REFERENCES

1. Bartlett JG, Mundy LM. Community-acquired pneumonia. N Engl J Med 1995;333:1618–1624.
   The authors present an excellent and concise review.

2. Boldy DAR, Skidmore SJ, Ayres JG. Acute bronchitis in the community: Clinical features, infective factors, changes in pulmonary function and bronchial reactivity to histamine. Respir Med 1990;84:377–385.

A prospective study was done of 42 episodes in 40 patients without underlying lung disease. An etiology was identified in 12 episodes (viral or mycoplasma in 11/12), and 37% of patients had reactive airways 6 weeks after presentation.

3. Fine MJ, Smith MA, Carson CA, Mutha SS, Sankey SS, Weissfield LA, Kapoor WN. Prognosis and outcomes of patients with community-acquired pneumonia: A meta-analysis. JAMA 1996;275:134–141.

From 122 studies, factors consistently associated with increased mortality included advanced age, male sex, diabetes mellitus, neurologic disease, neoplasia, pleuritic chest pain, hypothermia, tachypnea, hypotension, leukopenia, multilobar infiltrates on chest radiograph, bacteremia, and gram-negative or staphylococcal etiology.

4. Heckerling PS, Tape TG, Wigton RS, Hissong KK, Leiken JB, Ornato JP, Cameron JL, Racht EM. Clinical prediction rule for pulmonary infiltrates. Ann Intern Med 1990;113:664–670.

Among patients with acute respiratory complaints, the following were independent predictors of radiographic infiltrates: temperature greater than 37.8°C, pulse more than 100 beats per minute, rales, decreased breath sounds, and the absence of asthma.

5. Niederman MS, Bass JB, Campbell GD, Fein AM, Grossman RF, Mandell LA, Marrie TJ, Sarosi GA, Torres A, Yu VL. Guidelines for the initial management of adults with community-acquired pneumonia: Diagnosis, assessment of severity, and initial antimicrobial therapy. Am Rev Respir Dis 1993;148:1418–1426.

An official statement of the American Thoracic Society provides sensible guidelines with supporting rationale.

· ·

68 Asthma and Chronic Obstructive Pulmonary Disease

Problem

SHAWN J. SKERRETT

Definitions and Epidemiology. Asthma is a clinical syndrome of episodic symptoms associated with reversible airflow obstruction and bronchial hyperreactivity. Chronic obstructive pulmonary disease (COPD) is defined by progressive symptoms and irreversible airflow obstruction. The two major components of COPD are chronic bronchitis, defined by a productive cough on most days for at least 3 months of 2 consecutive years, and emphysema, defined anatomically by the destruction of alveolar walls and clinically by progressive airflow limitation, hyperexpansion, and reduced diffusing capacity for carbon monoxide. There is considerable overlap between asthma and COPD.

Asthma afflicts 3% to 5% of the adult population and accounts for 1% of outpatient visits. The mortality from asthma is rising, particularly among blacks and the elderly. COPD is found in 5% to 10% of the adult population, predominantly smokers, and is the fifth leading cause of death.

Symptoms and Signs. Most patients with asthma have episodes of cough, wheeze, chest tightness, and dyspnea, separated by symptom-free intervals. Some patients have chronic symptoms punctuated by exacerbations, and cough may be the only manifestation. Common precipitating factors include airborne allergens and nonspecific stimuli such as cold air, irritants, and exercise. COPD typically presents as gradually progressive dyspnea on exertion, chronic productive cough, or both. Many patients with COPD have periodic exacerbations of their symptoms, often associated with upper respiratory tract infections, changes in weather, or exposure to irritants.

The physical examination of the asthmatic patient with mild or absent symptoms may be normal. Diffuse wheezing is often apparent on chest auscultation, but it may be detectable only on forced exhalation. An inspiratory-to-expiratory ratio of less than 1 may be the only indication of airflow obstruction. Evidence of atopy may be present, including rashes, coryza, nasal polyps, postnasal drip, serous otitis media, and tenderness and opacification of the sinuses. Examination during an acute asthma attack reveals agitation and respiratory distress; the patient may be unable to speak in complete sentences. Somnolence or confusion indicates exhaustion and impending ventilatory failure. Tachycardia and tachypnea are typically present, and a pulsus paradoxus (a fall in systolic blood pressure of greater than 10 mm Hg during slow inspiration) suggests severe obstruction. The use of accessory muscles (sternocleidomastoids and intercostals) to assist in breathing is another sign of a severe attack. Auscultation of the chest in this setting usually reveals diffuse wheezing, but a quiet chest is ominous, indicating very little air movement.

The physical signs of COPD include evidence of chronic airflow obstruction and the sequelae of ventilatory fatigue and hypoxemia. The patient with severe COPD typically sits upright, leaning forward onto supporting arms to optimize lung mechanics and facilitate the use of accessory muscles. Pursed-lip breathing is common and serves to maintain positive pressure in the large airways, thereby reducing airway collapse during active exhalation. Muscular wasting may result from the high caloric expenditure associated with the work of breathing in COPD, coupled to poor oral intake. Cyanosis may be due to hypoxemia, and plethora suggests compensatory erythrocytosis. The hyperexpanded chest has an increased anteroposterior diameter, and percussion demonstrates hyperresonance and low diaphragms. Auscultation typically reveals diminished breath sounds, rhonchi (musical sounds), wheezes or prolonged exhalation, and coarse crackles. Heart sounds are often distant and disguised by lung sounds in COPD, but a loud P2 suggests pulmonary hypertension. Right ventricular failure is manifested by wide splitting of S2, parasternal gallops, and tricuspid regurgitation. Other signs of cor pulmonale include elevated jugular venous pressure, tender hepatomegaly (pulsatile with prominent tricuspid regurgitation), ascites, and peripheral edema.

Clinical Approach. In taking the history, the pattern of symptoms should be defined as progressive or intermittent, and any relation to time of day, day of week, or season should be noted. Precipitating factors, sensitivity to aspirin or other nonsteroidal anti-inflammatory medications, and potentially contributory conditions such as sinusitis and gastroesophageal reflux should be identified. Patients should be questioned regarding smoking habits and exposure to other airborne pollutants at work, home, or play. A history of atopy and a family history of lung disease also may be relevant.

All patients with suspected airflow limitation should undergo pulmonary function testing. The diagnosis of asthma can be confirmed by the demonstration of airflow obstruction that is reversible over time or in response to bronchodilators. In contrast, COPD is associated with airflow obstruction that is progressive and predominantly irreversible. Substantial overlap exists: some patients with asthma develop chronic airflow obstruction ("asthmatic bronchitis"), and some patients with COPD have partially reversible airflow obstruction, or an "asthmatic" component. A low diffusing capacity for carbon monoxide in association with airflow obstruction is suggestive of emphysema. In patients with episodic symptoms compatible with asthma but in whom no evidence of airflow obstruction is found at the time of spirometry, a therapeutic trial of bronchodilators can be given or methacholine challenge testing can be used to identify bronchial hyperreactivity. A suspicion of exercise-induced asthma can be confirmed by spirometry immediately after exercise. The use of a hand-held peak flowmeter at work and at home to record fluctuations in airflow throughout the day can be helpful in the diagnosis of occupational asthma and as a guide to management.

The chest radiograph may be of value in the evaluation of COPD. Flattened diaphragms, hyperlucency, and increased anteroposterior diameter are signs of airflow obstruction. Bullae and distal pruning of the vasculature suggest emphysema. Coarse reticular markings and peribronchial cuffing are consistent with chronic bronchitis. A descending right pulmonary artery greater than 16 mm in diameter suggests pulmonary hypertension, and an enlarged right ventricle and dilated azygos vein may be seen with cor pulmonale.

Blood studies in COPD may reveal erythrocytosis secondary to chronic hypoxemia or an elevated serum bicarbonate level in compensation for chronic respiratory acidosis. Eosinophilia is common in asthma. Arterial blood gases should be obtained in all patients with COPD and with a measured forced expiratory volume in 1 second (FEV_1) of less than 1 to 1.5 L or with clinical suspicion of hypoxemia or hypercarbia. Hereditary α_1-antitrypsin deficiency should be considered in nonsmoking patients with emphysema and smokers with accelerated or early-onset emphysema (fourth or fifth decade), particularly if the chest radiograph demonstrates bullous changes that are predominantly located in the lower lobes.

The differential diagnosis of cough, wheeze, and dyspnea includes acute bronchitis, cystic fibrosis, bronchiectasis, upper airway obstruction, focal bronchial obstruction, interstitial lung disease, mitral stenosis, congestive heart failure, and pulmonary embolism. Viral respiratory tract infection can cause bronchial hyperreactivity that is indistinguishable from asthma but resolves within 8 weeks. Cystic fibrosis and other forms of bronchiectasis can usually be separated from asthma by the chronicity of symptoms, the copious production of purulent sputum, and abnormal chest radiographs. Upper respiratory obstruction typically causes stridor, in which wheezing is audible during both inspiration and exhalation and can be differentiated from asthma in the pulmonary function laboratory by a flow-volume loop. Wheezing due to focal bronchial obstruction by tumor, foreign body, or stenosis is unilateral and often accompanied by radiographic abnormalities. Some interstitial lung diseases, such as sarcoidosis, eosinophilic granuloma, and lymphangioleiomyomatosis, may present with cough and wheeze, but these symptoms are usually accompanied by progressive dyspnea; auscultation of the chest often reveals crackles, the chest radiograph will show typical interstitial infiltrates, and pulmonary function tests will demonstrate a restrictive defect. Mitral stenosis and left ventricular failure usually can be distinguished from primary airway disease by cardiac examination and chest radiography, with confirmation by echocardiography. Wheezing is an uncommon manifestation of pulmonary embolism heralded by the abrupt onset of dyspnea and other clinical features.

Management. Asthma and COPD are not curable diseases. The goals of treatment are to relieve symptoms, improve functional status, prevent exacerbations, and prolong life. The components of management include (1) education regarding the nature of the disease and its treatment; (2) identification and avoidance of exacerbating factors such as allergens, irritants (including cigarette smoke and occupational exposures), drugs (such as aspirin and β-blockers), and infection; (3) medication; and (4) regular follow-up.

The bronchodilator and anti-inflammatory medications commonly given by inhalation to treat airflow obstruction are listed in Table 68–1. The effective administration of these medications requires that patients be instructed and repeatedly tested in the proper use of metered-dose inhalers. At the end of a normal tidal exhalation (functional residual capacity), the preshaken inhaler is held 4 cm from the open mouth and actuated once after initiation of a slow

Table 68–1. INHALED BRONCHODILATOR AND ANTI-INFLAMMATORY MEDICATIONS AVAILABLE IN METERED-DOSE INHALERS

Generic Name	Initial Dose	Brand Name	Cost ($ per Day)*
β₂-Adrenergic Agonists			
Epinephrine	2 puffs q4h	Primatene	0.33
Isoproterenol	2 puffs q4h	Isuprel	1.39
Isoetharine	2 puffs q4h	Bronkometer	1.39
Metaproterenol	2 puffs q4h	Alupent	1.20
Albuterol	2 puffs q4–6h	Proventil, Ventolin	0.92
Terbutaline	2 puffs q4–6h	Brethaire	0.55
Bitolterol	2 puffs q4–6h	Tornalate	0.91
Pirbuterol	2 puffs q4–6h	Maxair	0.61
Salmeterol	2 puffs q12h	Serevent	1.60
Anticholinergic			
Ipratropium	2 puffs q6h	Atrovent	1.13
Anti-inflammatory			
Cromolyn	2 puffs qid	Intal	2.42
Nedocromil	2 puffs qid	Tilade	1.81
Beclomethasone	2 puffs qid	Beclovent, Vanceril	1.20
Triamcinolone	2 puffs qid	Azmacort	1.39
Flunisolide	2 puffs bid	AeroBid	1.90

*Average wholesale price, lowest initial daily dose listed, 1995 *Drug Topics Red Book.*

deep inhalation. At the end of inspiration the breath is held for 5 to 10 seconds and tidal breathing is resumed. Each actuation (puff) should be separated by 1 minute. The use of a spacer should be considered in patients who have difficulty coordinating this procedure: the metered-dose inhaler is actuated into the spacer, then the patient takes a slow deep breath and holds at total lung capacity for 5 to 10 seconds.

Most patients with asthma can be treated with an inhaled β_2-adrenergic agonist such as metaproterenol or albuterol used in response to symptoms and in anticipation of symptoms (e.g., before exercise). An inhaled corticosteroid should be added if patients need to use β_2-adrenergic agonists on a daily basis and can be given in doses up to 2 mg/d. Irritation of the throat and oral thrush can be avoided if the mouth is rinsed after the use of these agents. Cromolyn or nedocromil can be helpful as additional or alternative agents to inhaled corticosteroids, particularly in patients with allergic or exercise-induced asthma. Patients with chronic symptoms may benefit from scheduled treatment with inhaled salmeterol, a long-acting β_2-adrenergic agonist. Patients using salmeterol must be supplied with short-acting β_2-adrenergic agonists for management of increasing symptoms and acute exacerbations and should be cautioned against increasing the prescribed dose of salmeterol. Further benefit may be achieved in some patients by the addition of inhaled ipratropium bromide, high-dose β_2-adrenergic agonists delivered by nebulizer, or oral bronchodilators. Oral β_2-adrenergic agonists and oral theophylline are more toxic and less effective than inhaled bronchodilators but have longer durations of action and may be particularly useful in patients with nocturnal symptoms. When symptoms are uncontrolled by the stepwise measures described earlier, oral prednisone (30–60 mg/d) should be added until full symptomatic recovery occurs, then tapered or stopped. If symptoms recur after discontinuation of corticosteroids, then prednisone should be maintained at the lowest effective daily or alternate-day dose, the dose of inhaled corticosteroids increased, and withdrawal of prednisone attempted at a later date. Patients who cannot be weaned from oral corticosteroids should be referred to an allergist or pulmonologist for evaluation and consideration of alternative anti-inflammatory therapy.

All asthmatics should be given specific, individualized guidelines for self-management of acute exacerbations. These may include directions for increasing use of bronchodilators, indications for starting systemic corticosteroids, and criteria for calling a physician or presenting to an emergency department. The use of a peak flowmeter can be very helpful in guiding home treatment, with values 50% to 80% of baseline indicating a moderate exacerbation and measurements less than 50% of baseline defining a severe episode.

Acute asthma attacks managed in the office or emergency department should be assessed by measurement of peak flow or FEV_1 and treated with oxygen and inhaled β_2-adrenergic agents delivered by nebulizer every 15 to 20 minutes. Subcutaneous epinephrine or terbutaline and inhaled anticholinergics may be effective in young adults who fail to respond to inhaled β_2-adrenergic agonists, but theophylline probably adds toxicity without improving outcome. After 1 hour of treatment, further decisions should be based on clinical assessment and measurements of airflow: if peak flow or FEV_1 improves to more than 70% of predicted, the patient can be discharged on bronchodilators; if airflow measurements are less than 70% of predicted, the patient should be given oral or parenteral corticosteroids equivalent to 60 mg of prednisone. Patients with continued severe obstruction (airflow measurements less than 40% of predicted) or evidence of ventilatory fatigue (e.g., somnolence or carbon dioxide retention) should be admitted. The decision to admit or continue outpatient treatment of patients with some clinical improvement and airflow measurements between 40% and 70% of predicted depends on the duration of the attack, the intensity of treatment before presentation, the severity of previous attacks, the time of day, and the reliability of supervision and follow-up.

Patients with COPD should be treated with inhaled bronchodilators on a regular schedule, even if no responsiveness to these agents is demonstrated by spirometry. Ipratropium bromide is a rational first choice in patients without a reversible component, but many patients prefer inhaled β_2-adrenergic agonists despite apparently fixed obstruction. The use of oral theophylline is controversial but probably helpful in some patients. If a trial of theophylline is given, patients should be warned about potential toxicity (such as gastrointestinal upset, palpitations, and agitation) and drug interactions (e.g., with cimetidine, erythromycin, phenytoin, and quinolones). Theophylline dosage should be adjusted to maximum symptomatic benefit without side effects, usually found at a serum level of 10 to 15 mg/dL. Systemic corticosteroids (given as described earlier for asthma) are beneficial in acute exacerbations of COPD and in a minority of patients with stable COPD, particularly those with a reversible component. Inhaled corticosteroids are less effective for COPD than for asthma but should be tried in patients who are responsive to prednisone. Supplemental oxygen is the only treatment for COPD proven to prolong life. Continuous oxygen should be prescribed if the room air PaO_2 is less than or equal to 55 mm Hg or arterial oxygen saturation (SaO_2) is less than or equal to 88%, or if the room air PaO_2 is less than or equal to 59 mm Hg or SaO_2 is less than or equal to 89% with cor pulmonale or polycythemia. Oxygen should be given part time if there is evidence of significant desaturation during sleep or ambulation that can be corrected with supplemental oxygen. The need for supplemental oxygen should be reassessed after 1 to 3 months of therapy. Antibiotics such as trimethoprim-sulfamethoxazole (160/800 mg twice daily), amoxicillin (250–500 mg three times a day), and doxycycline (100 mg twice daily) may be effective in acute exacerbations of chronic bronchitis associated with purulent sputum. Low doses of codeine (10–30 mg three times a day) may be helpful in relieving severe chronic dyspnea, but side effects are often limiting and there is a danger of depressed ventilatory drive.

Rehabilitation can assist patients with COPD in adapting to their progressive disability. Instruction in bronchial hygiene, pursed-lip breathing, and exercise conditioning; provision of devices such as shower chairs and electric carts to assist in daily activities; and attention to the psychosocial aspects of chronic disease can all be helpful. Smoking cessation is the single most important consideration in the management of COPD.

Follow-Up. The interval between office visits for asthma and COPD will depend on the severity of symptoms, the frequency of exacerbations, and the complexity of treatment. Symptom control, the use of medications, and inhaler technique should be reviewed regularly. Patients with COPD should be monitored for evidence of hypoxemia and cor pulmonale, and spirometry should be repeated annually.

Asthma follows an unpredictable clinical course. The prognosis of COPD depends on the severity of airflow obstruction and the rate of decline of the FEV_1. The 5-year survival of patients with an FEV_1 of less than 1 L is approximately 50%, but substantial variation precludes accurate predictions of survival in individual patients.

Cross-References: Adult Immunizations (Chapter 11), Smoking Cessation (Chapter 12), Screening for Occupational and Environmental Lung Disease (Chapter 59), Cough and Sputum (Chapter 63), Upper Respiratory Infection (Chapter 66), Pulmonary Function Testing (Chapter 69), Dysphagia and Heartburn (Chapter 96).

REFERENCES

1. Ferguson GT, Cherniack RM. Management of chronic obstructive pulmonary disease. N Engl J Med 1993;328:1017–1022.

   This is a concise and practical review.

2. Martin RJ, ed. Asthma. Clin Chest Med 1995;16:557–755.

   A dozen review articles cover many aspects of the subject.

3. Mayo PH, Richman J, Harris HW. Results of a program to reduce admissions for adult asthma. Ann Intern Med 1990;112:864–871.

   In an inner city population of repeatedly hospitalized asthmatics, randomized referral to a special clinic emphasizing education, inhaled corticosteroids, and access to health care providers markedly reduced emergency visits and hospital admissions.

4. McFadden ER, Gilbert IA. Asthma. N Engl J Med 1992;327:1928–1937.

   An excellent review is presented of pathophysiology and treatment.

5. Saint S, Bent S, Vittinghoff E, Grady D. Antibiotics in chronic obstructive pulmonary disease exacerbations: A meta-analysis. JAMA 1995;273:957–960.

   The evidence from nine studies favors a small but significant effect.

69 Pulmonary Function Testing

Procedure

SHAWN J. SKERRETT

Indications and Contraindications. Common indications for pulmonary function testing include (1) evaluation of patients with dyspnea, cough, or wheeze; (2) screening of smokers for occult airflow obstruction or accelerated decline in forced expiratory volume in 1 second (FEV_1) (markers for a high risk of developing chronic obstructive pulmonary disease [COPD]); (3) measuring bronchodilator responsiveness or the effect of corticosteroid treatment; (4) monitoring the course of obstructive or restrictive defects; (5) monitoring patients treated with potential pulmonary toxins, such as radiation or bleomycin; (6) preoperative evaluation; and (7) assessment of disability. The relative contraindications to pulmonary function testing include active airborne infection and recent massive hemoptysis or pneumothorax.

Rationale. Pulmonary function testing is used to identify airflow obstruction, restrictive defects in lung expansion, and abnormalities of the alveolar-capillary membrane. The measurements in common use include spirometry, peak expiratory flow rate, lung volumes, and the diffusing capacity of the lung for carbon monoxide (DL_{CO}). Normal values for pulmonary function tests are most accurately defined by the 95% confidence interval, or 1.64 standard deviations from the predicted norm, but are commonly estimated as within 20% of the predicted value. Normal values for flow rates and volumes are influenced by gender, age, height, and race.

Spirometry, the measurement of airflow over time, is the simplest and most reproducible of these tests, and a variety of devices are available for use in the clinic setting. Figure 69–1 shows a normal spirogram, illustrating tidal breathing, a deep inhalation, and complete exhalation. The most useful spirometric measurements are the vital capacity (VC), the volume of air expelled by a slow (SVC) or forced (FVC) complete exhalation after full inhalation; and FEV_1, the volume of air expelled in the first second of an FVC maneuver. Airflow obstruction is defined by a low FEV_1 and an FEV_1/FVC ratio less than 0.75. Reduction in FEV_1 and FVC with a normal FEV_1/FVC ratio is consistent with a restrictive process, but this pattern may be seen in airflow obstruction if compression of large airways during forced exhalation reduces FVC and FEV_1 to a similar extent; in this case the SVC usually exceeds the FVC. A significant bronchodilator response is defined as a 12% (at least 200 mL) improvement in FEV_1 or FVC 10 minutes after inhalation of a β-adrenergic agonist or 30 to 60 minutes after inhalation of ipratropium.

Hand-held peak flowmeters provide a simple and inexpensive way to

All of the material in Chapter 69 is in the public domain, with the exception of any borrowed figures and tables.

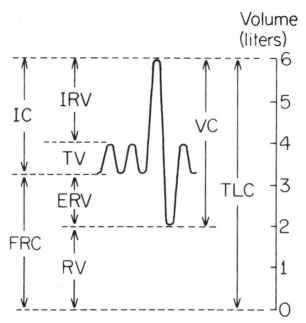

Figure 69–1. The normal spirogram and components of lung volume. RV = residual volume; ERV = expiratory reserve volume; TV = tidal volume; IRV = inspiratory reserve volume; TLC = total lung capacity; VC = vital capacity; FRC = functional residual capacity; IC = inspiratory capacity. (Reproduced with permission from Culver B, ed. The Respiratory System. Seattle, University of Washington Health Sciences Academic Series, 1990.)

monitor airflow obstruction at home and in the clinic. The peak expiratory flow rate is linearly related to FEV_1 but is more variable and effort dependent.

The measurement of lung volumes in the pulmonary function laboratory is required to define a restrictive defect. The four lung volumes and the four capacities they comprise are illustrated in Figure 69–1. These values are determined from spirometry and the measurement of functional residual capacity (FRC) by gas dilution or plethysmography. In the helium dilution method, the patient is connected to a closed circuit of helium at the end of a tidal breath (FRC) and allowed to breathe to equilibrium: the helium concentration of exhaled gas will be diluted by FRC. In the nitrogen washout technique, the patient is connected to 100% oxygen at FRC and allowed to breathe until nitrogen is no longer exhaled. FRC is calculated from the collected volume of expired nitrogen, assuming that nitrogen comprises 81% of alveolar gas. For plethysmography, the patient sits in an airtight chamber breathing through a mouthpiece, which is closed at FRC. The patient pants against the closed mouthpiece, and the resulting changes in thoracic volume and pressure are measured. The dilution methods measure communicating volume, which may underestimate total lung capacity (TLC) in the presence of severe airflow obstruction with air trapping or bullous lung disease. Plethysmography measures the total volume of compressible air in the chest and is more accurate. A reduced TLC defines a restrictive defect, found in interstitial lung disease, pulmonary resection, space-occupying intrathoracic abnormalities (e.g., pleural effusion, pneumonia, or tumor), chest wall defects, and neuromuscular disease. An elevated TLC, residual volume (RV), or RV/TLC ratio suggests air trapping.

The diffusing capacity for carbon monoxide (DLCO) is a useful indicator of alveolar-capillary gas exchange. The single-breath technique is most common: a known concentration of carbon monoxide is inhaled and held for 10 seconds, then the dilution of carbon monoxide in the expired gas is measured. The DLCO is low in conditions that reduce the surface area of the alveolar-capillary membrane (e.g., interstitial lung disease, pulmonary vascular disease, and emphysema) and when less hemoglobin is available for binding (as in anemia and in smokers with elevated carbon monoxide levels). An increased DLCO may be seen with erythrocytosis, an elevated pulmonary blood volume (as in atrial septal defect or pregnancy), and alveolar hemorrhage.

Other tests commonly available in pulmonary function laboratories include measurements of inspiratory and expiratory pressures and maximum voluntary ventilation to evaluate respiratory muscle strength; flow-volume loops to detect obstruction of the trachea and upper airway; methacholine challenge testing for the identification of bronchial hyperreactivity; and cardiopulmonary exercise testing to elicit oxygen desaturation, quantify impairment, and evaluate puzzling dyspnea.

Methods. Performance of the FVC maneuver with a spirometer should be explained and demonstrated. The patient then should be instructed to inhale fully to inspiratory capacity, place the lips around the mouthpiece, and blow out forcefully until an acceptable end is reached: a plateau in the volume-time curve for at least 2 seconds with an exhalation of at least 6 seconds; an exhalation lasting more than 15 seconds without reaching a plateau; or, in the judgment of the clinician, when the patient cannot or should not continue. Most patients will require exhortation to complete the test. The use of nose clips is encouraged. After a brief rest, the test should be repeated until three satisfactory tracings are obtained. The largest FEV_1 and FVC are recorded, even if they come from different curves. The best two efforts should not differ by more than 5%. Common sources of error include hesitation, coughing, Valsalva, early termination, air leak, and an obstructed mouthpiece.

The measurement of peak expiratory flow with a peak flowmeter requires a brief effort from full inhalation. The best of several measurements should be recorded.

Cost and Complications. Charges for spirometry range from $70 to $170, including interpretation. Charges for lung volumes and DLCO are each in the range of $100 to $150. The FVC maneuver may precipitate coughing or bronchospasm.

Cross-References: Determining Disability: The Primary Care Physician's Role (Chapter 5), Dyspnea (Chapter 19), Screening for Occupational and Environmental Lung Disease (Chapter 59), Asthma and Chronic Obstructive Pulmonary Disease (Chapter 68), Preoperative Pulmonary Problems (Chapter 221).

REFERENCES

1. American Thoracic Society. Lung function testing: Selection of reference values and interpretive strategies. Am Rev Respir Dis 1991;144:1202–1218.

This official statement by the American Thoracic Society includes a wealth of background material and detailed guidelines.

2. Crapo RO. Pulmonary-function testing. N Engl J Med 1994;331:25–30.

   A concise review of indications and interpretation is presented.

3. Nelson SB, Gardner RM, Crapo RO, Jensen RL. Performance evaluation of contemporary spirometers. Chest 1990;97:288–297.

   Only 35 of 62 devices were satisfactory; software problems were common.

4. Shapiro SM, Hendler JM, Ogirala RG, Aldrich TK, Shapiro MB. Evaluation of the accuracy of Assess and MiniWright peak flowmeters. Chest 1991;99:358–362.

   Two popular models performed well.

5. Zibrak JD, O'Donnel CR, Marton K. Indications for pulmonary function testing. Ann Intern Med 1990;112:763–771.

   A review of the role of pulmonary function testing in predicting postoperative outcomes is accompanied by a position paper from the American College of Physicians.

. . . .

70 Thoracentesis

Procedure

SHAWN J. SKERRETT

Indications and Contraindications. Diagnostic thoracentesis is indicated for the evaluation of pleural effusions of unknown etiology. Therapeutic thoracentesis is indicated for the reduction of large pleural effusions in dyspneic patients. The contraindications to thoracentesis include a bleeding diathesis, an uncooperative patient, infection of overlying skin, and a volume of pleural fluid too small to sample safely (less than 1 cm of fluid on a lateral decubitus radiograph). The major complication of thoracentesis is pneumothorax. Respiratory compromise from pneumothorax is particularly problematic in patients with one lung, bullous emphysema, or severe airflow obstruction.

Rationale. The accumulation of detectable fluid in the pleural space is invariably abnormal. Prompt diagnostic thoracentesis is indicated, except when pleural effusions are found in the presence of obvious volume overload, such as uncompensated congestive heart failure or massive ascites. Aspiration of pleural fluid can yield a specific diagnosis of malignancy (cytology), infection (stains, culture), systemic lupus erythematosus (antinuclear antibody, lupus erythematosus [LE] cells), and esophageal rupture (low pH, high amylase). The finding of blood (cancer, infarction, trauma), chyle (lymphoma, disruption of thoracic duct, lymphangioleiomyomatosis), or urine (hydronephrosis) in the pleural space also has strong diagnostic implications. Less specific information may support a presumptive diagnosis and exclude other considerations, such as identifying a parapneumonic effusion as a sterile exudate or proving an effusion to be transudative in a patient with heart failure. Diagnostic thoracentesis yields clinically helpful information in over 80% of cases. In one series of 86 patients, pleural aspiration yielded a specific diagnosis in 16%, a presumptive diagnosis in 51%, and useful but nondiagnostic information in 16%.

Therapeutic thoracentesis may be helpful in relieving acute dyspnea in patients with large pleural effusions, particularly if a mediastinal shift is apparent on the chest radiograph. In patients with volume overload due to heart, liver, or renal failure, removal of pleural fluid may provide symptomatic relief while awaiting the effects of diuretic therapy or dialysis. Therapeutic thoracentesis also may be of temporary benefit in patients with malignant pleural effusions. When malignant effusions reaccumulate slowly, repeated aspiration offers an alternative to tube thoracostomy and pleurodesis.

Methods. The patient should be seated on the side of the examination table with arms crossed over a pillow on a bedside table and feet supported by a stool. After review of the chest radiograph and physical examination, the clinician should select a site in the posterior midclavicular line one intercostal space below the upper level of dullness, but not below the eighth interspace. Wearing sterile gloves and a mask, the clinician then prepares the skin with an iodine solution and affixes a sterile drape. A skin wheal is raised with 1% lidocaine using a 25-gauge needle on a small syringe. Then, with a second syringe containing 10 to 15 mL of lidocaine, the skin is penetrated with a 22-gauge 1.5- to 2-inch needle directed perpendicularly to the superior border of the rib. After the periosteum is anesthetized, the needle is advanced over the rib (avoiding the neurovascular bundle under the adjacent rib), stopping every 1 to 2 mm to aspirate and inject. When pleural fluid is obtained, the needle is withdrawn. The track should be reentered with a 20- to 22-gauge 1.5- to 2-inch needle attached to a 50-mL syringe and 30 to 50 mL of fluid aspirated for analysis. The placement of a plastic catheter over or through the insertion needle before aspirating fluid is unnecessary for diagnostic thoracentesis and may be associated with a higher complication rate. After the needle is withdrawn, a sterile dressing should be applied and an expiration chest radiograph obtained to exclude a pneumothorax. The choice of pleural fluid studies will depend on the clinical situation but should always include protein, lactate dehydrogenase, glucose, white blood cell count, and differential. Cultures and stains for microorganisms, cytology, amylase, lipid studies, and pH are indicated in selected circumstances (see Chapter 65, Pleural Effusion).

Large-volume (therapeutic) thoracentesis is most safely performed with a plastic catheter, preferably using one of several commercially available kits that provide closed aspiration systems. Alternatively, therapeutic thoracentesis can be performed as follows. The site is prepared in the manner described earlier, but once pleural fluid is obtained with the anesthetizing needle, a sterile curved clamp is placed on the needle at the skin surface before withdrawal, to mark the depth of insertion. A second clamp is placed at the same point on a 14-gauge Intracath needle attached to a 10-mL syringe, and this needle is inserted with the bevel downward until pleural fluid can be aspirated. The syringe is then disconnected and the hub of the needle occluded with a finger to prevent entry of air into the pleural space. The 16-gauge internal catheter is then threaded, angling the needle slightly downward. When the catheter is fully inserted or when resistance is encountered, the needle is withdrawn and the needle guard mounted and taped to the chest. A 50-mL syringe with a three-way stopcock is attached to the catheter to aspirate fluid, which is then expelled through tubing connected to the side port of the stopcock (drainage may be accelerated by connecting the effluent tubing to a vacuum bottle). No more than 1 L should be removed at a time to avoid reexpansion pulmonary edema. When drainage is complete, the needle and catheter are removed together (withdrawing the catheter through the needle may shear it off), a sterile dressing is applied, and a chest radiograph is obtained.

Cost and Complications. Thoracentesis is a potentially dangerous procedure that should not be attempted without experience or supervision. Among procedures performed by housestaff, pneumothorax occurs in 10% to 15%; cough, retching, or vasovagal hypotension in 5% to 10%; and subjective symptoms such as pain and anxiety in 30% to 50%. Technical problems, such as a dry or traumatic tap, occur in 20% to 25%. Other potential complications include hemothorax, hemoperitoneum, and puncture of the liver or spleen. The complication rate is significantly reduced if thoracentesis is performed under direct ultrasound guidance. The added expense of ultrasonography is justified in patients with small or loculated effusions and in patients in whom a pneumothorax may be catastrophic, such as those with one lung or poor pulmonary reserve. The cost of thoracentesis will depend on the diagnostic studies that are ordered ($75–$300), the supplies that are used ($40–$120), the professional fee for the procedure ($100–$150), and the cost of radiographs or ultrasonography.

Cross-Reference: Pleural Effusion (Chapter 65).

REFERENCES

1. Collins TR, Sahn SA: Thoracentesis. Clinical value, complications, technical problems, and patient experience. Chest 1987;91:817–822.

   In a prospective study of 86 patients, thoracentesis yielded clinically useful information in 84% but complications were common.

2. Grogan DR, Irwin RS, Channick R, Raptopoulos V, Curley FJ, Bartter T, Corwin W: Complications associated with thoracentesis: A prospective, randomized trial comparing three different methods. Arch Intern Med 1990;150:873–877.

   Ultrasound guided aspiration was associated with fewer complications than "blind" thoracentesis using needle-only or needle-catheter techniques.

3. Kohan JM, Poe RH, Israel RH, Jennedy JD, Beazzi RB, Kallay MC, Greenblatt DW: Value of chest ultrasonography versus decubitus roentgenography for thoracentesis. Am Rev Respir Dis 1986;133:1124–1126.

   Sonography was helpful in choosing sites for aspirating small effusions.

4. Light RW: Pleural Diseases, 2nd ed. Philadelphia, Lea & Febiger, 1990:295–304.

   An illustrated description of the technique is provided.

5. Sahn SA: The pleura. Am Rev Respir Dis 1988;138:184–234.

   An exhaustive review provides a good discussion of the risks and benefits of thoracentesis.

71 Arterial Blood Sampling

Procedure

SHAWN J. SKERRETT

Indications and Contraindications. The most common indications for arterial blood sampling are suspected hypoxemia, hypercarbia, or acid–base disturbance. Common clinical settings include dyspnea, obtundation, cardiac arrhythmias, hypotension, vomiting, and renal failure. There are no absolute contraindications, but relative contraindications include a bleeding diathesis and severe peripheral arterial disease.

Rationale. Arterial blood is required for the accurate measurement of partial pressure of oxygen (PO_2), partial pressure of carbon dioxide (PCO_2), and pH. The PO_2 provides an indication of oxygen uptake by the blood but is an incomplete measure of oxygenation, which is determined by hemoglobin concentration, hemoglobin saturation, and tissue perfusion. Hypoxemia is usually defined as a PO_2 less than 80 mm Hg, but PO_2 normally falls with age. A simple approximation is to expect the PO_2 to be 1 mm Hg less than 80 for each year over 60. The PCO_2 accurately reflects the balance of carbon dioxide production and elimination (ventilation) and is normally 35 to 45 mm Hg. The pH of arterial blood reflects the acid–base balance, but electrolytes must be measured simultaneously to characterize acid–base disturbances. The normal arterial pH is 7.35 to 7.45.

Automated blood gas analyzers measure PO_2, PCO_2, and pH directly and calculate bicarbonate concentration. Most laboratories also measure hemoglobin concentration and estimate hemoglobin saturation. A co-oximeter is required for direct measurement of the various forms of hemoglobin, including oxyhemoglobin, deoxyhemoglobin, carboxyhemoglobin, and methemoglobin.

The most common sources of error in blood gas analysis occur in the collection and transportation of the sample. Active aspiration of blood during an attempted arterial puncture may result in venous admixture. If air bubbles are not removed, the partial pressures of gases in the blood will approach those of ambient air (PO_2 150 mm Hg and PCO_2 0 mm Hg), resulting in a fall in PCO_2 and associated rise in pH. Dilution of the blood with heparin will reduce the measured PCO_2 and the hemoglobin concentration. A time delay or failure to transport the specimen on ice will permit continued cellular metabolism, particularly in the presence of leukocytosis or thrombocytosis, resulting in oxygen consumption, carbon dioxide production, and acidification. The laboratory must be notified if the patient has hypothermia or fever, because blood gases are measured at 37°C and must be corrected for in vivo conditions.

Pulse oximetry is a noninvasive, inexpensive alternative to arterial blood sampling for the measurement of hemoglobin saturation. Current instruments are accurate at saturations above 70%. The technique is limited by conditions that diminish vascular pulsations, such as cold, hypotension, peripheral vascular disease, or use of vasoconstrictors.

Methods. Arterial blood should be drawn from the radial, brachial, or femoral artery, in descending order of preference. If the radial pulse is palpable, the adequacy of collateral circulation should be assessed with the modified Allen test. The patient should be instructed to expel blood from the hand by making a tight fist. The technician then compresses the radial and ulnar arteries simultaneously, then asks the patient to relax (but not fully extend) the hand. If, after releasing pressure from the ulnar artery, the color returns to normal within 10 seconds, then the ulnar artery alone can supply the hand.

For radial artery puncture, the hand should be positioned with the wrist extended, using a rolled towel or gauze for support, and the skin cleansed with alcohol or iodophor. A local anesthetic may be desirable if the technician is inexperienced or the patient is particularly anxious. At a site 1.5 to 2.5 cm proximal to the wrist fold a small wheal should be raised with 2% lidocaine, taking care not to obscure the pulse. Heparin is drawn into a glass or low-friction plastic syringe through a 20-gauge needle, wetting the walls of the syringe. The needle is then exchanged for a 23- or 25-gauge needle, and the heparin is expelled completely. Keeping two or three fingers on the pulse (to confirm location and direction), the technician punctures the skin at a 30- to 60-degree angle and advances the needle slowly until pulsatile blood fills the syringe (locating the artery is easier at a steeper angle, but through-and-through penetration and bleeding are less likely with a more oblique approach). The syringe should fill by arterial pressure, without aspiration. Once 2 to 3 mL of blood have been collected (sufficient to avoid significant dilution by residual heparin), the needle is withdrawn and firm pressure is applied to the artery for 5 to 10 minutes. Before transportation to the laboratory, the syringe should be free of air bubbles, sealed, and placed on ice.

Cost and Complications. The laboratory fee for blood gas analysis is in the range of $50 to $70, plus the charges for the procedure and supplies ($40 to $80). Local bleeding is common after inadequate compression. Distal ischemia and thrombosis are rare.

Cross-References: Dyspnea (Chapter 19), Sleep Apnea Syndrome (Chapter 64), Asthma and Chronic Obstructive Pulmonary Disease (Chapter 68), Hyperventilation Syndrome (Chapter 194).

REFERENCES

1. Hansen JE, Simmmons DH. A systematic error in determination of blood P_{CO_2}. Am Rev Respir Dis 1977;115:1061–1063.

   The effect of heparin is discussed.

2. Hess CE, Nichols AB, Hunt WB, Suratt PM. Pseudohypoxemia secondary to leukemia and thrombocytosis. N Engl J Med 1979;301:361–363.

   Another source of error is presented.

3. Raffin TA. Indications for arterial blood gas analysis. Ann Intern Med 1986;105:390–398.

   The author presents a thoughtful review.

4. Shapiro BA, Harrison RA, Cane RD, Templin R: Clinical Application of Blood Gases, 4th ed. Chicago, Year Book Medical Publishers, 1989:1–379.

   This book is a good source for technical aspects and clinical interpretation.

5. Vander Salm TJ. Arterial puncture. In Vander Salm TJ, Cutler BS, Wheeler HB, eds. Atlas of Bedside Procedures, 2nd ed. Boston, Little, Brown & Co, 1988:113–117.

   An illustrated description is provided.

SECTION VIII

Cardiovascular Disorders

··

72 Assessment of Physical Activity

Screening

RICHARD M. HOFFMAN and DEBORAH J. LIUM

Epidemiology. Approximately 24% of Americans are sedentary, and only 22% are active at levels adequate for cardiopulmonary benefit. The most active persons are men, younger adults, and persons of higher socioeconomic and educational levels. Surveys indicate that the most popular activities are walking, swimming, calisthenics, bicycling, and jogging. Activity levels often decline significantly in early adulthood and after marriage, job changes, moves, or recovery from serious illness or injury.

Rationale. Physical inactivity is a risk factor for coronary heart disease, hypertension, and obesity. Regular activity can help lower blood pressure; control weight gain and non–insulin-dependent diabetes mellitus; prevent osteoporosis in postmenopausal women; elevate high density lipoprotein cholesterol levels and lower triglyceride levels; and reduce anxiety and depression. Evidence suggests that the health benefits of physical activity derive from the total amount of activity performed and that the specific type, intensity, and duration of the activity are less important.

Physical activity, however, is not without risk. The chance of sudden death increases transiently during exercise, although the overall risk for sudden death is lower for the physically fit. Soft tissue injuries, tendinitis, and stress fractures occur more frequently with activity but are often preventable by avoiding excessive levels of activity, precipitous increases in activity, and poor exercise technique or equipment. Head injuries from falls can occur in the elderly, in individuals with autonomic neuropathy, and from the effects of medication. Female athletes can develop amenorrhea, especially when body fat drops below 16%. No studies have proven that physical activity accelerates the development of osteoarthritis.

Strategy. During all routine office visits, the physician should discuss the patient's present activity level and its medical implications. Men older than 40 years and women older than 50 years who plan vigorous activity or who have chronic illnesses or cardiovascular risk factors should consult their physician before beginning an exercise program. Appropriate baseline laboratory tests include determination of serum electrolyte levels and hematocrit, an electrocardiogram, and a chest radiograph, as indicated. Using graded exercise tests for screening purposes is controversial, particularly for asymptomatic persons, because false-positive rates are high and true-positive tests do not accurately predict cardiac arrest during exercise.

Action. Physicians should counsel all patients to be physically active. Aerobic weight-bearing exercises are the best types of activity. Healthy adults should perform 20 to 60 minutes of moderate- to high-intensity endurance exercise, 60% to 90% of the maximal heart rate (220 − age), at least three times a week. The first 4 to 6 weeks of an exercise program are the conditioning stage, with low-intensity training sessions. The next 4 to 5 months are the improvement stage, in which activity is increased by varying the intensity (moderate to high), frequency, or duration of exercise sessions. Finally, a maintenance stage is established based on the individual's fitness goals.

An expert panel from the Centers for Disease Control and Prevention and the American College of Sports Medicine issued recommendations encouraging *every* adult to perform 30 minutes of moderate-intensity activity, enough to expend about 200 calories, on most, if not all, days of the week. Even intermittent activity is beneficial; the 30 minutes of activity can be accumulated in short bouts throughout the day. Formal exercise programs are not necessary—lawn and garden work, home repairs, and walking are acceptable activities.

Sedentary and elderly persons should begin at lower levels and progress slowly. Patients on β-adrenergic blockers should use perceived exertion to estimate exercise intensity. Physical activity should be limited when the person is fatigued or has consumed alcohol or large meals or during very hot or cold weather. Physical activity should not be too vigorous; signs of overexertion include prolonged postexercise tachycardia, nausea, vomiting, light-headedness, confusion, claudication, angina, or excessive dyspnea.

Physicians can enhance patient compliance and influence behavior by presenting health risks and benefits, selecting appropriate activities, setting goals, encouraging social support, and providing positive reinforcement.

Cross-References: Periodic Health Assessment (Chapter 8), Chronic Nonspecific Pain Syndrome (Chapter 14), Obesity (Chapter 15), Essential Hypertension (Chapter 85), Exercise Tolerance Testing (Chapter 88), Osteoporosis (Chapter 116).

REFERENCES

1. American College of Sports Medicine. The recommended quantity and quality of exercise for developing and maintaining cardiorespiratory and muscle fitness in healthy adults. Med Sci Sports Exerc 1990;22:265–274.

   Guidelines for prescribing exercise are detailed.

2. Pate RP, Pratt M, Blair SN, et al. Physical activity and public health: A recommendation from

the Centers for Disease Control and Prevention and the American College of Sports Medicine. JAMA 1995;273:402–407.

The most recent recommendations are summarized with emphasis on the benefit of daily moderate-intensity exercise.

3. US Preventive Services Task Force. Counseling to promote physical activity. In Guide to Clinical Preventive Services, 2nd ed. Baltimore, Williams & Wilkins, 1996.

A critical review of the evidence that physical activity reduces the risk of morbidity and mortality from chronic conditions is presented.

....

73 Acute Chest Pain

Symptom

DAVID H. HICKAM and WILLIAM ABERNETHY

Epidemiology. Patients may describe chest discomfort as pain, pressure, tightness, fullness, or a burning sensation. Chest discomfort is more prevalent in older age groups. Identifiable syndromes of chest discomfort are defined by the pattern of occurrence. Acute chest pain, which often leads to hospital admission, is defined as pain of recent onset or as a recent increase in the intensity, frequency, or duration of recurrent pain.

Angina pectoris refers to a syndrome of pain that is usually substernal and brought on by physical exertion. It is more frequent in patients who have coronary artery disease but can occur with other diseases, such as esophageal disorders (see Chapter 78, Angina). Unstable angina is anginal chest pain that is of recent onset or has become more frequent or severe in patients with chronic symptoms.

Etiology. Causes of acute chest pain are classified into cardiovascular and noncardiovascular categories (Table 73–1). Several of these causes can be life threatening if not treated immediately, including acute myocardial infarction, unstable angina pectoris, aortic dissection, pulmonary embolism, and pneumothorax.

Among middle-aged and older adults who seek care for chest pain, approximately one third have cardiac ischemia as the cause of the discomfort, whereas in another one third the cause is esophageal disease. Because esophageal disorders are often associated with recurrent symptoms, they are discussed in Chapter 74, Recurrent Chest Pain.

Clinical Approach. The patient's history, physical examination findings, and initial electrocardiogram (ECG) must be used to estimate the probability that the pain is caused by cardiac ischemia. A study of emergency department patients with acute chest pain showed that initial decision-making can be based

Table 73–1. CAUSES OF ACUTE CHEST PAIN

Cardiovascular
Acute myocardial infarction
Atherosclerotic coronary artery disease, without acute infarction
Coronary artery spasm
Pericarditis
Pulmonary embolism

Noncardiovascular
Reflux esophagitis
Esophageal motor disorders
Pneumothorax
Pneumonia
Chest wall disorders
Anxiety disorders

on the ECG. Q waves or ST segment elevations (not known to be old) are specific enough for myocardial infarction that the physician should initiate management for this diagnosis when these findings are present, pending results of other tests. Although as many as 10% of patients with a normal ECG in the emergency department will subsequently be found to have a myocardial infarction, such patients are at low risk for serious complications.

If the ECG neither is completely normal nor shows the classic changes of an acute myocardial infarction, decisions should be based on the characteristics of the pain. Pain that is described as crushing, pressing, or tight is more likely to be ischemic than pain that is described as sharp or stabbing. Although vomiting occurs more frequently in transmural myocardial infarction than in unstable angina, the clinician should not try to distinguish these two syndromes on the basis of the history alone. Physical examination signs cannot reliably differentiate cardiac ischemia from other causes of chest pain. The probability of ischemia is lower in patients whose pain is fully reproduced by chest palpitation, but this sign is not specific enough to be relied on.

Single serum cardiac enzyme levels have limited value in the initial assessment of patients with acute chest pain. Although initial enzyme levels are more sensitive in patients who present more than 3 hours after the onset of pain, they cannot be used to exclude acute myocardial infarction. Furthermore, in patients whose symptoms suggest a low probability of cardiac ischemia, an elevated serum enzyme level is often a false-positive result (6% or greater). Serial ECGs and enzyme levels will establish whether the patient has acute myocardial infarction or unstable angina as the cause of ischemic-type chest pain.

Dissection of the thoracic aorta is rare but is often fatal. The most useful features of the history are patient age (the majority of patients are older than 50) and gender (more than 65% are male). Patients whose pain is located posteriorly have a higher probability of dissection. The most useful physical finding is hypertension; 70% of patients with dissection will have hypertension by history or on examination. Physical findings such as a murmur of aortic regurgitation, pulse deficits, and neurologic deficits are insensitive but moderately specific for dissection. Therefore, when one of these signs is present, the probability of aortic dissection is significantly increased. The finding of an increased aortic diameter on plain chest radiography has a sensitivity of approximately 70% for aortic dissection. The diagnosis can be confirmed by computed tomography, aortography, or transesophageal echocardiography.

Chest pain associated with pericarditis is often pleuritic, affected by body position, or described by the patient as sharp or stabbing. A pericardial friction rub is the most characteristic physical finding. The ECG often displays ST segment elevation in multiple leads, which can be confused with acute myocardial infarction, and PR segment depression. The echocardiogram often shows a pericardial effusion, but this test is not necessary to establish the diagnosis. An echocardiogram should be obtained if pericardial tamponade (in which a large pericardial effusion interferes with cardiac filling) is suspected.

Chest pain caused by pulmonary embolism is usually pleuritic and sharp. Pulmonary embolism may account for up to 20% of cases of pleuritic chest pain. Because the perfusion lung scan is highly sensitive for pulmonary embolism, a completely normal test excludes the diagnosis. However, owing to the high false-positive rate of lung scans, pulmonary arteriograms are considered the reference standard for confirming pulmonary embolism (see Chapter 61, Pleuritic Chest Pain).

When the cardiac causes of acute chest pain have been excluded, other causes may be considered. Chest pain can originate from various musculoskeletal sources. Although Tietze's syndrome refers to tender costochondral swelling, the more common chest wall syndromes are not associated with swelling but are characterized by localized chest wall tenderness and pain that is induced by chest wall movement. The diagnosis rests on reproducing the pain by palpation of the costochondral junctions. Results of laboratory tests and radiographic examinations are not helpful.

Management. The most important initial decision in managing acute chest pain is whether to admit the patient to the hospital. Admission to a coronary care unit is appropriate when the probability of acute ischemia is greater than 10% or when aortic dissection is suspected. If the initial ECG changes are minimal, patients with suspected myocardial infarction can be safely managed in an intermediate care unit.

Patients with acute myocardial infarction or unstable angina pectoris benefit from medical therapy that reduces cardiac workload and improves coronary perfusion. When ECG changes characteristic of acute myocardial infarction are present, the immediate use of aspirin also has been shown to improve survival. Thrombolytic medication is an important intervention that reduces mortality. If it can be performed expeditiously, percutaneous transluminal coronary angioplasty is an effective alternative.

Emergency treatment of the other causes of acute chest pain is quite variable. Patients with aortic dissection should receive medical therapy, including controlled treatment of hypertension, as soon as the diagnosis is considered. Pulmonary embolism also requires hospitalization for hemodynamic stabilization and initiation of anticoagulant therapy. Therapy for chest wall syndromes consists of reassurance, nonsteroidal anti-inflammatory drugs, stretching exercises, and warm packs. Local injections of corticosteroids and anesthetics may be useful in patients with persistent chest wall discomfort.

Follow-Up. If the patient is not admitted, outpatient follow-up should be scheduled for 2 to 3 days after the initial evaluation. Emergency department studies have found that approximately 5% of patients not hospitalized for acute chest pain will be found to have acute myocardial infarction on subsequent ECGs. If follow-up studies do not show myocardial infarction but the patient continues to have intermittent pain, the clinician should evaluate the patient for angina pectoris (see Chapter 78).

Cross-References: Pleuritic Chest Pain (Chapter 61), Recurrent Chest Pain (Chapter 74), Angina (Chapter 78), Exercise Tolerance Testing (Chapter 88), Dysphagia and Heartburn (Chapter 96).

REFERENCES

1. Goldman L, Cook EF, Brand DA, et al. A computer protocol to predict myocardial infarction in emergency department patients with chest pain. N Engl J Med 1988;318:797–803.

    An algorithm is presented for estimating the risk of acute myocardial infarction; it was developed from prospectively collected data on patients' symptoms and initial ECGs.

2. Hull RD, Raskob GE, Carger CJ, et al. Pulmonary embolism in outpatients with pleuritic chest pain. Arch Intern Med 1988;148:838–844.

    An approach to evaluating clinical characteristics and test results is described in suspected cases of pulmonary embolism.

3. Lee TH, Cook F, Weisberg MC, et al. Impact of the availability of a prior electrocardiogram on the triage of the patient with acute chest pain. J Gen Intern Med 1990;5:381–388.

    Data are provided on the clinical characteristics and relative usefulness of a prior ECG in patients who did and did not have acute myocardial infarction. A prior ECG improved the specificity of decisions to admit patients to the coronary care unit.

4. Lewis WR, Amsterdam EA. Evaluation of the patient with "rule out" myocardial infarction. Arch Intern Med 1996;156:41–45.

    This is a recent review of patient evaluation and diagnostic testing.

5. Senble EL, Wise CM. Chest pain: A rheumatologist's perspective. South Med J 1988;81:64–68.

    The authors present a useful review of syndromes and clinical approach.

6. Spittell PC, Spittell JA, Joyce JW, et al. Clinical features and differential diagnosis of aortic dissection: Experience with 236 cases (1980 through 1990). Mayo Clin Proc 1993;68:642–651.

    This report of a large case series includes detailed information about clinical findings and patient presentations.

74 Recurrent Chest Pain

Symptom

WILLIAM ABERNETHY and DAVID H. HICKAM

Epidemiology. Recurrent chest pain is episodic chest discomfort that occurs over a period of weeks or months. Ischemic heart disease is a frequent cause of recurrent chest pain (see Chapter 78, Angina), but recurrent chest pain often occurs in the absence of significant obstructive disease of the coronary arteries. In the United States, nearly 1 million new patients per year undergo coronary arteriograms, and normal coronary arteries are found in 20% or more of these patients. Thus, at least 200,000 new cases per year of recurrent chest pain are not associated with significant epicardial coronary artery disease. Despite an excellent prognosis, many patients continue to have episodic pain, limit their lifestyles, and believe they have undiagnosed heart disease.

Etiology. Recurrent chest pain has a large differential diagnosis. As in acute chest pain, cardiac disease is a major consideration, especially in patients with multiple cardiac risk factors (see Chapter 73, Acute Chest Pain, Table 73–1). Ischemic heart disease explains most cases of recurrent chest pain that follows a pattern typical of angina pectoris (see Chapter 78). In addition, both aortic stenosis and hypertrophic cardiomyopathy can cause anginal chest pain despite normal coronary arteries.

Microvascular angina refers to a syndrome of anginal or atypical chest pain, a positive exercise stress test, and no demonstrable coronary stenoses. Although some of these individuals probably have false-positive test results and noncardiac pain, others may suffer from a failure of the coronary arterioles to dilate adequately to meet increased myocardial oxygen demand in the setting of exercise or excitement. This diagnosis should be reserved for patients who have exertional chest pain, normal coronary arteriograms, and abnormal noninvasive testing (positive exercise electrocardiograms, reversible thallium perfusion defects, or left ventricular dysfunction in response to pharmacologic or physiologic stress).

Esophageal disorders constitute the most common cause of noncardiac chest pain and occur in as many as half of patients with chest pain and normal coronary arteries. Nearly 10% of patients with gastroesophageal reflux have chest pain as their only complaint. Reflux tends to occur after meals and to be exacerbated by bending forward or lying supine. Esophageal dysmotility (primarily nutcracker esophagus and nonspecific esophageal dysmotility) occurs in as many as 28% of patients with chest pain and normal coronary arteries, but many patients are pain free during abnormal esophageal contractions. Treatment of gastroesophageal reflux more frequently brings relief of symptoms than treatment of motility disorders.

A heightened sensitivity to normal or slightly noxious stimuli, called abnormal visceral nociception, has been demonstrated in patients with recurrent chest pain and normal coronary arteries. Low-level esophageal balloon distention, catheter manipulation within the right atrium, and injection of saline into a cardiac chamber catheter have been observed to be associated with characteristic chest pain in these patients. In addition, up to one third of patients with chest pain and normal coronary arteries meet criteria for panic disorder or the hyperventilation syndrome.

Clinical Approach. Whereas acute chest pain often requires urgent hospitalization and evaluation (see Chapter 73, Acute Chest Pain), chronic recurrent chest pain is usually managed in the outpatient clinic. The most important aspect of the evaluation is the history, focusing on characteristics of the chest pain (exertional, positional, quality, relation to food intake). The results of physical examination are often normal. Most importantly, cardiac disease must be excluded. The probability of ischemic heart disease depends on the characteristics of the pain, the patient's age and gender, and the presence of cardiac risk factors. The choice of tests to evaluate the patient for ischemia depends on the initial clinical evaluation (see Chapter 78, Angina).

Patients with associated symptoms of dysphagia, odynophagia, postprandial pain, or exacerbation of pain when recumbent likely have an esophageal disorder. Chest pain as an isolated symptom is unusual for esophageal strictures or cancer, and, unless the patient has dysphagia in addition to the chest pain, barium radiography is too insensitive to be useful. Endoscopy is the preferred test for esophagitis, but an empirical trial of acid-lowering therapy is often a reasonable alternative (see Chapter 95, Dyspepsia). For patients with persistent symptoms suggesting reflux who have normal findings on endoscopy and have failed a conventional trial of acid-lowering therapy, ambulatory 24-hour pH monitoring can be considered. Extensive esophageal dysmotility evaluations with manometry and provocative testing are of limited benefit, are quite costly, and should be used only in selected cases.

Patients with anxiety, depression, or panic disorders have often visited several physicians in search of a diagnosis and do not readily accept reassurance. Evidence of tension, excessive worry, feelings of helplessness, palpitations, paresthesias, or vegetative manifestations of depression supports these diagnoses.

Management. Controversies in the treatment of noncardiac chest pain reflect the intermittent nature of symptoms and uncertainty regarding the underlying cause. Recurrent chest pain frequently remains undiagnosed after subspecialty evaluations. For patients having negative cardiac evaluations, treatment should begin with reassurance. Although the pain is annoying, it is not life threatening, and the patient's prognosis is excellent. In a study of nearly 2000 such patients, 10-year follow-up revealed extremely low mortality (2%) from cardiac causes. Physicians should be supportive, acknowledge the patient's symptoms, firmly communicate the absence of heart disease, and encourage normal activity.

Empirical medication trials are often useful for patients with recurrent chest pain. For patients who meet the criteria for microvascular angina, a trial of antianginal drugs should be considered (see Chapter 78, Angina). In patients with symptoms suggesting reflux esophagitis and no signs of ischemia, an empirical trial of medical therapy for acid suppression is reasonable even in the absence of findings on endoscopy. Goals of an adequate trial should be to recommend lifestyle changes and medically suppress acid completely for 4 to 6 weeks and observe symptoms. If therapy relieves the symptoms, then the medication can be continued; no further diagnostic tests are needed.

Patients with esophageal motility disorders are often treated with smooth muscle relaxants. Nitrates and hydralazine have been successful in anecdotal reports, but these trials examined few patients and were not placebo controlled. Studies with calcium channel blockers in patients with esophageal dysmotility have yielded conflicting results. Cisapride, a promotility agent, is expensive and may be useful in selected patients. One of these agents may prove effective in the individual patient.

If symptoms of anxiety or depression are present, psychotropic drug therapy and behavioral programs may be the most helpful forms of management. The management approach is similar to that for a chronic visceral pain syndrome. Imipramine, 50 mg orally at bedtime, has been shown to decrease the frequency of symptoms in patients with noncardiac chest pain.

Cross-References: Chronic Nonspecific Pain Syndrome (Chapter 14), Acute Chest Pain (Chapter 73), Angina (Chapter 78), Exercise Tolerance Testing (Chapter 88), Dysphagia and Heartburn (Chapter 96), Myofascial Pain Syndromes (Chapter 122), Breast Pain in Nonlactating Women (Chapter 163), Panic Disorder (Chapter 191), Hyperventilation Syndrome (Chapter 194).

REFERENCES

1. Achem SR, Kolts BE. Current medical therapy for esophageal motility disorders. Am J Med 1992;92:98S–105S.

   Among current treatment options, none has emerged as the treatment of choice.

2. Beitman BD, et al. Follow-up of patients with angiographically normal coronary arteries and panic disorder. JAMA 1991;265:1545–1549.

   About 40% of patients with chest pain and normal coronary arteries have panic disorder and suffer more disability than those without panic disorder.

3. Cannon RO, et al. Imipramine in patients with chest pain despite normal coronary angiograms. N Engl J Med 1994;330:1411–1417.

   Sixty consecutive patients with chest pain and normal coronary arteries were randomized to imipramine, clonidine, or placebo. Patients receiving imipramine had a 52% reduction in symptoms. The response to imipramine occurred whether or not the patient had abnormal results on treadmill, esophageal, or psychiatric testing.

4. Papanicoban MN, et al. Prognostic implications of angiographically normal and insignificantly narrowed coronary arteries. Am J Cardiol 1986;58:1181–1187.

   Of 2000 patients, cardiac survival was 98% at 10 years.

75 Syncope

Symptom

WISHWA N. KAPOOR

Epidemiology. Syncope is defined as a sudden transient loss of consciousness and postural tone that spontaneously resolves without electrical or chemical cardioversion. Syncope should be differentiated from other conditions such as dizziness, vertigo, seizure, coma, and narcolepsy.

Syncope is a common problem in all age groups. It accounts for approximately 1% of hospital admissions and 3% of emergency department visits. Twelve percent to 48% of healthy young adults have experienced loss of consciousness (about one third of which are after trauma), although most do not seek medical attention. In persons older than age 75 years residing in long-term care institutions, the annual incidence of syncope is 6%, and 23% have had previous syncopal episodes.

Etiology. Although syncope has a large differential diagnosis, the etiology can be classified into four broad categories (Table 75–1). The first category is neurally mediated or neurocardiogenic syncope, which is loss of consciousness resulting from sudden reflex vasodilatation or bradycardia. The entities under this group include syndromes such as vasovagal, vasodepressor, situational (micturition, cough, defecation, and swallow), and carotid sinus syncope. A neurally mediated reflex mechanism is also implicated for syncope in association with exercise, especially immediately after exercise in individuals without structural heart disease. Neurally mediated syncope may also occur with drugs that decrease venous return to the heart in an upright position, such as nitroglycerin. Psychiatric disorders including generalized anxiety, panic disorder, and depression may also lead to neurally mediated syncope. Additionally, alcohol and drugs such as cocaine, hypnotics, and sedatives may cause syncope.

The second broad category is orthostatic hypotension, which may result from age-related physiologic changes, medications, volume depletion, and diseases affecting the autonomic nervous system. Postprandial syncope, a rare problem in the elderly, is due to hypotension after meals.

The third category is neurologic disorders, which are infrequent causes of syncope. These disorders include transient ischemic attacks (TIAs), migraines, and seizures. Syncope due to TIAs almost exclusively involves the vertebrobasilar territory. Migraines may be basilar artery related, or syncope may be a response to severe pain. Seizure-related syncope may be due to atonic, temporal lobe, or grand mal seizures.

The fourth category includes a large group of cardiac causes that can be divided into diseases associated with severe obstruction to cardiac output (due to lesions of the left or right side of the heart), ischemia, and arrhythmias.

Table 75–1. ETIOLOGY OF SYNCOPE

Neurally Mediated Syndromes

Vasovagal
Situational
  Micturition
  Cough
  Swallow
  Defecation
Carotid sinus syncope
Neuralgias
High altitude
Psychiatric disorders
Others (exercise, selected drugs)

Orthostatic Hypotension

Neurologic Diseases

Migraines
Transient ischemic attacks
Seizures

Decreased Cardiac Output

Obstruction to flow
  Obstruction to left ventricular outflow
    Aortic stenosis (hypertrophic obstructive cardiomyopathy)
    Mitral stenosis, myxoma
  Obstruction to right ventricular outflow
    Pulmonic stenosis
    Pulmonary embolism, pulmonary hypertension
    Myxoma
Other heart disease
  Pump failure
  Myocardial infarction, coronary artery disease, coronary spasm
  Tamponade, aortic dissection
Arrhythmias
  Bradyarrhythmias
    Sinus node disease
    Second- and third-degree atrioventricular block
    Pacemaker malfunction
    Drug-induced bradyarrhythmias
  Tachyarrhythmias
    Ventricular tachycardia
    Torsades de pointes (e.g., associated with congenital long QT syndromes or acquired QT
      prolongation)
    Supraventricular tachycardia

Adapted from Kapoor WN. Hypotension and syncope. In Braunwald E, ed. Heart Disease: A Textbook of Cardiovascular Medicine. Philadelphia, WB Saunders, 1996.

Clinical Approach. In studies of syncope from the 1980s, the most common causes were vasovagal syncope (25%), arrhythmias (14%), orthostatic hypotension (8%), seizures (less than 10%), and organic heart diseases (4%). Each of the other causes occurred in less than 5% of patients. A cause of syncope was not diagnosed in 34%. However, the proportion undiagnosed in the 1990s is probably substantially lower with wider use of event monitoring, tilt testing, electrophysiologic studies; greater attention to psychiatric illnesses; and greater recognition that syncope in the elderly may be multifactorial.

The history and physical examination identify a potential cause of syncope in approximately 45% of patients. Additionally, cardiac diseases causing syncope (e.g., pulmonary hypertension, aortic stenosis, pulmonary embolism) are usually suspected clinically and can be confirmed by specific testing in an additional 8%.

Results of routine blood tests and glucose tolerance testing are rarely abnormal and rarely diagnostically helpful in patients with syncope.

DIAGNOSIS OF ARRHYTHMIAS. Arrhythmias are diagnosed by electrocardiography (ECG), Holter monitoring, intermittent loop event records, and electrophysiologic studies. Causes of syncope are diagnosed in less than 5% of patients by ECG and rhythm strip. However, an ECG is recommended in most patients with syncope because abnormalities found on ECG (such as bundle branch block) may guide further evaluation; or if a specific diagnosis is made, the findings can be important in immediate decision-making.

In studies of ambulatory (Holter) monitoring, approximately 4% of patients had symptoms concurrently with arrhythmias. In another 17% of patients, symptoms were reported but no arrhythmias were found, thus potentially excluding arrhythmias as a cause of symptoms. In approximately 79% of patients there were no symptoms during monitoring, but brief arrhythmias were found in 13% of the 79%. In the absence of symptoms during monitoring, finding brief or no arrhythmias does not exclude arrhythmic syncope. Brief arrhythmias are nonspecific and can be found in asymptomatic healthy individuals. Additionally, absence of arrhythmias on monitoring does not exclude arrhythmic syncope because arrhythmias are episodic and may not occur during monitoring. In patients with a high pretest probability of arrhythmias, such as brief sudden loss of consciousness without prodrome, patients with an abnormal electrocardiogram, or those with structural heart disease, further evaluation is needed for the diagnosis of arrhythmias as a cause of syncope. Ambulatory monitoring (for 24 hours) is recommended for patients with high pretest likelihood of arrhythmias as defined previously.

Loop event recorders are likely to capture a rhythm during syncope after the patient has regained consciousness because at least 4 to 5 minutes of retrograde recording is possible and monitors can be worn for several weeks. Arrhythmias with symptoms are found in 8% to 20% of patients, and in an additional 27% there are symptoms without concurrent arrhythmias. This test is recommended in patients with recurrent syncope when there is a low probability of events during a brief monitoring period.

Patients should be considered for electrophysiologic testing only after thorough clinical and noninvasive evaluation using history, physical examination, ECG, ambulatory monitoring, and other noninvasive, directed tests. Results of electrophysiologic studies are abnormal primarily in patients with recurrent unexplained syncope who have organic heart disease (left ventricular dysfunction, coronary or valvular diseases, or hypertrophic cardiomyopathy) or an abnormal ECG (e.g., bundle branch block). Abnormal electrophysiologic test results are found in approximately 50% of patients studied and mainly constitute ventricular tachycardia and conduction system disease. The sensitivity and the specificity of electrophysiologic testing for detection of bradyarrhythmias are low. It is recommended that patients with structural heart disease or an abnormal ECG undergo electrophysiologic testing if clinical assessment is suggestive of arrhythmic syncope and noninvasive testing with Holter or loop monitoring has not been diagnostic.

UPRIGHT TILT TESTING. Maintaining the patient in an upright position for a brief duration on a tilt table has become a common method of testing for predisposition to vasovagal syncope. Approximately 50% of patients with unexplained syncope have a positive response to passive tilt testing (without using chemical stimulation). With use of isoproterenol during tilt testing, overall positive responses are approximately 64%. Specificity of passive testing is approximately 90% (range: 0%–100%). The overall specificity of tilt testing with isoproterenol is approximately 75% (range: 35%–100%). In patients with positive results (showing symptoms identical to spontaneous symptoms in association with hypotension or bradycardia), therapy can be planned with β-blockers, disopyramide, anticholinergic agents, or fludrocortisone plus salt.

OTHER TESTS. Cardiovascular testing such as echocardiography, stress testing, ventricular function studies, and cardiac catheterization can clarify specific findings noted on history and physical examination. The use of myocardial band isoenzyme of creatine kinase (CK-MB) is useful when myocardial infarction is suspected. Signal-averaged ECG for detection of low amplitude signals (late potentials) has a sensitivity of 73% to 89% and a specificity of 80% to 90% for prediction of induced sustained ventricular tachycardia in patients with syncope. This test does not establish a diagnosis but may occasionally help select a group of patients more likely to have ventricular tachycardia.

Autonomic function studies are generally not needed in patients with orthostatic hypotension because clinical evaluation often provides clues to its etiology. Electroencephalography and head computed tomography (CT) scans are rarely useful in determining a cause of syncope. They may be valuable when seizure is suspected clinically or when focal neurologic symptoms are associated with syncope.

Management. Most syncope patients presenting to primary care physicians can be evaluated and treated as outpatients. Patients are admitted to the hospital if a rapid diagnostic evaluation is deemed necessary mainly because of concerns about serious arrhythmias, sudden death, newly diagnosed serious cardiac disease (e.g., aortic stenosis, myocardial infarction), new onset of seizure, or stroke. Patients with evidence of possible acute ischemia or infarction on ECG, with chest pain, or with congestive heart failure and those taking medications capable of provoking malignant arrhythmias should be admitted. Occasionally, admission may also be needed for treatment when etiology is clear (e.g., management of dehydration or subarachnoid hemorrhage). In the large group of patients with unexplained syncope after initial history, physical examination, and ECG, risk stratification for arrhythmias and sudden death should guide the admission decision. Factors related to these two outcomes include presence of structural heart disease and an abnormal ECG.

Elderly patients are often hospitalized for rapid workup because of concern about the presence of underlying asymptomatic heart disease (especially coronary disease).

Follow-Up. Patients with cardiac causes of syncope have markedly higher mortality and sudden death rates at 1 and 5 years as compared with patients with noncardiac causes or syncope of unknown origin. Thus, determining which patients have a cardiac etiology is important for prognosis and management. Recurrence rates for syncope of 12% to 15% per year are reported. The rates are not significantly different in patients with cardiac causes as compared with other groups. Neurocardiogenic syncope has an excellent long-term prognosis, although recurrences are common and are a major reason patients seek medical care. Similarly, syncope associated with psychiatric disease has no increased mortality but has a 1-year recurrence rate of 26% to 50%.

Cross-References: Diagnosis and Management of Drug Abuse (Chapter 9), Alcohol Problems (Chapter 10), Dizziness (Chapter 20), Aortic Stenosis (Chapter 80), Chronic Ventricular Arrhythmias (Chapter 83), Ambulatory Cardiac Monitoring (Chapter 87), Cerebrovascular Disease (Chapter 146), Somatization (Chapter 188), Panic Disorder (Chapter 191).

REFERENCES

1. Kapoor WN. Evaluation and outcome of patients with syncope. Medicine 1990;69:160–175.

   In a large prospective study of syncope, history and physical examination led to diagnoses in the majority of patients. Patients with cardiac causes had higher mortality.

2. Kapoor WN. Evaluation and management of the patients with syncope. JAMA 1992;268:2553–2560.

   An in-depth review of diagnostic tests for evaluation of syncope is presented.

3. Kapoor WN, Smith M, Miller NL. Upright tilt testing in evaluating syncope: A comprehensive literature review. Am J Med 1994;97:78–88.

   A summary of studies of tilt testing in patients with syncope provides specific recommendations on various protocols.

4. Kapoor WN, Fortunato M, Hanusa BH, Schulberg HC. Psychiatric illnesses in patients with syncope. Am J Med 1995;99:505–512.

   Psychiatric illnesses are commonly found in patients with syncope. Patients with psychiatric illnesses have higher rates of recurrence.

76 Palpitations

Symptom

BARBARA E. WEBER and WISHWA N. KAPOOR

Epidemiology. Palpitations, the awareness of one's own heartbeat, are produced by a change in the rate, rhythm, or strength of cardiac contraction. Patients may describe palpitations as "fast heartbeats," "irregular heartbeats," "skipped heartbeats," "irregular heart rate," or "heart pounding." The incidence of this symptom in general medical practice is not accurately known but may range from less than 1% to 8% per year.

Etiology. The causes of palpitations range from isolated benign processes to serious cardiac diseases (Table 76–1). In a prospective cohort study of 190 patients with a chief complaint of palpitations, a cause could be determined in 84% (cardiac 43%, psychiatric 31%, and miscellaneous 10%).

Table 76–1. ETIOLOGY OF PALPITATIONS

Habits	Pacemaker
Alcohol	Diaphragmatic flutter
Caffeine	Paced beats
Cocaine	Prosthetic heart valve
Tobacco	Other cardiac diseases
Medications	Cardiomegaly
Sympathomimetic	Mitral valve prolapse
Anticholinergic	Myxoma
Vasodilator	Arrhythmias
Dehydration	Isolated single palpitation
Psychiatric	Premature beats (atrial or ventricular)
Anxiety	The beat after a compensatory pause
Panic attack/disorder	The beat following a blocked beat
Somatization	Paroxysmal episodes
Emotional stress	Regular rhythm
Metabolic	Supraventricular tachycardia
Hypoglycemia	Ventricular tachycardia
Thyrotoxicosis	Sick sinus syndrome
Pheochromocytoma	Sinus bradycardia
High-output states	Irregular rhythm
Anemia	Paroxysmal atrial fibrillation
Fever	Paroxysmal atrial tachycardia
Paget's disease	Multifocal atrial tachycardia
Pregnancy	Frequent premature ventricular
Increased stroke volume	contractions or premature atrial
Valvular heart disease	contractions
Exertion	
Cardiac and noncardiac arteriovenous shunts	

Clinical Approach. The clinical features of palpitations, such as the rapidity of onset and the frequency, duration, and regularity of the heartbeat, as well as any associated symptoms, help to characterize the cause and severity of the problem. For example, isolated forceful heartbeats following a pause frequently represent premature atrial or ventricular contractions. Abrupt runs of strong heartbeats suggest a paroxysmal reentrant tachycardia. A gradual onset and termination is more often associated with sinus (physiologic) tachycardia. Patients who can terminate palpitations by coughing, drinking ice water, or massaging their neck (vagal maneuvers) probably have supraventricular tachycardia.

The patient should be questioned about symptoms related to disorders that may cause palpitations (see Table 76–1), including psychiatric illnesses such as anxiety and panic disorders. The clinician should identify high-risk patients who may require more intensive evaluation and management. Patients with underlying organic heart disease (coronary artery disease, congestive heart failure, valvular heart disease, hypertrophic cardiomyopathy) who experience recurrent palpitations are more likely to have arrhythmias. Although cohort studies of patients with palpitations are not available, patients with heart disease and complex ventricular ectopy appear to be at higher risk for sudden death.

Even though a patient's palpitations may have resolved, the vital signs may provide clues to their cause. Orthostatic hypotension may indicate volume depletion. A fast, regular heart rate suggests supraventricular or sinus tachycardia, atrial flutter, or ventricular tachycardia. A rapid regular rate of 100 to 140 beats per minute suggests sinus tachycardia, and 150 beats per minute suggests atrial flutter. A fast irregular rate may represent multifocal atrial tachycardia, atrial fibrillation, or atrial flutter with variable atrioventricular block. A slow heart rate results from sinus bradycardia, junctional rhythm, or complete heart block. Occasional irregularity of an otherwise regular pulse may represent premature contractions or atrial fibrillation.

When a diagnosis is not evident after clinical examination, helpful laboratory tests include a serum glucose test and determination of electrolyte and hemoglobin levels. If these results are normal, specialized tests such as thyroid function tests, serum and urine catecholamine levels, or echocardiography may be required to diagnose hyperthyroidism, pheochromocytoma, or underlying heart disease, respectively.

Although the yield of a 12-lead electrocardiogram and rhythm strip is low, it may show specific arrhythmias (e.g., atrial fibrillation or premature ventricular contractions) or conduction system disease that prompts further evaluation such as electrophysiologic studies. The electrocardiogram may show evidence of myocardial ischemia or infarction. If symptoms occur with exertion, an exercise electrocardiogram may be diagnostic.

Ambulatory electrocardiographic monitoring is often used to evaluate palpitations, despite a sensitivity of only 10% to 69% for symptomatic arrhythmias. Other limitations include a poor correlation between symptoms and arrhythmias, the frequent detection of brief asymptomatic arrhythmias unrelated to palpitations, and failure of intermittently symptomatic arrhythmias to occur during the monitoring period (see Chapter 87, Ambulatory Cardiac Monitoring). Patient-activated transtelephonic monitoring (e.g., with loop monitors) is more likely to capture a rhythm during palpitations.

Invasive electrophysiologic studies may be warranted in patients with unexplained recurrent palpitations who have organic heart disease, preexcitation syndrome, or conduction system disease (on 12-lead electrocardiogram) or to evaluate specific arrhythmias detected by noninvasive means.

In our study, for those patients discovered to have a cause for their palpitations, the cause was determined by history and physical examination, electrocardiography, or laboratory data in 40%.

Management. Treatment of underlying disease should lead to resolution of the symptoms. Hospitalization is unnecessary unless symptoms are severe or arrhythmias are diagnosed or highly likely.

Follow-Up. Depending on the cause of palpitations and the existence of co-morbid conditions, the prognosis in patients with palpitations and no underlying cardiac disease is generally favorable. Although 1-year rates of stroke and death are negligible, there are both a high rate of recurrent symptoms and a moderate impact on productivity.

REFERENCES

1. Barsky AJ, Cleary PD, Coeytaux RR, Ruskin JN. Psychiatric disorders in medical outpatients complaining of palpitations. J Gen Intern Med 1994;9:306–313.

   In this cohort study of patients with palpitations referred for Holter monitoring, almost half have a psychiatric disorder, more than one fourth have lifetime panic disorder, and one fifth had panic attacks in the month before monitoring.

2. Diamond TH, Smith R, Myburgh DP. Holter monitoring: A necessity for the evaluation of palpitations. S Afr Med J 1983;63:5–7.

   Symptomatic correlation was achieved in 44% of patients with palpitations referred for Holter monitoring.

3. Kinlay S, Leitch JW, Neil A, Chapman BL, Hardy DB, Fletcher PJ. Cardiac event recorders yield more diagnoses and are more cost-effective than 48-hour Holter monitoring in patients with palpitations. A controlled clinical trial. Ann Intern Med 1996;124(1 Pt 1):16–20.

   Holter monitoring is a poor diagnostic test for intermittent palpitations. Event recorders provide better data and are more cost-effective. Event monitors were twice as likely to provide a diagnostic rhythm strip electrocardiogram during symptoms as 48-hour Holter monitoring (67% vs. 35%). Event monitors result in a cost savings of $213 for each additional diagnostic rhythm strip obtained while the patient has symptoms.

4. Knudson MP. The natural history of palpitations in a family practice. J Fam Pract 1987;24:357–360.

   In this retrospective cohort study of young family practice patients with palpitations, an incidence of less than 1% and no increased risk of cardiac morbidity or mortality were suggested when compared with a control population.

5. Weber BW, Kapoor WN. Evaluation and outcomes of patients with palpitations. Am J Med 1996;100:138–148.

   The authors present a prospective cohort study of 190 inpatients and outpatients with a chief complaint of palpitations.

77 Edema

Symptom

STEVEN R. McGEE

Epidemiology. In one survey of healthy subjects older than age 65, 16% had swelling of the ankles and lower calves that, with firm pressure from an examiner's finger, pitted to a depth of 1 cm or more.

Etiology. Swelling of an extremity may result from increased capillary hydrostatic pressure (e.g., congestive heart failure), increased capillary permeability (e.g., inflammation), decreased oncotic pressure (e.g., hypoalbuminemia), reduced lymph removal (lymphedema), or increased amounts of normal tissues (lipedema). Table 77–1 is a list of the causes of unilateral and bilateral edema. In one study of 245 consecutive patients older than age 65 with edema (mean duration of 7.5 months), the final diagnoses were chronic venous insufficiency (63%), congestive heart failure (15%), drug-induced edema (14%), and other (8%). Chapter 130 (Painful and Swollen Calf) includes a discussion of acute unilateral swelling of the lower extremity.

Table 77–1. ETIOLOGY OF EDEMA

Bilateral
  Congestive heart failure
  Pulmonary hypertension from lung disease
  Hepatic cirrhosis
  Nephrotic syndrome
  Acute glomerulonephritis
  Hypoalbuminemia
  Lipedema
  Primary lymphedema
  Medications
    Antihypertensive drugs
      Nifedipine
      Guanethidine
      Prazosin
    Nonsteroidal anti-inflammatory medications
Unilateral
  Acute*
    Deep venous thrombosis
    Cellulitis
    Baker's cyst
    Muscle hematoma
  Chronic
    Chronic venous insufficiency
    Primary or secondary lymphedema

*Discussed in Chapter 130, Painful and Swollen Calf.

The ease of pitting reflects the protein content of the edema fluid. Edema due to low-protein fluids (hypoalbuminemia, cardiac and venous edema) has low viscosity, pits easily with local pressure, and recovers promptly when the pressure is removed. High-protein fluids (cellulitis edema, lymphedema) have high viscosity, resist pitting, and, once pitted, recover slowly ("brawny" or "woody" edema). Leg elevation and diuresis increase the protein content of the edema and make it more firm on examination. All edematous conditions are aggravated by high environmental heat, perhaps because of vasodilation and increased capillary transudation of fluid.

The edema of *chronic venous insufficiency* is worse at the end of the day and is often associated with the sensation of leg heaviness and the findings of superficial venous varicosities, brown pigmentation about the ankle, and, in some, a pruritic dermatitis and ulceration.

Lymphedema is painless and firm and, in contrast to venous edema, varies little throughout the day. Squaring of the toes is characteristic, and ulceration is rare unless the edema is complicated by trauma or infection. Lymphedema of the lower extremity that begins before age 40 usually results from congenitally abnormal lymphatics ("primary" lymphedema), may be bilateral, and is much more common in women. Lower extremity lymphedema beginning after age 40 is "secondary" to malignancy or recurrent cellulitis; 95% of cases are unilateral. When secondary to malignancy, prostate cancer is the most common diagnosis in men, and lymphoma is most often found in women. Lymphedema of the upper extremity is almost always due to breast cancer, either from the tumor itself or from combined treatment by surgery and irradiation.

Lipedema results from increased deposition of fat in the lower extremities, occurs exclusively in obese women, does not pit, and, unlike lymphedema, spares the feet.

Clinical Approach. The patient interview should determine the distribution of edema, how quickly it developed, and whether there is associated trauma or pain. Edema that develops quickly over days excludes lymphedema and lipedema. Generalized edema involving the face or sacrum, or associated with abdominal swelling or shortness of breath (anasarca), suggests renal disease, hepatic disease, congestive heart failure, or severe pulmonary hypertension from lung disease. Severe pain is uncommon in anasarca, lymphedema, and lipedema, unless complicated by infection, ulceration, or thrombosis.

Physical examination—which focuses on the neck veins, chest, abdomen, and pelvis—may reveal lymphadenopathy (inflammation, lymphedema), a prostatic or pelvic mass (lymphedema), elevated neck veins (congestive heart failure or pulmonary hypertension), or findings of hepatic disease (spider telangiectasia, gynecomastia, palmar erythema). The clinician should determine how easily the edema pits. Routine laboratory tests in patients with bilateral edema include a chemistry profile, complete blood cell count, creatinine, urinalysis, and chest radiograph. Computed tomography of the abdomen and pelvis is indicated in cases of suspected secondary lymphedema.

Management. General principles in treating edema include (1) elevation of the involved extremity; (2) use of elastic stockings or custom-made gradient stockings to reduce dependent edema (unless the patient has severe arterial insufficiency); (3) treatment of the underlying cause (e.g., lymphedema may resolve with treatment of the underlying malignancy); (4) monitoring for and prompt treatment of any cellulitis or ulceration (see Chapter 133, Leg Ulcers); (5) avoidance of offending medications if possible (see Table 77–1); and (6) use of diuretics (see Chapter 79, Congestive Heart Failure) when the edema is refractory to more conservative measures. Potential complications of all diuretics include saline depletion, hypokalemia, hyponatremia, and renal insufficiency.

Therapy for generalized edematous disorders (cardiac, renal, or hepatic diseases) includes dietary salt restriction, diuretics, and specific treatments tailored to the underlying disorder (e.g., surgery for valvular heart disease, corticosteroids for some causes of the nephrotic syndrome). Most patients with acute or severe generalized edema are best hospitalized for enforced bed rest (which promotes diuresis) and diagnostic tests.

Cross-References: Eczema (Chapter 28), Congestive Heart Failure (Chapter 79), Painful and Swollen Calf (Chapter 130), Leg Ulcers (Chapter 133), Proteinuria (Chapter 181).

REFERENCES

1. Ciocon JO, Galindo-Ciocon D, Galindo DJ. Raised leg exercises for leg edema in the elderly. Angiology 1995;46:19–25.

   Prospective analysis is provided of the causes of edema in a geriatric population and their management.

2. Henry JA, Altmann P. Assessment of hypoproteinaemic oedema: A simple physical sign. BMJ 1978;1:890–891.

   The ease with which edema pits on examination and the rapidity with which the pitting recovers correlates with the inverse of the serum albumin value.

3. Smith RD, Spittell JA, Schirger A. Secondary lymphedema of the leg: Its characteristics and diagnostic implications. JAMA 1963;185:80–82.

   The clinical features of 80 cases are reviewed.

4. Young JR. The swollen leg: Clinical significance and differential diagnosis. Cardiol Clin 1991;9:443–456.

   This is a comprehensive and well-organized review of the differential diagnosis of edema (with 21 accompanying photographs illustrating the various clinical features).

78 Angina

Problem

DAVID H. HICKAM

Epidemiology and Etiology. Angina is the syndrome of recurrent chest pain in adults. Classically, angina pectoris refers to a characteristic pain that occurs intermittently for a few minutes at a time, is located substernally, radiates to the neck or arms, is described as tight or pressing, is brought on by exertion and relieved by rest, and is severe enough to cause the patient to stop all activities. However, many patients' symptoms lack some of these features, leading to the use of terms such as *atypical angina, variant angina, nonanginal chest pain,* and *noncardiac chest pain.* Angina, particularly in less typical variants, can be caused by any of the causes of chest pain (see Chapter 73, Acute Chest Pain, Table 73–1).

Many studies of patients undergoing coronary arteriography have found that patients with classic angina pectoris are more likely to have obstructive disease of the coronary arteries than those with less typical pain. Other risk factors for coronary artery disease (CAD)—male sex, older age, hypertension, hypercholesterolemia, diabetes mellitus, smoking history—increase the likelihood that an individual will have anginal pain and that the pain is caused by CAD. Among women with typical angina, the prevalence of CAD is lower, and the characteristics of the pain are less useful in women than in men for predicting the likely cause.

Studies of patients with angina and negative tests for CAD have found evidence of esophageal motor disorders in 28% and reflux esophagitis in 10% to 20%. However, it is possible that the esophageal disorders were not actually the cause of pain in some of these patients.

Symptoms and Signs. Because the degree to which a patient's pain is typical of angina correlates with the probability that CAD is present, specific criteria should be used to classify pain as typical anginal, atypical anginal, or nonanginal. The most important criterion is whether the pain is brought on by exertion and relieved by rest. Approximately 80% of patients with exertional chest pain have CAD. Relief of the pain with nitroglycerin is also a helpful characteristic. Pain caused by CAD is usually relieved within 3 minutes. The specificity of this criterion decreases as the time accepted as defining relief is lengthened. Because nitroglycerin relaxes esophageal smooth muscle, esophageal motor disorders should be considered in patients whose pain is relieved by nitroglycerin but who do not have CAD on further evaluation.

Approximately half of patients with the syndrome of atypical angina are found to have CAD on coronary arteriography. Patients should be considered as having atypical angina when there is an inconsistent relationship of the pain to exertion (e.g., when a certain level of exercise brings on pain only some of the time or when mild activities cause the pain but other more strenuous activities do not). It is also appropriate to consider anginal pain atypical if it is consistently exertional but other characteristics are atypical, such as a location in the lateral chest, a pleuritic quality, or inconsistent relief achieved with nitroglycerin.

Approximately 20% of patients whose pain was classified as nonanginal have CAD on arteriography. Nonanginal chest pain is not exertional, is not relieved by nitroglycerin, is usually located in the lateral chest, and is often aggravated by deep breaths or other chest movement.

A clinician's estimate of the probability that a patient's chest pain is caused by CAD should take into account other patient characteristics. CAD is rare in patients younger than age 40 unless there are significant risk factors such as a severely elevated cholesterol level or use of cigarettes or cocaine. Patients with a known history of myocardial infarction are more likely to have CAD. The physical examination is of little use, however, because most patients with CAD have no specific physical findings.

The clinician should resist using evidence of other diseases to influence the estimate of the probability of CAD. For example, murmurs suggesting mitral valve prolapse are probably as common in patients with CAD as in those without CAD. Some patients with CAD have chest wall tenderness. Relief of pain by antacids (suggesting reflux esophagitis) does not reliably exclude CAD.

Clinical Approach. The reference standard test is coronary arteriography, though rare patients may have ischemia caused by small-vessel obstructions not visible on arteriography. Tests other than arteriography are commonly referred to as noninvasive studies. For all the noninvasive tests, the clinician must estimate the pretest probability of CAD, then use the test result to convert the pretest estimate to a post-test probability (see Chapter 7, Principles of Screening).

The resting electrocardiogram (ECG) is easy to perform, can be interpreted by the average clinician, and should be obtained in all patients except those with a very low pretest probability of CAD. Its greatest value is in detecting Q waves indicative of prior myocardial infarction. If Q waves are absent, the test should be considered positive if there are T-wave inversions or ST segment depression of 1 mm or greater. These findings have a sensitivity for CAD of 25% in men and 40% in women, with a specificity of approximately 75%. Thus, the resting ECG is not sensitive enough to exclude CAD in patients with an intermediate pretest probability.

In patients with a high pretest probability of CAD, no diagnostic testing other than the ECG is necessary. If the ECG shows new changes or significant ST segment depressions or elevations, immediate hospitalization should be considered. Otherwise, the patient should be started on medical therapy for CAD pending further evaluation (see later).

The three most commonly used cardiac stress tests are exercise ECG, thallium scintigraphy, and exercise echocardiography. These tests are based on recordings made before, during, and after the patient undergoes a graded exercise load, usually on a treadmill. On average, the exercise ECG has a sensitivity of 0.70 and a specificity of 0.70 for any CAD. Thallium scintigraphy has a sensitivity of approximately 0.85 and a specificity of approximately 0.80.

Exercise echocardiography has a sensitivity of approximately 0.75 and a speci- ficity of approximately 0.80. The specificity of exercise echocardiography is somewhat higher in patients having normal resting left ventricular contractility. With the exception of using echocardiography in patients with normal left ventricular function at rest, the specificity of none of these tests is high enough to be used reliably to exclude CAD in patients with a high pretest probability (see Chapter 86, Echocardiographic and Nuclear Assessment of Cardiac Func- tion, and Chapter 88, Exercise Tolerance Testing).

There are two situations in which stress tests are most useful clinically. The first is to help make a diagnosis in patients with an intermediate pretest probability of CAD, such as middle-aged men with atypical angina. A positive exercise test result moves the patient's probability to the high range, and a negative result moves the probability to the low range. Because exercise ECG is less expensive and easier to perform than the other studies, it is preferable for most patients.

The second major clinical indication for stress tests is to help plan manage- ment in patients with a high probability of CAD. Some subgroups of these patients may have better long-term outcomes when treated with either coronary bypass surgery or coronary angioplasty. For example, a patient with a single high-grade proximal coronary lesion may be greatly improved by angioplasty. Patients with left main coronary disease, multiple vessel disease, or poor left ventricular function may have improved survival with bypass surgery. If the exercise test is abnormal, the consulting cardiologist may choose to proceed with arteriography to guide the patient's further treatment.

If CAD has been excluded, tests for esophageal disorders can be consid- ered, although these tests are expensive and uncomfortable for the patient. The only definitive test for reflux esophagitis is endoscopy. Barium esophagog- raphy is insensitive for motor disorders and lacks specificity for reflux. Thus, the diagnosis of esophageal disease is often based on clinical grounds (atypical chest pain and previous history of peptic disease) rather than on testing.

Management. Successful reduction of symptoms in CAD is associated with better long-term outcomes in these patients. Three major classes of medications are available to treat symptoms of CAD: nitrates, β-blockers, and calcium channel blockers (Table 78–1). The major pharmacologic action of all three classes is to reduce cardiac workload. Whereas drugs in two of the classes (nitrates and calcium channel blockers) may improve coronary perfusion through dilation of coronary arteries, this probably is a minor effect in patients other than those having coronary artery spasm. Because the pharmacologic effects differ across the three classes, patients often benefit from treatment with more than one medication.

Nearly all patients with CAD should be given sublingual nitroglycerin, which usually brings rapid relief when symptoms occur. It sometimes is useful to instruct the patient to take nitroglycerin prophylactically just before engag- ing in strenuous activity, though longer-acting drugs are generally of greater value for preventing episodes of pain. Any of the three classes can be chosen for initial therapy. Nitrates cause reduced ventricular volume through venous pooling and are relatively free of side effects. β-blockers reduce heart rate, ventricular contractility, and blood pressure, making them particularly appro-

Table 78–1. MEDICATIONS USED TO REDUCE THE FREQUENCY OF ANGINAL CHEST PAIN IN PATIENTS WITH CORONARY ARTERY DISEASE

Generic Name	Brand Name	Starting Dose	Maximal Dose
*Sublingual Nitrates**			
Nitroglycerin	Nitrostat	0.3 mg prn	0.8 mg prn
*Topical Nitrates**			
Transdermal nitroglycerin	Nitro-Dur	0.2 mg/h	0.8 mg/h
	Transderm-Nitro		
Nitroglycerin ointment, 2%	Nitrol	1 inch qhs	6 inches qhs
*Oral Nitrates**			
Isosorbide dinitrate	Isordil	5 mg qid	40 mg qid
	Sorbitrate		
Isosorbide mononitrate	Ismo	20 mg bid	20 mg bid
Pentaerythritol tetranitrate	Peritrate	10 mg qid	60 mg qid
Erithrityl tetranitrate	Cardilate	10 mg qid	40 mg q4h
β-Blockers†			
Propranolol	Inderal	20 mg qid	60 mg qid
Metoprolol	Lopressor	50 mg bid	100 mg qid
Atenolol	Tenormin	50 mg qd	200 mg qd
Nadolol	Corgard	40 mg qd	240 mg qd
Timolol	Blocadren	10 mg bid	30 mg bid
Calcium Channel Blockers‡			
Nifedipine	Adalat	10 mg tid	40 mg qid
	Procardia		160 mg tid
Verapamil	Calan	40 mg tid	160 mg tid
	Isoptin		
Diltiazem	Cardizem	30 mg tid	120 mg qid

*All the nitrate preparations have similar side effects, including headache, hypotension, and tachycardia. Individual patients may tolerate some preparations better than others.

†All the β-blockers in this table can cause any of the side effects of this class of medications. The "cardioselective" agents (atenolol and metoprolol) are slightly less prone than the other β-blockers to cause bronchoconstriction, cold extremities, and insulin-mediated hypoglycemia. The "lipophilic" agents (atenolol, nadolol, and timolol) are slightly less prone to cause fatigue and sleep disorders. All of these β-blockers have similar tendencies to cause bradycardia and left ventricular depression. Other β-blockers having intrinsic sympathomimetic activity (acebutolol, carteolol, pindolol) are commonly used to treat hypertension but are not primary agents for the treatment of ischemic heart disease.

‡The three calcium channel blockers vary in their side effect profiles. Nifedipine is more likely than the other agents to cause headache and hypotension but it is less likely to cause problems attributable to bradycardia or left ventricular depression. Verapamil has a greater tendency than nifedipine and diltiazem to cause gastrointestinal symptoms.

priate in hypertensive patients. They can cause bronchoconstriction and are relatively contraindicated in patients with pulmonary disease. Calcium channel blockers reduce ventricular contractility and peripheral vascular resistance, making them a useful alternative to β-blockers in patients with hypertension.

Medication doses should be increased and additional medications added until the patient has adequate reduction of angina frequency or has achieved maximal hemodynamic effects of the drugs. Doses of β-blockers usually should not be increased if the resting heart rate is less than 60 beats per minute or the heart rate with moderate exercise is less than 90 beats per minute. Calcium channel blocker doses should not be increased if the systolic blood pressure is less than 100 mm Hg. Nitrates are ineffective at single doses larger than approximately 60 mg for isosorbide dinitrate and comparable doses for the other agents.

Either calcium channel blockers or nitrates can be used for patients with esophageal motor disorders. Chapter 96, Dysphagia and Heartburn, is a review of the management of reflux esophagitis.

Follow-Up. Patients with suspected CAD should be seen frequently in the clinic to assess their initial response to treatment. Patients who do not respond to treatment should undergo further diagnostic evaluation. Patients should be instructed to seek care immediately if an episode of pain does not respond to nitroglycerin. If the frequency of a patient's anginal episodes increases while on medical therapy, hospitalization for intensive treatment of unstable angina should be considered.

Cross-References: Acute Chest Pain (Chapter 73), Recurrent Chest Pain (Chapter 74), Essential Hypertension (Chapter 85), Echocardiographic and Nuclear Assessment of Cardiac Function (Chapter 86), Exercise Tolerance Testing (Chapter 88), Dysphagia and Heartburn (Chapter 96), Preoperative Cardiovascular Problems (Chapter 218).

REFERENCES

1. Goldman L, Lee TH. Noninvasive tests for diagnosing the presence and extent of coronary artery disease: Exercise electrocardiography, thallium scintigraphy, and radionuclide ventriculography. J Gen Intern Med 1986;1:258–265.

   This article is a good review of noninvasive testing, with strategies for testing in various clinical syndromes.

2. Katz PO, Dalton CB, Richter JE, et al. Esophageal testing of patients with noncardiac chest pain or dysphagia: Results of three years' experience with 1161 patients. Ann Intern Med 1987;16:593–597.

   Data on prevalence of esophageal disorders are presented along with the yield of tests for these disorders.

3. Landenheim ML, Kotler TS, Pollock BH, et al. Incremental prognostic power of clinical history, exercise electrocardiography and myocardial perfusion scintigraphy in suspected coronary artery disease. Am J Cardiol 1987;59:270–277.

   The authors provide useful algorithms for using test results to classify patients' risk of complications of coronary artery disease.

4. Mark DB, Hlatky, MD, Harrell FE, et al. Exercise treadmill score for predicting prognosis in coronary artery disease. Ann Intern Med 1987;106:793–800.

   Additional data on estimating the risk of adverse events in coronary artery disease are presented.

5. Ryan T, Vasey CG, Presti CF, et al. Exercise echocardiography: Detection of coronary artery disease in patients with normal left ventricular wall motion at rest. J Am Coll Cardiol 1988;11:993–999.

   This is a useful discussion of the use of exercise echocardiography in the diagnosis of suspected coronary artery disease.

79 Congestive Heart Failure

Problem

DAWN E. DeWITT and STEVEN R. McGEE

Epidemiology. The prevalence of congestive heart failure (CHF) in the United States is 1% overall, rising to 10% in persons older than age 75. Mortality is 200,000 per year, and about half of these are sudden deaths, presumably due to arrhythmias. Five-year survival rates for patients with CHF are 60% for men and 45% for women; for patients with New York Heart Association class IV disease, 1-year mortality is 50%. Major risk factors for CHF include hypertension; coronary artery disease; rheumatic, valvular, or congenital heart disease; and diabetes mellitus.

Symptoms and Signs. Table 79–1 lists the symptoms and signs of CHF. Shortness of breath, traditionally regarded as a symptom of left atrial hypertension associated with pulmonary interstitial edema, may also result from low cardiac output (respiratory muscle fatigue, tachypnea of Cheyne-Stokes respiration) or right atrial hypertension (hydrothorax, ascites).

An S3 early diastolic filling sound, if present after age 40, is pathologic and signifies rapid diastolic filling, usually from elevated atrial pressures or atrioventricular (AV) valve regurgitation. Additional important physical findings include (1) an abnormal abdominojugular test—midabdominal pressure elevates the jugular venous pressure for longer than 10 seconds—which reflects pulmonary wedge pressures greater than 15 mm Hg (in the absence of right ventricular infarction or isolated right ventricular failure); (2) an apical impulse diameter greater than 3 cm, measured in the left lateral decubitus position, which predicts an abnormally elevated left ventricular end-diastolic volume (sensitivity = 92%, specificity = 75%); and (3) an abnormal Valsalva response (square wave response, absence of phase IV overshoot), detected with a sphyg-

Table 79–1. CONGESTIVE HEART FAILURE: SYMPTOMS AND SIGNS

Hemodynamics	Symptom	Sign
Low cardiac output	Fatigue, syncope, angina, dyspnea	Cheyne-Stokes respiration, peripheral cyanosis, cool extremities
High right atrial pressure	Edema, abdominal swelling, dyspnea, anorexia	Elevated central venous pressure, edema, ascites, right ventricular S3
High left atrial pressure	Dyspnea, orthopnea, paroxysmal nocturnal dyspnea, cough	Lung crackles,* left ventricular S3

*More sensitive in acute than chronic congestive heart failure.

momanometer, which correlates with a depressed ejection fraction and an elevated left-ventricular end-diastolic pressure.

Clinical Approach. Recently, CHF has been reclassified into systolic versus diastolic dysfunction with symptomatic and asymptomatic categories in each class. This classification, based on pathophysiology, is useful for both prognosis and treatment. Characteristic symptoms, signs, and chest radiographic findings (large heart, redistribution of blood flow to upper zones, pleural effusions, pulmonary edema) support the diagnosis of CHF. Echocardiography provides an estimate of ejection fraction (< 0.35–0.40 is considered systolic dysfunction) or may reveal a normal ejection fraction (> 0.40) with clinical evidence of pulmonary venous hypertension and congestion, suggesting a diagnosis of diastolic dysfunction (up to one third of patients with CHF have normal systolic function). Echocardiography also provides information about valvular function. Although radionuclide ventriculography is less operator dependent, its usefulness is limited to assessing systolic function. In addition, patients found by echocardiogram to have systolic dysfunction with reduced ejection fraction or hypertrophic or hypertensive cardiomyopathy, even in the absence of symptoms, benefit from treatment.

The clinician should always attempt to clarify the cause of the patient's cardiomyopathy using the patient interview, physical examination, laboratory evaluation, chest radiography, electrocardiography, and echocardiography, because the specific treatment for many patients depends on a precise diagnosis. Table 79–2 lists etiologies of CHF and the causes of unstable CHF.

Management. Management goals include reducing symptoms, preventing complications, and improving survival. All patients should follow a no-added-salt

Table 79–2. ETIOLOGIES AND PRECIPITATING
CAUSES OF CONGESTIVE HEART FAILURE

Etiology		Precipitating Causes
Dilated	*Nondilated*	
Low Output	*Restrictive*	Hyperthyroidism
Ischemic	Amyloidosis	New drug added (β-blocker, nonsteroidal
Hypertension	Sarcoidosis	anti-inflammatory, alcohol, verapamil,
Viral/human	Hemochromatosis	disopyramide, group I antiarrhythmic)
immunodeficiency virus		Myocardial ischemia
Valvular	*Hypertrophic*	Dietary noncompliance
Metabolic: Ca, Mg, K, P	Hypertrophic obstructive	Bradyarrhythmia or tachyarrhythmia
Familial	cardiomyopathy	Anemia
Medications	Hypertension	Renal failure
Idiopathic	Aortic stenosis	Fever
		Uncontrolled hypertension
High Output	*Constrictive/Pericardial*	
Thyrotoxicosis	Surgery	
Anemia	Tuberculosis	
Atrioventricular fistula	Rheumatologic	
Vascular lesions	Malignancy	
Infection	Viral	
Paget's disease		
Beriberi		

diet (3–4 g/day), weigh themselves daily, stay as active as possible (submaximal exercise), and avoid cigarettes and alcohol. Most drug treatments for CHF require careful monitoring of blood pressure, serum electrolyte levels, and renal function.

In general, multiple randomized trials during the past decade show that for patients with systolic dysfunction with or without symptoms, angiotensin-converting enzyme (ACE) inhibitors decrease morbidity and mortality, are first-line agents in patients with mild CHF, should be given to all patients with CHF in combination with diuretics unless contraindicated, and benefit post–myocardial infarction patients with decreased ejection fractions. Digoxin should be added if patients remain symptomatic on full-dose ACE inhibitors and diuretics. Patients with diastolic dysfunction often benefit from β-blockers, diltiazem, or verapamil.

VASODILATOR (ACE INHIBITOR) THERAPY. Arterial and venous beds constrict when the cardiac output decreases, maintaining blood pressure and increasing preload. In CHF this physiologic response can be maladaptive. Reversal of vasoconstriction with vasodilators, originally by hydralazine plus isosorbide (Veterans Administration Cooperative Study) and subsequently with ACE inhibitors (Cooperative North Scandinavian Enalapril Survival Study: Study of Left Ventricular Dysfunction [SOLVD]), improves not only exercise duration, dyspnea, and fatigue but also survival. Enalapril reduces mortality and decreases hospitalizations for CHF, and enalapril and captopril improve functional status. Other ACE inhibitors likely to have similar effects include lisinopril, but this has not yet been proven. ACE inhibitors also reduce mortality in asymptomatic patients with decreased systolic function (< 35%–40%). In addition, mortality is reduced by 17% to 27% in post–myocardial infarction patients with clinical CHF or ejection fractions less than 40% (begin therapy after 24 hours).

Hydralazine and isosorbide cause more side effects and are less effective than ACE inhibitors in reducing mortality (25% mortality vs. 18% mortality, respectively) but should be used when ACE inhibitors are not tolerated. After assessment for volume depletion, the initial dose of an ACE inhibitor should be small (Table 79–3); if well tolerated, the dose may be increased every several days, while blood pressure and renal function are monitored. ACE inhibitors may cause significant hypotension and renal insufficiency, especially in patients who have previously received large doses of diuretics or who have hyponatremia or severe CHF. In these patients, ACE inhibitors are best initiated during a hospitalization; if they are given in the outpatient setting, the clinician should monitor the patient's orthostatic blood pressure frequently after the first dose until the peak effect period has passed (3 hours for captopril, 6 hours for enalapril). Some side effects—hypotension, worsening renal function, and hyperkalemia—occur more often with long-acting agents (e.g., enalapril) and may be minimized by diuretic reduction. Other side effects of ACE inhibitors include dysgeusia, rash, angioedema (an absolute contraindication), and cough. In one trial (SOLVD), cough was reported in 37% of patients on enalapril versus 31% of those on placebo. Only 1% of patients discontinued therapy because of cough. Increasing diuretics may help because cough may be due to CHF rather than the medication. Although not yet fully evaluated, angiotensin II receptor blockers (e.g., losartan) may be better tolerated in patients with ACE inhibitor–induced cough.

Table 79–3. DRUG THERAPY OF CONGESTIVE HEART FAILURE

Drug	Starting Oral Dose (mg)	Usual Maintenance Oral Dose (mg)	Cost ($ per month)*
Thiazide Diuretics			
Hydrochlorothiazide	25 qd	25–50 qd	1.05–1.08
Metolazone	2.5 qd	2.5–10 qd	12.85–17.50
Loop Diuretics			
Furosemide	20 qd	20–160 qd–bid	1.20–6.90
Potassium-sparing Diuretics			
Triamterene	100 qd	100–200 qd	12.30–24.60
Spironolactone	50 qd	50–200 qd	4.35–12.00
Vasodilators			
Direct-acting			
Hydralazine	25 q8h	50–100 q6–8h	4.25–11.30
Isosorbide dinitrate	10 q8h	20–80 q6–8h	4.10–21.80
Angiotensin-converting enzyme inhibitor			
Captopril	6.25 q8h	25–50 q8h	62.80–176.31
Enalapril	2.5 qd	10–20 bid	57.45–81.70
Lisinopril	2.5 qd	2.5–20 qd	15.12–25.10
Digoxin	0.125 qd	0.125–0.5 qd	3.40–6.80

*Average wholesale price, 1995 *Drug Topics Red Book*, for dose range under Usual Maintenance Oral Dose.

Doses should be increased to those proven to be maximally therapeutic (e.g., 50 mg of captopril three times daily or 10 mg of enalapril twice daily). Diuretics should be tapered as needed to reach these goals. In patients who remain symptomatic, the dose should be increased weekly to a systolic blood pressure greater than 85 to 90 mm Hg as long as the serum creatinine level remains below 1.8 mg/dL and the potassium level remains below 5.0 mg/dL.

DIURETICS. Most patients with CHF have sodium and water (volume) overload. Diuretics reduce atrial pressures, and therefore symptoms, more rapidly and effectively than any other oral drug available for CHF (see Table 79–3). Treatment of patients without diuretics (e.g., with vasodilators alone) may result in recurrent pulmonary edema. Diuretics should be titrated to achieve a jugular venous pressure less than 8 cm H_2O and absent abdominojugular reflex, but their use should not prevent adequate dosing of ACE inhibitors. Single doses of loop diuretics are more effective than divided doses (e.g., use furosemide as a single dose until greater than 160 mg/d, then divide). Hypokalemia is common with thiazide and loop diuretics and requires treatment if (1) the potassium level is below 4.0 mEq/L (care should be taken in patients on ACE inhibitors) or (2) the patient is taking digoxin. Other complications of diuretics include saline depletion, magnesium depletion, hypotension, renal insufficiency, and increased neurohormonal activation (e.g., increased serum catecholamines that increase heart rate). This last complication has led to suggestions that diuretics should not be used alone.

DIGOXIN. Digoxin decreases renin activity, increases vagal tone, and is a positive inotrope and mild vasodilator. Digoxin benefits patients with dilated hearts who have an S3 and poor systolic function and is the drug of choice for patients with CHF and atrial fibrillation. In these patients, serum trough digoxin levels of 1.2 to 1.7 ng/mL result in less dyspnea, increased exercise tolerance and functional class, and decreased heart size; withdrawal of digoxin may result in worsening CHF. However, digoxin has not been shown to alter the progression of CHF and should be instituted only in those patients who are symptomatic on diuretics and ACE inhibitors. Digoxin produces no benefit in patients with normal-sized hearts and normal systolic function (e.g., hypertrophic cardiomyopathy, pericardial diseases). Patients with digoxin toxicity may experience bradyarrhythmias or tachyarrhythmias, confusion, visual disturbances, anorexia, nausea, or vomiting. Digoxin blood levels help predict digoxin toxicity, but there is considerable overlap between toxic and therapeutic levels. Decreased renal function, hypokalemia, myocardial disease, and hypothyroidism all predispose patients to digoxin toxicity.

β-BLOCKERS. Neurohormonal activation, specifically increased plasma norepinephrine, is strongly associated with increased mortality in CHF. Although still controversial, β-blockers decrease mortality in post–myocardial infarction patients, decrease sudden death in post–myocardial infarction patients with CHF, decrease heart rate, increase left ventricular ejection fraction, increase exercise tolerance, and delay the need for heart transplant. Carvedilol, an α- and β-blocker with weak calcium channel blocking effects, appears promising. Patients should be referred to a cardiologist for treatment. Most patients tolerate small doses (e.g., 5 mg metoprolol twice daily), which can be increased slowly over months.

VENTRICULAR ARRHYTHMIAS. Up to 90% of CHF patients may demonstrate complex ventricular ectopy. *Symptomatic* ventricular tachycardia requires treatment (see Chapter 83, Chronic Ventricular Arrhythmias). Treatment of *asymptomatic* ventricular arrhythmias is controversial, because (1) evidence that treatment improves survival is scant and some drugs actually increase mortality, (2) some antiarrhythmic drugs depress cardiac output and potentially have proarrhythmic effects, and (3) prospective identification of patients at high risk for sudden death is imprecise.

Amiodarone has been shown to suppress asymptomatic, nonsustained ventricular arrhythmias and improve left ventricular function. Trials have not shown significant mortality benefits but have demonstrated safety and trends toward survival benefit. Thus, amiodarone appears to be the safest antiarrhythmic drug and should be considered first-line therapy for suppression of ventricular arrhythmias.

ANTICOAGULATION. In nonrandomized retrospective studies of patients with dilated cardiomyopathy and normal sinus rhythm, anticoagulation reduced the risk of systemic embolism from 3.5 episodes per 100 patient-years to zero. Without anticoagulation, the lifetime risk of systemic embolism is estimated at 10% to 18%. If no contraindications exist, many authorities recommend anticoagulation. Although echocardiography documents left ventricular mural thrombi in 40% of patients with dilated cardiomyopathy, clinically evident emboli may occur just as frequently when this finding is present as when it is not. Warfarin (international normalized ratio, range: 2–3) should be considered for patients who have a left ventricular ejection fraction less than or equal to 25%.

ANTIDEPRESSANTS. Some patients with CHF require treatment for depression. Selective serotonin-reuptake inhibitors (e.g. paroxetine, sertraline) are the drugs of choice due to favorable side-effect profiles. Although tricyclic antidepressants possess antiarrhythmic properties and do not affect cardiac output, they may cause severe orthostatic hypotension in CHF patients. Hypotension may occur even with low doses but is least problematic with nortriptyline. If preexisting bundle branch block exists, tricyclic therapy produces second- or third-degree heart block in 25%; these patients require extremely close follow-up by experienced personnel.

REFRACTORY CHF. Possible reasons for refractory CHF include (1) poor absorption of drug (documented in uncontrolled CHF), (2) poor compliance with a low-salt diet, (3) concomitant nonsteroidal anti-inflammatory drug use, (4) renal insufficiency (if the glomerular filtration rate is less than 25 mL/min, thiazide diuretics alone are ineffective), (5) uncontrolled precipitating cause of CHF (see Table 79–2), and (6) the patient's dyspnea is not due to elevated left atrial pressure and therefore should not respond to diuresis (e.g., dyspnea from low cardiac output or chronic obstructive lung disease).

Some patients with refractory CHF benefit from combined loop and thiazide diuretics. Initiation of such therapy may require hospitalization because of the risk of profound hypokalemia, hypotension, and renal insufficiency. Hospitalization of patients with refractory CHF also enforces bed rest (which increases diuresis) and provides the opportunity for parenteral diuretic therapy. For the few patients with severe refractory CHF (ejection fraction < 30%, CHF functional class III or IV despite optimal therapy), cardiac transplantation is the only effective alternative.

Follow-Up. Patient education regarding diet, exercise, sodium restriction, and medication compliance is key. Medication noncompliance ranges from 20% to 58% among patients with CHF. Patients should weigh themselves daily and contact their health care provider if their weight increases by 2 to 4 lb. Many patients can follow a self-adjustable diuretic regimen with home monitoring of blood pressures and weekly or bimonthly determination of serum electrolyte levels. Patients should be educated regarding thirst and cough as symptoms of CHF to avoid noncompliance with diuretics and ACE inhibitors.

Major causes of death include progressive CHF (40%), sudden death (40%), infection, pulmonary embolus, and myocardial infarction. Poor prognostic signs include severe symptoms (the 1-year mortality for patients with class IV CHF exceeds 50%), poor ejection fraction, hyponatremia, and ventricular arrhythmias.

Cross-References: Pleural Effusion (Chapter 65), Aortic Stenosis (Chapter 80), Other Valvular Disease (Chapter 81), Atrial Fibrillation (Chapter 82), Echocardiographic and Nuclear Assessment of Cardiac Function (Chapter 86), Chronic Anticoagulation (Chapter 201), Preoperative Cardiovascular Problems (Chapter 218).

REFERENCES

1. Baker DW, Konstam MA, Bottorff M, Pitt B. Management of heart failure: I. Pharmacologic treatment. JAMA 1994;272:1361–1366.
   Comprehensive review of pharmacologic treatment of CHF due to left ventricular systolic dysfunction emphasizes ACE inhibitors for all patients. Specific dosing and follow-up guidelines are provided for all major therapies. See also part II, in the next issue, on counseling and lifestyle modifications.

2. Ertl G, Neubauer S, Gaudron P, Horn M, et al. Beta-blockers in cardiac failure. Eur Heart J 1994;(suppl C):16–24.

   The authors review the clinical trials and pathophysiology of this controversial treatment.

3. Gaasch WH. Diagnosis and treatment of heart failure based on left ventricular systolic or diastolic dysfunction. JAMA 1994;271:1276–1280.

   A new classification of left ventricular dysfunction is developed with treatment strategies based on systolic versus diastolic dysfunction with stratification of prognosis and treatment by symptoms.

4. Nishimura RA, Tajik AJ. The Valsalva maneuver and response revisited. Mayo Clin Proc 1986;61:211–217.

   Utility of Valsalva response in CHF is discussed. A normal Valsalva response correlates with an ejection fraction of 69% ± 11%, an absent phase IV overshoot with an ejection fraction of 48% ± 15%, and a square wave response with an ejection fraction of 29% ± 11%. The specificity of the test decreases if the patient is taking β-blockers.

5. Tsevat J, Eckman MH, McNutt RA, Pauker SG. Warfarin for dilated cardiomyopathy: A bloody tough pill to swallow? Med Decision Making 1989;9:162–169.

   Decision analysis supports chronic anticoagulation, but authors conclude that any such recommendation should consider the effects of anticoagulation on the patient's quality of life.

■ ■

80 Aortic Stenosis

Problem

CATHERINE M. OTTO

Epidemiology. Valvular aortic stenosis is the most common indication for valvular surgery in adults, with more than 20,000 aortic valve replacements performed annually in the United States. The clinician must exclude severe valvular obstruction in elderly adults with symptoms that may be due to aortic stenosis and a systolic murmur on examination.

Etiology. In adults, valvular aortic stenosis is most often due to degenerative calcification of a trileaflet valve, with clinical symptoms occurring at ages 70 to 80 years. Secondary calcification and fibrosis of a congenital bicuspid valve (occurring in about 1% of the population) results in severe aortic stenosis at ages 50 to 60 years. The prevalence of postinflammatory rheumatic aortic stenosis, always accompanied by rheumatic mitral valve disease, is declining. Valvular aortic stenosis must be distinguished from fixed (membrane or muscular ridge) or dynamic (hypertrophic obstructive cardiomyopathy) subaortic obstruction.

Clinical Approach. In the patient with suspected aortic stenosis, the history should determine whether typical symptoms are present, including exertional angina, heart failure (dyspnea on exertion is the usual initial symptom), and exertional dizziness or syncope. Physical examination is helpful when the systolic murmur is accompanied by a thrill (grade IV/VI), the carotid upstroke rises slowly with a reduced systolic impulse, the pulse pressure is reduced, and A2 is absent (a split S2 excludes severe aortic stenosis in adults). However, physical examination can be misleading in that most adults with severe aortic stenosis have a softer murmur (grade II/III) and often have a normal carotid upstroke and pulse pressure. The absence of left ventricular hypertrophy on electrocardiography does not exclude aortic stenosis in adults.

When aortic stenosis is suspected on clinical grounds, further evaluation with two-dimensional and Doppler echocardiography is indicated. Two-dimensional imaging confirms the diagnosis, defines the cause of disease, measures any coexisting aortic regurgitation, and excludes subvalvular obstruction. In addition, left ventricular hypertrophy, chamber dimensions, and systolic function can be assessed. Doppler echocardiography allows accurate calculation of the transaortic pressure gradient and valve orifice area.

Management decisions may be based on echocardiographic findings in most cases. Cardiac catheterization should be employed to evaluate the severity of the stenosis only if the echocardiographic findings are discordant with the clinical impression. Because of the high prevalence (50%) of coexisting coronary disease in patients with aortic stenosis, coronary angiography is usually indicated before aortic valve replacement and may be indicated to define an alternative cause for the patient's symptoms in mild to moderate aortic stenosis.

Management. The prognosis of medically treated severe *symptomatic* valvular aortic stenosis is extremely poor, with a 3-year survival rate of only 25%. Aortic valve replacement can be performed, even in the elderly, with an acceptable operative mortality (10% for patients older than 70 years of age). Left ventricular systolic function typically improves after valve replacement (due to afterload reduction). Percutaneous balloon aortic valvuloplasty is not an effective treatment for aortic stenosis in adult patients, nor have valve débridement or repair procedures been successful. Coronary bypass grafting can be performed concurrently at the time of valve replacement, if needed, with little increase in the operative risk.

In contrast, the prognosis for *asymptomatic* aortic stenosis is no different than that for age-matched controls. Regardless of hemodynamic severity, valve replacement can be deferred until symptoms occur. Medical management in asymptomatic patients should include (1) confirmation of the diagnosis and degree of obstruction with a baseline Doppler echocardiographic study, (2) endocarditis prophylaxis for dental and other procedures, (3) discussion with the patient regarding the eventual need for valve replacement, and (4) counseling the patient to recognize typical symptoms and seek medical attention promptly, because the risk of sudden death is high once symptoms become apparent.

Follow-Up. Symptomatic patients with aortic stenosis need medical follow-up after surgery to monitor anticoagulation (for mechanical prostheses), for endocarditis prophylaxis, and for medical treatment of residual cardiac symptoms. An echocardiogram should be obtained 2 to 3 months after surgery to serve as a baseline should prosthetic valve dysfunction be suspected in the future.

Asymptomatic patients should receive endocarditis prophylaxis and be observed closely for development of symptoms. The frequency of follow-up echocardiography (every 1 to 3 years) is based on the initial severity of disease and on intervening changes in clinical status.

Cross-References: Recurrent Chest Pain (Chapter 74), Echocardiography (Chapter 89), Preoperative Cardiovascular Problems (Chapter 218), Preoperative Infectious Disease Problems (Chapter 222).

REFERENCES

1. Brener SJ, Duffy CI, Thomas JD, Stewart WJ. Progression of aortic stenosis in 394 patients: Relation to changes in myocardial and mitral valve dysfunction. J Am Coll Cardiol 1995;25:305–310.

   In 394 patients with aortic stenosis the rate of progression of valvular obstruction was predictable: the mean transaortic pressure gradient increased by an average of 6.3 mm Hg/y and valve area decreased by 0.14 cm²/y. Typically, increased valvular obstruction was accompanied by increased left ventricular hypertrophy but preserved systolic function.

2. Judge KW, Otto CM. Doppler echocardiographic evaluation of aortic stenosis. Cardiol Clin 1990;8:203–216.

   Echocardiographic evaluation of aortic stenosis is reviewed with a description of methodology and emphasis on limitations.

3. O'Keefe JH Jr, Shub C, Rettke SR. Risk of noncardiac surgical procedures in patients with aortic stenosis. Mayo Clin Proc 1989;64:400–405.

   Forty-eight patients (mean age 73) with severe aortic stenosis underwent noncardiac surgery with careful diagnostic evaluation and hemodynamic monitoring. There were no intraoperative deaths, although operative morbidity occurred in 9% (transient events in all but one patient).

4. Otto CM, Pearlman AS. Doppler echocardiography in adults with symptomatic aortic stenosis: Diagnostic utility and cost-effectiveness. Arch Intern Med 1988;148:2553–2560.

   Diagnostic approach to symptomatic patients with aortic stenosis is discussed: a jet velocity greater than 4.0 m/s confirms severe aortic stenosis and need for valve replacement; a velocity less than 3.0 m/s excludes severe aortic stenosis; a velocity of 3.0 to 4.0 m/s requires valve area calculation and assessment of coexisting aortic regurgitation.

5. Selzer A. Changing aspects of the natural history of valvular aortic stenosis. N Engl J Med 1987;317:91–98.

   The natural history of valvular aortic stenosis is reviewed.

81 Other Valvular Disease

Problem

CATHERINE M. OTTO

Epidemiology and Etiology. *Mitral regurgitation* is the second most common type of valvular disease in adults requiring surgical intervention (aortic stenosis is the most common). It may be due to abnormalities of the leaflets themselves (myxomatous mitral valve disease, rheumatic disease, or endocarditis) or to abnormalities of the supporting structures (annular calcification, papillary muscle dysfunction due to myocardial infarction, left ventricular dilation, and systolic dysfunction of any cause). The cause of *mitral stenosis* is nearly always rheumatic, although an occasional patient may have functional mitral stenosis due to severe degenerative annular and leaflet calcification. The prevalence of rheumatic mitral stenosis has been steadily declining in the past few years as a consequence of the earlier decline in acute rheumatic fever, and rheumatic mitral stenosis is now reported most often in recent immigrants. *Aortic regurgitation* may be due to a congenital bicuspid valve, endocarditis, or aortic root dilation (e.g., hypertension, Marfan's syndrome, aortic dissection, annuloaortic ectasia). *Tricuspid regurgitation* may be due to congenital anomalies (Ebstein's anomaly), endocarditis, rheumatic disease, or carcinoid syndrome or may be secondary to pulmonary hypertension of any cause. *Tricuspid stenosis* is rare. Hemodynamically significant pulmonic valve disease is uncommon in adults.

Clinical Approach. The most important methods for detecting valvular heart disease remain a careful history and physical examination. If the physical examination reveals a pathologic murmur or if the clinical presentation suggests significant valvular disease (a mitral stenosis murmur may be difficult to appreciate on auscultation), echocardiography should be performed. Echocardiography provides definitive information on valve anatomy and dynamics, the cause of valvular disease, the presence and severity of stenosis or regurgitation, compensatory chamber dilation, pulmonary artery pressure, and ventricular function. Cardiac catheterization may be needed to evaluate the degree of coronary artery disease but rarely is needed for evaluation of valvular disease per se.

It is important to distinguish between *acute* and *chronic* valvular regurgitation. With acute regurgitation (e.g., mitral regurgitation due to papillary muscle rupture after myocardial infarction or aortic regurgitation due to endocarditis), both compensatory chamber enlargement and the classic physical findings may be absent. A high level of suspicion based on the patient's history and prompt echocardiography are needed to diagnose acute regurgitation.

Management. Medical management includes the appropriate use of diuretics to relieve pulmonary congestion, endocarditis prophylaxis for dental and other procedures, treatment of associated arrhythmias, and careful follow-up. In

253

mitral stenosis with atrial fibrillation, chronic anticoagulation with warfarin is indicated to prevent left atrial thrombus formation and systemic embolization. For chronic valvular regurgitation, afterload reduction with a calcium channel blocker or an angiotension-converting enzyme inhibitor is beneficial.

In symptomatic patients with severe valvular disease, surgical intervention—valve repair for mitral regurgitation, percutaneous valvuloplasty for mitral stenosis, or valve replacement—is indicated. The timing of valve replacement in asymptomatic patients with chronic valvular regurgitation is controversial insofar as irreversible left ventricular systolic function can occur before symptoms develop.

Follow-Up. Patients with significant valvular regurgitation should be carefully followed with cardiac imaging at 6-month to 1-year intervals (depending on ventricular size and systolic function at entry). Echocardiography is the preferred follow-up method with sequential measurement of left ventricular end-systolic dimension and assessment of left ventricular systolic function. In some settings, resting and exercise radionuclide ventriculography may be useful. Patients should be referred to a cardiologist when they become symptomatic, for severe regurgitation regardless of left ventricular size and function, for any evidence of deteriorating left ventricular systolic function, or when left ventricular end-systolic dimension exceeds 45 mm.

Cross-References: Dyspnea (Chapter 19), Echocardiography (Chapter 89), Chronic Anticoagulation (Chapter 201), Preoperative Cardiovascular Problems (Chapter 218), Preoperative Infectious Disease Problems (Chapter 222).

REFERENCES

1. Biem HJ, Detsky AS, Armstrong PW. Management of asymptomatic chronic aortic regurgitation with left ventricular dysfunction: A decision analysis. J Gen Intern Med 1990;5:394–401.

   Decision analysis (with references to previous literature) of timing of valve replacement in asymptomatic aortic regurgitation is accompanied by an editorial.

2. Cheitlan MD. The timing of surgery in mitral and aortic valve disease. Curr Probl Cardiol 1987;12:69–149.

   The author presents a well-referenced review of the diagnosis, natural history, and treatment of valvular disease.

3. Lin M, Chiang H-T, Lin S-L, Shang M-S, Chiang B-N, Kuo H-W, Cheitlin MD. Vasodilator therapy in chronic asymptomatic aortic regurgitation: Enalapril versus hydralazine therapy. J Am Coll Cardiol 1994;24:1046–1053.

   A randomized trial was performed of 76 patients with asymptomatic mild-to-moderate aortic regurgitation. At 1 year, the enalapril group had reduced left ventricular end-diastolic and end-systolic volume and left ventricular mass indexes compared with the hydralazine group.

4. Scognamiglio R, Rahimtoola SH, Gasoli G, Nistri S, Dalla Volta S. Nifedipine in asymptomatic patients with severe aortic regurgitation and normal left ventricular function. N Engl J Med 1994;331:689–694.

   A randomized trial is reported of nifedipine versus digoxin in 143 patients with severe asymptomatic aortic regurgitation. By 6 years, $15 \pm 3\%$ of the nifedipine group underwent valve replacement compared with $43 \pm 6\%$ of the digoxin group (P < .001).

82 Atrial Fibrillation

Problem

JOYCE E. WIPF

Epidemiology and Etiology. Atrial fibrillation, the most common atrial arrhythmia, may be chronic or paroxysmal. The prevalence of atrial fibrillation is 0.4% in adults, increasing with age to 2% to 4% among those older than age 60. Paroxysmal atrial fibrillation becomes chronic in about one third of cases. Although rheumatic mitral valve disease was once the most common cause, coronary artery disease, hypertension, and congestive heart failure now account for over 40% of cases and hyperthyroidism accounts for 15%. Up to 15% of cases of chronic atrial fibrillation occur in otherwise healthy adults with no identifiable risk factors, a condition called "lone" atrial fibrillation. Paroxysmal atrial fibrillation may be precipitated by alcohol ("holiday heart"), stress, caffeine, or intercurrent acute illnesses such as pneumonia or pulmonary embolism.

Atrial fibrillation not only causes immediate hemodynamic effects but increases the potential risk of thromboembolism to the brain and other organs. Compared with subjects with normal sinus rhythm, the risk of stroke is 17 times higher for patients with rheumatic heart disease and chronic atrial fibrillation, 5 times higher for patients with chronic nonrheumatic atrial fibrillation, and 2 times higher for patients with paroxysmal atrial fibrillation. Carefully defined, lone atrial fibrillation (i.e., no underlying cardiovascular disease, including hypertension) poses a low risk of embolism. Over 20% of patients with atrial fibrillation and a history of stroke will have another embolic event during the first year. The lifetime risk of recurrence is 30% to 75% without anticoagulation.

Symptoms and Signs. Atrial fibrillation often produces no symptoms and is discovered incidentally on electrocardiography or by detecting an irregularly irregular pulse on examination. Those with a rapid ventricular rate may experience palpitations, lightheadedness, fatigue, angina, and dyspnea, with hypotension and signs of congestive heart failure. Because the atrial contraction contributes approximately 10% of the cardiac output, patients with underlying left ventricular dysfunction may become symptomatic even at relatively normal heart rates. Patients with thyrotoxicosis may experience anxiety, restlessness, and diarrhea, although atrial fibrillation without symptoms may be the sole clue to apathetic hyperthyroidism in the elderly.

Clinical Approach. The two major questions in the diagnostic workup of newly noted atrial fibrillation are (1) What is the etiology? and (2) Has the patient had an embolic event? Both help to determine subsequent therapy and the patient's risk of embolism.

Physical examination focuses on vital signs, thyroid palpation, and evaluation for valvular heart disease and congestive heart failure.

Routine laboratory tests include thyroid function tests and echocardiography, which may disclose abnormal heart valves, left ventricular dysfunction, or a cardiac thrombus. Left atrial size does not accurately predict successful cardioversion or maintenance of sinus rhythm. Patients who are acutely symptomatic require hospital admission and evaluation for myocardial ischemia, pulmonary embolism, or pneumonia.

Among patients with acute strokes, 15% to 25% are in atrial fibrillation; of these, 75% have had an embolism originating from an atrial thrombus. There is no reference standard for determining whether a stroke is cardiogenic, but supporting features include the presence of an atrial thrombus, infarcts in multiple vascular distributions, the sudden onset of a maximal deficit without prior transient ischemic attacks, and absence of significant atherosclerotic carotid stenoses. Cardiogenic strokes are more likely to be hemorrhagic. To detect carotid stenosis, noninvasive duplex ultrasonography should be performed irrespective of the finding of carotid bruits on examination. Other helpful diagnostic studies include computed tomography of the brain and echocardiography.

Management. Patients with rapid atrial fibrillation and acute symptoms should be hospitalized for evaluation, cardiac monitoring, and treatment. Patients with acute atrial fibrillation and hemodynamic compromise (angina, hypotension, pulmonary edema) require emergency electrical cardioversion to normal sinus rhythm. No anticoagulation is required for arrhythmias present less than 48 hours. If the patient has a rapid ventricular rate but is hemodynamically stable, the physician should lower the rate with antiarrhythmic medications; digoxin is the usual agent of choice unless a preexcitation syndrome (e.g., Wolff-Parkinson-White syndrome) is present. Decisions about cardioversion or antiarrhythmic agents should be made in consultation with a cardiologist if possible. Patients with asymptomatic chronic atrial fibrillation can usually be evaluated as outpatients until they are admitted for cardioversion. Stable patients who are not candidates for cardioversion or anticoagulation may be treated with digoxin alone for rate control.

Because cardioversion carries a 1% to 5% risk of embolism, stable patients with chronic atrial fibrillation should be anticoagulated with warfarin (prothrombin time ratio of 1.3:1.7, or international normalized ratio of 2.0–3.0) before the procedure. The usual initial dose of warfarin is 2.5 to 5 mg/d; the prothrombin time should be checked weekly (see Chapter 201, Chronic Anticoagulation). Once therapeutically anticoagulated for 3 weeks, the patient is admitted and chemical cardioversion attempted with a type 1A antiarrhythmic agent such as procainamide or quinidine before electrical cardioversion. Anticoagulation should be continued for 3 to 4 weeks after cardioversion, because left atrial function may not return to normal for several weeks after conversion to sinus rhythm and embolic events have been documented up to 10 days after the procedure. Patients are more likely to remain in sinus rhythm if the atrial fibrillation had been present for less than 1 year and if they are placed on chronic antiarrhythmic therapy. There is, however, evidence that chronic treatment with quinidine may increase overall mortality. Newer drugs such as amiodarone and sotalol may now be the antiarrhythmic agents of choice.

A controversial and complex issue is whether to chronically anticoagulate patients in whom cardioversion fails and who remain in chronic atrial fibrillation. Multiple randomized trials have shown that warfarin anticoagulation reduces embolic risk but is associated with major bleeding complications in 2% to 4% of patients. Data suggest that 325 mg/d of aspirin reduces the stroke risk in atrial fibrillation patients younger than age 75. Presently, aspirin is considered less beneficial than warfarin but also less risky. If the patient is a low-risk anticoagulation candidate, warfarin is indicated. Aspirin is reasonable primary stroke prevention for individuals not considered candidates for warfarin therapy. Age alone is not a contraindication to anticoagulation, although elderly individuals need to be carefully assessed for risk of falls, cognitive impairment, and noncompliance with medications. Absolute and relative contraindications to anticoagulation appear in Chapter 201 (Chronic Anticoagulation).

Patients with chronic atrial fibrillation and valvular heart disease, prosthetic heart valves, or a history of embolism should be anticoagulated. A randomized trial of secondary stroke prevention in patients with atrial fibrillation and a recent history of transient ischemic attack or stroke found that warfarin significantly reduced the stroke risk over placebo, with aspirin benefit similar to placebo. In patients with acute nonhemorrhagic stroke whose blood pressure is controlled, the risk of converting a nonhemorrhagic to a hemorrhagic stroke by anticoagulation is low. Anticoagulation is also recommended for atrial fibrillation with associated cardiovascular disease in the absence of contraindications (Table 82–1).

Follow-Up. After successful cardioversion, patients need follow-up within a few weeks to evaluate whether sinus rhythm is maintained and to monitor antiarrhythmic drug levels and potential side effects of antiarrhythmic therapy.

Table 82–1. GUIDELINES FOR ANTICOAGULATION IN CHRONIC ATRIAL FIBRILLATION

Anticoagulation Indicated in Atrial Fibrillation

Associated with rheumatic heart disease
History of embolic event
Short-term before and after cardioversion
Prosthetic mitral valve of any type

Anticoagulation Recommended If No Relative Contraindications

Cardiomyopathy with poor left ventricular function
Nonvalvular heart disease
Cardiac thrombus

Unclear Relative Risk and Benefit

Recent onset of atrial fibrillation
Lone atrial fibrillation in the elderly
Thyrotoxicosis and atrial fibrillation
Documented long-standing uncomplicated atrial fibrillation

Anticoagulation Not Recommended

Lone atrial fibrillation in patients younger than 65
Paroxysmal atrial fibrillation without history of embolism

If cardioversion is unsuccessful or atrial fibrillation recurs, the clinician must decide whether to reattempt cardioversion (if drug levels are subtherapeutic or atrial fibrillation is poorly tolerated) or to initiate chronic anticoagulation. Follow-up of anticoagulated individuals is described in Chapter 201 (Chronic Anticoagulation). Sixty percent to 80% of individuals treated chronically with antiarrhythmic agents will be in sinus rhythm 1 year after cardioversion. Use of alcohol increases the likelihood of recurrence of atrial fibrillation.

Cross-References: Palpitations (Chapter 76), Congestive Heart Failure (Chapter 79), Echocardiography (Chapter 89), Cerebrovascular Disease (Chapter 146), Common Thyroid Disorders (Chapter 153), Chronic Anticoagulation (Chapter 201).

REFERENCES

1. AF Investigators. Risk factors for stroke and efficacy of antithrombotic therapy in atrial fibrillation: Analysis of pooled data from five randomized controlled trials. Arch Intern Med 1994;154:1449–1457.

   Risks for stroke in atrial fibrillation include increasing age, previous stroke or transient ischemic attack, diabetes mellitus, and hypertension. These researchers showed that elderly patients with lone atrial fibrillation had an annual stroke rate of 3.0%. Warfarin efficacy is confirmed; evidence for aspirin is less consistent than that for warfarin.

2. Albers G. Atrial fibrillation and stroke: Three new studies, three remaining questions. Arch Intern Med 1994;154:1443–1448.

   The safety of anticoagulation in the elderly is discussed, along with efficacy of aspirin and identification of risk factors for stroke. Although the elderly are at greater risk for bleeding, warfarin should be considered given the high stroke risk.

3. European Atrial Fibrillation Trial Study Group. Secondary prevention in non-rheumatic atrial fibrillation after transient ischemic attack or minor stroke. Lancet 1993;342:1255–1262.

   This is the only randomized trial of secondary stroke prevention in atrial fibrillation: 1007 patients with atrial fibrillation and transient ischemic attack or minor stroke within the previous 3 months were randomized to aspirin, 300 mg, versus warfarin. The annual incidence of stroke was significantly reduced from 12% in the placebo group to 4% in the warfarin group. Aspirin had no notable benefit over warfarin. Warfarin risk of major bleeding was under 3% per year, with no intracranial hemorrhages.

4. Kannel WB, Abbott RD, Savage DD, McNamara PM. Epidemiologic features of chronic atrial fibrillation: The Framingham Study. N Engl J Med 1982;306:1018–1022.

   This is the classic epidemiologic study of 5200 residents of Framingham, Massachusetts, followed prospectively for development of cardiovascular disease. The risk of stroke was increased in both valvular and nonvalvular atrial fibrillation.

5. Wipf JE. Anticoagulation and atrial fibrillation: Putting the results of clinical trials into practice. West J Med 1995;163:145–152.

   Literature review of data on embolic risk of chronic and paroxysmal atrial fibrillation and the relative benefit and risk of anticoagulation and aspirin therapy includes algorithms for the management of atrial fibrillation and guidelines for anticoagulation.

83 Chronic Ventricular Arrhythmias

Problem

MARYE J. GLEVA

The management of ventricular tachycardia (VT) and ventricular fibrillation (VF) changed markedly in the past decade. Suppression of premature ventricular complexes after myocardial infarction in an attempt to decrease the risk of sustained ventricular arrhythmias is no longer a goal. Contemporary care of the patient with VT or VF involves a team composed of the primary internist, cardiologist, cardiac electrophysiologist, and possibly a cardiac surgeon.

Epidemiology. VT most commonly arises in patients who have suffered a prior myocardial infarction. An initial episode of VT may be experienced years after the myocardial infarction. Sustained VT indicates that the duration of tachycardia is more than 30 seconds. VF is the most frequent arrhythmia found in the 250,000 to 400,000 patients in the United States who experience sudden cardiac death each year. Patients who present with VF are less likely to have had a prior myocardial infarction, depressed left ventricular function, and inducible ventricular arrhythmias at electrophysiologic study when compared with patients with VT. VF is the first presentation of coronary artery disease in approximately 30% of patients who experience sudden cardiac death.

Although coronary artery disease is the most common underlying cause of left ventricular dysfunction, other causes are also associated with malignant ventricular arrhythmias. Idiopathic dilated cardiomyopathy, valvular heart disease, repaired congenital heart disease, and alcoholic cardiomyopathy not infrequently result in decreased left ventricular systolic function. Sarcoidosis, hemachromatosis, postpartum cardiomyopathy, and endocardial fibroelastosis are rare causes of left ventricular dysfunction.

Signs and Symptoms. VT may present clinically as an incidental finding in an awake and alert patient with a stable blood pressure or as cardiovascular compromise and collapse. Patients with VF present with cardiac arrest requiring resuscitation.

Clinical Approach. Physical examination is used to evaluate the cardiovascular system for an underlying pathologic process, especially myocardial ischemia. Laboratory examination should include drug and electrolyte levels. As with supraventricular tachycardia, an electrocardiogram should be obtained during hemodynamically stable tachycardia. VT is a monomorphic or polymorphic wide complex rhythm at heart rates that range from 100 to 270 beats per minute. VT should be differentiated from supraventricular tachycardia with aberrancy because treatment and prognosis are different.

Management. Current therapies for VT and VF are focused on secondary prevention. No clear recommendations exist for primary prevention other than general guidelines for prevention of coronary artery disease. The acute management of a patient with a wide complex tachycardia determined to be VT is described in the Advanced Cardiac Life Support (ACLS) guidelines. Hospitalization is necessary to evaluate for myocardial ischemia. Cardiac catheterization to evaluate the severity of coronary artery disease and nuclear, angiographic, or echocardiographic assessments of left ventricular function are routine. Electrophysiologic studies characterize the tachycardia mechanism and the response to pharmacologic and nonpharmacologic intervention such as overdrive pacing.

The Cardiac Arrhythmia Suppression Trials, which were randomized placebo-controlled trials, were undertaken to evaluate the effect of suppression of premature ventricular contractions after myocardial infarction on the incidence of malignant ventricular arrhythmias. The drugs evaluated were flecainide, encainide, and moricizine. All three treatment arms were associated with increased mortality compared with placebo. Amiodarone and implantable cardioverter-defibrillators suppress and treat arrhythmia recurrence, respectively.

The optimal initial management of VT is prompt defibrillation. Hemodynamic stabilization and hospitalization in a cardiac intensive care unit with evaluation for ischemia and exclusion of inciting electrolyte or drug abnormalities follows. VF in the context of an acute myocardial infarction carries a better prognosis than VF without an acute myocardial infarction, for which the 1-year recurrence risk approaches 25%.

Long-term management of the VF survivor depends on cardiac function and the degree of neurologic recovery. The likelihood of awakening after cardiac arrest is predicted by initial serum glucose concentration, presence of spontaneous eye movements, pupillary light response, and motor response. As in patients with VT, coronary artery anatomy and left ventricular function must be evaluated. Surgical revascularization is considered in patients with three-vessel coronary artery disease. The first randomized trial of antiarrhythmic drugs in VF survivors was the Cardiac Arrest in Seattle: Conventional versus Amiodarone Drug Evaluation (CASCADE). Participants were randomized to the best conventional drug as determined by electrophysiologic studies or Holter monitoring or empirical administration of amiodarone. Cardiac survival at 2 years was 82% in the amiodarone group versus 69% in the conventionally treated group. Automatic implantable cardioverter-defibrillators have evolved over the past decade from shock-only devices that require open chest procedures for placement to tiered-therapy devices that are placed transvenously in the pectoral region. Newer devices provide antitachycardia and antibradycardia pacing capabilities, sophisticated detection algorithms, and increased memory. Randomized trials currently underway are comparing implantable cardioverter-defibrillators with antiarrhythmic drugs in patients who have survived VT or VF.

Follow-Up. Patients treated with amiodarone should have twice-yearly thyroid function tests, liver function tests, pulmonary function tests, and chest radiographs. Patients with implantable cardioverter-defibrillators require follow-up visits at intervals specified by the device manufacturers. During these visits, lead system integrity, monitoring of battery voltage, and capacitor reformation are assessed.

Cross-References: Dizziness (Chapter 20), Syncope (Chapter 75), Palpitations (Chapter 76), Congestive Heart Failure (Chapter 79), Ambulatory Cardiac Monitoring (Chapter 87), Preoperative Cardiovascular Problems (Chapter 218).

REFERENCES

1. Cardiac Arrhythmia Suppression Trial (CAST) Investigators. Preliminary report: Effect of encainide and flecainide on mortality in a randomized trial of arrhythmia suppression after myocardial infarction. N Engl J Med 1989;21:406–412.

   Patients were randomized to best drug or placebo. Drug therapy was associated with a greater than threefold increase in relative risk of death.

2. CASCADE Investigators. Randomized antiarrhythmic drug therapy in survivors of cardiac arrest. Am J Cardiol 1993;72:280–287.

   In this study, 228 cardiac arrest survivors were enrolled to evaluate amiodarone versus conventional therapy. No differences were found in causes of mortality, but cardiac survival improved in the amiodarone-treated group.

3. Mason JW for the Electrophysiologic Study versus Electrocardiographic Monitoring Investigators. A comparison of seven antiarrhythmic drugs in patients with ventricular tachyarrhythmias. N Engl J Med 1993;329:452–458.

   In this trial 296 patients with ventricular arrhythmias underwent serial drug evaluation and then were observed over 4 years. Patients treated with sotalol had fewer deaths. β-blockers and amiodarone were not included in the trial.

4. Sweeny MO, Ruskin JN. Mortality benefits and the implantable cardioverter-defibrillator. Circulation 1994;89:1851–1858.

   A review is presented of implantable cardioverter-defibrillator survival data (nonrandomized to date) with commentary on defining appropriate patient subgroups for future mortality and economic studies.

5. Wellens HJJ, Bar FWHM, Lie KI. The value of the electrocardiogram in the differential diagnosis of a tachycardia with a widened QRS complex. Am J Med 1978;64:27–33.

   In this seminal paper the authors differentiate VT from supraventricular tachycardia with aberrancy.

· ·

84 Supraventricular Arrhythmias

Problem

MARYE J. GLEVA

Epidemiology. Supraventricular tachycardias are common outpatient problems seen in patients of all ages. Certain supraventricular arrhythmias, notably atrial fibrillation, increase in incidence with increasing age. It is estimated that 2% to 4% of patients 60 years or older have atrial fibrillation.

Signs and Symptoms. Patients with supraventricular arrhythmias may be asymptomatic or may experience palpitations, chest pain, dyspnea, near-syncope, or frank syncope. Physical examination may be normal or may reveal murmurs indicating valvular disease; gallops, heaves, elevated jugular venous pressure, hepatomegaly, or lower extremity edema in patients with underlying ventricular dysfunction; or goiter in patients with thyroid disease. The pulse is rapid if an arrhythmia is ongoing.

Clinical Approach and Management. Supraventricular arrhythmias arise in the conduction system above the level of the bundle branches. The 12-lead electrocardiogram facilitates diagnosis and directs therapy. Supraventricular tachycardias can be classified as regular or irregular based on the pattern of the RR intervals on the electrocardiogram. The QRS complex duration during tachycardia may be normal at 0.08 second or may reflect aberrant conduction if 0.12 second or longer.

Supraventricular tachycardias with irregularly irregular RR intervals include atrial fibrillation and multifocal atrial tachycardia. *Atrial fibrillation* is characterized by continuous atrial activity with the absence of discrete P waves in limb leads II and III and precordial lead V_1. It is either paroxysmal or chronic and is seen in patients with underlying heart disease due to atherosclerosis, hypertension, valvular problems such as rheumatic mitral valve disease, or cardiomyopathies. Atrial fibrillation in Wolff-Parkinson-White syndrome is rapid with a wide and bizarre-appearing QRS complex. In this disorder, atrial impulses conduct to the ventricle over an accessory atrioventricular pathway. Atrial fibrillation in the absence of underlying heart disease or hypertension in patients younger than 60 years old is termed *lone atrial fibrillation*. Noncardiac causes of atrial fibrillation include thyrotoxicosis, pneumonia, and pulmonary embolism.

Treatment goals for patients with atrial fibrillation include stroke prevention with anticoagulation and control of the ventricular response. Anticoagulation with warfarin or aspirin in selected patients can be started on an outpatient basis. The ventricular response in atrial fibrillation can be controlled with medications such as β-blockers, calcium channel blockers, and digoxin, singularly or in combination. Diltiazem, 30 mg three or four times daily; atenolol, 25 or 50 mg/d; and metoprolol, 50 mg twice daily are reasonable empirical starting doses. Digoxin may be less effective in controlling the ventricular response. Rarely, mechanical rate control through radiofrequency ablation of the atrioventricular junction and concomitant single-chamber rate-responsive pacemaker placement is necessary.

The decision to attempt to restore a sinus rhythm must be based on a patient's symptoms and underlying heart function. The choice of antiarrhythmic medication is closely coupled to left ventricular function because all antiarrhythmic drugs with the possible exception of amiodarone are negative inotropes. Drug options include quinidine, procainamide, disopyramide, propafenone, flecainide, sotalol, and amiodarone, which optimally are begun in the hospital with continuous telemetry monitoring.

Surgical or catheter-based procedures to achieve normal sinus rhythm are reserved for severely symptomatic patients when the standard medical therapies have failed. The restoration of sinus rhythm has not been shown to decrease the incidence of stroke nor to improve mortality.

Multifocal atrial tachycardia is characterized by three or more discrete P wave morphologies and PR intervals as seen on the electrocardiogram. It occurs in patients with underlying chronic lung disease or digoxin or theophylline toxicity. Calcium channel blocking agents such as diltiazem and verapamil are the drugs of choice for treatment of this tachycardia, assuming that left ventricular function is adequate.

There are six common types of regular supraventricular tachycardia: atrial flutter, atrioventricular node reentry tachycardia, orthodromic reciprocating tachycardia, accelerated junctional tachycardia, ectopic atrial tachycardia, and sinus tachycardia. The electrical circuit, electrocardiographic characteristics, associated disease states, and acute therapeutic interventions are shown in Table 84–1. A discussion of other forms of supraventricular tachycardia is beyond the scope of this chapter.

Chronic treatment for any of the arrhythmias in Table 84–1 includes therapy for any underlying condition as well as rate control with β-blockers and calcium channel blockers (Table 84–2). Rapid tachycardia rates, presyncope, or multiple drug failures warrant an invasive evaluation in the electrophysiology laboratory with consideration of radiofrequency catheter ablation.

Cross-References: Alcohol Problems (Chapter 10), Dizziness (Chapter 20), Syncope (Chapter 75), Palpitations (Chapter 76), Atrial Fibrillation (Chapter

Table 84–1. COMMON SUPRAVENTRICULAR ARRHYTHMIAS

Arrhythmia	Location of Electrical Circuit	Electrocardiographic Characteristics	Associated Conditions	Acute Arrhythmia Management
Atrial flutter	Posterior/inferior right atrium or around prior surgical scar	Flutter waves in inferior leads, with typical rates of 300 beats per minute	Atherosclerotic coronary artery disease, surgically corrected congenital heart disease	Ventricular rate control with calcium blockers or β-blockers; electrical cardioversion if unstable
Atrioventricular node reentrant tachycardia	Zones of differing conduction in the atrioventricular node	Narrow complex tachycardia without discernible P waves	Typically seen in patients without structural heart disease	Adenosine, 6–12 mg IV; electrical cardioversion if unstable
Orthodromic reciprocating tachycardia	Atrioventricular node with accessory bypass tract	Narrow complex tachycardia with retrograde P waves; baseline electrocardiogram may have a delta wave	Structurally normal hearts, Ebstein's anomaly, atrial septal defect	Adenosine, 6–12 mg IV; electrical cardioversion if unstable
Atrial tachycardias	Right or left atrial tissue	P waves with nonsinus morphology and axis	Atherosclerotic coronary artery disease, dilated cardiomyopathies, pulmonary disease	Control of ventricular rate with calcium blockers or β-blockers
Sinus tachycardia	Sinus node	Rate > 100 beats per minute with sinus P wave morphology and axis	Pain, fever, sepsis, hypotension, anxiety	Not indicated
Accelerated junctional rhythm	Atrioventricular node	No P waves	Digoxin toxicity, sepsis, intravenous ionotropes	Treat underlying cause

Table 84–2. COMMON ANTIARRHYTHMIC DRUGS

Class	Drug	Dose	Cost ($ per month)
Calcium channel blocker	Diltiazem	30–120 mg q8h	31.91–91.92
	Diltiazem, sustained release	120–300 mg qd	31.32–68.94
	Verapamil	40–120 mg tid–qid	24.40–36.90
	Isoptin SR	120–240 mg qd–bid	25.75–74.60
Cardiac glycoside β-blocker	Digoxin	0.125–0.5 mg qd	3.40–6.80
	Inderal LA	10–80 mg q6h	8.20–25.75
		60–160 mg qd–bid	23.00–87.40
	Metoprolol	50–100 mg q12h	27.56–41.42
	Metoprolol, sustained release	50–200 mg qd	13.39–40.24
Nucleoside sodium channel blocker	Adenosine	6–12 mg IV bolus	26.97/6-mg vial
	Quinidine sulfate	200–400 mg q4–6h	18.90–37.80
	Quinidine gluconate	324–648 mg q8–12h	26.10–52.20
	Procainamide	250–1000 mg q4h	14.95–39.60
	Procan SR	500–1500 mg q6h	72.85–216.25
	Disopyramide	100–200 mg q6–8h	49.10–98.20
	Norpace CR	150–400 mg bid	46.60–78.80
	Flecainide	50–200 mg q12h	38.05–138.20
	Moricizine	200–300 mg q8h	25.15–35.20
Sodium channel blockade with prolongation of action potential	Amiodarone	100–400 mg qd	43.90–175.60
β-blockade with prolongation of action potential duration	Sotalol	160–320 mg qd (divided bid)	92.20–153.70

*Average wholesale price, from 1995 *Drug Topics Red Book*.
Medications listed are commonly used to treat cardiac arrhythmias. Electrophysiologic properties, generic names, common dosages, and representative average wholesale prices are given. Administered PO unless otherwise indicated.

82), Ambulatory Cardiac Monitoring (Chapter 87), Common Thyroid Disorders (Chapter 153), Preoperative Cardiovascular Problems (Chapter 218).

REFERENCES

1. Jackman WM, Wang X, Friday KJ, Roman CA, Moulton KP, Beckman, KJ, McClelland JH, Twidale N, Hazlitt HA, Prior MJ, Margolis PD, Calame JD, Overholt ED, Lazzara R. Catheter ablation of accessory atrioventricular pathways (Wolff-Parkinson-White syndrome) by radiofrequency current. N Engl J Med 1991;324:1605–1611.

   This first large trial of radiofrequency energy was done in 166 patients with Wolff-Parkinson-White syndrome and had a 99% success rate and no mortality.

2. Jackman, WM, Beckman KJ, McClelland JH, Wang X, Friday KJ, Roman CA, Moulton KP, Twidale N, Hazlitt HA, Prior MJ, Oren J, Overholt ED, Lazzara R. Treatment of supraventricular tachycardia due to atrioventricular nodal reentry by radiofrequency catheter ablation of slow pathway conduction. N Engl J Med 1992;327:313–318.

   Eighty patients with atrioventricular nodal reentry tachycardia underwent ablation with 100% success; one patient developed complete heart block and required dual-chamber pacing, and one patient had a pulmonary embolus.

3. Ganz LI, Friedman PL. Supraventricular tachycardia. N Engl J Med 1995;332:162–173.

   This comprehensive review includes acute and chronic medical therapy.

85 Essential Hypertension

Problem

JOHN F. STEINER

Epidemiology. Two aspects of the epidemiology of hypertension have major implications for the clinical diagnosis of the disease. First, about 95% of patients with elevated blood pressure in primary care settings have essential hypertension. Extensive diagnostic workups for secondary hypertension are rarely justified in the absence of characteristic signs or symptoms, onset of disease at the extremes of age, or hypertension refractory to medications. Second, establishing a diagnosis of hypertension requires consistently elevated blood pressure readings over time and in multiple settings, particularly in patients with stage I (mild) hypertension at screening (systolic blood pressure 140 to 159 mm Hg or diastolic blood pressure 90 to 99 mm Hg). Blood pressure readings outside the clinician's office can identify patients who have an exaggerated pressor response to office visits ("white coat" hypertension), whereas readings over a period of weeks to months can identify patients whose blood pressure elevations are transient.

Clinical Approach. Individuals with hypertension are generally unaware that their blood pressure is elevated. The lack of symptoms complicates diagnosis and treatment, because many individuals seek care or take medications only when they believe their blood pressure is high. The patient's understanding of the causes, symptoms, and treatment of hypertension ("illness model") should be discussed directly and nonjudgmentally to enhance the therapeutic alliance.

The medical history should focus on a personal or family history of hypertension and its complications, the duration of the hypertension, the prior treatment, the reasons for any lapses from treatment, the presence of other cardiovascular risk factors such as smoking or hyperlipidemia, and the use of medications that can raise blood pressure. In addition, the clinician should inquire about symptoms that suggest a cause of secondary hypertension, such as the headaches and palpitations of pheochromocytoma or the hirsutism, myopathy, and menstrual disorders of Cushing's syndrome. During the initial physical examination the physician should (1) use an appropriately sized sphygmomanometer to confirm the presence of hypertension in both arms with the patient supine (or seated) and upright; (2) seek evidence of existing cardiovascular disease (e.g., atherosclerosis or congestive heart failure); and (3) search for evidence of a secondary cause of hypertension (e.g., renal artery bruits, the body habitus of Cushing's syndrome, and blood pressure discrepancies between extremities suggestive of aortic coarctation).

Most hypertensive patients require only limited laboratory testing to screen for cardiovascular risk factors and to establish baseline values for tests to be monitored during treatment. Some of these tests also serve to screen for secondary causes of hypertension, such as hypokalemia associated with primary hyperaldosteronism and elevated creatinine levels in renal parenchymal disease. A reasonable initial evaluation includes an electrocardiogram; urinalysis; determination of serum lipids, potassium, calcium, creatinine, uric acids, hemoglobin and hematocrit; and a plasma glucose (preferably fasting).

Management. In patients with stage I hypertension, nonpharmacologic measures should be first-line therapy, particularly for those with diastolic blood pressure below 100 mm Hg. Nonpharmacologic therapy is additive to antihypertensive medications and can facilitate subsequent reduction of medications. Weight reduction in obese patients is the most consistently effective nonpharmacologic measure, reducing systolic blood pressure by 1 to 4 mm Hg and diastolic blood pressure by 1 to 2 mm Hg per kg of weight loss. Dietary sodium restriction to 2 g/d or less induces a substantial fall in blood pressure for "salt-sensitive" hypertensive patients, but patients who will respond cannot easily be distinguished prospectively from those who will not. Because consumption of more than 1 oz of ethanol a day (2 oz of 100-proof whiskey, 8 oz of wine, or 24 oz of beer) exerts a pressor effect, reduction or cessation of alcohol use can obviate or reduce the need for antihypertensive medications. Finally, regular isometric exercise can also lower blood pressure independent of its effect on weight and helps to lower overall cardiovascular risk. Like medications, nonpharmacologic measures pose compliance difficulties and have potential costs and impacts on lifestyle that should be discussed with the patient.

If the blood pressure remains uncontrolled or if stage II to IV hypertension is present (i.e., systolic blood pressure $\geq$ 160 mm Hg or diastolic blood pressure $\geq$ 100 mm Hg), medications are generally necessary. Studies of hypertensive patients, including the elderly, have shown that a long-term reduction in diastolic blood pressure of as little as 5 to 6 mm Hg led to a 38% reduction in strokes and a 16% reduction in coronary heart disease. Most clinical trials of drug therapy have attempted to reduce diastolic blood pressure to below 90 mm Hg or to achieve at least a 10-mm Hg fall in patients with initial values below 100 mm Hg. The merits of more stringent blood pressure control are debated; at present, a target blood pressure of less than 140/90 mm Hg is a reasonable guideline for clinical practice. Studies have also demonstrated the benefits of reducing isolated systolic hypertension (systolic blood pressure > 160 mm Hg with diastolic blood pressure < 90 mm Hg). Although diuretics, adrenergic blockers, calcium antagonists, and angiotensin-converting enzyme inhibitors all have been shown to control blood pressure in 50% to 60% of individuals, only diuretics and β-adrenergic blockers are proven to reduce the incidence of stroke and cardiovascular disease. Thus, drugs from these classes should be the choice for most individuals (Table 85–1). In some cases, special characteristics of the drug (such as patient tolerance, side effects, cost, drug–drug or drug–disease interactions) or the patient (Table 85–2) require selection of drugs from other therapeutic classes.

General principles in initiating antihypertensive therapy include the following:

1. Begin treatment with a low dose of a single drug.
2. Minimize the frequency of doses to enhance compliance.

3. Consider drug pharmacokinetics, complications, and potential interactions when choosing medications.
4. Select drugs that potentially benefit the patient's other illnesses (e.g., consider a β-adrenergic blocker in a patient also requiring prophylaxis for migraine).
5. Choose drugs that minimize the costs of treatment.

Follow-Up. After beginning antihypertensive drugs, patients should be seen at intervals of 2 to 4 weeks until the blood pressure is controlled. Patients should be encouraged to begin monitoring their own blood pressure outside the office. Mercury sphygmomanometers and anaeroid manometers are generally more accurate than digital readout devices and automated machines (such as those in pharmacies and supermarkets). All home monitoring devices require intermittent calibration to ensure accuracy. The patient should be taught that the pattern of blood pressure readings over time is more important than the results of any single blood pressure determination. Office visits are best spent in counseling about nonpharmacologic management, drug side effects, and compliance. If the patient's blood pressure is still above the target range, the dose of the initial drug can be gradually increased. Most medications reach a plateau of effectiveness in the middle of the recommended dosage range; maximal doses often confer little additional benefit but magnify side effects.

If the blood pressure remains elevated despite reasonable doses of a single antihypertensive drug, the clinician must decide whether the failure to attain blood pressure control is due to noncompliance, inadequate dosage, or true drug resistance. Fifty percent to 80% of patients with uncontrolled hypertension are not compliant with medication regimens. Strategies for assessing and treating noncompliance are discussed in Chapter 4. If the patient is compliant, the physician should consider switching to an antihypertensive drug with a different mechanism of action. If monotherapy with a range of drugs is unsuccessful, moderate doses of drugs with complementary mechanisms of action should be added to the treatment regimen. When multidrug therapy is ineffective despite good compliance, problems with measurement of blood pressure ("white coat" hypertension or "pseudohypertension" due to sclerotic, poorly compressible brachial arteries), drug–drug interactions (e.g., with oral contraceptives), failure to adequately reduce intravascular volume, and secondary causes of hypertension must be considered.

After the patient attains normal blood pressure, office visits can become less frequent. Some patients benefit from regular reevaluation and counseling to maintain adherence, whereas others are able to manage their medications, monitor their own blood pressure, and visit their physician infrequently. Ongoing home monitoring of blood pressure should be encouraged to enlist the patient as a participant in his or her own care and to detect discrepancies between home and office blood pressure readings. For drugs such as diuretics and angiotensin-converting enzyme inhibitors, which have potentially serious metabolic effects, determination of serum electrolyte levels and serum creatinine should be repeated after the first month of therapy. After the patient attains a stable treatment regimen, laboratory tests may be monitored as infrequently as once a year.

After the blood pressure has been under good control for a year or more,

Table 85–1. USUAL DAILY DOSAGES, SIDE EFFECTS, AND COSTS OF REPRESENTATIVE ANTIHYPERTENSIVE DRUGS

Drug	No. of Doses/Day	Usual Minimum Dose (mg/d)	Usual Maximum Dose (mg/d)	Common Side Effects	Cost*	Other Considerations
Diuretics						
Hydrochlorothiazide	1	12.5	50.0	Hypokalemia, hyperuricemia, hyperglycemia, may worsen lipid profile	1+	Ineffective if creatinine > 2.5 mg/dL
Furosemide	2	20.0	320.0	Hypokalemia	1+	Useful in chronic renal failure
β-Adrenergic Blockers						
Atenolol	1	25.0	100.0	Bradycardia, may worsen lipid profile	2+	Avoid in patients with congestive heart failure, claudication: may block gluconeogenesis in diabetics; β_1-selective
Pindolol	2	10.0	60.0		3+	"Intrinsic sympathomimetic activity" attenuates effects on heart rate, lipids
Propranolol	2+	40.0	240.0	Bradycardia, fatigue, insomnia, nightmares, bronchospasm, may worsen lipid profile	1+	As for atenolol: nonselective for β-receptors
Combined α- and β-Blocker						
Labetalol	2	200.0	1200.0	Fatigue, dizziness, bronchospasm	3+	As for atenolol
Central α_2-Agonists						
Clonidine	2+	0.1	1.2	Drowsiness, dry mouth, depression	1+	Rapid withdrawal may cause rebound hypertension
Peripheral Adrenergic Antagonists						
Reserpine	1	0.1	0.25	Nasal stuffiness, depression	1+	Long duration of action

Drug	Relative cost			Side effects		Comments
α₁-Adrenergic Blocker						
Prazosin	2	1.0	20.0	Orthostatic hypotension, especially with first dose	2+	Lowers serum lipids
Vasodilators						
Hydralazine	2	50.0	300.0	Tachycardia, fluid retention; drug-induced lupus syndrome	1+	Used with diuretic and β-blocker
Minoxidil	2	2.5	20.0	Tachycardia, fluid retention, hypertrichosis	2+	Used for refractory hypertension with loop diuretic and β-blocker
Calcium Channel Blockers						
Nifedipine	3	30.0	120.0	Tachycardia, fluid retention	2+	
long-acting form	1	30.0	90.0		4+	
Diltiazem	3–4	90.0	360.0		2+	Reduces cardiac output; avoid with high-grade atrioventricular block, congestive heart failure
long-acting form	1–2	120.0	360.0		4+	As for diltiazem
Verapamil	2	120.0	480.0	Constipation	2+	
long-acting form	1–2	120.0	480.0		4+	
Angiotensin-Converting Enzyme Inhibitors						
Captopril	2	12.5	150.0	Cough, rash, angioedema, hyperkalemia, acute renal failure	4+	Reduces proteinuria and progression of renal failure
Enalapril	1	2.5	40.0	As for captopril	4+	As for captopril
Lisinopril	1	5.0	40.0	As for captopril	4+	As for captopril
Angiotensin II Receptor Blockers						
Losartan	2	25.0	100.0	Little long-term experience	4+	No cough (vs. angiotensin-converting enzyme inhibitors); limited clinical experience

*Relative cost estimated from 1995 *Drug Topics Red Book*, using average wholesale price across manufacturers.
†Long-acting forms also available.

Table 85–2. CONSIDERATIONS IN CHOOSING ANTIHYPERTENSIVE DRUGS FOR SPECIAL POPULATIONS

Population	Drugs to Consider*	Reasons	Drugs to Avoid*	Reasons
Elderly patients	Thiazides	Demonstrated efficacy (most have low renin); low cost	Centrally acting adrenergic inhibitors	Increased risk of central nervous system side effects
Black patients	Thiazides	Demonstrated efficacy (most have low renin)	β-Adrenergic blockers	Less effective as monotherapy
Smokers			β-Adrenergic blockers	Less effective
Diabetes	Angiotensin-converting enzyme inhibitors	Retard progression of nephropathy (but may cause hyperkalemia in patients with hyporeninemic hypoaldosteronism)	Thiazides	May worsen glucose tolerance (especially if hypokalemic)
			β-Adrenergic blockers	May impair metabolic response to hypoglycemia
Hyperlipidemia	α_1-Adrenergic blockers	Reduce serum lipids	Thiazides	May raise total cholesterol and low-density lipoproteins, lower high-density lipoproteins
			β-Adrenergic blockers without sympathomimetic activity	May raise very low-density lipoproteins and lower high-density lipoproteins
Asthma			β-Adrenergic blockers	Cause bronchospasm
Bradycardia, heart block, sick sinus syndrome			β-Adrenergic blockers, verapamil, diltiazem	Increase atrioventricular block
Congestive heart failure	Angiotensin-converting enzyme inhibitors	Efficacy for both congestive heart failure and hypertension	β-Adrenergic blockers, verapamil, diltiazem	Negative inotropic effect
	Furosemide	Promotes sodium excretion		
Renal failure	Angiotensin-converting enzyme inhibitors	Slow progression of disease	Thiazides	Ineffective if serum creatinine > 2.5 mg/dL
				Monitor for early reduction in renal function
Coronary artery disease	β-Adrenergic blockers	Also treat angina pectoris; prevent reinfarction after myocardial infarction	Thiazides	May worsen lipids; hypokalemia may provoke arrhythmias unless potassium-sparing diuretic prescribed
	Calcium channel blockers	Also treat angina pectoris		
Benign prostatic hypertrophy	α_1-Adrenergic blockers	Improve bladder emptying	Thiazides	May worsen frequency and nocturia
			Loop diuretics	
Pregnancy	Methyldopa	Proven effectiveness and safety	Angiotensin-converting enzyme inhibitors	Possible teratogenesis
	Hydralazine	Proven effectiveness and safety		
	β-Adrenergic blockers	Also effective and appear safe		

*Few of these recommendations are absolute. Individual patients vary in their response to any drug.

consideration should be given to a trial of treatment reduction. Few patients in whom hypertension is properly diagnosed are able to stop medications permanently, but many can reduce drug dosages. Such "stepdown" of antihypertensive medications is most often successful in patients with blood pressure lower than the usual target range and in those who have successfully instituted nonpharmacologic measures of blood pressure control.

Hypertensive Crises. Patients with a diastolic blood pressure above 120 to 130 mm Hg are at substantially increased short-term risk of complications and must be treated immediately. If the patient manifests end-organ disease of the central nervous system (encephalopathy, focal neurologic deficits), cardiovascular system (angina pectoris, myocardial infarction, pulmonary edema, aortic dissection), renal failure, or eclampsia in pregnancy, prompt hospital admission and the use of parenteral antihypertensive agents are recommended. If blood pressure elevations are severe but end-organ disease is absent, treatment can be instituted promptly in the outpatient department with oral medications. The goal of immediate therapy is to produce a *gradual* reduction in blood pressure to a target diastolic blood pressure of 100 to 110 mm Hg; more rapid lowering of the blood pressure may lead to hypoperfusion of end organs because of changes in autoregulation of blood flow. The drugs most commonly used to treat hypertensive "urgencies" in primary care are clonidine and nifedipine. Oral clonidine loading can be accomplished with an initial dose of 0.1 to 0.2 mg orally, followed by repeated doses of 0.05 to 0.1 mg every hour until the blood pressure reaches the target range or a total of 0.6 to 0.7 mg has been given. Nifedipine can be administered either orally or sublingually, with an initial dose of 10 mg, repeated once if necessary. Patients should be observed for several hours after either mode of therapy to ensure that the blood pressure does not fall excessively. When the blood pressure is stable, patients should leave the clinic with a prescription for medications and should receive frequent follow-up, as often as daily, to ensure that the blood pressure is coming under control.

Cross-References: Compliance (Chapter 4), Periodic Health Assessment (Chapter 8), Alcohol Problems (Chapter 10), Obesity (Chapter 15), Assessment of Physical Activity (Chapter 72), Congestive Heart Failure (Chapter 79).

REFERENCES

1. Gifford RW. An algorithm for the management of resistant hypertension. Hypertension 1988;11 (suppl II):II-101–II-105.

   A sequential method is shown for evaluating patients whose blood pressure appears refractory to three-drug antihypertensive therapy.

2. Gifford RW. Management of hypertensive crises. JAMA 1991;266:829–835.

   This is a practical review of the clinical syndromes and management of hypertensive emergencies and urgencies.

3. Hebert PR, Moser M, Mayer J, Glynn RJ, Hennekens CH. Recent evidence on drug therapy of mild to moderate hypertension and decreased risk of coronary heart disease. Arch Intern Med 1993;153:578–581.

   Meta-analysis of hypertension treatment trials includes more recent studies in elderly hypertensives and those with isolated systolic hypertension.

4. Neaton JD, Grimm RH, Prineas RJ, Stamler J, Grandits GA, Elmer PJ, et al. Treatment of Mild Hypertension Study: Final results. JAMA 1993;270:713–724.

A comparison of monotherapy with five different drugs (diuretics, β-blockers, α-blockers, angiotensin-converting enzyme inhibitors, calcium channel blockers) demonstrating divergent metabolic effects but comparable declines in blood pressure and left ventricular mass and improvements in quality of life.

5. The 1993 Joint National Committee. The fifth report of the Joint National Committee on Detection, Evaluation and Treatment of High Blood Pressure (JNC V). Arch Intern Med 1993;153:154–183.

This report by the most authoritative consensus panel on hypertension management emphasizes a practical approach for ambulatory care, based on initial pharmacotherapy with diuretics or β-adrenergic blockers.

· ·

86 Echocardiographic and Nuclear Assessment of Cardiac Function

Procedure

JAMES R. REVENAUGH and DAWN E. DeWITT

Indications. Nuclear and echocardiographic imaging techniques are indicated to evaluate for the presence and severity of underlying coronary artery disease (CAD), to guide preoperative cardiac assessment, and to detect myocardium at risk in patients with known CAD (Table 86–1). They are also indicated in patients who have congestive heart failure or suspected structural abnormalities. In patients with underlying electrocardiographic abnormalities, in whom conventional exercise tolerance testing (ETT) has suboptimal predictive value, techniques that combine exercise or pharmacologic stress such as dobutamine or intravenous vasodilators such as adenosine or dipyridamole with these imaging modalities offer more accurate assessment of CAD.

ASSESSMENT OF CARDIAC STRUCTURE AND FUNCTION. Both transthoracic echocardiography and radionuclide ventriculography assess ventricular function and size. Radionuclide methods, which are less dependent on image acquisition technique than echocardiography, are often used when serial assessment of ventricular function and size is of interest, as in a patient undergoing chemotherapy with cardiotoxic agents. In patients in whom congestive heart failure is newly diagnosed, echocardiography offers assessment of valvular integrity and hemodynamics in addition to ventricular function and cardiac structure.

ASSESSING THE PRESENCE OR SIGNIFICANCE OF CAD. A major goal of noninvasive diagnosis of CAD is to identify patients for whom more invasive testing is

Table 86–1. ECHOCARDIOGRAPHIC AND NUCLEAR IMAGING TESTS

Test	Sensitivity/ Specificity*	Cost†	Advantages	Disadvantages
Exercise tolerance	68% (23–100)/ 77% (17–100)	$308	Provides important prognostic information inexpensively	Less accurate in women, patients with bundle branch blocks
Exercise nuclear imaging (e.g., thallium or sestamibi)	84% (78–96)/ 87% (74–100)	$1300	Better accuracy in women, locates ischemia	Contraindications (see text), expensive, false-negative results (see text)
Nuclear imaging with pharmacologic stress (e.g., dipyridamole)	88% (83–98)/ 85% (64–100)	$1800	Useful in patients who cannot exercise	Contraindications (see text), false-positive results (see text)
Exercise echocardiography	88% (84–100)/ 80% (64–93)	$800	Allows assessment for exercise-induced mitral regurgitation, structural information	Contraindications (see text), requires skilled ultrasonographer
Echocardiography with pharmacologic stress (e.g., dobutamine)	88% (86–96)/ 84% (66–95)	$820	Useful in patients who cannot exercise	Contraindications (see text)

*Sensitivity and specificity data from Chou TM, Amidon TM. Evaluating coronary artery disease noninvasively—which test for whom? West J Med 1994; 161:173–180.
†Cost based on fees at the University of Washington, 1996.

indicated, such as those with physiologically significant coronary stenosis or disease involving the left main coronary artery. Conventional exercise tolerance testing without nuclear or echocardiographic imaging is indicated in patients with a normal resting electrocardiogram who can exercise to a heart rate at or above 85% of predicted rate, based on age. In patients with uncomplicated myocardial infarction (no congestive heart failure, ventricular dysrhythmias, or postinfarction angina), low-level exercise stress testing before hospital discharge generally provides adequate information regarding the need for coronary angiography. However, both echocardiographic and nuclear stress imaging add independent diagnostic information to that obtained by standard ETT in patients with chest pain suggestive of angina in whom the risk of CAD is at least moderate. Because only a *regional* flow disparity is detected using conventional nuclear techniques (without exercise or pharmacologic stress), perfusion imaging has the potential to miss "balanced" three-vessel CAD; bundle branch blocks also diminish the diagnostic accuracy. In patients with known CAD (with or without recent myocardial infarction) and recurrent chest pain, stress imaging provides information that may aid in identifying the (perhaps one of many) coronary lesion contributing to the patient's symptoms and thus may help direct the interventional cardiologist or cardiac surgeon in revascularization. In patients in whom exercise is not possible or in whom the resting electrocardiogram is abnormal, pharmacologic stress provides diagnostic accuracy similar to exercise stress testing.

PREOPERATIVE RISK ASSESSMENT. When used in conjunction with exercise or pharmacologic stress, a positive radionuclide or echocardiographic study is 85% to 90% accurate in predicting cardiac complications. Because the relative merits of nuclear perfusion imaging versus echocardiographic stress techniques are controversial, the ultimate choice depends in large part on availability and the experience of the facility in which the procedure is performed.

Contraindications. Contraindications to exercise imaging evaluation are identical to those of conventional, symptom-limited ETT (see Chapter 88). Intravenous vasodilator stress should not be administered to patients in whom ETT is contraindicated, in the setting of reactive airway disease, or if the patient is taking methylxanthines or oral dipyridamole. Adenosine should not be used in the setting of underlying conduction system disease (atrioventricular block). Dobutamine stress should not be performed when ETT is contraindicated and should be avoided in the setting of ventricular dysrhythmias or concurrent use of β-blockers. There are no absolute contraindications to resting nuclear or transthoracic echocardiographic evaluations.

Rationale. Nuclear cardiac scintigraphy and echocardiography enable extensive structural and functional evaluation. Stress imaging techniques are designed to induce either controlled myocardial ischemia or a regional blood flow disparity, which are then visualized directly (nuclear perfusion imaging), or the postexercise functional impairment is visualized (e.g., echocardiogram). Exercise is the preferred method of stress because it allows assessment of exercise tolerance and correlation of symptoms with activity and because exercise performance provides independent prognostic information.

Indications for the use of exercise echocardiography or radionuclide exercise testing include patients in whom standard exercise treadmill testing is nondiagnostic, those with a high likelihood of a false-positive ETT (e.g., women), patients with electrocardiographic abnormalities that render ETT uninterpretable (e.g., digitalis, bundle branch blocks), or patients in whom the location and extent of disease needs to be evaluated. In patients in whom underlying noncardiac medical conditions preclude the use of vigorous exercise, pharmacologic stress agents are used. Vasodilator stress agents such as dipyridamole and adenosine induce a regional blood flow disparity without markedly increasing myocardial oxygen consumption and have been used with both echocardiography (in high doses) and nuclear imaging. Dobutamine stress induces physiologic coronary vasodilation by increasing myocardial oxygen demand and is also used as a pharmacologic stress agent with both imaging modalities. Radionuclide methods can be used to assess ventricular function, regional myocardial blood flow, and myocardial viability. Tracer techniques (e.g., radiolabeled red blood cell studies) can be used to assess intracardiac shunts, and labeled monoclonal antibodies can detect underlying inflammation, such as in patients after acute myocardial infarction or in cardiac transplant patients with acute cardiac rejection.

Nuclear perfusion scintigraphy is performed with thallium-201 or similar radiolabeled tracers of myocardial blood flow. A gamma camera detects the location of radioactivity; the reconstructed images allow for comparison of regional tracer concentration and are usually viewed in multiple imaging planes. Perfusion tracers are initially taken up in viable myocardial tissue in direct proportion to the regional myocardial blood flow. Imaging after injection of the tracer at peak physical or pharmacologic stress can detect physiologically significant atherosclerotic coronary stenoses because, unlike normal vessels, stenotic areas are unable to dilate in response to exercise or pharmacologic stress. Stress images of *normal* myocardium are characterized by avid and uniform radiotracer uptake; regions of *hypoperfused* or *infarcted* myocardium appear as areas of diminished or absent radiotracer activity, respectively. Delayed or rest images similarly reflect the resting perfusion state of myocardium. Areas of viable but hypoperfused myocardium appear as diminished radiotracer uptake during stress that improves at rest; infarcted myocardium is characterized by absent or severely reduced radiotracer uptake during stress without change on rest imaging.

Equilibrium radionuclide ventriculography requires radiolabeling the patient's red blood cells, which are then reinjected and remain in the intravascular space, allowing for imaging of the ventricular cavity and generation of a computerized composite image of one cardiac cycle. Evaluation during rest and with supine bicycle exercise delineates resting function as well as the ventricular response to exercise.

Stress echocardiography relies on the observation that regional wall motion abnormalities occur during ischemia. Echocardiography allows for direct visualization of cardiac structure and ventricular function; gives information about hemodynamics, valvular structure and function, intracardiac shunts, or congenital abnormalities; and provides estimates of right-sided (and sometimes left-sided) heart pressures. Although helpful in assessing the size and physiologic significance of pericardial effusion, assessment of pericardial thickness is generally suboptimal. Good images can be obtained in most patients; conditions such as emphysema and obesity can limit a thorough assessment when the transthoracic approach is used. As with nuclear techniques, stress images are compared with those obtained at rest. The regional myocardial wall motion in patients without physiologically significant coronary stenoses appears uniformly hyperdynamic during stress in comparison with rest images. Abnormalities in regional wall motion and wall thickening are seen in areas of viable myocardium subserved by significantly diseased coronary vessels, and irreversible thinning with akinesis at stress and rest is seen in regions where infarcted tissue is present. Cardiac wall motion is analyzed at each stage of exercise, and judgments are made regarding ischemia or infarction. Treadmill or bicycle ergometer (allows imaging during exercise) testing may be done. Rapid recovery of wall motion abnormalities may lead to false-negative results when treadmill testing with postexercise imaging is done. CAD can be predicted correctly by exercise echocardiography in approximately 75% of patients with an ambiguous or false-negative treadmill test. Furthermore, in women, in whom false-positive test results are common, 82% to 85% of exercise echocardiogram tests are accurate, even in those with atypical symptoms and nondiagnostic stress ETTs.

Methods. Exercise and pharmacologic stress cardiac evaluations require continuous electrocardiographic and blood pressure monitoring, intravenous access for administration of radiotracer or pharmacologic stress agent, and exercise equipment such as a bicycle ergometer or treadmill. Studies are performed in close proximity to the imaging equipment. If echocardiography is used, the rest study is usually performed before stress to define optimal imaging views. In the case of nuclear perfusion imaging, stress studies are generally performed first, and if these results are *completely* normal, the resting study may be omitted.

Rest nuclear imaging is performed in the majority of cases, as indicated by the results of the stress imaging study.

Cross-References: Assessment of Physical Activity (Chapter 72), Recurrent Chest Pain (Chapter 74), Angina (Chapter 78), Exercise Tolerance Testing (Chapter 88), Preoperative Cardiovascular Problems (Chapter 218).

REFERENCES

1. Chou TM, Amidon TM. Evaluating coronary artery disease noninvasively—which test for whom? West J Med 1994;161:173–180.

   Available testing is summarized along with the sensitivity and specificity of each test (lists the sources); recommendations are given for choosing tests.

2. Fletcher G, Froelicher V, et al. Exercise standards: A statement for health professionals from the American Heart Association. Circulation 1990;82:2286–2319.

   This article is an excellent review of standard exercise testing and exercise prescription.

3. Marwick T, Willemart B, et al. Selection of the optimal nonexercise stress for the evaluation of ischemic regional myocardial dysfunction and malperfusion: Comparison of dobutamine and adenosine using echocardiography and ^{99m}Tc-MIBI single photon emission computed tomography. Circulation 1993;87:345–354.

   Vasodilator and inotropic pharmacologic stress testing using both echocardiographic and nuclear imaging is compared with angiography.

4. Ritchie JL, et al. Guidelines for clinical use of cardiac radionuclide imaging. Report of the American College of Cardiology/American Heart Association Task Force on Assessment of Diagnostic and Therapeutic Cardiovascular Procedures (Committee on Radionuclide Imaging). J Am Coll Cardiol 1995;25:521–547.

   Indications for use of positron emission tomography are included.

5. Ryan T, Feigenbaum H. Exercise echocardiography. Am J Cardiol 1992;69:82H–89H.

   The diagnostic accuracy of the test is reviewed, and exercise echocardiography is compared with other imaging modalities.

Position statements and practice guidelines pertaining to echocardiography and nuclear stress imaging are also available through the Internet at the American College of Cardiology Home Page: http://www.acc.org/

87 Ambulatory Cardiac Monitoring

Procedure

WISHWA N. KAPOOR

Indications. Ambulatory electrocardiographic (ECG) monitoring is used in the following circumstances:

1. To evaluate symptoms possibly due to arrhythmias. Ambulatory monitoring is indicated in the evaluation of syncope, presyncope, dizziness, and palpitations of unexplained etiology after initial clinical assessment and baseline laboratory tests.
2. To guide antiarrhythmic therapy.
3. To identify and treat high-risk groups. Although ventricular arrhythmias identify high-risk patients after acute myocardial infarction, in hypertrophic cardiomyopathy, and in certain other conditions (see later), there is no evidence of improved outcomes after therapy for arrhythmias.
4. To detect silent ischemia.
5. To detect marked bradycardia in patients with sleep apnea, to evaluate pacemaker function, and, rarely, to evaluate sudden dyspnea or fatigue when paroxysmal arrhythmias are clinically suspected.

Rationale. Results of ambulatory monitoring are often difficult to interpret when used for the diagnostic evaluation of patients with syncope and dizziness. The major problems are lack of a gold standard for diagnosis of arrhythmias and the rarity of symptoms during monitoring. One way to assess the usefulness of ambulatory monitoring is to use presence or absence of symptoms during monitoring. By using studies that included patients who were monitored for 12 hours or more and who kept symptom diaries, researchers found approximately 4% had symptoms concurrently with arrhythmias. In another 17% of patients, symptoms were reported but no arrhythmias were found, thus potentially excluding arrhythmias as a cause of symptoms. In approximately 79% of patients there were no symptoms, but *brief* arrhythmias were found in 13% of these patients. Finding brief (e.g., sinus pauses less than 2 seconds or three beats of ventricular tachycardia) or no arrhythmias without symptoms during monitoring does not exclude arrhythmias as a cause of symptoms. Brief arrhythmias are nonspecific and can be found in asymptomatic healthy individuals. Absence of arrhythmias on monitoring does not exclude episodic arrhythmic syncope because this may not be captured during monitoring. In patients with high pretest probability of arrhythmias, such as brief sudden symptoms without prodrome, patients with abnormal electrocardiograms, or those with structural heart disease, further testing for arrhythmias may be needed. Generally, 24 hours of monitoring is sufficient in the initial evaluation of patients with unexplained symptoms when arrhythmias are suspected clinically. Extending the duration of monitoring to 48 to 72 hours has not been shown to increase the detection of symptomatic arrhythmias.

Event loop recorders provide the capability of ECG recording during a symptomatic period. Studies of loop monitoring show that arrhythmias with symptoms (syncope and dizziness) are found in 8% to 20% of patients. In an additional 27%, symptoms are present without concurrent arrhythmias. This test is recommended in patients with recurrent symptoms when there is a high probability of a recurrent event during the monitoring period. Loop monitoring is complementary to Holter monitoring and has not eliminated the need for initial Holter monitoring for the evaluation of unexplained syncope. In patients with palpitations, ambulatory monitoring using event loop recorders is an excellent means of achieving symptomatic correlation when symptoms are clinically unexplained.

Ambulatory monitoring has been used extensively to document suppression of ventricular and supraventricular arrhythmias after initiation or change in dosage of antiarrhythmic drugs. An 80% to 90% decrease in the frequency of arrhythmia compared with baseline is generally considered adequate suppression. However, a gold standard for adequate suppression is not available. Asymptomatic patients treated with antiarrhythmic drugs for ventricular ectopy have not been shown to have an improved outcome. Increased mortality has been reported with encainide or flecainide and is a concern with quinidine and procainamide owing to proarrhythmic drug effects.

Electrophysiologic studies are an alternative approach to the management of tachyarrhythmias. However, these arrhythmias may not be inducible with ventricular stimulation in up to 50% of patients with spontaneous ventricular tachyarrhythmias. Additionally, there is little evidence to suggest improved outcome with therapy guided by electrophysiologic studies as compared with ambulatory monitoring. Thus, using ambulatory monitoring as a guide to antiarrhythmic therapy is an acceptable alternative.

Frequent (> 10/h) or repetitive ventricular ectopy is associated with increased incidence of sudden death, cardiac mortality, and total mortality in patients with recent myocardial infarction. This increased risk can also be predicted from other variables (cardiomegaly, ejection fraction, extent of myocardial necrosis, ST segment depression, prior myocardial infarction, exercise testing). Therapy for asymptomatic ventricular ectopy has not been shown to improve outcome. Therefore, routine ambulatory monitoring is not recommended in asymptomatic survivors of myocardial infarction.

Ventricular tachycardia is reported in up to 25% of patients with hypertrophic cardiomyopathy, and nonsustained ventricular tachycardia is a predictor of sudden death. However, the routine use of this test for screening in patients with hypertrophic cardiomyopathy is not established, and studies are not available to show that therapy alters outcome.

In patients with known coronary artery disease (but not acute myocardial infarction), congestive heart failure, or chronic obstructive lung disease, ventricular arrhythmias have not generally been shown to be an independent predictor of mortality or sudden death. Thus, routine use of ambulatory monitoring is not supported.

In patients with coronary disease, ST segment changes on Holter monitoring may indicate episodes of ischemia. Frequency of silent ischemia during daily activities in patients with coronary artery disease is as much as 8 to 10 times that of symptomatic periods. Prolonged and frequent episodes of silent ischemia identify high-risk patients with increased future cardiac event rates. Because stress ECG also provides prognostic information, the additional value of ambulatory monitoring for prognosis is not clear. Ambulatory ECG is currently not widely used for diagnosis of coronary artery disease, determination of its prognosis, or monitoring of antianginal therapy.

Methods. The traditional system uses a battery-powered tape recorder to record two ECG leads continuously over a 24- to 48-hour period. The only restriction involves bathing and swimming during the recording period. The patient is instructed to keep a diary of symptoms to determine whether symptoms occur concurrently with an arrhythmia. The recorded information is analyzed by computer comparing each QRST complex with a series of templates already classified and determined to be normal, aberrant supraventricular, or ventricular. All questionable signals are analyzed by an operator to eliminate artifacts. Other types of devices include patient-activated event recorders, which are useful for infrequent arrhythmias in patients who have recurrent symptoms. A loop ECG recording is a noninvasive test enabling patients to be monitored for prolonged period of times (such as for a month or more). Loop monitors generally use two chest ECG leads that are continuously worn and connected to a small recorder. Loop monitors can be activated after symptoms, and recording of 4 to 5 minutes of retrograde rhythm strip is possible. Tracings can be transmitted by telephone.

Cost. Cost for standard Holter monitoring ranges from $250 to $350 per 24 hours. The charges for cardiac loop ECG recorders are similar, with the major advantage of increasing the observational period to several weeks. There are no studies on cost-effectiveness of ambulatory cardiac monitoring.

Cross-References: Dizziness (Chapter 20), Syncope (Chapter 75), Palpitations (Chapter 76), Chronic Ventricular Arrhythmias (Chapter 83), Supraventricular Arrhythmias (Chapter 84).

REFERENCES

1. American College of Physicians. Ambulatory ECG (Holter) monitoring: Position paper. Ann Intern Med 1990;113:77–79.

    This is a review of recommendations by the American College of Physicians for use of ambulatory Holter monitoring.

2. DiMarco JP, Philbrick JT. Use of ambulatory electrocardiographic (Holter) monitoring. Ann Intern Med 1990;113:53–68.

    This is a thoughtful review of efficacy of ECG monitoring and guidelines for its use in clinical practice.

3. Fisch C, DeSanctis RW, Dodge HT, Reeves TJ, Weinberg SL. Guidelines for ambulatory electrocardiography. J Am Coll Cardiol 1989;13:249–258.

    This is the report of the American College of Cardiology and American Heart Association Task Force on ambulatory ECG monitoring.

4. Stern S, Cohn PF, Pepine CJ. Silent myocardial ischemia. Curr Probl Cardiol 1993;18:301–360.

    This is an overview of silent ischemia with a summary of studies on the use of ambulatory monitoring and other tests for ischemia.

88 Exercise Tolerance Testing

Procedure

STEVEN R. McGEE

Indications and Contraindications. Exercise testing adds useful information in three common clinical settings: (1) diagnosis of chest pain in patients with an intermediate pretest probability of coronary artery disease, (2) evaluation of prognosis in patients with known coronary artery disease, and (3) prediction of future coronary events after uncomplicated myocardial infarction. Less frequent indications include evaluation of pulmonary disease and exercise-induced arrhythmias.

Contraindications include acute myocardial infarction during the previous 10 to 14 days, unstable angina, severe aortic stenosis (exercise-induced vasodilatation causes syncope), uncompensated congestive heart failure, acute systemic illness, uncontrolled hypertension, and significant cardiac arrhythmias.

Rationale

DIAGNOSIS OF CORONARY ARTERY DISEASE. Abnormal exercise test ST segment responses (greater than 1 mm horizontal or downsloping depression) predict anatomic coronary artery disease with a sensitivity of 50% to 70% and a specificity of 90%. Table 88–1 lists causes of false-positive and false-negative results. The physician should address the patient's age, quality of chest pain, and risk factors to determine the pretest likelihood of coronary artery disease. Diagnostic exercise testing benefits those patients with intermediate pretest probability (40%–60%) (Table 88–2). Most patients with high pretest likelihood of coronary artery disease and negative test results actually have coronary artery disease (false negative); most with low pretest likelihood and positive results do not have disease (false positive). Easy-to-use nomograms simplify these calculations.

Table 88–1. CAUSES OF FALSE-POSITIVE AND FALSE-NEGATIVE EXERCISE TESTS

False-Positive Tests

Digoxin
Left ventricular hypertrophy
Left bundle branch block
Preexcitation syndromes
Hyperventilation

False-Negative Tests

Antianginal medication
Single-vessel disease
Test limited by noncardiac symptoms (claudication, fatigue)

All of the material in Chapter 88 is in the public domain, with the exception of any borrowed figures and tables.

Table 88–2. PRETEST AND POST-TEST PROBABILITY
OF CORONARY ARTERY DISEASE

Patient Example	Pretest Likelihood	Post-test Likelihood	
		Positive	Negative
45-year-old woman with nonanginal chest pain	0.05 (low)	0.24	0.02
50-year-old man with atypical angina	0.50 (intermediate)	0.86	0.31
60-year-old man with typical angina	0.90 (high)	0.98	0.80

Exercise thallium scintigraphy, with its higher sensitivity (80%), or exercise echocardiography, which allows assessment of cardiac structure and function (success rates of 85% with sensitivity of 74% to 100%, depending on study criteria), is preferable (see Chapter 86, Echocardiographic and Nuclear Assessment of Cardiac Function) when the physician anticipates false-positive conventional exercise test results (see Table 88–1). When poor patient effort or inability to exercise is anticipated, use of medications rather than exercise (e.g., dipyridamole [Persantine] or dobutamine stress tests) is indicated.

PROGNOSIS IN CORONARY ARTERY DISEASE. Three variables predict prognosis: (1) duration of exercise (testing stopped early because of abnormal findings signifies higher risk), (2) presence of angina during testing, and (3) abnormal ST segment response. Simple arithmetic scores identify patients at high, moderate, and low risk who have respective 5-year myocardial infarction–free survivals of 63%, 86%, and 93% with medical treatment. Exercise-induced hypotension, in the absence of obstructive cardiomyopathy or valvular heart disease, is highly specific for left main or triple-vessel disease (sensitivity, however, is less than 20%). Exercise-induced premature beats add little independent information. In low-risk patients, medical treatment may be safely continued, because survival benefit with surgery is difficult to demonstrate. Higher-risk patients are most likely to benefit from cardiac catheterization, which may further define those who will benefit from revascularization or angioplasty.

PROGNOSIS AFTER MYOCARDIAL INFARCTION. Low-level exercise testing 2 to 3 weeks after uncomplicated myocardial infarction stratifies patients into low- and high-risk groups. Exercise testing is not appropriate when patients experience early recurrent angina or severe heart failure, because risk of future cardiac events in these patients is already high. Of the remaining 80% who safely may undergo exercise testing, two thirds have normal results and subsequent 1-year mortality of 2.6%. Medical therapy is appropriate for these low-risk patients. The one third of patients with abnormal results (ST segment changes, poor exercise duration, or angina) have a 1-year mortality of 20% and account for 80% of posthospitalization deaths. Cardiac catheterization in this high-risk group may identify disease amenable to angioplasty or bypass surgery. Exercise-induced hypotension in the first few weeks after myocardial infarction is a nonspecific self-limited finding and does not signify severe myocardial ischemia as it does in those without recent infarction.

ASYMPTOMATIC PATIENTS. Exercise testing in asymptomatic patients is inappropriate for two reasons: (1) even though positive test results (abnormal ST

Table 88–3. REASONS TO TERMINATE EXERCISE TESTING

Symptoms

Progressive angina
Extreme fatigue or dyspnea

Signs

Fall in systolic blood pressure
Confusion, staggering gait
Pallor, clammy skin

Electrocardiographic Criteria

Arrhythmia (frequent ventricular salvos, ventricular tachycardia, heart block, supraventricular tachycardia)
Excessive ST segment change (criteria vary, usually > 3 mm ST segment depression or > 2 mm ST segment elevation)

segment change) increase the asymptomatic patient's risk for future coronary events (death, myocardial infarction, angina) fivefold, the overwhelming majority of positive results are false positive because of very low pretest probability of disease (see Table 88–2); and (2) the initial cardiac event during follow-up is usually angina (potentially reversible), not myocardial infarction or sudden death.

Methods. Patients progressively increase exercise workload at regularly timed intervals, or stages, while the physician monitors the patient's symptoms, signs, and physiologic responses. Treadmill testing, the most popular form of exercise testing, increases either treadmill speed or grade at each stage. Exercise testing after myocardial infarction employs modified protocols, which change workload more gradually.

Exercise testing begins after informed consent, history, physical examination, and resting electrocardiogram. During testing the physician watches for endpoints listed in Table 88–3. Low-level modified protocols usually include heart rate as an endpoint (determined to be 70% to 75% maximal heart rate or 120 to 130 beats per minute).

Cost and Complications. The risk of death, which usually occurs because of acute myocardial infarction or arrhythmia, is 0.5 per 10,000 during exercise testing. Although this is extremely low, resuscitation equipment and skills must be nearby. Cost of treadmill exercise testing is $308.*

Cross-References: Assessment of Physical Activity (Chapter 72), Acute Chest Pain (Chapter 73), Angina (Chapter 78), Echocardiographic and Nuclear Assessment of Cardiac Function (Chapter 86).

REFERENCES

1. DeBusk RF. Specialized testing after recent acute myocardial infarction. Ann Intern Med 1989;110:470–481.

*Based on 1996 University of Washington hospital and professional fees.

This excellent review, with accompanying American College of Physicians position paper, compares the role of exercise testing, radionuclide testing, Holter monitoring, and echocardiography after myocardial infarction.

2. Mark DB, Hlatky MA, Harrel FE, Lee KL, Califf RM, et al: Exercise treadmill score for predicting prognosis in coronary artery disease. Ann Intern Med 1987;106:793–800.

The derivation and testing of an arithmetic treadmill score that adds prognostic information independent from coronary anatomy and left ventricular function is discussed.

3. McHenry PL, O'Donnell J, Morris SN, Jordan JJ. The abnormal exercise electrocardiogram in apparently healthy men: A predictor of angina pectoris as an initial coronary event during long-term follow-up. Circulation 1984;70:547–551.

Among 916 asymptomatic Indiana State patrolmen, 34% with ST changes during exercise testing developed a cardiac event (angina, infarction, or sudden death) during a mean of 12 years follow-up, compared with 5% of those with negative test results (i.e., although exercise tolerance testing identified increased risk, most positive results were false negative).

4. Patterson RE, Eng C, Horowitz SF. Practical diagnosis of coronary artery disease: A Bayes' theorem nomogram to correlate clinical data with noninvasive exercise tests. Am J Cardiol 1984;53:252–256.

Nomograms that incorporate patient's age, sex, risk factors, and treadmill and thallium testing results are used to define post-test likelihood of anatomic coronary artery disease.

5. Schlant RC, Blomqvist CG, Brandenburg RO, DeBusk R, Ellestad MH, et al. Guidelines for exercise testing. J Am Coll Cardiol 1986;8:725–738.

Recommendations for exercise testing were prepared by the American College of Cardiology/American Heart Association task force.

• •

89 Echocardiography

Procedure

CATHERINE M. OTTO

Indications. *Standard transthoracic echocardiography* is useful for evaluating a broad range of cardiac diseases (Table 89–1). Echocardiography is *not* routinely indicated in the evaluation of supraventricular arrhythmia or to search for a source of embolism unless the history or physical examination suggests the possibility of structural heart disease.

Stress echocardiography (either exercise or pharmacologic) has a high diagnostic yield for the presence and extent of coronary artery disease, particularly in patient groups with a low diagnostic yield on exercise electrocardiographic testing (e.g., women or patients with resting electrocardiographic abnormalities). This procedure is indicated in patients with suspected coronary artery disease (including those being evaluated preoperatively for noncardiac procedures), to evaluate the extent of ischemia and the results of revascularization,

Table 89–1. INDICATIONS FOR ECHOCARDIOGRAPHY

Clinical Problem	Information Obtainable by Echocardiography	Limitations	Alternative Diagnostic Tests
Valvular disease	Valve anatomy Transvalvular pressure gradients and valve areas Regurgitant severity PA pressures Chamber enlargement Ventricular function	Possible underestimation of stenosis severity. Prosthetic valve dysfunction requires TEE.	If echocardiographic data are of good quality, cardiac catheterization is rarely needed. TEE if LA thrombus suspected
Pericardial disease	Presence, size, distribution of effusion Evidence of tamponade physiology Possible evidence of pericardial constriction (difficult diagnosis)	Not all patients with acute pericarditis have an effusion. The diagnosis of tamponade requires correlation with clinical findings.	Cardiac catheterization and CT (pericardial thickness) may be needed to diagnose constriction.
Cardiomyopathy	Chamber sizes, wall thickness LV systolic function Outflow obstruction in hypertrophic cardiomyopathy PA pressures LV thrombus RV systolic function Associated valve dysfunction		Coronary angiography if indicated Radionuclide or contrast angiographic ejection fraction (does not provide assessment of valve function, wall thickness, etc.)
Ischemic heart disease Acute myocardial infarction	Bedside evaluation of global and segmental LV function Extent of myocardium at risk Complications: acute MR or VSD, pericarditis, LV thrombus, aneurysm, RV infarct	Direct visualization of coronary anatomy is not feasible.	Coronary angiography
Angina	LV systolic function Resting wall motion abnormalities Stress echocardiography for ischemia and myocardial viability	Wall motion may be normal at rest despite severe coronary disease.	Exercise testing with radionuclide perfusion imaging Coronary angiography

Cardiac masses			
LV thrombus	High sensitivity (95%) and specificity (86%) for detection of LV thrombus	Technical artifacts can be misleading	Radionuclide and contrast angiography have a low sensitivity for LV thrombus.
LA thrombus	Transthoracic echo has a low sensitivity (33%–50%) for diagnosis of LA thrombus although specificity is high (99%–100%).	TEE is needed to detect LA thrombus reliably (sensitivity > 95%).	TEE
Cardiac tumors	Size, location, physiologic consequences of tumor mass		CT with cardiac gating, MRI
Endocarditis	Detection of vegetations Evaluation of valve regurgitation Chamber sizes LV systolic function	Detection of paravalvular abscess often requires TEE. Vegetation may persist after the acute episode.	Blood cultures and clinical examination are key features of the diagnosis of endocarditis.
Aortic dissection	Aortic root, arch, and descending thoracic aortic size Imaging of dissection flap Detection of severity and mechanism of aortic regurgitation Detection of pericardial effusion	TEE often needed for adequate images Cannot assess distal vascular beds	Aortography, CT, MRI
Congenital heart disease	Detection and assessment of anatomic abnormalities Quantitation of physiologic abnormalities Chamber enlargement Ventricular function		Echocardiography is the initial diagnostic test of choice for congenital heart disease. Cardiac catheterization by an experienced operator may be needed.

CT, computed tomography; LA, left atrium; LV, left ventricle; RV, right ventricle; MR, mitral regurgitation; MRI, magnetic resonance imaging; PA, pulmonary artery; TEE, transesophageal echocardiography; VSD, ventricular septal defect.

and to detect myocardial viability in patients with known coronary artery disease.

Transesophageal echocardiography (TEE) provides improved images of posterior cardiac structures, especially when standard images are suboptimal. TEE is essential for evaluation of suspected prosthetic mitral valve dysfunction, left atrial thrombus, and paravalvular abscess. Many centers use TEE as the procedure of choice for diagnosis of acute aortic dissection. TEE also provides valuable clinical data in patients with endocarditis, congenital heart disease, valvular heart disease, and suspected cardiogenic emboli and in other situations in which transthoracic images are nondiagnostic.

Rationale. Echocardiography uses ultrasound waves (nonionizing radiation) to generate two-dimensional images of cardiac structures in motion and to display intracardiac blood flow information in a variety of formats. Echocardiography has no known adverse effects, is noninvasive (except for TEE), is portable, and can be performed quickly and repeatedly.

Methods. Standard transthoracic echocardiographic data are obtained with the ultrasound transducer placed on the patient's chest while using a water-soluble acoustic coupling gel. Because ultrasound waves do not transmit well through air or bone, the major limitation to echocardiography is suboptimal data quality in some patients owing to poor tissue penetration. TEE provides superior images of posterior cardiac structures owing to the absence of interposing lung (containing air) and the decreased distance of cardiac structures from the ultrasound transducer. Stress echocardiography is performed by recording digital cine-loop images of the left ventricle at baseline and after an intervention (such as exercise or a graded dobutamine infusion) to increase myocardial oxygen demand.

Two-dimensional echocardiography provides detailed tomographic cardiac images in a dynamic (real-time) format that allows assessment of both normal anatomy (ventricular endocardial motion and wall thickening, valve anatomy and motion) and abnormal intracardiac structures (e.g., tumor, vegetation, thrombus). These images also provide accurate measurements of wall thickness, chamber dimensions, and great-vessel diameters and allow calculation of left ventricular volumes, mass, and ejection fraction. Not all laboratories quantitate left ventricular systolic function by two-dimensional echocardiography because of the laborious task of tracing endocardial borders, but as automated methods become available, this will become routine. When carefully measured, echocardiographic, angiographic, and radionuclide procedures are equally accurate. In general, echocardiography is the procedure of choice, even if only a qualitative estimate of left ventricular function is reported, because of the additional clinically relevant information obtained with this technique.

A Doppler examination typically includes three different modalities—pulsed, continuous-wave, and color flow Doppler imaging. Pulsed Doppler measures blood flow velocity at specific intracardiac sites and is useful for evaluation of left ventricular diastolic filling and for calculation of stroke volume and cardiac output. Continuous-wave Doppler study accurately measures high velocities and is useful in determining pressure gradients across stenotic valves, pulmonary artery systolic pressure (based on the tricuspid regurgitant jet velocity), and other intracardiac hemodynamics. Color flow

Doppler study displays mean velocity information superimposed on the two-dimensional image in a real-time format and is most useful for detecting intracardiac shunts and for evaluating valvular regurgitation.

Cost and Complications. There are no known adverse effects of standard transthoracic echocardiography. The risk of stress echocardiography is related to the presence of underlying coronary artery disease. The risk of TEE is low, with potential complications similar to those of upper endoscopy, including aspiration (patients are fasting), bleeding, and, rarely, esophageal perforation (a careful swallowing history is taken and a barium swallow or screening upper endoscopy is performed if indicated). The cost of echocardiography is lower than alternative cardiac imaging procedures. Costs vary geographically and with the extent of the procedure performed, but total costs (procedure and professional fees) for a comprehensive two-dimensional and Doppler study range from $500 to $1000.

Cross-References: Congestive Heart Failure (Chapter 79), Aortic Stenosis (Chapter 80), Other Valvular Disease (Chapter 81), Echocardiographic and Nuclear Assessment of Cardiac Function (Chapter 86).

REFERENCES

1. Feigenbaum H. Echocardiography. In Braunwald E, ed. Heart Disease: A Textbook of Cardiovascular Medicine, 4th ed. Philadelphia, WB Saunders, 1996.

   This provides a comprehensive review of M-mode and two-dimensional echocardiography.

2. Fisher EA, Goldman ME. Transesophageal echocardiography: A new view of the heart. Ann Intern Med 1990;113:91–93.

   This editorial summarizes techniques and indications for transesophageal echocardiography; 20 references are included.

3. Otto CM, Pearlman AS. Textbook of Clinical Echocardiography. Philadelphia, WB Saunders, 1995.

   This concise, clinically oriented textbook describes the technique of echocardiography, clinical indications, and application in various disease states.

4. Popp RL. Echocardiography. N Engl J Med 1990:323:101–109, 165–172.

   Indications for and the principle of echocardiography are reviewed briefly, including more than 150 references.

Gastrointestinal Disorders

· ·

90 Colorectal Cancer Screening

Screening

STEPHAN D. FIHN

Epidemiology. Colorectal cancer is the second most common cancer in the United States, with 150,000 new cases diagnosed each year. The lifetime risk of colorectal cancer is 5%. Fifty percent of cases are fatal, accounting for more than 60,000 deaths annually. The mean age at diagnosis is 69. Well-established risk factors include a family history of colorectal cancer or familial polyposis; prior colorectal, endometrial, breast, or ovarian cancer; adenomatous polyps; and long-standing ulcerative colitis.

Rationale. Colorectal cancer is a significant cause of pain and suffering as well as death. Although early cancers are amenable to surgical extirpation, most cancers are detected at a late stage for which therapy is unsatisfactory. Most cancers are thought to arise from polyps that have a long preclinical phase. Recent studies have shown that routine screening with either fecal occult blood testing or periodic flexible sigmoidoscopy reduces mortality from colorectal cancer by approximately one third, largely by enabling detection of neoplasms at an earlier stage when surgical cure is possible. Definitive studies demonstrating an advantage of sigmoidoscopy versus fecal occult blood testing or more invasive approaches such as colonoscopy in terms of both cost and effectiveness are not available.

Less than 10% of cancers occur within 8 cm of the anal verge, making digital examination exceedingly insensitive. Testing for fecal occult blood is based on the fact that early colorectal neoplasms add 1 to 2 mL of blood to the 0.7 mL normally excreted in the stool each day. The amount of blood loss is directly proportional to the size of the tumor. Thus, occult blood testing is more sensitive for larger lesions. It also is more sensitive for distal lesions because hemoglobin released into the proximal colon can be diluted or degraded by peroxidases in the stool.

The sensitivity of fecal occult blood testing in various studies has ranged between 50% and 90%, while the specificity is 90% to 98%. When performed in mass screening programs involving persons older than 50 years of age, 1%

to 2.4% of participants are found to have at least one positive slide, and the predictive value of a positive test for cancer is 2% to 10%. Several studies suggest that occult blood testing performed every 1 to 2 years can reduce mortality from colorectal cancer by 25% to 43%. Screening less often appears much less beneficial.

Unfortunately, fecal occult blood testing has several drawbacks. It misses 30% to 50% of cancers. It must be done annually, and up to 50% of patients fail to return the test cards. Because the positive predictive value is so low, 90% to 98% of persons with a positive test will undergo expensive and uncomfortable examinations of the colon for no benefit. If detection of adenomatous polyps is included, the predictive value of a positive test is 30% to 54%. However, because 10% to 33% of older adults are found to have adenomas at autopsy, only a fraction of such lesions can be assumed to progress to clinically significant malignancies. The US Congressional Office of Technology Assessment estimated that offering occult blood testing to all Medicare beneficiaries would cost $1.5 billion, translating into $35,000 per life saved.

For these reasons, screening proctosigmoidoscopy has been proposed as a better screening test. This approach enables removal of potentially malignant polyps. The sensitivity of sigmoidoscopy is directly related to the length of the instrument. Modern 35-cm (short bundle) sigmoidoscopes disclose 30% to 40% of cancers, whereas longer 60-cm instruments disclose 50% to 60%. During the examination polyps are also removed. It has been postulated that such prophylactic polypectomies prevent the development of cancer. Many patients find this procedure unpleasant, uncomfortable, and costly. A single examination costs $100 to $200. Moreover, there is a very small risk of colonic perforation or bleeding after biopsy.

Based on currently available evidence, some authorities now recommend combining occult blood testing and flexible sigmoidoscopy.

Action. The US Preventive Services Task Force currently recommends annual screening for fecal occult blood in asymptomatic patients over age 50, sigmoidoscopy (frequency unspecified), or both. Clinicians who decide to offer screening sigmoidoscopy often select an interval of every 5 to 10 years, especially for persons with one or more risk factors for colorectal cancer. Patients with strong risk factors for colorectal cancer, including prior detection of a polyp, should be advised to undergo periodic colonoscopy. All patients to whom screening is offered should be carefully advised of the potential costs, risks, and benefits.

Cross-References: Principles of Screening (Chapter 7), Periodic Health Assessment (Chapter 8), Sigmoidoscopy and Colonoscopy (Chapter 104).

REFERENCES

1. Frame PS. Screening flexible sigmoidoscopy: Is it worthwhile? An opposing view. J Fam Pract 1987;25:604–607.

   To adhere to American Cancer Society recommendations, a typical family physician with 1000 patients over age 50 would have to perform five sigmoidoscopies daily for initial screening and two per day thereafter.

2. Herrington LJ, Selby JV, Friedman GV, Quesenberry CP, Weiss NS. Case-control study of digital-

rectal screening in relation to mortality from cancer of the distal rectum. Am J Epidemiol 1995;142:961–964.

A case-control study in a large HMO population failed to demonstrate any reduction in mortality from rectal cancer as a result of screening with digital rectal examination.

3. Ransohoff DF. The case for colorectal cancer screening. Hosp Pract (Office Edition) 1994;29:25–32.

This review concludes that an optimal strategy for reducing the mortality of colorectal cancer by as much as 70% would be flexible sigmoidoscopy every 5 to 10 years for persons aged 50 to 75 but acknowledges the panoply of barriers to implementation of this policy.

4. Ransohoff DF, Lang CA, Kuo HS. Colonoscopic surveillance after polypectomy. Considerations of cost effectiveness. Ann Intern Med 1991;114:177–182.

This cost-effectiveness analysis suggests that regular colonoscopic surveillance following removal of adenomatous polyps may be very expensive and of limited benefit.

5. Selby JV, Friedman GV, Quesenberry CP, Weiss NS. A case-control study of screening sigmoidoscopy and mortality from colorectal cancer. N Engl J Med 1992;326:653–657.

An earlier study from the same group of investigators working in the same population showed dramatic (31%–75%) reductions in risk of death from colorectal cancer among persons who had screening sigmoidoscopy within the previous 10 years.

<hr>

91 Diarrhea

Symptom

DEBORAH L. GREENBERG

Epidemiology. Diarrhea is a major cause of morbidity and mortality worldwide. It is defined as an increase in stool water or a stool weight greater than 200 g/d. Patients report frequent bowel movements, loose stools, or an increase in stool volume. The incidence of diarrhea in adults in the United States is 1.5 to 1.7 episodes per person per year. More than 8 million Americans seek medical advice for diarrhea annually at a projected cost of $23 billion. Most episodes of diarrhea are self-limited, require no diagnostic evaluation, and are treated symptomatically with oral hydration. Diarrhea that persists longer than 4 weeks is considered chronic.

Etiology. The average person consumes 2 L of fluid daily, whereas the small bowel and colon secrete 8 L and absorb 9.9 L of fluid. Diarrhea results from increased electrolyte and fluid secretion into the bowel lumen, decreased water absorption, or both. Increased secretion is usually caused by mediators (e.g., bacterial enterotoxins, neurohormonal agents, laxatives, fatty acids, bile acids) that alter intracellular second messengers (e.g., cyclic adenosine monophosphate), leading to decreased sodium chloride absorption and increased chloride secretion. Decreased water absorption results from mucosal abnormalities, the ingestion of a poorly absorbed solute (e.g., carbohydrates), or altered bowel motility. Disruption of the mucosal surface by inflammation (e.g., inflammatory bowel disease, invasive microorganisms, ischemia) generally involves the colon and produces small-volume bloody diarrhea accompanied by fever and abdominal pain. Noninflammatory processes (e.g., viruses, enterotoxigenic bacteria, lactose intolerance) primarily affect the small bowel, causing hypersecretion of fluid and electrolytes that results in large-volume (i.e., > 500 mL/24 h) watery diarrhea accompanied by nausea, vomiting, and abdominal cramps. In general, inflammatory processes cause more severe disease and often require further evaluation and treatment.

Infections cause most acute diarrhea. Viruses (e.g., Norwalk agent, rotavirus) are the most common pathogens, but bacteria and parasites cause significant disease (Table 91–1). Transmission occurs by means of the fecal-oral route, ingestion of food or water contaminated with microorganisms, or sexual activity. Normal host defense mechanisms including gastric acid and intestinal motility prevent gastrointestinal infection after inoculation. Patient populations at particular risk for acute infectious diarrhea include children in day care centers

Table 91–1. COMMON CAUSES OF ACUTE INFECTIOUS DIARRHEA IN UNITED STATES

Agent	Exposure	Incubation Period	Associated Symptoms	Treatment
Noninvasive				
Viral	Person to person, day care	24–72 h	N, V, C, HA, malaise	Symptomatic
Staphylococcus aureus	Pastries, meat	2–8 h	N, V, C	Symptomatic
Clostridium perfringens	Warmed food, especially meats	8–24 h	C	Symptomatic
Clostridium botulinum	Canned foods	12–36 h	V, paralysis	Antitoxin
Bacillus cereus	Fried rice, pasta	6–16 h	V, C	Symptomatic
Enterotoxigenic *Escherichia coli*	Travel	24–72 h	N, C	Symptomatic
Giardia lamblia	Day care, camping, travel	1–4 wk	N, C, flatulence	See Table 92–4
Cryptosporidium parvum	Day care, water	5–21 d	C	Symptomatic
Invasive				
Salmonella species (not *typhi*)	Eggs, poultry, meat, travel	6–48 h	N, V, C, F	Symptomatic
Shigella species	Fecal-oral, day care, travel	12–72 h	C, F	See Table 92–4
Campylobacter jejuni	Pets, day care, poultry	2–7 d	HA, F, myalgias	Symptomatic See Table 92–4
Yersinia enterocolitica	Meat, dairy	1–3 d	C, F, A, mesenteric adenitis	
Enteroinvasive *E. coli*	Cheese, meat	24–48 h	F	See Table 92–4
Clostridium difficile	Hospital, antibiotics	1–10 d (up to 8 wk)	F, A	See Table 92–4
Vibrio parahaemolyticus	Shellfish	12–48 h	C, V, HA	Symptomatic See Table 92–4
Entamoeba histolytica	Travel, sexual contact	Days to months	C	

A, abdominal pain; C, cramps; F, fever; HA, headache; N, nausea; V, vomiting.

and their household contacts (e.g., from rotavirus, *Shigella, Campylobacter, Giardia*), travelers (e.g., from *Escherichia coli, Shigella, Salmonella, Giardia, Campylobacter*), patients with recent antibiotic use, institutionalization, or hospitalization (e.g., from *Clostridium difficile*), immunocompromised persons (see Chapter 203, HIV Infection: Disease Prevention and Antiretroviral Therapy; Chapter 204, HIV Infection: Office Evaluation; Chapter 205, HIV Infection: Evaluation of Common Symptoms), and participants in anal sexual activity (e.g., from *Chlamydia, Neisseria,* herpesvirus).

Other causes of acute diarrhea include medication side effects (Table 91–2), inflammatory bowel disease, ischemic colitis, radiation injury, fecal impaction, narcotic withdrawal, pelvic inflammation, diverticulitis, and gastrointestinal bleeding.

A wide variety of disease processes cause chronic diarrhea (Table 91–3). Three of the more common causes, lactose intolerance, infection with *Giardia lamblia,* and irritable bowel syndrome, are difficult to distinguish clinically. Lactose intolerance, due to an acquired lactase deficiency, has a prevalence of 70% to 75% in blacks, 85% in Asians, and 5% to 20% in whites. Unabsorbed lactose causes an osmotic diarrhea along with flatulence and bloating caused by the bacterial breakdown of the carbohydrate. *Giardia* can cause acute, foul-smelling steatorrhea or intermittent, chronic flatulence and abdominal pain. Irritable bowel syndrome is associated with poorly characterized disturbances in intestinal motility and visceral sensitivity. Patients often report intermittent abdominal pain, diarrhea, and constipation.

Clinical Approach.   The history and physical examination identify those patients who need further diagnostic testing or treatment. The history should explore risk factors, including underlying diseases, food intake during the previous 72 hours, medications, personal contacts (e.g., day care, living situation, work, sexual history), and recent travel. The clinician should elucidate the patient's normal stool pattern, onset (e.g., abrupt, gradual) and duration of symptoms, frequency and pattern of bowel movements (e.g., postprandial, nocturnal, or with fasting), and character of stools (e.g., large volume, mucus, blood). A description of associated symptoms (e.g., fever, thirst, postural dizziness, viral prodrome, abdominal pain or cramps, nausea, vomiting, weight loss, tenesmus) is also important.

Physical examination should focus on vital signs, orthostatic blood pressure and pulse, mucous membranes, and mental status to assess the degree of

---

Table 91–2. COMMON MEDICATIONS CAUSING DIARRHEA

Antibiotics: ampicillin, cephalosporins, clindamycin
Antacids: magnesium containing
Antihypertensives: furosemide, hydralazine, propranolol, reserpine, methyldopa
Cardiac medications: digitalis, quinidine
Nonsteroidal anti-inflammatory analgesics
Antimetabolites: colchicine
Alcohol
Antidepressants: fluoxetine, paroxetine, sertraline
Laxatives: lactulose, phenolphthalein, bisacodyl, docusate sodium, senna, ricinoleic acid, cascara, danthron
Caffeine

Table 91–3. CAUSES OF CHRONIC DIARRHEA

Inflammatory Diarrhea

Chronic infection: *Entamoeba histolytica, Clostridium difficile*
Inflammatory bowel disease: ulcerative colitis, Crohn's disease, collagenous colitis
Ischemic colitis
Radiation colitis

Malabsorptive Diarrhea

Carbohydrate malabsorption (e.g., lactose, sucrose, sorbitol, gluten, fructose, mannitol)
Laxatives (magnesium-containing antacids)
Bile acid malabsorption: intestinal resection, ileal disease, vagotomy, cholecystectomy

Malabsorptive Diarrhea with Steatorrhea

Intraluminal malabsorption: pancreatic insufficiency, bacterial overgrowth, chronic liver disease
Mucosal malabsorption: infection (e.g., *Giardia*), celiac sprue, lymphoma

Secretory Diarrhea

Medications (see Table 91–2)
Hormone-producing tumors (e.g., VIPomas, carcinoid, gastrinoma)
Villous adenomas

Motility Disorders

Irritable bowel syndrome
Dumping syndrome (e.g., postvagotomy, postgastrectomy)

Other

Hyperthyroidism
Diabetes
Addison's disease
Collagen vascular disease
Colon cancer

volume depletion and clinical toxicity. The abdomen is examined for tenderness, rebound, organomegaly, or masses. A rectal examination is done looking for skin lesions, to confirm the gross appearance of the stool, and to test for occult blood.

After the history and physical examination, most patients with acute diarrhea need only reassurance and education about oral rehydration therapy (Fig. 91–1). Patients with significant illness due to diarrhea (e.g., severe volume depletion, peritonitis) or evidence of clinically important diarrhea (e.g., fever, duration greater than 3 days, bloody stools, immunocompromised host) require further attention. Selective diagnostic evaluation based on the patient's particular circumstances should be done if test results are likely to affect management or outcome. Many tests are available, and their indiscriminate use is both ineffective and costly. For example, routine stool cultures in all patients with diarrhea are positive only 1.5% to 2.4% of the time, resulting in a cost of $952 to $1200 per positive stool culture. More selective testing increases diagnostic yield and cost-effectiveness (i.e., $30–$264 per positive test).

Patients who have been hospitalized, who are residents of a chronic care facility, or who have received antibiotics during the previous 8 weeks should have a stool assay for *Clostridium difficile* toxin. *C. difficile* accounts for 25% of

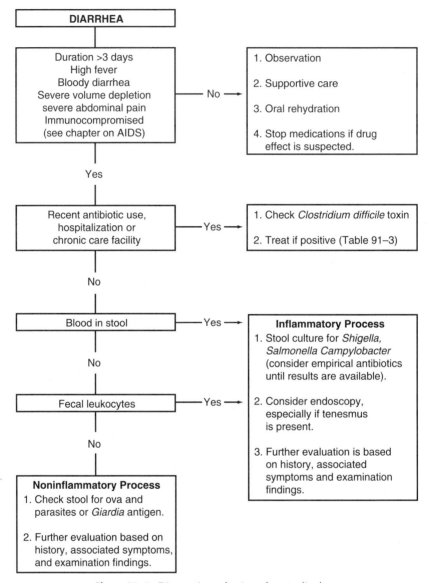

Figure 91–1. Diagnostic evaluation of acute diarrhea.

antibiotic-associated diarrhea and can produce mild to severe symptoms. Detection of the *C. difficile* toxin is needed to differentiate asymptomatic colonization (3% of adults, 10%–20% of hospitalized adults) from clinical disease. The toxin assay has a false-negative rate of roughly 10%.

Examination of the stool for fecal leukocytes and blood is done next to distinguish inflammatory from noninflammatory processes and direct further workup. A small amount of fresh stool is diluted with saline and then put on a microscope slide. A few drops of Gram stain or methylene blue are added, and a coverslip is placed over the mixture. After 2 or 3 minutes the preparation is examined for leukocytes. At least three white blood cells in four or more high-power fields is suggestive of an inflammatory process. Because this test is less reliable for stored or transported samples, other leukocyte markers, such as lactoferrin, are being developed.

If an inflammatory process is suspected either historically or by examination of the stool, fecal culture for *Salmonella, Shigella,* and *Campylobacter* is performed. *Campylobacter jejuni* is the most common invasive organism. Endoscopy should be performed if the patient has prominent rectal symptoms or if the culture is negative in a patient with inflammatory diarrhea.

In patients at risk for *Giardia* or other parasitic infections, stool examination for ova and parasites should be performed. For *Giardia,* the sensitivity of three properly obtained fresh stool specimens for ova and parasites is 65% to 80%. An enzyme-linked immunosorbent assay for stool *Giardia* antigen is 92% to 96% sensitive and 95% to 100% specific.

Patients whose diarrhea persists more than 4 weeks (i.e., chronic diarrhea) require further evaluation. Unless obvious, the presence of diarrhea should be confirmed because 40% of patients referred for diarrhea have normal fecal weights (i.e., less than 200 g/d). Initial screening laboratory tests including complete blood cell count, erythrocyte sedimentation rate, electrolyte levels, albumin level, and stool test for occult blood, fecal leukocytes, and ova and parasites help differentiate inflammatory, malabsorptive, and secretory mechanisms of disease and direct further workup. Evidence of malabsorption (e.g., weight loss, anemia, low albumin, ecchymoses, peripheral neuropathy) should prompt a quantitative fecal fat analysis and investigation into diseases of the pancreas and small bowel. Patients with signs of inflammation (e.g., fever, prominent pain, bloody diarrhea, fecal leukocytes, leukocytosis, elevated sedimentation rate) should undergo endoscopy as the next diagnostic step. An empirical trial of a lactose-free diet is reasonable in patients with associated bloating and cramps and no epidemiologic risk factors or symptoms pointing toward a specific disease. Many other tests are available, and their judicious use should be guided by the individual patient's history and objective findings.

Management. Diarrhea causes illness primarily through loss of fluids and electrolytes. Therapy focuses on replacement of these losses and treatment of a specific etiology, if identified. Patients with mild volume depletion can replace their losses with any caffeine-free beverage containing glucose. Patients with moderate volume depletion require replacement with glucose and electrolytes in appropriate proportions. Oral rehydration solutions are available commercially or can be made easily at home. One such replacement fluid contains ¾ teaspoon salt, 4 tablespoons sugar, 1 teaspoon baking soda, 1 cup orange juice or two bananas, and 1 L clean water. Patients should drink 1 to 2 L initially and then 1 to 2 L/d to replace stool losses. Patients with severe salt and water depletion or vomiting should be hospitalized for intravenous fluid replacement.

Antibiotics are not required in most cases of acute infectious diarrhea. Exceptions include those organisms for which antibiotics have been shown to reduce fecal excretion, hasten recovery, or resolve persistent infection (Table 91–4). Antibiotic treatment of *Shigella* shortens the illness from 3 to 7 days to

Table 91–4. ANTIMICROBIAL THERAPY FOR ACUTE DIARRHEA

Pathogen	Medication	Cost ($)*
Clostridium difficile	Metronidazole, 250 mg PO qid × 10 days	5.60
	Vancomycin, 125 mg PO qid × 10 days	189.00
Enteroinvasive Escherichia coli	Ciprofloxacin, 500 mg PO × 1	3.20
Salmonella typhi	Trimethoprim-sulfamethoxazole, 1 DS PO bid × 5 days	1.45
Shigella species	Trimethoprim-sulfamethoxazole, 1 DS PO bid × 3–5 days	0.90–1.45
	Ciprofloxacin, 500 mg PO bid × 3 days	19.20
Yersinia enterocolitica	Ciprofloxacin, 500 mg PO q12H × 3 days	19.20
	Doxycycline, 100 mg PO bid × 3 days	1.05
Giardia lamblia	Metronidazole, 250 mg PO tid × 7 days	2.90
Entamoeba histolytica	Metronidazole, 750 mg PO tid × 5–10 days	6.25–12.50
	Iodoquinol, 650 mg PO tid × 21 days	25.40

*Average wholesale price, 1995 *Drug Topics Red Book*, generic if available.

1 to 2 days and decreases excretion of the organism. Treatment of traveler's diarrhea can reduce the severity and duration of illness. Patients with *Salmonella* gastroenteritis or *C. difficile* diarrhea should be given antibiotics only if there is evidence of moderate to severe disease (e.g., high fever, leukocytosis, frequent stools) because routine treatment can prolong the carrier state in some patients. Amebic dysentery requires prolonged therapy to eliminate the cyst form of the organism.

Several types of medications are available for the symptomatic treatment of diarrhea (Table 91–5). Preparations such as kaolin or pectin adsorb factors in the intestinal lumen that cause diarrhea (e.g., bacterial endotoxin). Bismuth subsalicylate has intraluminal antibacterial and anti-inflammatory properties as well as antisecretory action. This drug can reduce the number of unformed stools by 50%. Opiate derivatives, diphenoxylate and loperamide, slow small- and large-intestinal motility, allowing more time for fluid absorption, and can reduce the number of stools by 80%. These agents may be used cautiously to reduce abdominal cramping and stool frequency. Antimotility agents can prolong the course of diarrhea from invasive bacteria.

Follow-Up. Patients are instructed to contact their physician if their diarrhea worsens, they develop fever, or they are unable to keep down adequate fluids. Many of the invasive organisms have a significant relapse rate. *C. jejuni* often

Table 91–5. SYMPTOMATIC ANTIDIARRHEAL AGENTS

Drug	Mechanism	Dosage	Cost ($)*
Kaolin (Kaopectate)	Adsorbent	60 mL once; repeat after each unformed stool	7.50 (720 mL)
Bismuth subsalicylate (Pepto-Bismol)	Antisecretory	2 tablets or 30 mL q30 min up to eight doses per 24 h	2.65 (24 tabs)
			8.00 (720 mL)
Loperamide (Imodium A-D)	Decreased motility	2–4 mg q4h up to 16 mg/24 h	8.85 (24 tabs)
			12.40 (240 mL; 1 mg/mL)
Diphenoxylate-atropine (Lomotil)	Decreased motility	2.5–5.0 mg q4h up to 20 mg/24 h	0.80 (24 tabs)
			12.60 (120 mL; 2.5 mg/mL)

*Average wholesale price, 1995 *Drug Topics Red Book*, generics.

resolves spontaneously; however, it has a relapse rate up to 20%. Relapse of *Giardia* also occurs in approximately 20% of patients and often responds to retreatment. *C. difficile* has a relapse rate of 10% to 25%, generally within 3 weeks of therapy. Patients who develop *C. difficile* diarrhea with the use of a particular antibiotic are not at increased risk for recurrence on reexposure to the same agent. Patients whose diarrhea persists for more than 4 weeks should undergo a repeat history, physical examination, and diagnostic evaluation focusing on chronic causes of diarrhea. Referral to a gastroenterologist—for endoscopic procedures and for treatment of conditions such as inflammatory bowel disease—is indicated for patients in whom the cause of documented diarrhea is unclear.

Cross-References: Inflammatory Bowel Disease (Chapter 97), Sigmoidoscopy and Colonoscopy (Chapter 104).

REFERENCES

1. Bennett RG, Greenough WB. Approach to acute diarrhea in the elderly. Gastroenterol Clin North Am 1993;22:517–533.

   Epidemiologic risk factors, presentation, and diagnostic workup of acute diarrhea specific to elderly patients are discussed.

2. Caputo GM, Weitekamp MR, Bacon AE, Whitener C. *Clostridium difficile* infection: A common problem for the general internist. J Gen Intern Med 1994;9:528–532.

   Clinical presentation, diagnostic evaluation, and treatment of C. difficile infection, including treatment of symptomatic relapse, is reviewed.

3. Donowitz M, Kokke FT, Saidi R. Evaluation of patients with chronic diarrhea. N Engl J Med 1995;332:725–729.

   This article is a more detailed review of an outpatient workup of chronic diarrhea as well as a discussion of diarrhea of undetermined origin.

4. Fine KD, Krejs GJ, Fordtran JS. Diarrhea. In Sleisenger MH, Fordtran JS, eds. Gastrointestinal Disease, 5th ed. Philadelphia, WB Saunders, 1993:1043–1072.

   The chapter in this book is a good review of pathophysiology and an explanation of diagnostic tests, including fecal fat, electrolyte, and osmolality measurements.

92 Jaundice

Symptom

JOHN SEKIJIMA

Epidemiology. Jaundice or icterus results from the excessive deposition of bilirubin pigment in the skin, sclerae, and mucous membranes. In general, the classic yellow hue of clinical jaundice does not become grossly apparent until the serum bilirubin level exceeds 3.0 mg/dL. Viral hepatitis is the most frequent cause of jaundice in young adults, whereas biliary obstruction from either stone disease or malignancy is more likely in older patients.

Etiology. Bilirubin production begins with the phagocytosis of senescent red blood cells and breakdown of heme by the reticuloendothelial system. Unconjugated bilirubin is released into the circulation and taken up by the hepatocyte, where it is conjugated (glucuronidated) before being secreted into the canaliculus.

Unconjugated hyperbilirubinemia results from either a relative increase in bilirubin production (hemolysis, transfusions, hematoma resorption, ineffective erythropoiesis) or a decrease in bilirubin conjugation (i.e., Gilbert's syndrome or the Crigler-Najjar syndrome) (Table 92–1). Gilbert's syndrome, which affects 3% to 8% of the general population, appears to be caused by a defect in the hepatic uptake of bilirubin and, to a lesser degree, by a partial impairment of bilirubin conjugation. Bilirubin levels are usually less than 3 mg/dL but may rarely rise to 5 to 6 mg/dL with illness, stress, alcohol, or prolonged fasting.

Conjugated hyperbilirubinemia may be associated with primary hepatocellular injury (e.g., due to viral hepatitis, drug toxicity, ischemia), cholestatic disease, or both (Table 92–2). Cholestasis results from either the impaired secretion of bile (intrahepatic cholestasis) or the mechanical disruption of bile flow by a stone, tumor, or stricture (extrahepatic cholestasis/obstruction). The bile ducts proximal to a blockage are dilated unless it is very early in the process or the ducts are scarred (sclerosing cholangitis) or rendered nondistensible by surrounding fibrotic parenchyma (cirrhosis). Obstructive jaundice may also be caused by malignancy, including pancreatic carcinoma, cholangiocarcinoma, gallbladder cancer, hepatoma, metastatic disease, and encroaching malignant lymph nodes.

Table 92–1. UNCONJUGATED HYPERBILIRUBINEMIA

Increased Production	Decreased Conjugation
Hemolytic anemia	Gilbert's syndrome
Red cell transfusions	Crigler-Najjar syndrome
Hematoma resorption	Newborn jaundice
Ineffective erythropoiesis	

Table 92–2. ETIOLOGY OF CONJUGATED HYPERBILIRUBINEMIA

Intrahepatic Cholestasis	Extrahepatic Cholestasis
Hepatocellular disease	Intrinsic biliary disease
Viral hepatitis	Choledocholithiasis
Chronic active hepatitis	Biliary stricture
Alcoholic hepatitis	Cholangiocarcinoma
Cirrhosis	Sclerosing cholangitis
Drug-induced cholestasis	Extrinsic disease
Infiltrative liver disease	Pancreatic carcinoma
Malignancy	Acute pancreatitis
Amyloidosis	Chronic pancreatitis
Granulomatous hepatitis	Metastatic disease
Familial syndromes	
Primary biliary cirrhosis	
Sepsis and postoperative states	

Symptoms and Signs. The patient interview should focus on the onset and duration of symptoms. Acute upper or right upper quadrant abdominal pain suggests choledocholithiasis and when accompanied by fever and shaking chills indicates cholangitis. Obstructive malignancy is a concern when the patient has had significant weight loss and anorexia for several weeks before presentation. Prodromal symptoms of fever, arthralgias, and rash are suggestive of viral hepatitis and should prompt an inquiry into a previous history of transfusions, injection drug use, raw shellfish ingestion, recent travel, sexual preference, and exposures.

The history should also include alcohol consumption, toxin exposure, prior biliary surgery, family history of liver diseases, and a careful review of all medications, emphasizing those with hepatotoxicity.

Cachexia, temporal wasting, and a palpable gallbladder or epigastric mass suggest an intra-abdominal malignancy. A yellow discoloration of the skin in the absence of true scleral icterus is consistent with high carotene intake, uremia, or quinacrine ingestion rather than jaundice. Stigmata of chronic liver disease include palmar erythema, spider angiomas, ascites, prominent collateral veins on the abdominal wall, gynecomastia, splenomegaly, and asterixis. The liver may be firm and shrunken in cirrhosis or enlarged, nodular, and rock-hard with metastatic involvement.

Clinical Approach. Combining a history, physical examination, and routine laboratory tests leads to the accurate differentiation of obstructive from nonobstructive jaundice in approximately 80% of cases. Initial laboratory tests should include a complete blood cell count, total and direct bilirubin level determination, and study of hepatocellular enzyme levels.

When unconjugated hyperbilirubinemia is present (usually less than 5 mg/dL), the two primary causes to consider are Gilbert's syndrome and hemolysis. These diagnoses may be distinguished by comparing the bilirubin levels in the fasting and nonfasting states (fasting levels are higher in Gilbert's syndrome) as well as by evaluating the reticulocyte count, lactate dehydrogenase level, peripheral smear, and haptoglobin levels, as indicated (abnormal in hemolysis).

If the bilirubin is predominantly conjugated, the next step is to distinguish between a hepatocellular and a cholestatic pattern of injury. When the alanine aminotransferase (ALT) and aspartate aminotransferase (AST) levels are characteristic of primary liver cell injury, viral serologic studies should be done and offending medications or toxins discontinued if present.

The AST, ALT, and alkaline phosphatase levels are important in distinguishing between a primary hepatocellular process (liver cell injury) and cholestasis. Hepatocellular damage is characterized by marked elevations of ALT and AST, generally exceeding 5 times the normal values, and alkaline phosphatase levels that are mildly elevated (less than 2 to 3 times normal). In contrast, cholestatic disease is characterized by alkaline phosphatase levels often greater than three times normal and ALT and AST levels less than threefold to fivefold higher than normal. A notable exception to these generalizations is the passage of a common duct stone, which, on occasion, exhibits transient but strikingly high aminotransferase levels on the order of 10 to 20 times normal. Obstruction due to gallstones rarely causes bilirubin levels over 10 mg/dL, and values above this level make malignant obstruction more likely. Very high alkaline phosphatase levels out of proportion to the degree of jaundice favor the diagnosis of intrahepatic cholestasis over extrahepatic obstruction. Finally, aminotransferase levels less than 350 IU/L with AST/ALT ratios greater than 2 are most consistent with alcoholic hepatitis.

When the biochemical tests are consistent with cholestasis, an imaging study, usually ultrasonography, should be obtained to identify biliary obstruction or infiltrating liver lesions. Ultrasonography is quite sensitive and specific for detecting biliary obstruction (85%–95%). However, although ultrasonography is highly sensitive for cholelithiasis (95%), it is not sensitive for choledocholithiasis (30%–50%). Other possible limitations include operator inexperience, poor technical quality in obese patients, and overlying bowel gas obscuring the distal common duct and pancreas. For jaundiced patients in whom malignancy is likely (e.g., patients of advanced age, patients with weight loss, patients with or without abdominal or back pain), computed tomography rather than ultrasonography may be preferable (Fig. 92–1). Although often equivalent to ultrasonography in detecting common duct stones, computed tomography often provides greater detail regarding the presence of pancreatic pathology, distant metastases, lymph node involvement, and potential tumor resectability.

If there is no clear evidence of biliary obstruction or drug liver injury, the clinician should attempt to rule out specific disease entities. Antimitochondrial antibodies to test for primary biliary cirrhosis should be obtained when there is marked intrahepatic cholestasis. A liver biopsy may be necessary to establish the diagnosis of infiltrative liver pathology such as sarcoidosis, tuberculosis, amyloidosis, and malignancy.

When the pattern of injury is mixed or if cirrhosis is a consideration, the following laboratory studies should be obtained, as appropriate: iron indices (hemochromatosis), hepatitis B and C serologic studies, ceruloplasmin (Wilson's disease), antinuclear and anti–smooth muscle antibody titers (autoimmune hepatitis), and α_1-antitrypsin (α_1-antitrypsin deficiency). A subsequent liver biopsy may also be required to confirm the diagnosis.

Direct visualization of the biliary tree, usually by means of endoscopic

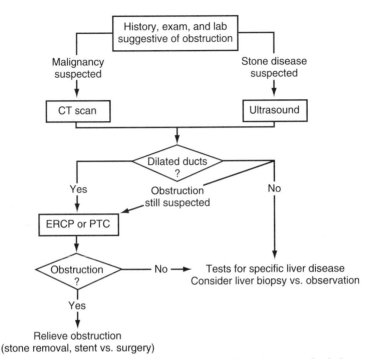

Figure 92–1. Evaluation of cholestatic jaundice. ERCP = endoscopic retrograde cholangiopancreatography; PTC = percutaneous transhepatic cholangiography.

retrograde cholangiopancreatography (ERCP), should be pursued when the bile ducts are dilated. Endoscopic therapy with stone extraction, stent placement, and tissue sampling can be accomplished simultaneously, or the patient can be sent to subsequent surgery as necessary. Direct cholangiography may also be useful when the ultrasonographic or computed tomographic scan is normal or equivocal but the clinical suspicion of obstruction remains high. Examples include a patient presenting with acute upper abdominal pain, mild jaundice, and nondilated ducts or an individual with possible sclerosing cholangitis.

ERCP enables close inspection of the major papillae and direct cannulation of both the common bile and pancreatic ducts. Stricture dilatation, brushings, biopsies, stent placement, and sphincterotomy with stone extraction can be performed in appropriate circumstances. Percutaneous transhepatic cholangiography (PTC) is a suitable alternative to ERCP and allows access to the biliary tree by a direct transhepatic puncture of a peripheral bile duct. Depending on local expertise, PTC may be preferred if the patient has had previous biliary surgery or if there is a proximal hilar obstruction. PTC has rates of complications similar to those of ERCP; and therapeutic maneuvers including balloon dilatation, stone retrieval, and internal/external stent drainage can also be accomplished.

Clinical Approach. Management should be directed at the underlying disease whenever possible. The course of Gilbert's syndrome is always benign, and the patient should be educated and reassured. Patients with hepatocellular injury or cholestasis should have all potentially offending medications stopped and should be followed closely to ensure that biochemical tests revert to normal. Patients with jaundice due to alcoholic cirrhosis or viral hepatitis can usually be managed in the primary care setting unless severe complications occur.

Severe, chronic cholestasis causes pruritus. The use of oral antihistamines, cholestyramine, or ursodeoxycholic acid may provide variable relief, and reports suggest that agents such as naloxone and rifampin may also be of benefit.

In most cases, biliary tract disease requires the expertise of a gastroenterologist, particularly if diagnostic procedures might be indicated.

Follow-up is dependent on the underlying cause of the jaundice.

Cross-References: Alcohol Problems (Chapter 10), Pruritus (Chapter 23), Abdominal Pain (Chapter 94), Biliary Tract Disease (Chapter 98), Viral Hepatitis (Chapter 100), Interpretation of Serologic Tests (Chapter 123), Anemia (Chapter 199).

REFERENCES

1. Fran BB. Clinical evaluation of jaundice: A guideline of the Patient Care Committee of the American Gastroenterology Association. JAMA 1989;262:3031–3034.

   This article provides a useful discussion on the use of appropriate diagnostic studies based on their relative sensitivities and specificities.

2. Van Ness MM, Diehi AM. Is liver biopsy useful in the evaluation of patients with chronically elevated liver enzymes? Ann Intern Med 1989;111:473–478.

   Data are presented to support the utility of liver biopsy in correctly establishing the diagnosis of overlooked or misdiagnosed treatable causes of liver disease.

3. Zimmerman HJ. Hepatotoxicity. Dis Mon 1993;39:675–787.

   This is a very thorough and well-written overview by a preeminent expert in the field.

93 Constipation

Symptom

SHOBA KRISHNAMURTHY

Epidemiology. Constipation is one of the most common chronic digestive complaints, affecting 1 in every 50 persons. Although there is no universally accepted or precise definition of this complaint, one objective definition is passage of fewer than three stools per week. Subjective definitions (small or hard stools, difficult passage of stools, or a feeling of incomplete evacuation) are difficult to quantify or assess. Various national surveys suggest a prevalence of 2%, with 2.5 million physician visits per year for constipation. It is more common in persons older than 65 years of age, in women, and affects nonwhites more than whites.

Etiology. It is widely believed that inadequate intake of dietary fiber is a common cause of constipation, despite the lack of evidence that constipated individuals consume less fiber. Constipation can be caused by gastrointestinal disorders (primarily colonic and anorectal disorders); drugs; and metabolic, endocrine, and neurologic disorders (Table 93–1). Although inactivity and suppression of the urge to defecate are often considered causes of constipation, these factors have not been adequately studied.

Irritable bowel syndrome is the most common functional gastrointestinal disorder associated with constipation. The onset is usually before age 35, and affected women outnumber men 2 to 1. This syndrome, which is characterized by disordered intestinal motility, causes abdominal pain; passage of small, hard stools; bloating; and a sense of incomplete evacuation. In 50% of cases, symptoms are induced by stress and associated with psychologic disorders such as depression, anxiety, and somatization. Up to 50% of affected women have a history of being victims of sexual and physical abuse. The diagnosis depends on a long duration of symptoms beginning at a young age in the absence of weight loss, nocturnal abdominal pain, hematochezia, and laboratory or radiologic abnormalities. *Diverticular disease* is present in 50% of patients older than 60 years of age, with symptoms similar to those of irritable bowel syndrome. Diverticulitis and stricture formation can cause or exacerbate constipation.

Colon carcinoma must be considered in any patient older than age 40 with a new history of recent constipation. Associated hematochezia; weight loss; a history of colon polyps or ulcerative colitis; and a family history of colon cancer or familial polyposis support this diagnosis. *Hirschsprung's disease* is an uncommon disorder (1 in 5000 live births) caused by the absence of ganglion cells along a variable length of the distal colon. This diagnosis should be considered in patients with a history of constipation from birth or infancy. *Neuromuscular disorders* affecting either the colonic smooth muscle or the colonic

Table 93–1. CAUSES OF CONSTIPATION

Medications

Analgesics/opiates*
Antacids (calcium and aluminum)
Anticholinergics*
Anticonvulsants
Antidepressants*
Antihypertensives
Antiparkinson agents
Iron
Heavy metal poisoning (lead, mercury,
    arsenic)
Calcium channel blockers*
Sucralfate
Barium sulfate

Metabolic Disorders

Diabetes*
Porphyria
Amyloidosis
Uremia
Hypokalemia
Hypercalcemia

Endocrine Disorders

Panhypopituitarism
Hypothyroidism*
Pheochromocytoma
Pregnancy
Glucagonoma

Gastrointestinal Disorders

Colonic obstruction
    Extraluminal (tumors, chronic volvulus,
        hernias)
    Luminal (tumors,* benign strictures)
Abnormalities of colonic motor function
    Irritable bowel syndrome*
    Diverticular disease*

Gastrointestinal Disorders Continued

Pseudo-obstruction
    Disorder of intestinal muscle (scleroderma,
        hollow visceral myopathy)
    Disorders of myenteric nerves (visceral
        neuropathy, paraneoplastic neuropathy,
        Chagas' disease, neuronal intestinal
        dysplasia, Hirschsprung's disease)
Rectal disorders
    Rectocele
    Intussusception
    Prolapse
    Rectosphincter dyssynergia
Anal problems
    Stenosis
    Fissures

Neurologic Disorders

Brain
    Parkinson's disease
    Tumors
    Cerebrovascular accidents*
Other
    Trauma to nervi erigentes and lumbosacral
        cord
    Cauda equina tumor
    Meningocele
    Autonomic insufficiency
    Tabes dorsalis
    Multiple sclerosis

*Most common causes.

myenteric plexus can cause severe constipation and a prolonged colonic transit that responds poorly to laxatives.

Diabetes frequently causes constipation, affecting 80% to 90% of patients with autonomic and peripheral neuropathy and 30% of patients without neuropathy. Constipation may be the only symptom of *hypothyroidism*, which commonly causes constipation and is sometimes associated with a megacolon (an enlarged and dilated colon on abdominal radiographs).

Constipation is common in patients with *Parkinson's disease*, and megacolon is present in 10%. Antiparkinsonian medications may also cause constipation. About 40% of patients with *multiple sclerosis* complain of constipation.

Clinical Approach. The patient interview should focus on the exact nature of the patient's complaint and include a detailed account of drug intake and symptoms of metabolic, endocrine, and neurologic disease. A history of sexual and physical abuse should also be obtained. A careful physical examination of the gastrointestinal and neurologic systems is mandatory. Anorectal and perineal examination should include a search for perineal disease, rectal prolapse, and anal fissure. A digital rectal examination may detect a rectal mass, tenderness of a fissure, or anal stenosis.

Routine laboratory tests include a complete blood cell count, fecal occult blood test, thyroid function tests, blood urea nitrogen, serum calcium, electrolyte, and fasting blood glucose determinations, as indicated. Patients with recent onset of symptoms or especially severe symptoms should undergo sigmoidoscopy and barium enema examination to look for colorectal neoplasms, strictures, diverticula, megacolon, or a narrowed distal segment with dilated proximal colon (suggesting Hirschsprung's disease).

If the above evaluation is entirely normal, the patient should be started on a high-fiber diet (20–30 g/d of fiber, generally in the form of 1 cup of All-Bran cereal or 1 to 2 tbsp of psyllium) for 30 days. If constipation resolves, no further workup is required. In patients with persistent constipation who complain primarily of infrequent defecation, a colonic transit study on a high-fiber diet is indicated. Although many transit studies are described, it is most simply done by having the patient ingest 20 radiopaque markers (5-mm pieces cut from a No. 16 French nasogastric tube or commercially available markers), which are taken on day 0, the day after the patient has had a bowel movement. Plain abdominal radiographs are obtained on days 5 and 7. Normal subjects pass 80% of markers by day 5 and 100% by day 7. The patient should avoid laxatives or enemas during the test. This is an excellent way of objectively confirming prolonged colonic transit time. An abnormal test suggests a neuromuscular disorder ("colonic inertia"). These patients are best referred to a gastroenterologist for further evaluation and management. A normal colonic transit study in a patient who complains of severe constipation may suggest a psychiatric disorder, and referral for evaluation should be considered.

In the patient with persistent constipation, referral for studies such as anorectal manometry, rectal biopsy, and defecography may be helpful.

Management. Although appropriate treatment of constipation depends on the underlying cause, there are several important principles: (1) An increase in fiber intake to 20 to 30 g/d in the form of dietary fiber or supplemental fiber (psyllium, calcium polycarbophil, or cellulose) benefits most patients. Of the dietary fibers, wheat bran is most effective in increasing stool weight, followed by fruits and vegetables, oats, mucilage, corn, cellulose, soya, and pectin. (2) Routine use of laxatives over long periods should be discouraged. There are a great number of laxatives available, and the choice of a laxative may depend on patient preference and tolerance. However, it would be reasonable to start with a milder laxative such as milk of magnesia (magnesium hydroxide) or mineral oil. The other saline laxatives such as magnesium sulfate and citrate are more potent. Stool softeners (docusate salts) are widely used but generally not effective. Hyperosmolar laxatives (lactulose, sorbitol) have the disadvantages of causing excessive bloating and flatulence. If the milder laxatives are ineffective, the next choice of agents would be stimulant laxatives such as anthraquinones (senna, cascara, danthron), castor oil, phenolphthalein (Ex-

Lax), and bisacodyl (Dulcolax). Polyethylene glycol solutions (Colyte, Go-LYTELY) can be used but are generally more expensive.

Suppositories and enemas can be used for treatment when prompt, immediate relief is desired. Habit training (i.e., having a scheduled time each day for bowel movements, usually after a meal) and contingency management (i.e., using a cleansing enema if defecation does not occur after 2 days) have been used in the management of constipation in children but have not been adequately studied in adults.

Cross-References: Colorectal Cancer Screening (Chapter 90), Abdominal Pain (Chapter 94), Multiple Sclerosis (Chapter 141), Parkinsonism (Chapter 145), Common Thyroid Disorders (Chapter 153).

REFERENCES

1. Devroede G. Constipation. In Sleisinger MH, Fordthan JS, eds. Gastrointestinal Disease: Pathophysiology, Diagnosis and Management. Philadelphia, WB Saunders, 1993:837–887.
   A detailed review is provided in this chapter.

2. Wald A. Approach to the patient with constipation. In Yamada T, ed. Textbook of Gastroenterology. Philadelphia, JB Lippincott, 1995:864–880.
   This chapter is a comprehensive, practical review of the subject.

94 Abdominal Pain

Symptom

CHARLES E. POPE, II

Acute abdominal pain and chronic recurrent abdominal pain differ substantially in terms of causation, evaluation, and treatment.

Epidemiology

ACUTE ABDOMINAL PAIN. The frequency of acute abdominal pain depends on the setting. In the emergency department, evaluations for acute abdominal pain account for 5% of all visits. In this population, the majority of individuals are female because of the frequency of obstetric and gynecologic problems. The incidence of acute abdominal pain of lesser intensity in private medical offices is poorly documented but is probably higher than 5%.

CHRONIC ABDOMINAL PAIN. Population studies suggest that 15% to 20% of individuals in Western countries suffer from chronic recurrent abdominal pain, although many never seek formal medical attention for this syndrome. Those

Table 94–1. EMERGENCY DEPARTMENT VISITS FOR ABDOMINAL PAIN

Undiagnosed acute abdominal pain	25%
Gastrointestinal tract problems	26%
Obstetric-gynecologic problems	12%
Urinary tract problems	12%
Miscellaneous problems	25%

Modified from Powers RD, Guertler AT. Abdominal pain in the ED: Stability and change over 20 years. Am J Emerg Med 1995;13:301–303.

that do represent 40% to 60% of the patients seen by gastroenterologists. Cultural factors may determine whether medical help is sought. In Western countries, female patients predominate; in India, males are more likely to seek medical assistance.

Etiology

ACUTE ABDOMINAL PAIN. Among the many different agents and processes that produce acute abdominal pain are inflammation, smooth muscle contractions, metabolic processes, and chemical and physical agents. The data from one university hospital emergency department provide a rough estimate of the relative incidences of the main causes of acute abdominal pain and are presented in Table 94–1; undiagnosed abdominal pain predominates.

CHRONIC ABDOMINAL PAIN. An estimate of the distribution of causes of chronic abdominal pain can be inferred from a large group of patients referred to a Scottish hospital for evaluation of dyspepsia. Abdominal pain was present in 91% (Table 94–2). The clinician's degree of certainty in the final diagnosis was lowest for irritable bowel syndrome and functional dyspepsia. The prevalence of peptic ulcer disease might be less in other Western medical centers.

Clinical Approach

ACUTE ABDOMINAL PAIN. At the outset, the intensity of acute abdominal pain should be estimated based on historical and observational features. A complaint of severe pain accompanied by an obviously distressed patient with fever or hypotension leads to immediate hospitalization, perhaps to the intensive care unit, where resuscitation will likely precede an evaluation that includes not only careful clinical examination but also laboratory and imaging procedures. The intensity of the pain determines the speed and sequence of other information gathering. Low-intensity pain allows an extensive history to be obtained. High-intensity pain may lead more rapidly to physical examination and imaging studies.

Table 94–2. COMMON ETIOLOGIES OF CHRONIC ABDOMINAL PAIN

Peptic ulcer disease	42%
Gastric carcinoma	3%
Other specific diseases	8%
Irritable bowel syndrome	16%
Functional bowel syndrome	6%

Modified from Crean GP, Holden RJ, Knill-Jones RP, Beattie AD, James WB, Marjoribanks FM, Spiegelhalter DJ. A database on dyspepsia. Gut 1994;35:191–202.

Demographic characteristics such as age, gender, and ethnic origin may focus diagnostic efforts in specific directions. For example, cancer is rarely a cause for acute abdominal pain in very young persons but is more common in those older than 65 years of age.

Descriptions of the character of the pain may or may not be helpful. Adjectives such as "sharp," "stabbing," "burning," or "aching" are rarely of discriminative value. More valuable are features such as relationship to meals, sleep, menstrual cycle, or exercise. The anatomic location and radiation of the pain help to narrow the diagnostic possibilities. Classically, visceral pain tends to be less precisely localized by the patient than pain from the abdominal wall or from irritation of the parietal peritoneum. Other descriptions of location can also be of some help. Is the discomfort shallow or deep? Is it localized to a point or is the pain felt diffusely throughout the abdominal cavity? Does it radiate through to the back, up to the chest, or down into the legs?

Knowledge of recent travel, exposure to job-related toxins, previous abdominal surgery, or abdominal trauma may be helpful. A careful inquiry into the social history and the presence of stress in the patient's life is often essential. The temporal characteristics of pain are important; does the level of pain rise and fall on a regular basis? The patient may assist by drawing a graph of the intensity of pain versus time. Information on intake of coffee, alcohol, and medications may also be helpful.

Also important are other symptoms or signs associated with the pain. A jaundiced patient with shaking chills may have a biliary tract infection, whereas a jaundiced patient with ascites and stigmata of liver disease may have a completely different problem, such as spontaneous bacterial peritonitis. Nausea, vomiting, obstipation, weight loss, and other constitutional symptoms help to direct the search.

The physical examination begins with observation of the patient during the history taking. Does the patient seem acutely ill? Is the patient sweating, tachypneic, or flushed? Does the patient remain quiet or is he or she in constant motion? Are there signs of weight loss or other evidence of systemic illness?

First the examiner should inspect the abdomen in a good light. An enlarged gallbladder is sometimes more easily seen than felt. Grouped vesicles may herald an attack of herpes zoster. Auscultation is performed next so that the abdomen is undisturbed and the patient is reassured that the examination will be gentle. Rushes of bowel sounds coincident with the patient's discomfort or high-pitched tinkles signal a partial bowel obstruction. An abdominal bruit is uncommonly heard but may suggest investigation of the aorta (for an aneurysm) or some of its branches (for an insufficiency syndrome).

Palpation is the last and most useful step. The patient is asked where the discomfort is localized, and the examination is begun as far away from this point as possible. The first circuit around the abdomen should be done with extremely light pressure. Not much will be learned, but the patient will again be reassured that the examiner will be gentle. The hand should be moved in a circular pathway, with special attention paid to the indicated areas of discomfort. Is there guarding or tenderness? Are there any masses? When trying to assess the liver o. spleen, the hand is placed parallel to the rib margin and the patient is asked to take slow deep breaths. The depth of palpation can be increased during each inspiration without moving the hand. Inspiration moves the liver or the spleen down to the waiting hand.

Palpation affords the most direct method of detecting peritoneal irritation. The classic method for determining whether peritoneal irritation is present is to seek for rebound tenderness by pressing deeply into the abdomen and then snapping the hand briskly away. This is often unnecessarily painful when peritoneal inflammation does exist, and the same information can be gained less traumatically by having the patient cough gently. If peritoneal irritation is present, the patient will wince after coughing and discomfort will be localized to the area of inflammation.

Urinalysis, white blood cell count, hematocrit, and amylase concentrations are generally the first tests ordered. Supine and upright films of the abdomen can demonstrate abnormal collections of gas. However, plain radiographs are highly limited and newer methods of imaging are often more helpful. Ultrasonography is able to detect gallbladder wall thickening, pericholecystic collections of fluid, gallstones, dilation of the renal pelvis, aortic aneurysm, ascites, and masses in the liver. Computed tomography is useful and should be obtained urgently if a leaking aneurysm or a process causing thickened bowel wall is suspected.

CHRONIC ABDOMINAL PAIN. The good news about patients with chronic recurrent pain is that they rarely have a life-threatening problem that requires immediate diagnosis and therapy. The bad news is that usually the pain has resisted the diagnostic or therapeutic efforts of physicians. First, one must determine whether the pain pattern fits that usually seen in defined illnesses such as peptic ulcer or inflammatory bowel disorders. That is, is the pain accompanied by relief with antacids or is it associated with diarrhea? If symptoms suggest a specific syndrome, the physician must reassess whether the correct diagnostic methods have been performed. A diagnosis of irritable bowel syndrome should be based on the presence of the appropriate disturbances of bowel habit, including constipation, diarrhea, or alternating bowel habit; straining at stool or a sensation of incomplete evacuation; or relief of pain with defecation. Inflammatory bowel disease or cancer of the colon is ruled out by appropriate barium or endoscopic studies. However, these studies need not be repeated by every new clinician who sees the patient if an adequate examination has been done in the recent past. The practitioner must recognize that many patients with chronic recurrent abdominal pain do not fit into a definite diagnostic category.

Management

ACUTE ABDOMINAL PAIN. Management of acute abdominal pain is dependent on the diagnostic information that has been obtained and response to interventions (e.g., removal of a fecal impaction, treatment of a urinary tract infection, or removal of a gallbladder full of stones). However, even after obtaining a full history and completing physical and laboratory investigations, many cases of acute abdominal pain will not be found to have a definitive cause. The decision must then be made whether to admit the patient for further evaluation and observation. In a large series from the emergency department, this was necessary in 18% of the cases. When no cause is found, the chance that serious illness is present is small and the pain usually resolves.

CHRONIC ABDOMINAL PAIN. Management of chronic pain is often the test of a clinician's patience and skill. If the diagnostic impression is irritable bowel syndrome, or if extensive investigation has made the diagnosis of functional bowel syndrome more likely, then explanation and reassurance are essential. Symptomatic measures to control diarrhea or constipation are in order, and a trial of bulking agents (e.g., psyllium) is often helpful. If these measures are not helpful and if the patient remains extremely uncomfortable, referral to a gastroenterologist is often in order. Consultation and perhaps more specialized tests will often aid with the patient's management.

Follow-Up

ACUTE ABDOMINAL PAIN. Follow-up depends on both medical and social factors. If a specific cause for the pain has been found and a specific treatment recommended, then the patient should be told what to expect and to return if those expectations are not met. If the results of psychological evaluation or the patient's social circumstances cause concern, then either hospitalization or visiting nurse supervision might be entertained. Most undiagnosed acute abdominal pain is self-limited. The patient should be told to return if the pain persists for more than 2 or 3 days.

CHRONIC ABDOMINAL PAIN. Follow-up is necessary until both the patient and clinician are convinced that they understand the situation and that the therapeutic interventions tried are helping the patient cope with this often ongoing situation. Frequency of visits will be determined by the comfort of the patient. Knowledge that help is available on request allows the patient to space out the visits. The patient–clinician relationship is often paramount.

The astute clinician should always be on the alert for symptoms and signs that do not fit usual patterns of disease. When a diagnosis has been made, the clinician should not hesitate to reevaluate this diagnosis if the clinical course is atypical. Some final advice is quoted by deDombal, "Very young? Very old? Very odd? Be very careful!"

Cross-References: Chronic Nonspecific Pain Syndrome (Chapter 14), Jaundice (Chapter 92), Constipation (Chapter 93), Dyspepsia (Chapter 95), Inflammatory Bowel Disease (Chapter 97), Biliary Tract Disease (Chapter 98), Diverticulitis (Chapter 101), Peptic Ulcer Disease (Chapter 102), Sigmoidoscopy and Colonoscopy (Chapter 104), Upper Gastrointestinal Endoscopy (Chapter 105), Diabetes Mellitus (Chapter 154), Pelvic Pain in Women (Chapter 160), Pelvic Inflammatory Disease (Chapter 166), Nephrolithiasis (Chapter 174), Urinary Tract Infections in Women (Chapter 175), Somatization (Chapter 188).

REFERENCES

1. Camilleri M, Prather CM. The irritable bowel syndrome: Mechanisms and a practical approach to management. Ann Intern Med 1992;116:1001–1008.

   In combination with Reference 4, this article gives a thorough approach to diagnosis and therapy of irritable bowel syndrome.

2. Crean GP, Holden RJ, Knill-Jones RP, Beattie AD, James WB, Marjoribanks FM, Spiegelhalter DJ. A database on dyspepsia. Gut 1994;35:191–202.

   Of 1540 patients referred to a university hospital for evaluation of dyspepsia, 1100 had abdominal pain. This is a very thorough discussion as to the usefulness of symptoms in predicting diagnosis.

3. deDombal FT. Acute abdominal pain in the elderly. J Clin Gastroenterol 1994;19:331–335.

The twilight years of life present significant problems in the recognition of intra-abdominal problems.

4. Drossman DA, Thompson WG. The irritable bowel syndrome: Review and a graduated multicomponent treatment approach. Ann Intern Med 1992;116:1009–1016.

   In combination with Reference 1, this article is an excellent discussion of irritable bowel syndrome and includes recommendations for recognition, treatment, and when to refer the patient to a gastroenterologist.

5. Powers RD, Guertler AT. Abdominal pain in the ED: Stability and change over 20 years. Am J Emerg Med 1995;13:301–303.

   This second report of characterization of emergency department visits for abdominal pain shows the following: 5% of all visits are for abdominal pain, women are affected more than men, and undiagnosed pain is the most common discharge diagnosis.

■ ■

95 Dyspepsia

Symptom

DAVID C. DUGDALE

Epidemiology. *Dyspepsia* is defined as chronic or recurrent upper abdominal discomfort not related to exertion and not associated with jaundice, bleeding, or dysphagia. Common symptoms include postprandial fullness, bloating, belching, early satiety, anorexia, nausea, vomiting, and heartburn or regurgitation. Research has defined categories of dyspepsia, including *reflux-like* (prominent heartburn and regurgitation), *ulcer-like* (localized epigastric pain, relief of pain by food and antacids, and a pattern of remission and relapse), *dysmotility-like* (prominent bloating, early satiety, and poorly localized discomfort), but their usefulness has not been fully validated. Because an important question is often whether a patient has a duodenal or gastric ulcer, *nonulcer dyspepsia* (dyspepsia without an ulcer or gastritis) is often used, but its usage in the literature is inconsistent. The point prevalence rate for dyspepsia approaches 30%, although only 25% of affected patients seek medical attention.

Etiology. In studies of general practice patients with dyspepsia conducted in the United Kingdom, esophagogastroduodenoscopy (EGD) revealed duodenal ulcer in 13% of patients, gastric ulcer in 7%, gastritis or duodenitis in 21%, esophagitis in 24%, and gastric cancer in 2%. In 34% of patients, EGD findings were normal. In other smaller studies the cause of dyspepsia has varied with age. In persons younger than age 25, ulcers were found in about 40%, with no cases of gastric cancer; in persons older than 70, ulcers were found in about 60%, and cancer (gastric and other sites) was found in 33%. Some patients with nonulcer dyspepsia experience symptoms typical of reflux esophagitis and benefit from antireflux therapy despite normal findings on EGD. Others may describe biliary pain that usually appears suddenly in the right hypochondrium or epigastrium, is severe and constant, and fades gradually over hours. Medications such as potassium chloride, digoxin, iron supplements, antibiotics, or nonsteroidal anti-inflammatory agents as well as alcohol may provoke dyspepsia.

The etiology of most cases of nonulcer (nonorganic or functional) dyspepsia remains unknown. Proposed mechanisms include gastric acid hypersecretion, motility disorders, and *Helicobacter pylori* gastritis. Acid hypersecretion probably plays a minor role. *H. pylori* is recovered from the stomachs of as many as 70% of patients with nonulcer dyspepsia and does correlate with histologic evidence of gastritis, but successful treatment of the bacterium does not significantly improve symptoms. Motility disturbances may play a role, especially when dyspepsia involves symptoms such as bloating, nausea, distention, or early satiety or when irritable bowel syndrome symptoms are present. Manometric studies document abnormalities such as antral hypomotility in about 80% of patients with nonulcer dyspepsia.

Clinical Approach and Management. Nocturnal pain and pain relieved by food, milk, or antacids favor peptic ulcer disease. Pain provoked by meals and pain insufficient to influence daily activities favor nonulcer dyspepsia. No symptom, however, reliably distinguishes nonulcer dyspepsia from ulcer disease or gastric cancer. Epigastric tenderness, though reproducible, occurs just as often in nonulcer dyspepsia as in that from other causes. All causes of dyspepsia may produce weight loss.

The physical examination should search for complications of peptic ulcer disease and gastric cancer. Weight loss, abdominal masses, gastrointestinal bleeding, obstruction, or jaundice should prompt diagnostic evaluation. The approach to patients without such complications may include avoidance of potentially offending agents (including alcohol and cigarettes), empirical therapy with antacids, H_2 blockers, or sucralfate; or early EGD. Patients who do not respond to 7 to 10 days of empirical therapy, or who have recurrent symptoms after withdrawal of empirical therapy, should undergo diagnostic evaluation. Patients who develop dyspepsia while taking a nonsteroidal anti-inflammatory drug and whose symptoms do not resolve promptly after stopping the drug should also have diagnostic evaluation because of their increased risk of gastric ulcer. EGD is preferred over an upper gastrointestinal radiographic series because of better accuracy and the opportunity to sample suspicious lesions.

The empirical approach has been the traditional path of therapy. Its safety is predicated on the following principles: (1) the treatment for all organic causes of dyspepsia, except gastric cancer, is the same (antacid or acid secretion inhibitor therapy); (2) gastric cancer is rare in general practice; (3) refractory ulcers and gastric cancer, if symptomatically improved on empirical therapy, will recrudesce after withdrawal of therapy; and (4) there is no evidence demonstrating increased complications from an 8-week diagnostic delay. However, the knowledge that 95% of duodenal ulcers and 70% of gastric ulcers are associated with *H. pylori* infection has changed the approach of many physicians. *H. pylori*–related peptic disease is a chronic condition, and relapse is expected without eradication of the bacteria. However, antibiotic therapy directed against *H. pylori* does not help persons with nonulcer dyspepsia and should not be given. Furthermore, because acid reduction therapy is minimally effective for persons with nonulcer dyspepsia, it represents cost without benefit. Better results for this category of patients (especially if "dysmotility-like" dyspepsia is present) are obtained by using metoclopramide, 10 mg three or four times a day, or cisapride, 5 to 10 mg three times a day. Cisapride appears more effective than metoclopramide. A randomized trial comparing the strategies of early EGD versus initial empirical therapy found no difference in symptom relief and other clinical outcomes but lower costs in the early EGD group. The lower cost hinged on withholding acid-reduction drug treatment from patients with nonorganic dyspepsia and including time lost from work in the assessment of the cost.

Follow-Up. Over 70% of peptic ulcers respond to 8 weeks of acid-reduction therapy, but the relapse rate is 50% to 80% at 1 year without maintenance therapy. In patients with nonulcer dyspepsia, although the risk of subsequent peptic ulcer and life-threatening complications is low, 70% of patients continue to experience intermittent symptoms over a 2- to 7-year follow-up period. In the absence of a change of clinical features, additional medical evaluation, such as repeated EGD, has a very low yield of an organic diagnosis. Small studies suggest that psychologic assessment and intervention may be beneficial in persons with recurrent symptoms.

Cross-References: Alcohol Problems (Chapter 10), Smoking Cessation (Chapter 12), Abdominal Pain (Chapter 94), Peptic Ulcer Disease (Chapter 102), Upper Gastrointestinal Endoscopy (Chapter 105).

REFERENCES

1. Bytzer P, Hansen JM, Schaffalitzky de Muckadell OB. Empirical H_2-blocker therapy or prompt endoscopy in management of dyspepsia. Lancet 1994;343:811–816.

   Results of a randomized trial of two strategies are presented. Prompt endoscopy is favored.

2. Haug TT, Wilmelmsen I, Svebak S, Berstad A, Ursin H. Psychotherapy in functional dyspepsia. J Psychosom Res 1994;38:735–744.

   Short-term cognitive psychotherapy was found beneficial for dyspeptic symptoms.

3. Talley NJ. Drug treatment of functional dyspepsia. Scand J Gastroenterol 1991;26(suppl 182):47–60.

   This is a comprehensive review of drug trials for dyspepsia; prokinetic drugs were most effective globally, especially for the dysmotility-like dyspepsia subgroup.

4. Talley NJ. A critique of therapeutic trials in *Helicobacter pylori*–positive functional dyspepsia. Gastroenterology 1994;106:1174–1183.

   In this review the author concluded that H. pylori treatment does not help dyspepsia unless ulcer disease is present.

5. Thompson WG. Dyspepsia: Is a trial of therapy appropriate? Can Med Assoc J 1995;153:293–299.

   Data are summarized regarding empirical therapy versus early endoscopy; the conclusion favored early endoscopy.

96 Dysphagia and Heartburn

Symptom

SUSAN A. EGAAS and STEVEN R. McGEE

DYSPHAGIA

Epidemiology and Etiology. Dysphagia, defined as difficulty swallowing, is traditionally classified into disorders occurring above the cricopharyngeal muscle in the mouth or pharynx (oropharyngeal dysphagia) and those occurring below the cricopharyngeal muscle in the esophagus (esophageal dysphagia). Table 96–1 lists the important causes of dysphagia. Neuromuscular disorders cause 75% of the cases of oropharyngeal dysphagia. Structural abnormalities cause 85% of cases of esophageal dysphagia.

Clinical Approach. Dysphagia is always associated with the act of swallowing. The globus sensation, in contrast, is a constant tightness or lump in the middle of the throat that is sometimes relieved by swallowing. In some patients, globus results from reflux esophagitis. Odynophagia, or painful swallowing, usually

Table 96–1. ETIOLOGY OF DYSPHAGIA

Oropharyngeal dysphagia (above the cricopharyngeal muscle)	Esophageal Dysphagia (below the cricopharyngeal muscle)
Neuromuscular disease	Neuromuscular (motility) disorder
Central nervous system*	Achalasia*
CNS depression from any cause	Scleroderma/CREST syndrome
Stroke	Diffuse esophageal spasm
Parkinson's disease	Amyloidosis
Multiple sclerosis	Nonspecific motility disorders*
Amyotrophic lateral sclerosis	Obstructive disease
Peripheral nervous system	Intrinsic
Guillain-Barré syndrome	Peptic stricture*
Bulbar poliomyelitis	Esophageal carcinoma*
Neuromuscular junction	Lower esophageal (Schatzki's) ring*
Botulism	Webs
Myasthenia gravis	Stricture secondary to caustic ingestion
Myopathies	Extrinsic
Polymyositis/dermatomyositis	Mediastinal blood vessels or tumors
Muscular dystrophy	
Obstructive disease	
Cancer	
Zenker's diverticulum	
Surgical resection	
Radiation therapy	
Tracheostomy	

*Most common causes.

results from an inflammatory process such as infectious esophagitis (e.g., *Candida*, herpesvirus, cytomegalovirus), caustic ingestion (e.g., lye), severe reflux, or pill-induced esophagitis.

Acute dysphagia requires urgent evaluation usually with endoscopy because it may be caused by a foreign body requiring removal. Chronic dysphagia is commonly evaluated in the outpatient setting. The history should initially distinguish oropharyngeal from esophageal dysphagia. Patients with oropharyngeal dysphagia have difficulty initiating a swallow (especially of liquids or dry solids such as biscuits), may experience immediate coughing or nasopharyngeal regurgitation with liquid swallows, and usually exhibit other symptoms of neuromuscular disease (e.g., ptosis, diplopia, muscle fasciculations, proximal muscle weakness, incoordination, tremor, or other movement disorders). Esophageal dysphagia lacks these features; instead, soon after initiation of the swallow, the bolus "sticks."

In patients with esophageal dysphagia, the history helps distinguish obstructive from motility disorders. Patients with obstructive disorders have more trouble with solid boluses than liquid, are not affected by the temperature of the food, and usually have regurgitation with subsequent bolus impaction. Those with motility disorders, in contrast, have equal difficulty with solids and liquids; may have more trouble with cold liquids; and, after bolus impaction, may eventually swallow the food by maneuvers such as swallowing more liquids or hyperextending the neck.

Dysphagia from esophageal rings is intermittent, with months between episodes; dysphagia from strictures progresses gradually over months; and dysphagia from cancer progresses over weeks, often with associated weight loss. Achalasia leads to continuous dysphagia without heartburn, scleroderma leads to continuous dysphagia with heartburn, and diffuse esophageal spasm leads to intermittent dysphagia with chest pain.

Although the patient interview accurately defines the cause of dysphagia in 80% of cases, the patient's opinion of the site of a lesion, demonstrated with a finger pointed on the chest, is often inaccurate.

A barium esophagram reliably identifies strictures, esophageal cancers, and, if a marshmallow is swallowed during the test, esophageal rings. Esophagography should precede endoscopy in evaluation of oropharyngeal dysphagia because it is better for evaluating the pharynx and upper esophagus. Patients with esophageal dysphagia should be referred for endoscopy because (1) many require biopsy and (2) treatment for many cases (e.g., dilation for stricture) can be initiated during the diagnostic procedure. Most patients with human immunodeficiency virus infection and odynophagia have esophagitis due to *Candida.* These patients should be given empirical antifungal therapy. If they do not respond, endoscopy is indicated to determine a specific etiology and guide treatment. Patients with persistent unexplained dysphagia or whose esophagrams suggest motility disorders should be referred for manometry.

Management. An experienced speech pathologist best determines the safety of swallowing in patients with oropharyngeal dysphagia. In general, patients should be alert, be able to elevate the larynx with a dry swallow and to sit up for 20 minutes after a meal, and have a clear voice and a good cough. Severe cases may require a temporary nasogastric tube or feeding gastrostomy (placed percutaneously by endoscopy).

Gastroenterologists manage esophageal rings, strictures, and achalasia with esophageal dilation. Inoperable esophageal cancer may require placement of an esophageal stent.

HEARTBURN

Epidemiology. Heartburn, a hallmark symptom of gastroesophageal reflux disease (GERD), is a substernal burning sensation that radiates toward the mouth, decreases with antacids, and is provoked by factors that transiently reduce lower esophageal sphincter (LES) pressure, such as bending over, lying down, lifting heavy objects; and ingesting particular substances (alcohol, caffeine, peppermint, acidic foods, chocolate) and certain medications (calcium channel blockers, narcotics, and tricyclic antidepressants). The syndrome of GERD includes both symptoms and pathologic changes of mucosa caused by reflux. It is estimated that more than 60 million people in the United States experience symptoms of GERD. In one survey of hospital workers, heartburn occurred daily in 7% and at least monthly in 36%. Other than during pregnancy, when 25% of women have daily heartburn, there is no age or sex predilection. Up to 20% of patients with GERD develop complications (e.g., hemorrhage, dysphagia, stricture, or Barrett's esophagus).

Symptoms and Signs. Other symptoms that may be associated with GERD include acid regurgitation (effortless appearance of bitter fluid in the mouth without nausea), retrosternal chest pain, nocturnal asthma, dysphagia (even without stricture), episodic hypersalivation, and hoarseness.

The correlation between the severity of heartburn and the endoscopic grade of esophagitis is poor. In endoscopic surveys of patients with heartburn, about 50% have esophagitis, 35% have normal findings, and 15% have peptic ulcer disease. Cancer is rare (< 1%). GERD is a chronic disease with a relapsing course.

Clinical Approach. Patients with classic heartburn and no complications should receive empirical treatment for GERD without further testing. Early diagnostic evaluation is indicated when (1) complications are present, such as dysphagia, severe nausea and vomiting, weight loss, or gastrointestinal bleeding, (2) the patient fails to respond to empirical therapy, or (3) the heartburn worsens with exercise, suggesting angina.

Barium radiography is less expensive and often more available than endoscopy, and accurately demonstrates esophageal strictures and peptic ulcer disease. Endoscopy is preferred by many practitioners, however, because it has superior diagnostic sensitivity for esophagitis and is the only test that identifies Barrett's esophagus, a precursor of esophageal adenocarcinoma found in 0% to 20% of endoscopic examinations undertaken for persistent heartburn. The "gold standard" of diagnosis for GERD is 24-hour ambulatory pH monitoring, which can be helpful in diagnosing patients with a clinical history consistent with GERD but with normal results of radiography or endoscopy.

Management. Treatment is directed at decreasing the amount of reflux and making the refluxed substance less noxious to the esophagus. All patients should elevate the head of the bed (replacing casters with 6-inch wooden blocks), avoid troublesome foods, refrain from eating 3 hours before bedtime, stop smoking, limit alcohol intake, and use antacids as needed. This conservative approach alone may be effective in mild cases and is the backbone of all more aggressive therapies. Because GERD is a chronic disease, patients should be strongly encouraged to continue these lifestyle modifications indefinitely.

Patients with mild to moderate symptoms should additionally receive H_2-receptor antagonists or a prokinetic drug (Table 96–2). Patients with severe or refractory symptoms usually benefit from a proton pump inhibitor and should be referred for endoscopy. In most patients, symptoms dramatically improve during the first 2 weeks of therapy. Whatever medical therapy is chosen should continue for a total of 6 to 8 weeks, after which it is withdrawn. Although some patients experience relapse (up to 50% of those with severe disease), many experience no further symptoms. In controlled trials, elevation of the head of the bed and the use of H_2-receptor antagonists or omeprazole effectively reduce heartburn and heal esophagitis. Omeprazole is superior to H_2-receptor antagonists with faster rates of healing and relief of symptoms in erosive esophagitis. It has been approved for long-term maintenance treatment of healed erosive esophagitis. Antiulcer maintenance doses of H_2-receptor antagonists (see Chapter 102, Peptic Ulcer Disease) are not effective for preventing recurrent esophagitis. Patients on long-term omeprazole should have vitamin B_{12} levels monitored every 3 years.

Complications of GERD include esophageal stricture, Barrett's esophagus, and, rarely, gastrointestinal bleeding. Although antireflux therapy improves the symptoms of those with Barrett's esophagus, there is no evidence that Barrett's epithelium regresses or that the risk of cancer is reduced. Periodic endoscopic surveillance is recommended for patients with Barrett's esophagus, but the timing is controversial. Surgical treatment of GERD may be considered in lieu of long-term medical therapy in young patients or in patients who fail medical therapy.

Cross-References: Alcohol Problems (Chapter 10), Smoking Cessation (Chapter 12), Acute Chest Pain (Chapter 73), Recurrent Chest Pain (Chapter 74), Dyspepsia (Chapter 95), Peptic Ulcer Disease (Chapter 102), Upper Gastrointestinal Endoscopy (Chapter 105).

Table 96–2. THERAPY FOR GASTROESOPHAGEAL REFLUX DISEASE

Drug	Dose	Cost ($ per Day)*
H₂ blockers		
Cimetidine	300 mg PO qid	3.08
Ranitidine	150 mg PO bid	3.30
Famotidine	20 mg PO bid	3.08
Nizatidine	150 mg PO bid	3.08
Proton pump inhibitors		
Omeprazole	20 mg PO qd or bid	3.63 or 7.26
Lansoprazole	15 mg PO qd or bid	3.25 or 6.50
Prokinetic agent		
Cisapride	20 mg PO bid	2.44

*Average wholesale price, 1995 *Drug Topics Red Book.*

REFERENCES

1. Edwards DAW. Discriminatory value of symptoms in the differential diagnosis of dysphagia. Clin Gastroenterol 1976;5:49–57.

   This is an overview of the importance of the patient interview, based on evaluation of more than 1200 cases of dysphagia (see also J R Coll Phys 1975;9:257–263).

2. Kitchin LI, Castell DO. Rationale and efficacy of conservative therapy for gastroesophageal reflux disease. Arch Intern Med 1991;151:448–454.

   Evidence is reviewed that supports conservative antireflux treatments: head of bed elevation, selective food and medicine avoidance, smoking cessation, and antacids.

3. Pope CE. Acid-reflux disorders. N Engl J Med 1994;331:656–660.

   The author presents a thorough review of the pathophysiology and clinical approach to reflux disorders.

4. Vigneri S, et al. A comparison of five maintenance therapies for reflux esophagitis. N Engl J Med 1995;333:1106–1110.

   A randomized trial evaluating 175 patients with endoscopy confirmed esophagitis, which was treated for 12 months and reevaluated by endoscopy. Omeprazole alone or in combination with cisapride is more effective than ranitidine alone or cisapride alone, and the combination of omeprazole and cisapride is more effective than ranitidine plus cisapride.

97 Inflammatory Bowel Disease

Problem

EDWARD J. BOYKO and DAVID R. PERERA

Epidemiology. Idiopathic inflammatory bowel disease (IBD) refers to three chronic gastrointestinal diseases of unknown etiology (*ulcerative colitis, ulcerative proctitis,* and *Crohn's disease*) that afflict about 1 in 1000 persons in the United States. These diseases share a peak incidence between ages 20 and 40 years, no clear sex predominance, and higher incidence in whites, Jews, and possibly residents of developed countries. Smoking may increase the risk of Crohn's disease and decrease the risk of ulcerative colitis. There is little evidence that stress and psychiatric disorders cause these diseases.

Symptoms and Signs. The most common presentation of ulcerative colitis or ulcerative proctitis is bloody diarrhea. Other presenting features include fever, weight loss, or extraintestinal manifestations, including large-joint arthritis, ankylosing spondylitis, erythema nodosum, pyoderma gangrenosum, iritis, thromboembolic events, and several hepatobiliary disorders (fatty liver, pericholangitis, chronic active hepatitis, cirrhosis, granulomatous hepatitis, sclerosing cholangitis, cholangiocarcinoma, and gallstones).

About one half of patients with Crohn's disease have colonic involvement and present with bloody diarrhea. Small-bowel disease (about 40% of patients) leads to chronic diarrhea, weight loss, bowel obstruction, or fever. Because Crohn's disease may affect any part of the gastrointestinal tract from mouth to anus, initial symptoms may include dysphagia, oral complaints, or gastric outlet obstruction. The extraintestinal events seen in ulcerative colitis also occur with Crohn's disease, except that ankylosing spondylitis and thromboembolic events are less frequent in Crohn's disease.

Several clinical features distinguish ulcerative colitis from Crohn's disease. Ulcerative colitis spares the small intestine and, in contrast to Crohn's disease, rarely causes malabsorption, bowel obstruction, or intestinal fistulae. The transmural Crohn's disease process may produce fistulae with other loops of bowel or adjoining organs such as bladder, vagina, or skin. Severe perirectal fissures, fistulae, or abscesses are much more common in Crohn's disease than ulcerative colitis.

Clinical Approach. Most patients will present with diarrhea (see Chapter 91, Diarrhea). If fecal leukocytes and diarrhea persist beyond 3 weeks without an identifiable pathogen, the diagnosis of IBD should be pursued with sigmoido-scopic examination. Friable, erythematous mucosa extending proximally from the rectum without interruption suggests the diagnosis of ulcerative colitis. If normal mucosa appears above the abnormal mucosa, the patient probably has ulcerative proctitis. Areas of erythema, friability, or ulceration separated by normal mucosa suggest Crohn's disease. Normal rectal mucosa excludes active ulcerative colitis but should lead to further investigation for Crohn's disease, including colonoscopy or air-contrast barium enema, and upper gastrointestinal series with small-bowel followthrough (to examine the terminal ileum).

Because the initial symptoms of IBD may appear identical to those of self-limited infectious diarrhea and because misdiagnosis of chronic disease may inflict psychologic damage on patients, the clinician should refrain from diag-nosing IBD until duration criteria for disease are satisfied. Although 6 weeks of diarrhea establishes the diagnosis of IBD in clinical studies, self-limited diarrhea without an identifiable pathogen may persist longer than 6 weeks, as has been reported in recent Third World travelers or in community outbreaks of chronic diarrhea linked to untreated water or unpasteurized milk. Diagnostic restraint in these settings is advised. Rectal or colonic biopsy and clinical course will help to substantiate the diagnosis of IBD.

Management. A gastroenterologist should see all patients with IBD soon after diagnosis to confirm the diagnosis, measure the extent of disease, and help plan a course of rational therapy. Although primary care physicians may man-age quiescent and mild disease (particularly ulcerative proctitis), moderate to severe symptoms probably require continuing care by a gastroenterologist in concert with the primary care physician. Fewer than four bowel movements per day, occasional blood in the stool, normal hemoglobin, and absence of fever and extraintestinal manifestations would be considered mild IBD. Anemia, fever, more frequent bowel movements, extraintestinal complications, and fre-quent blood in the stool would be considered at least moderately severe disease. For Crohn's disease, presence of bowel obstruction, fistulae, or severe perianal disease would be considered more severe disease.

Mild ulcerative proctitis usually responds to hydrocortisone enemas, 100 mg/60 mL at bedtime for 2 to 3 weeks, followed by an every other night taper for 2 to 3 weeks. Further treatment is unnecessary for patients who respond rapidly and completely.

Patients with relapsing ulcerative proctitis or ulcerative colitis with mild symptoms should in addition receive sulfasalazine, 2 to 4 g/d in divided doses. Mesalamine (5-aminosalicylic acid) in an oral, enema, or rectal suppository preparation is available to treat ulcerative proctitis in patients who are intolerant to sulfasalazine or hydrocortisone enemas. More severe symptoms, such as fever, weight loss, and six to eight stools per day, necessitate prednisone, 40 mg/d for 2 to 4 weeks followed by a slow taper. Very ill patients with ulcerative colitis require hospitalization for intensive treatment, including bowel rest and observation for the development of toxic megacolon. Anticholinergic agents increase the risk of this life-threatening condition and are contraindicated. Colectomy cures severe ulcerative colitis refractory to medical treatment but need not always result in a permanent ileostomy. An ileorectal anastomosis with rectal mucosectomy and formation of a pouch from the terminal ileum may obviate the need for a permanent ileostomy. After resolution of acute symptoms, both sulfasalazine, 2 to 4 g/d, and oral mesalamine reduce the relapse rate. Immunosuppressive agents may play a role in both the treatment and maintenance of remission in corticosteroid-dependent patients with ulcerative colitis.

Fewer treatment options exist for Crohn's disease. Sulfasalazine, 2 to 4 g/d, is an effective treatment for mild colonic Crohn's disease. Oral mesalamine may also be efficacious in colonic and possibly small-bowel Crohn's disease. Metronidazole, 20 mg/kg in divided doses, is an alternative treatment, particularly if severe perirectal disease is present. Sulfasalazine does not consistently benefit Crohn's disease of the small bowel. Severe disease activity requires prednisone treatment as described earlier and hospitalization if severe diarrhea (more than six to eight stools per day), brisk intestinal bleeding, bowel obstruction, signs of abdominal abscess or fistulae, or another serious condition is present. Disease unresponsive to medical therapy can be managed surgically, but recurrences are frequent. Sulfasalazine does not reduce the relapse rate of Crohn's disease. Azathioprine, 6-mercaptopurine, intravenous cyclosporine, and methotrexate may reduce the corticosteroid dose required to control disease activity. Oral mesalamine may prolong remission in patients with Crohn's disease who previously responded to an aminosalicylate.

A summary of drug treatment options for IBD according to disease severity is shown in Table 97–1. Aminosalicylate refers to sulfasalazine (which is split by colonic bacteria into sulfapyridine and mesalamine) and mesalamine. When an oral aminosalicylate is indicated, sulfasalazine should be tried first. Up to 30% of patients taking sulfasalazine, 4 g/d, have side effects (headache, nausea, fatigue, rash, fever, hemolytic anemia, bone marrow suppression, folate malabsorption). If intolerable side effects occur, then oral mesalamine should be substituted by virtue of its lower incidence of side effects, although the daily cost is much higher ($5 versus $1) for a typical regimen (4 g/d). Of the aminosalicylates, only mesalamine is available for rectal administration as a suppository or enema.

Table 97-1. DRUG TREATMENT OPTIONS FOR INFLAMMATORY BOWEL DISEASE

Severity	Ulcerative Proctitis	Ulcerative Colitis	Crohn's Disease
Mild	Rectal corticosteroid Oral or rectal aminosalicylate	Oral aminosalicylate	Oral aminosalicylate if colon involved Metronidazole
Moderate	Oral corticosteroid Rectal corticosteroid	Oral corticosteroid	Oral corticosteroid Azathioprine or 6- mercaptopurine
Severe	Oral corticosteroid Rectal corticosteroid	Intravenous corticosteroid Intravenous cyclosporine	Intravenous corticosteroid Intravenous cyclosporine
Remission	Oral or rectal aminosalicylate Oral azathioprine or 6- mercaptopurine	Oral aminosalicylate Oral azathioprine or 6- mercaptopurine	Oral mesalamine if previously responsive to oral aminosalicylate

Follow-Up. Ulcerative proctitis progresses to pancolitis in 5% to 10% of patients after 10 years. The disease is usually more severe in the first 5 years and often "burns out" after 10 to 15 years. Colon cancer risk is slightly higher in ulcerative proctitis and left-sided ulcerative colitis, especially if disease began before age 30 years. Because pancolitis results in a 40% cumulative incidence of colon cancer after a disease duration of 35 years, patients with long-standing, extensive disease should be screened for colon cancer with colonoscopy and biopsy. Time to initiation of screening in patients with pancolitis has not been determined from randomized trials, but screening should probably not commence until 10 years after disease onset.

Crohn's disease of the small bowel leads to surgical resection in 50% of patients; postsurgical recurrences occur in about 40%. Colonic Crohn's disease probably increases the risk of acquiring colorectal carcinoma, but not to the same degree as ulcerative colitis. It is not clear whether cancer surveillance is warranted.

Cross-References: Colorectal Cancer Screening (Chapter 90), Diarrhea (Chapter 91), Abdominal Pain (Chapter 94), Sigmoidoscopy and Colonoscopy (Chapter 104), General Approach to Arthritic Symptoms (Chapter 106).

REFERENCES

1. Ekbom A, Helmick C, Zack M, Adami HO. Ulcerative colitis and colorectal cancer—a population-based study. N Engl J Med 1990;323:1228–1234.

   This article lists the results of the largest and most methodologically sound study of colorectal cancer risk and ulcerative colitis performed to date.

2. Hanauer SB. Drug therapy: Inflammatory bowel disease. N Engl J Med 1996;334:841–848.

   Treatments for inflammatory bowel disease had not changed much since the 1940s until recently. This article reviews the efficacy of old and new treatments for these chronic disorders.

3. Kirsner JB, Shorter RG. Inflammatory Bowel Disease, 4th ed. Philadelphia, Lea & Febiger, 1995.

   A comprehensive and up-to-date textbook covering all aspects of inflammatory bowel disease includes epidemiology, etiology, clinical course, medical and surgical treatment, and psychosocial issues.

4. Sartor B. Differential diagnosis and treatment of Crohn's disease. Gastrointest Dis Today 1995;4:1–10.

   This is a recent review of the epidemiology, diagnosis, and treatment of Crohn's disease.

98 Biliary Tract Disease

Problem

ANDREW K. DIEHL

Epidemiology. Gallstones occur in 5% to 15% of white women younger than age 50 and in 25% of older women. For men, prevalences range from 4% to 10% in those younger than age 50 to 10% to 15% thereafter. Hispanics of Mexican origin have rates roughly twice those of other whites. In contrast, blacks are at substantially lower risk. Almost 90% of those affected have cholesterol or mixed-composition stones, whereas the remainder harbor pigment stones. The most important risk factors are advancing age and female gender. Obesity, upper-body fat distribution, childbearing, parental history of stones, and rapid weight loss increase the risk of gallstone development. Moderate alcohol intake is associated with a lower risk. Whether diet influences gallstone formation remains controversial.

Choledocholithiasis (the presence of stones in the cystic or common bile duct) is seen most commonly in older patients with gallbladder stones. Retained or recurrent common duct stones occur in up to 3% of older patients after cholecystectomy. Gallbladder cancer is strongly associated with gallstones, and stones are an important cause of acute pancreatitis. Acute cholecystitis is usually linked to gallstones. However, acute acalculous cholecystitis may occur in the settings of major burns, trauma, extensive surgery, and rarely extensive atherosclerotic disease of outpatients. The condition is characterized by a high mortality.

Symptoms and Signs. The majority of persons with gallstones remain unaware of their presence for many years. The symptom most closely linked to stones is severe epigastric or right upper quadrant pain (biliary "colic") that characteristically begins abruptly and persists for 30 minutes to several hours before resolving gradually. Pain attacks are episodic and infrequent. The pain is typically steady in intensity (i.e., not fluctuating) and severe enough to interrupt everyday activities. It radiates to the upper back in a minority of patients. It often occurs at night, may follow meals (but by more than 1 hour), and is accompanied by nausea. However, fatty food intolerance, bloating, belching, and heartburn are no more common in those with gallstones than in normal persons. Physical examination during an attack may reveal local abdominal tenderness. Patients with lower abdominal symptoms or signs are significantly less likely to have gallstones.

Acute cholecystitis is characterized by prolonged biliary pain accompanied by fever, leukocytosis, or guarding on physical examination. Vomiting is commonly reported. Murphy's sign (tenderness in the area of the gallbladder that halts the patient's inspiration) is found in a fourth of affected patients, and mild jaundice may occur. Those with choledocholithiasis may also develop jaundice. Severe upper abdominal pain with hypoactive bowel sounds may represent acute pancreatitis, which is often related to gallstones. Rarely, stones may erode into the small intestine, resulting in gallstone ileus and fistula formation. Gallbladder cancer presents insidiously as abdominal pain, weight loss, and jaundice.

Nevertheless, the symptoms and signs of biliary tract disease are nonspecific, and judgments based on the clinical assessment alone are unreliable. Imaging studies are required to confirm the diagnosis.

Clinical Approach. Patients whose presentation suggests biliary tract disease should first undergo gallbladder ultrasonography. This test, which requires only that the patient be fasting, has a sensitivity for gallstones of 88% to 90% and a specificity of 97% to 98%. Stones as small as 3 mm diameter can be detected. Oral cholecystography has comparable specificity but lower sensitivity, requires more time and patient preparation, and has many inconclusive results. Computed tomography is also relatively insensitive. Plain abdominal radiographs occasionally suggest pigment stones but rarely establish a diagnosis. Liver chemistry tests are of no value in distinguishing uncomplicated cholelithiasis from other conditions.

Patients with severe abdominal pain and fever may have acute cholecystitis. Leukocytosis is often present. Ultrasonography can demonstrate gallstones and gallbladder wall thickening, as well as the "sonographic Murphy's sign" (tenderness over the gallbladder elicited by the ultrasonic transducer). Its sensitivity is estimated to be 91%, with a specificity of 79%. Indeterminate evaluations can be clarified by use of technetium-99m iminodiacetic acid scans, which have an estimated sensitivity of 97% and a specificity of 90% for acute cholecystitis. Although more accurate than ultrasonography, radionuclide scanning involves some radiation, takes longer to complete, is less widely available on nights and weekends, and is more costly.

Patients with evidence of biliary obstruction should be evaluated for common duct stones. Endoscopic retrograde cholangiopancreatography or percutaneous transhepatic cholangiography is recommended in this circumstance because ultrasonography is insensitive for this condition. Serum amylase and lipase levels are usually elevated in gallstone pancreatitis. Gallbladder cancer can be detected by ultrasonography but generally only in late stages when it is incurable. However, patients with calcification of the gallbladder wall on plain radiography ("porcelain gallbladder") or with a stone 30 mm diameter or larger are at substantially increased risk for cancer.

Oral cholecystography is required before consideration of most nonsurgical treatments because it provides more accurate information on physiologic function, stone number, and stone dimensions than does ultrasonography.

Management. Patients found to have asymptomatic gallstones should usually be observed, because fewer than half will develop definite symptoms within 20 years of diagnosis, and even fewer will present with complications. Patients with a high risk of gallbladder cancer, for whom prophylactic cholecystectomy may be advisable, are exceptions. Patients with diabetes should be considered for treatment even in the absence of symptoms because of their higher mortality when complications do occur. In many patients, close observation is an acceptable alternative.

In general, patients with definite gallstone symptoms should be treated, because the risks of further symptoms and complications usually outweigh the risks of surgery. Moreover, immediate surgery is associated with overall gains in life expectancy, especially for patients ages 50 years and younger. Cholecystectomy remains the treatment of choice because of its high success rate and low mortality. The laparoscopic approach is now the standard because of its lower morbidity.

Nonsurgical approaches, although less efficacious than cholecystectomy, are indicated for symptomatic patients who are at high risk for surgery. Oral dissolution therapy with ursodiol can be attempted for those with radiolucent stones under 20 mm in diameter, but complete dissolution occurs in only 20% to 30% within 2 years. Gallstone lithotripsy is most successful in those with a solitary radiolucent stone under 20 mm, but complete dissolution is seen in only 35% after 6 months. Percutaneous gallbladder lavage with methyl-*tert*-butyl ether is performed in only a few centers. Both lithotripsy and ether treatments require subsequent treatment with ursodiol until dissolution of the stones is complete.

Follow-Up. Patients who have successfully undergone cholecystectomy do not require long-term follow-up and may eat a normal diet. Recurrent gallstones after nonsurgical treatments occur at a rate of 10% annually, less often in those who had small solitary stones. Although ursodiol or aspirin may prevent recurrent stones in such patients, most recurring stones will respond to repeat dissolution therapy.

Cross-References: Jaundice (Chapter 92), Abdominal Pain (Chapter 94).

REFERENCES

1. Diehl AK. Epidemiology and natural history of gallstone disease. Gastroenterol Clin North Am 1991;20:1–19.

   This is a comprehensive review of prevalence, risk factors, time trends, and possibilities for preventive interventions.

2. Diehl AK. Symptoms of gallstone disease. Baillières Clin Gastroenterol 1992;6:635–657.

   Evidence linking symptoms to gallstones is reviewed, along with a description of the natural history of asymptomatic and symptomatic stones and a discussion of the medical management of biliary pain.

3. Ransohoff DF, Gracie WA. Treatment of gallstones. Ann Intern Med 1993;119:606–619.

   This comprehensive, evidence-based review of issues surrounding the management of gallstones includes decision analyses examining surgical versus expectant treatment of patients with symptomatic and asymptomatic stones.

4. Shea JA, Berlin JA, Escarce JJ, Clarke JR, Kinosian BP, Cabana MD, Tsai WW, Horangic N, Malet PF, Schwartz JS, Williams SV. Revised estimates of diagnostic test sensitivity and specificity in suspected biliary tract disease. Arch Intern Med 1994;154:2573–2581.

   This is a meta-analysis of diagnostic tests for gallstones and acute cholecystitis.

99 Cirrhosis and Chronic Liver Failure

Problem

M. CONNIE MORANTES

Epidemiology. Cirrhosis is an end-stage condition resulting from a wide variety of chronic, progressive liver diseases that scar the liver. Alcohol toxicity and viral hepatitis are the most common causes of cirrhosis in the United States. The liver is able to regenerate and continue functioning until the hepatic parenchymal reserve is exceeded (about 20% functioning parenchymal cells), after which clinically overt cirrhosis and liver failure ensue. The complications of chronic liver disease and cirrhosis result from two major processes: (1) impaired parenchymal function and (2) portal hypertension.

Symptoms and Signs. Fatigue is often a presenting symptom, along with other nonspecific complaints such as anorexia, weight loss, weakness, nausea, vomiting, and jaundice. Physical signs of chronic liver disease include spider telangiectases, palmar erythema, parotid and lacrimal gland hypertrophy, nail changes, Dupuytren's contractures, clubbing, gynecomastia, testicular atrophy, amenorrhea, and signs of portal hypertension (e.g., splenomegaly, ascites, and prominent superficial veins of the abdominal wall). The physical examination may reveal an enlarged firm liver, although a nonpalpable shrunken and hard liver is common late in the disease. Personality changes, defiant behavior, confusion, or the presence of asterixis suggests encephalopathy.

Clinical Approach. Metabolic complications result from both portal hypertension and synthetic dysfunction. These include hyperbilirubinemia, hypoalbuminemia, osteodystrophy, abnormalities in thyroid function, glucose intolerance early in the course, and hypoglycemia in later stages. Common hematologic manifestations include anemia caused by blood loss, folate deficiency, or hemolysis; leukopenia; and thrombocytopenia from hypersplenism. Coagulopathy can result both from decreased synthesis of clotting factors and from decreased vitamin K absorption due to malnutrition or cholestasis.

Because specific diagnostic studies and therapy are available for several of the causes of cirrhosis, the clinician should attempt to identify the underlying cause. Table 99–1 is a list of diseases that may lead to cirrhosis and the corresponding diagnostic studies.

Management. The cardinal objective is to prevent further liver injury. Patients with alcohol-related cirrhosis who stop drinking have a significantly better 5-year survival rate than those who continue to drink. Toxin or drug-induced cirrhosis also may improve after removing the offending agent. Adequate caloric intake of 2000 to 3000 kcal/d should be maintained, potentially hepato-

Table 99–1. CAUSES OF CIRRHOSIS AND DIAGNOSTIC TESTS

Etiology	Initial Evaluation
Alcoholism	History, γ–glutamyltranspeptidase (GGT)
Viral hepatitis	Hepatitis B surface antigen, hepatitis B surface antibody, antibody to hepatitis C virus, antibody to hepatitis delta virus
Autoimmune chronic active hepatitis	Antinuclear antibody, anti–smooth muscle antibody
Primary biliary cirrhosis	Antimitochondrial antibody
Genetic hemochromatosis	Iron saturation, ferritin
Wilson's disease	Ceruloplasmin, serum copper, slit-lamp examination
α_1-Antitrypsin deficiency	α_1-Antitrypsin levels
Drugs and toxins	History
Hepatic venous outflow obstruction	Abdominal ultrasonography
Cryptogenic	Diagnosis of exclusion

Adapted from Chung RT, Jaffe DL, Friedman LS. Complications of chronic liver disease. Crit Care Clin 1995;11:431–463.

toxic agents should be avoided, and the use of tranquilizers and sedatives should be minimized.

Complications of cirrhosis include portal hypertension and its consequences (e.g., esophagogastric varices, ascites, and hepatic or portosystemic encephalopathy), spontaneous bacterial peritonitis, hepatorenal syndrome, coagulopathy, and hepatocellular carcinoma.

Patients with new-onset *ascites* should undergo diagnostic ultrasonography (to confirm ascites, identify hepatic masses, and detect portal vein thrombosis) and diagnostic paracentesis (to exclude infection or malignancy). A serum ascites–albumin gradient greater than or equal to 1.1 g/dL correctly identifies the presence of portal hypertension in 95% of patients. Initial management of ascites should include withdrawal of offending agents and adequate dietary protein intake. If these measures are insufficient, the clinician should prescribe a 1- to 2-g-sodium diet while monitoring serum sodium and potassium levels and restricting water intake to 1.5 L/d if hyponatremia ensues. If ascites persists despite adequate sodium restriction, diuretic therapy may be initiated with the aldosterone antagonist spironolactone (starting dose, 100 mg/d). The dose should be increased by 100 mg every 3 to 5 days until the urinary sodium concentration is twice the urinary potassium concentration or a maximum dose of 400 mg/d is reached. Furosemide (starting dose 40 mg/d) can be added, but at the risk of volume depletion and hepatorenal syndrome. Patients with high urinary sodium excretion (> 10 mEq/L) on a spot urine sample are more responsive to diuretics and may not need combination therapy. For patients without edema, the goal is to lose no more than 0.5 to 0.75 kg/d, whereas patients with edema may lose up to 1 to 2 kg/d without significant risk of volume depletion. All patients require frequent monitoring of postural blood pressure, weight, and serum electrolytes. Ascites that is refractory to dietary and diuretic therapy may respond to repeated large-volume paracentesis. The routine use of intravenous albumin in all patients undergoing large-volume paracentesis is not cost-effective. Peritoneovenous shunts have not been shown to improve survival when compared with conventional therapy and are associated with an increased risk of infection and consumptive coagulopathy.

Although complicated by increased hepatic encephalopathy, transjugular intra-hepatic portosystemic shunt (TIPS) has been reported in uncontrolled trials to improve refractory ascites.

Spontaneous bacterial peritonitis occurs in roughly 25% of patients with ascites and should be considered whenever the condition of a patient with cirrhosis deteriorates without obvious explanation (e.g., worsening encephalopathy, increased liver failure, fever, or abdominal pain). Diagnostic paracentesis demonstrating more than 250 polymorphonuclear leukocytes per cubic millimeter is considered positive and should prompt hospital admission for administration of broad-spectrum parenteral antibiotics. The use of bedside inoculation of blood culture bottles with ascitic fluid increases the yield of positive cultures. The most common causative agents are *Escherichia coli*, streptococci, and *Klebsiella*. The treatment of choice is a 10- to 14-day course of a third-generation cephalosporin (e.g., cefotaxime, 1 g every 8 hours). Aminoglycosides should be avoided, given the high risk of nephrotoxicity in this setting. Patients with low ascitic fluid protein are at risk for spontaneous bacterial peritonitis. In these patients, prophylactic antibiotic use decreases the recurrence rate of spontaneous bacterial peritonitis as well as the risk of acquiring the disorder while hospitalized. However, the recommendation of using prophylactic antibiotics (e.g., norfloxacin, 400 mg/d; trimethoprim-sulfamethoxazole, 1 double-strength tablet 5 days/wk) in all outpatients with low-protein ascites cannot be made until further information on the long-term benefits and risks of prophylaxis is available.

Bleeding from ruptured *esophagogastric varices* is a serious complication of portal hypertension and carries a high mortality. Up to 40% to 70% of persons who bleed from varices die of their initial variceal hemorrhage. Because one third to one half of cirrhotic patients with upper gastrointestinal hemorrhage are bleeding from sources other than varices, it is essential to confirm the source of bleeding by endoscopy as soon as hemodynamic stability is achieved. Endoscopic sclerotherapy has been established as first-line therapy for the treatment of acute variceal hemorrhage and prevention of recurrent variceal hemorrhage. It has been shown that endoscopic variceal ligation is at least as effective as endoscopic sclerotherapy and is associated with a lower rate of complications. TIPS has been introduced for the treatment of refractory acute variceal bleeding. Given the serious complications associated with TIPS (e.g., development of new-onset or worsening encephalopathy, rebleeding due to shunt stenosis), this procedure is reserved for individuals who have failed endoscopic and medical management and who are poor surgical risks. Although effective in helping to control acute variceal bleeding, acute pharmaco-therapy (e.g., vasopressin, octreotide) has not shown any beneficial effect on survival. The use of nonselective β-blockers (e.g., propranolol) in a dose sufficient to reduce the resting pulse by about 25% has been shown to decrease the rate of bleeding in patients with portal hypertension.

Portosystemic *encephalopathy* is a reversible metabolic cerebral dysfunction that results from inability of the liver to remove various neurotoxins or to synthesize certain protective substances. Encephalopathy is often precipitated by gastrointestinal bleeding, infection, increased dietary protein intake, volume contraction and resulting alkalosis, azotemia, diuresis-related hyponatremia or hypokalemia, or injudicious use of sedatives or narcotics. Therapy includes limiting dietary protein to less than 50 g/d, maintaining standard caloric intake with fat and carbohydrate, and giving the nonabsorbable disaccharide lactulose. The dose of lactulose is titrated to induce two or three loose bowel movements per day (usually 60–120 mg/d). Neomycin, 2–6 g/d orally, an inexpensive second-line agent, may cause nephrotoxicity and ototoxicity.

Liver transplantation is now an established treatment for many patients with chronic progressive liver disease for whom no other effective therapy is available. Indications for liver transplantation include primary biliary cirrhosis, sclerosing cholangitis, toxin-induced injury, alcoholic liver disease, and some cases of chronic viral hepatitis. Referral for a liver transplant should be considered as soon as the patient begins to experience the serious complications of liver disease such as refractory ascites, variceal bleeding, and hepatic encephalopathy.

Cross-References: Alcohol Problems (Chapter 10), Viral Hepatitis (Chapter 100), Upper Gastrointestinal Endoscopy (Chapter 105).

REFERENCES

1. Buckley SE, Herrera JL. Management of ascites. Compr Ther 1995;21:195–199.

   Analysis of ascitic fluid and treatment options for ascites are summarized.

2. Chung RT, Jaffe DL, Friedman LS. Complications of chronic liver disease. Crit Care Clin 1995;11:431–463.

   This detailed discussion focuses on management and treatment of complications.

3. Ochs A, Rossle M, Haag K, et al. The transjugular intrahepatic portosystemic stent-shunt procedure for refractory ascites. N Engl J Med 1995;332:1192–1197.

   An uncontrolled prospective study found that TIPS was an effective treatment for refractory ascites; a 74% response rate was noted.

4. Ring EJ, Lake JR, Roberts JP, et al. Using transjugular intrahepatic portosystemic shunt stenting to control variceal bleeding before liver transplantation. Ann Intern Med 1992;116:304–309.

   Results are presented of a prospective uncontrolled trial using TIPS in 13 patients with refractory variceal bleeding.

100 Viral Hepatitis

Problem

M. CONNIE MORANTES

Epidemiology. Viral hepatitis is a systemic illness that causes hepatic inflammation and hepatic cell necrosis. Hepatitis A virus (HAV), hepatitis B virus (HBV), hepatitis C virus (HCV), hepatitis D virus (delta agent), and hepatitis E virus (HEV) cause the majority of clinical cases of viral hepatitis (Table 100–1). Less common causes of viral hepatitis include Epstein-Barr virus, herpes simplex virus, cytomegalovirus, and rubella virus.

In the United States, HAV accounts for about 50% of clinically apparent cases of acute viral hepatitis; however, the majority of cases are subclinical. Personal contact with an infected person is the most commonly reported risk factor. Other risk factors include employment or attendance at a day care center, a history of injection drug use, recent international travel, or association with a suspected food-borne or water-borne infection. By age 50, 70% of adults in the United States will be seropositive for anti-HAV antibodies.

Hepatitis B virus is a major cause of acute and chronic hepatitis, cirrhosis, and hepatocellular carcinoma worldwide. In the United States, an estimated 1 to 1.25 million persons have chronic HBV infection. Routes of transmission for HBV include sexual activity with an infected person, injection drug use, blood-borne exposure (e.g., hemodialysis, needlesticks), and vertical (mother to infant) transmission. Transmission by blood transfusions is rare in the United States due to current screening practices. Thirty percent to 40% of cases of HBV in the United States cannot be associated with an identifiable risk factor. Co-infection with the delta agent (which requires the presence of HBV to replicate) often results in fulminant hepatitis and can be fatal. Eighty percent of patients with chronic hepatitis delta infection will develop cirrhosis.

Table 100–1. CLINICAL FEATURES OF VIRAL HEPATITIS

	Hepatitis A Virus	Hepatitis B Virus	Hepatitis Delta Virus	Hepatitis C Virus	Hepatitis E Virus
Genome	RNA	DNA	RNA	RNA	Unknown
Mean incubation time	25 days	75 days	35 days	50 days	27 days
Transmission mode	Fecal-oral, sexual	Parenteral, sexual	Parenteral in United States, sexual	Parenteral	Fecal-oral
Acute mortality	0.1%–0.2%	0.2%–1.0%	1%–20%	0.2%–1.0%	1%–2%
Risk of chronicity	None	1%–10%	1%–80%	50%	None
Risk of hepatocellular carcinoma	No	Yes	Unknown	Yes	No

Hepatitis C virus is also a major cause of acute and chronic hepatitis, cirrhosis, and hepatocellular carcinoma. More than 60% of those infected with HCV will develop chronic liver disease. Transmission through injection drug use or transfusion accounts for almost half of reported cases of acute symptomatic HCV infection. Although the seroprevalence of anti-HCV among persons with multiple sexual partners seems to be elevated, the risk of transmission through sexual contact appears to be much lower than in HBV. Transmission through household contact appears to be rare.

Hepatitis E hepatitis (also known as enteric non-A, non-B hepatitis) is endemic to Southeast and Central Asia, the former Soviet Union, Africa, and Mexico. Confirmed cases in the United States have been limited to travelers returning from endemic regions. Mortality rates are high (> 20%) in infected pregnant patients.

Symptoms and Signs. The spectrum of acute viral hepatitis ranges from asymptomatic anicteric infection to fulminant hepatic necrosis and death. Patients classically present with acute malaise, fatigue, fever, anorexia, and nausea, followed by diffuse or right upper quadrant abdominal discomfort. Jaundice, pruritus, dark-colored urine, and light-colored stools are characteristic of the icteric phase.

Fulminant hepatitis rarely occurs in HAV infection. Acute HBV infection is subclinical in two thirds of cases. Some patients with HBV infection have findings due to circulating antigen–antibody complexes (rash, neuralgia, arthralgia, arthritis, and vasculitis) before jaundice develops. Although acute HBV infection usually resolves completely, about 10% of patients develop chronic hepatitis or the asymptomatic carrier state. Acute hepatitis delta infection causes a more severe illness than the other hepatitis viruses. Acute HCV infection is usually asymptomatic.

Many patients with chronic hepatitis B or C are asymptomatic. Symptomatic patients usually seek medical attention for complaints of fatigue, anorexia, nausea, and sometimes right upper quadrant pain. Occasionally patients present with evidence of advanced liver disease (e.g., bleeding esophageal varices, ascites, encephalopathy).

Clinical Approach. The diagnosis of viral hepatitis relies on the recognition of symptoms suggestive of acute inflammation of the liver, the elimination of other obvious considerations in the differential diagnosis (e.g., drug reaction, alcohol use, ischemic liver injury), and the serologic confirmation of acute infection. The patient's history including previous travel, injection drug use, known exposure, or other risk factors should guide the choice of studies.

Table 100–2 summarizes the serologic tests for viral hepatitis. As many as 10% of individuals with acute HBV infection have a negative hepatitis B surface antigen (HBsAg) and negative IgM anti-hepatitis B serologies but positive IgM anti–hepatitis B core assays. Infection with HCV virus is detected by enzyme immunoassay measurements of antibodies to any of three viral antigens. These assays cannot differentiate acute from chronic infection. Development of a detectable serologic response to HCV may take up to 6 months (mean: 11 weeks) after onset of clinically evident hepatitis. False-negative tests can occur if testing is done too early in the course or if the patient is immunosuppressed or on hemodialysis. False-positive tests occur in patients with autoimmune

Table 100–2. SEROLOGIC TESTS FOR VIRAL HEPATITIS

Test	Interpretation of Positive Result
Hepatitis A IgM antibody (IgM anti-HAV)	Current or recent acute hepatitis A; detectable IgM persists for 4–6 mo after infection but can persist for up to 12 mo
Hepatitis A total antibody (total anti-HAV)	Current or previous HAV infection; test detects IgM and IgA early in course and predominantly IgG thereafter
Antibody to hepatitis B surface antigen (anti-HBS)	Previous exposure to HBV and no active liver disease, *or* Previous hepatitis B vaccination, *or* Recent hepatitis B immune globulin prophylaxis, *or* When present with HBsAg (unusual), indicates ineffective antibody and chronic hepatitis B
Hepatitis B surface antigen (HBsAg)	Acute or chronic hepatitis B; patient is infectious through sexual contact and blood exposure
Hepatitis B e antigen (HBeAg)	Acute or chronic hepatitis B with active viral replication
Antibody to hepatitis B e antigen (anti-HBe)	Suppression of hepatitis B viral replication
Hepatitis B core IgM antibody (IgM anti-HBc)	Current or recent hepatitis B (past 4–6 mo), *or* Chronic hepatitis B with active viral replication (less common)
Hepatitis B core total antibody (total anti-HBc)	Previous hepatitis B; timing and chronicity unknown if both HBsAg and anti-HBs are not detected
Hepatitis B DNA (HBV DNA)	Acute or chronic hepatitis B
Hepatitis C antibody by enzyme immunoassay (anti-HCV by enzyme immunoassay)	Chronic hepatitis C (rarely detectable in acute hepatitis C)
Hepatitis C antibody by recombinant immunoblot assay (anti-HCV by RIBA)	Chronic hepatitis C (useful for evaluating suspected false-positive anti-HCV enzyme immunoassay)
Hepatitis C RNA by polymerase chain reaction (HCV RNA by PCR)	Acute or chronic hepatitis C

RIBA, recombinant immunoblot assay; PCR, polymerase chain reaction.
Adapted from Neuschwander-Tetri BA. Common blood tests for liver disease: Which ones are most useful? Postgrad Med 1995;98:49–63.

disease or hypergammaglobulinemia. Patients who are positive for anti-HCV with no identifiable risk factors should undergo further evaluation with recombinant immunoblot assay or with polymerase chain reaction to test for HCV RNA in the serum.

Management. Initial management of acute viral hepatitis is supportive. Patients should be instructed to avoid alcohol and other hepatotoxins. Nausea and vomiting may respond to prochlorperazine, 5–10 mg orally three or four times a day). Pruritus may respond to antihistamines or cholestyramine.

Fulminant viral hepatitis occurs rarely but is associated with a mortality of 70% to 80%. Patients presenting with altered mentation require immediate attention by physicians experienced in managing fulminant hepatic failure. Orthotopic liver transplantation may be lifesaving.

The use of recombinant interferon alfa for chronic hepatitis B has shown an initial response rate of 40% to 50% with a return to normal of serum aminotransferase levels and a sustained loss of viral replication. Interferon alfa is less effective in the treatment of chronic HCV infection, with only 40% of patients showing an initial response and less than 20% having a sustained response.

As in other infectious diseases, the most effective approach to treatment is the prevention of infection through the use of vaccines. An inactivated whole-virus vaccine for HAV, approved for use in the United States, is targeted for travelers to endemic areas and other high-risk persons. Recombinant HBV vaccine has proved highly useful for the prevention of infection in high-risk groups, including health care workers. Universal vaccination of children is being practiced in hopes of decreasing the incidence of chronic liver disease.

Follow-Up. Patients with acute HAV infection need no specific follow-up after their symptoms resolve. Follow-up of patients with acute hepatitis B, C, or delta virus infection is mandatory owing to the possibility of chronic infection. Patients should be seen at 1- to 2-month intervals during the first 6 months to document that the serum transaminase levels return to normal. In patients with HBV infection, clinicians should monitor serial HBsAg and anti-HBsAg titers until anti-HBsAg antibody is present.

Cross-References: Jaundice (Chapter 92), Abdominal Pain (Chapter 94), Cirrhosis and Chronic Liver Failure (Chapter 99).

REFERENCES

1. Becherer PR. Viral hepatitis: What have we learned about risk factors and transmission? Postgrad Med 1995;98:65–74.

   This review article focuses on epidemiology and prevention.

2. Neuschwander-Tetri BA. Common blood tests for liver disease: Which ones are most useful? Postgrad Med 1995;98:49–63.

   A nice summary of serologic tests for viral hepatitis and interpretation of positive results is presented.

3. Olynyk JK, Bacon BR. Hepatitis C: Recent advances in understanding and management. Postgrad Med 1995;98:79–92.

   This up-to-date summary of HCV includes a discussion on new treatment strategies.

4. Werzberger A, Mensch B, Kuter B, et al. A controlled trial of a formalin-inactivated hepatitis A vaccine in healthy children. N Engl J Med 1992;327:453–457.

   A double-blind, placebo-controlled trial randomized 1037 children to receive a single intramuscular dose of inactivated vaccine versus placebo; the efficacy equaled 100%.

101 Diverticulitis

Problem

RAVI MOONKA and HUBERT N. RADKE

Epidemiology. Diverticulitis results from obstruction and inflammation of a colonic diverticulum. Most colonic diverticula develop with age: one third of persons in the United States have diverticula by age 50, and two thirds have them by age 80. Ninety-five percent of patients with diverticulosis have disease confined to or including the sigmoid colon. Twenty percent to 30% of people with colonic diverticula develop diverticulitis during their lifetime, usually in the sigmoid colon.

Symptoms and Signs. The patient's presentation depends on the severity of the disease. Generally, patients with mild disease complain of poorly localized lower abdominal pain accompanied by constipation or diarrhea. Localized left lower quadrant pain, focal abdominal tenderness, or guarding suggests worsening inflammation with intramural or microscopic perforation. Systemic signs of fever, anorexia, and nausea may also be present. Progression of inflammation to pericolic tissues results in severe or complicated diverticulitis, with possible abscess formation, obstruction, diffuse peritonitis from free perforation, or fistula formation between the colon and adjacent structures (including bladder, bowel, uterus, or abdominal wall). In such cases sepsis, distention, pyuria, or pneumaturia can overshadow or obscure the diagnosis of diverticulitis. Gross colonic bleeding is virtually never a complication of diverticulitis but does occur in patients with diverticula that are not inflamed.

Clinical Approach

MILD DISEASE. The evaluation of a patient suspected of having diverticulitis is predicated on the severity of the disease. In mild cases, when pain, change in bowel habits, and minimal to no tenderness are the only findings, the differential diagnosis includes constipation, infectious enterocolitis, urinary tract infections, inflammatory bowel disease, and carcinoma. Although performing a white blood cell count and urinalysis often constitutes an adequate initial workup, computed tomography (CT) or barium enema examination should be performed within 1 to 2 weeks to exclude carcinoma and other causes of colon pathology and to document the presence of diverticulitis should surgery be considered subsequently. Tests delayed beyond this period may fail to reveal the subtle but characteristic abnormalities of diverticulitis.

A barium enema is more sensitive than CT for mucosal abnormalities caused by inflammatory bowel disease, cancer, and ischemia, as well as those due to diverticulosis and mild diverticulitis. Although CT better defines extraluminal extension of disease, this is uncommon in patients with mild symptoms. Endoscopy can document diverticulosis and sometimes diverticulitis but, more

333

importantly, can help eliminate other worrisome diagnoses. Ultrasonongraphy may be helpful but is extremely operator dependent, and its precise role is yet to be defined.

In mild cases, therapy includes oral fiber supplementation (a low fiber diet is thought to be important in the development of diverticulosis and diverticulitis) and mild analgesics such as acetaminophen or ibuprofen (narcotics, especially morphine, are contraindicated). Antibiotics, when indicated, should cover both anaerobic and gram-negative enteric pathogens. Common regimens include a combination of trimethoprim-sulfamethoxazole and metronidazole or amoxicillin/clavulanate. If the patient is reliable and can be followed closely, outpatient therapy is satisfactory.

MODERATE AND SEVERE DISEASE. In moderate cases, patients have significant abdominal pain and left lower quadrant tenderness, with varying degrees of bowel dysfunction, fever, and leukocytosis. Plain abdominal radiographs may reveal an ileus, a mass effect from an abscess, or an alternative explanation for the patient's pain. Upright chest radiography may, rarely, detect free peritoneal air. After these initial studies, the diagnosis of diverticulitis is generally made presumptively, and treatment consists of bowel rest, hydration, surgical consultation, and parenteral antibiotics. The combination of an aminoglycoside and metronidazole or clindamycin or, alternatively, a second-generation cephalosporin with anaerobic coverage such as cefoxitin or cefotetan used alone is an effective regimen.

Patients who fail to improve or whose condition deteriorates after 24 to 48 hours often have complicated diverticulitis. Diffuse peritonitis indicates likely free perforation and necessitates emergency surgery. Should focal peritonitis develop or fever and leukocytosis persist, CT can identify a diverticular abscess or other source for intra-abdominal infection and guide percutaneous abscess drainage. Although patients who develop an abscess eventually require surgery, percutaneous drainage can decrease the urgency and obviate the need for a temporary colostomy. If a patient is not improving and CT-guided percutaneous drainage is not possible, surgery must be strongly considered. In patients with diabetes, those on chronic glucocorticosteriod therapy, or those who are immunocompromised, the clinical presentation frequently underestimates the severity of disease, accelerating the need for CT scanning and surgical consultation.

FOLLOW-UP. Most episodes of treated diverticulitis resolve without invasive intervention, and only 25% of patients have a second attack. Elective surgery after a single past episode is therefore not indicated unless the patient is younger than 45 years old, is immunosuppressed, is diabetic, develops an abscess, or has had two documented episodes of diverticulitis. These groups suffer high rates of complicated or recurrent disease. Surgery is also indicated in instances in which carcinoma cannot be excluded.

Cross-References: Constipation (Chapter 93), Abdominal Pain (Chapter 94), Sigmoidoscopy and Colonoscopy (Chapter 104).

REFERENCES

1. Freeman SR, McNally PR. Diverticulitis. Med Clin North Am 1993;77:1149–1167.
   A comprehensive review of the presentation, diagnosis, and management of complicated and uncomplicated diverticulitis is presented.

2. Rothenberger DA, Wiltz O. Surgery for complicated diverticulitis. Surg Clin North Am 1993;73:975–992.

   The management of severe diverticulitis is discussed from a surgical perspective.

3. Smith TR, Cho KC, Morehouse HT, Kratka PS. Comparison of CT and contrast enema evaluation of diverticulitis. Dis Colon Rectum 1990;33:1–6.

   A retrospective study highlights the relative strengths of each test.

4. Tyau ES, Prystowsky JB, Joehl RJ, Nahrwold DL. Acute diverticulitis: A complicated problem in the immunocompromised patient. Arch Surg 1991;126:855–859.

   An analysis of diverticulitis in an immunocompromised cohort is followed by an interesting discussion.

102 Peptic Ulcer Disease

Problem

MICHAEL B. KIMMEY

Epidemiology. The lifetime prevalence of peptic ulcer is approximately 10%; at any one time, between 1% and 2% of adults have an ulcer. Although ulcer disease used to be more frequent in men, and duodenal ulcers more common than gastric ulcers, the prevalence of gastric and duodenal ulcers is now approximately equal, with little sex difference. Over 90% of duodenal ulcers and 70% of gastric ulcers are associated with gastric mucosal infection with *Helicobacter pylori*. Most of the other ulcers are found in patients taking nonsteroidal anti-inflammatory drugs (NSAIDs). Cigarette smoking increases the risk of duodenal ulcer in patients with *H. pylori* infection, and glucocorticoids increase the risk of gastric ulcers in those who are on NSAIDs. NSAID treatment also increases the risk of ulcer bleeding and perforation. Other causes of ulcer disease, including gastrinoma and Crohn's disease, are uncommon.

Symptoms and Signs. Although many patients are asymptomatic, the cardinal symptom of ulcer disease is epigastric pain. Duodenal ulcer pain typically occurs 1 to 2 hours after a meal and during the night and is relieved by antacids or food. Gastric ulcer pain is also felt in the epigastrium but is less clearly related to meals and is not always relieved by antacids. Ulcers associated with NSAID consumption are frequently painless. Although some patients with ulcers have nausea and vomiting, this may reflect the complication of gastric outlet obstruction. Epigastric tenderness has no predictive value for the diagnosis of ulcer.

Clinical Approach. The clinician must first determine whether the patient has an ulcer complication, such as gastric outlet obstruction, acute or chronic gastrointestinal bleeding, weight loss, or unusually severe or prolonged pain. Patients with suspected complications from ulcers should undergo immediate diagnostic evaluation with either upper gastrointestinal radiography or upper endoscopy. If no complications are present, an empirical 2-week trial of oral H_2-receptor antagonist therapy is indicated. If the pain completely resolves within 2 weeks and there are no other signs of complications, a 6-week course of these drugs is appropriate, and further diagnostic workup is unnecessary. If ulcer pain does not resolve after 2 weeks of H_2-receptor antagonist therapy, diagnostic testing is indicated (see Chapter 95, Dyspepsia).

The decision whether to perform upper gastrointestinal radiography or upper endoscopy to diagnose an ulcer should be individualized. An upper gastrointestinal series costs about half as much as upper endoscopy and is more readily available to the primary care physician. The sensitivity of endoscopy in detecting superficial ulcers is greater than that of upper gastrointestinal radiography. However, high-quality air-contrast barium radiographs reveal over 90% of chronic gastric and duodenal ulcers. Endoscopy is preferred in patients with gastrointestinal bleeding, because barium will confound further attempts at endoscopic or angiographic therapy. If an upper gastrointestinal series demonstrates a gastric ulcer with radiographic signs suggestive of malignancy, the patient should be referred for endoscopy and biopsy. Because 2% to 4% of benign-appearing gastric ulcers are actually ulcerated gastric cancers, gastric ulcer healing should be documented after treatment. Endoscopy is preferred for this indication because biopsy samples can be taken if the ulcer has not healed. Endoscopy is also preferred in patients who have a history of ulcers or prior gastric surgery because scarring may interfere with accurate diagnosis using contrast radiography.

All patients with a documented ulcer or history of an ulcer should be tested for *H. pylori* infection. Endoscopic biopsy for a rapid urease test or histologic evaluation is over 90% sensitive and specific for *H. pylori* infection. For those patients not undergoing endoscopy, serologic testing is preferred and is 90% to 95% sensitive and specific for prior *H. pylori* infection. Antibody titers may persist for years after successful treatment of the infection, however. A radiolabeled urea (^{13}C or ^{14}C) breath test is the test of choice for confirming the efficacy of antibiotic treatment. Testing for eradication should be delayed for 1 month after completion of antibiotics.

A serum gastrin level is a good screening test for the presence of gastrinoma, a neoplastic condition that results in acid hypersecretion. The gastrin level should be checked when duodenal ulcers are multiple, are recurrent, are found distal to the duodenal bulb, recur after ulcer surgery, or resist standard treatment. Gastrin levels should also be obtained in patients with duodenal ulcers who are not infected with *H. pylori* or taking NSAIDs.

Management. The advent of specific drug therapy that promotes ulcer healing has limited the roles for diet, lifestyle changes, and surgery in management of peptic ulcer disease. There is little evidence that specific dietary components, including caffeinated beverages, dairy products, and fiber, affect ulcer healing.

Even with antiulcer medications, cigarette smoking impairs ulcer healing. Smoking also favors an earlier recurrence after the ulcer has healed and antiulcer therapy is stopped. Even if smoking cannot be stopped, reducing cigarette consumption to fewer than 10 cigarettes per day benefits ulcer healing. Because NSAIDs impair healing of gastric but not duodenal ulcers, they should be stopped if possible during treatment of gastric ulcers.

Most gastric and duodenal ulcers respond to antacids, H_2-receptor antagonists, or proton-pump inhibitors. H_2-receptor antagonists and proton-pump inhibitors are favored over antacids because they can be given once daily with fewer side effects. Because the various H_2-receptor antagonists are equally efficacious and have similar side effects (Table 102–1), the choice of therapy depends primarily on cost. However, in patients who are also taking theophylline, warfarin, or phenytoin, famotidine is preferred because it is less likely to inhibit hepatic drug metabolism. Alternatively, the proton-pump inhibitors omeprazole or lansoprazole can be given for 4 weeks with healing rates comparable to those after 6 to 8 weeks of H_2-receptor antagonists.

Patients with duodenal ulcers may be treated with a single dose of an H_2-receptor antagonist at bedtime. Because gastric ulcers are more difficult to heal, twice-daily therapy with H_2-receptor blockers may offer a slight therapeutic advantage. Sucralfate is as effective as H_2-receptor antagonists in treating duodenal ulcers but is less effective in treating gastric ulcers. Although misoprostol, a synthetic prostaglandin, may promote healing of gastric ulcers when NSAIDs are continued, significant diarrhea and abdominal cramping has limited its clinical usefulness. Omeprazole or lansoprazole are especially useful for treating refractory ulcers, for treating gastric ulcers when NSAIDs must be continued and when used in conjunction with antibiotics to eradicate *H. pylori* infection.

Eradication of *H. pylori* infection reduces the risk of ulcer recurrence after 1 year from 70% to less than 5%. There are several options for eradicating *H. pylori* (Table 102–2). The selection of antibiotic regimens for an individual patient depends on several factors, including compliance (especially important with three- and four-drug regimens), prior antibiotic exposure (resistance to metronidazole is found in up to 30% of patients with previous metronidazole exposure), and cost of treatment.

Patients with ulcer complications such as upper gastrointestinal hemorrhage or perforation should be hospitalized. Perforation is managed surgically by oversewing the ulcer. Hemorrhage can usually be managed with endoscopic

Table 102–1. STANDARD ANTIULCER REGIMENS

Drug	Dosage	Cost ($ per day)*	Cost ($ per 6 weeks)*
Mylanta suspension	30 mL qid	1.40	59
Maalox suspension	30 mL qid	1.45	61
Riopan suspension	30 mL qid	1.38	58
Cimetidine (generic)	800 mg hs†	2.24	94
	400 mg bid†	2.52	106
Ranitidine	300 mg hs	3.00	126
	150 mg bid	3.36	141
Nizatidine	300 mg hs	2.92	123
	150 mg bid	3.10	130
Famotidine	40 mg hs	2.92	123
	20 mg bid	3.02	127
Sucralfate	1 g qid	2.96	124
Omeprazole	20 mg qd	3.63	102‡
Lansoprazole	30 mg qd	3.25	91‡

*Average wholesale price, 1995 *Drug Topics Red Book.*
†Actual price is often lower because of contract buying.
‡Four weeks of therapy.

**Table 102–2. ANTIBIOTIC REGIMENS FOR THE TREATMENT
OF *HELICOBACTER PYLORI* INFECTION**

Drugs	Dosage	Duration (days)	Efficacy	Comments
Bismuth subsalicylate + metronidazole + tetracycline	2 tablets qid 500 mg qid 500 mg qid	14	90%	Poor compliance with taking multiple pills reduces efficacy.
Above plus omeprazole or lansoprazole	20 mg bid 30 mg bid	7	95%	Shorter course than triple therapy alone.
Clarithromycin + omeprazole or lansoprazole	500 mg tid 20 mg bid 30 mg bid	14	75%	Most costly of the regimens listed.
Amoxicillin + omeprazole	1 g bid 20 mg bid	14	60%	US studies did not reproduce the higher success rates achieved in European trials.
Metronidazole or amoxicillin + clarithromycin + omeprazole or lansoprazole	500 mg bid 1 g bid 500 mg bid 20 mg bid 30 mg bid	7–10	90%	Early European trials with these regimens need confirmation in United States.

injection or coagulation therapy. Although it is rarely necessary, some patients with intractable pain, failed healing, or gastric outlet obstruction may require surgical treatment with selective vagotomy or gastric resection.

Follow-Up. In most patients, pain resolves within 1 week of beginning therapy with antacids, H$_2$-receptor antagonists, or proton-pump inhibitors. Nevertheless, these treatments should be continued for a total of 6 to 8 weeks with antacids and H$_2$-receptor antagonists and 4 weeks for proton-pump inhibitors to ensure ulcer healing. Patients with duodenal ulcers need no documentation of ulcer healing. Patients with gastric ulcers should have follow-up endoscopic documentation of healing, unless biopsies at the time of diagnosis were benign.

Maintenance ulcer therapy with full-dose H$_2$-receptor antagonists is advisable for patients with ulcer complications such as hemorrhage or perforation until confirmation of *H. pylori* eradication is obtained. Recurrent ulcer bleeding is seen in 30% of bleeding ulcer patients within 1 year unless *H. pylori* is eradicated. Confirmation of *H. pylori* eradication is usually not necessary in patients with uncomplicated ulcers.

Patients who have had ulcers associated with NSAID use require special consideration if NSAIDs must be resumed. It is unknown whether treatment of concomitant *H. pylori* infection reduces the risk of recurrent ulcers if NSAIDs are resumed. Acetaminophen has no ulcer risk and is preferred if only an analgesic is needed. A nonacetylated salicylate (salsalate or choline magnesium trisalicylate) has anti-inflammatory properties with a lower risk of ulcer. Nabumetone also appears to have a lower risk of inducing ulcers. Misoprostol has been shown to reduce the frequency of ulcers and ulcer complications attributed to NSAIDs and should be considered for the highest risk groups (previous ulcer or ulcer complication or concomitant glucocorticoid or anticoagulant therapy).

Cross-References: Smoking Cessation (Chapter 12), Abdominal Pain (Chapter 94), Dyspepsia (Chapter 95), Upper Gastrointestinal Endoscopy (Chapter 105).

REFERENCES

1. Brown KE, Peura DA. Diagnosis of *Helicobacter pylori* infection. Gastroenterol Clin North Am 1993;22:105–115.

   Diagnostic tests for H. pylori *infection are reviewed.*

2. Feldman M, Burton ME. Histamine 2-receptor antagonists: Standard therapy for acid-peptic diseases. N Engl J Med 1990;323:1672–1680, 1749–1755.

   A comprehensive review of the H_2-receptor antagonists is presented.

3. Peterson WL. *Helicobacter pylori* and peptic ulcer disease. N Engl J Med 1991;324:1043–1048.

   This spiral-shaped bacterium causes gastritis and contributes to the pathogenesis of ulcer disease and ulcer recurrence.

4. Silverstein FE, Graham DY, Senior JR, et al. Misoprostol reduces serious gastrointestinal complications in patients with rheumatoid arthritis receiving nonsteroidal anti-inflammatory drugs. A randomized, double-blind, placebo-controlled trial. Ann Intern Med 1995;123:241–249.

   Misoprostol reduces NSAID-associated ulcer complications by 40%.

5. Walan A, Bodey JP, Classen M, et al. Effects of omeprazole and ranitidine on ulcer healing and relapse rates in patients with benign gastric ulcer. N Engl J Med 1989;320:69–75.

   Omeprazole heals gastric ulcers more rapidly than ranitidine, even when NSAIDs are continued during treatment.

103 Hemorrhoids and Anal Fissures

Problem

STEVEN R. McGEE

Epidemiology. In the United States the prevalence of hemorrhoids is 4.4%, although only one third of affected patients seek medical attention. Hemorrhoids affect whites more than blacks, are rare in persons younger than the age of 20 years, have a peak incidence between ages 45 and 65, and diminish in frequency after age 65 years. Despite traditional teachings, hemorrhoids are not more prevalent in patients with portal hypertension. Anal fissures, common in middle-aged patients, represent the most common cause of anal pain.

Symptoms and Signs. Hemorrhoids consist of anatomically normal vascular anal cushions, oriented in the left lateral, right anterior, and right posterior position, which have lost their fibromuscular support and become trapped by the anal sphincter in the prolapsed position. Common symptoms include bright-red bleeding after defecation (85%–90%), prolapse (40%–60%), anal discomfort (15%–50%), and pruritus (20%–50%). Severe pain is uncommon and suggests thrombosed external hemorrhoids, which appear as tender blue swellings at the anal verge and usually occur after strenuous effort such as heavy lifting. Hemorrhoids are traditionally classified both by stage (stage 1—no prolapse; stage 2—prolapse reducing spontaneously; stage 3—prolapse requiring manual reduction; and stage 4—irreducible prolapse) and by whether they are external or internal (depending on whether involved tissue is below or above the dentate line). This classification has limited value, however, because most symptomatic hemorrhoids involve both internal and external tissues and move between different stages over hours or days.

Fissures cause acute severe anal pain, sometimes accompanied by bright-red blood, immediately after passage of hard stool or, less commonly, after explosive diarrhea. Pain from fissures, in contrast to other common causes of anal pain (thrombosed external hemorrhoid and perirectal abscess), decreases between bowel movements. All fissures are visible during examination as tears in the anal mucosa located below the dentate line in the posterior (90% women, 98% men) or anterior midline. Fissures that are not anterior or posterior should suggest Crohn's disease, syphilis, or tuberculosis.

Clinical Approach. Most patients with anal discomfort or bleeding believe they have hemorrhoids, although the differential diagnosis includes tumors, inflammatory bowel disease, and infections (herpes, syphilis, gonorrhea, chlamydia, perirectal abscess). The patient interview should identify risk factors for trauma and infection (e.g., anal intercourse), any self-prescribed medications (some nonprescription anesthetics cause contact dermatitis), and family history of Crohn's disease, ulcerative colitis, polyps, and cancer. No symptom, however, reliably distinguishes hemorrhoids from cancer; even bright-red blood on top of the stool, the traditional symptom of hemorrhoids, may be the result of cancer. Most patients with concurrent anemia and hemorrhoids have separate, often serious, causes for the anemia.

The recommended minimal clinical approach in all patients with perirectal bleeding or discomfort is digital rectal and rigid or flexible sigmoidoscopy examination. In addition, the following groups of patients with perirectal symptoms should undergo examination of the entire colon (double-contrast barium enema or colonoscopy): (1) patients older than 40 years; (2) patients with hemorrhoids identified but no response to several weeks of conservative treatment; (3) patients with a family history of cancer, polyps, or inflammatory bowel disease; or (4) patients whose sigmoidoscope examination identifies blood in the stool above the sigmoidoscope. In one study of elderly men with hematochezia and hemorrhoids identified during anoscopy, other important lesions were identified during colonoscopy in 35% (e.g., carcinomatous polyps, villous adenoma, tubular adenoma).

In contrast, the physical examination does differentiate among the causes of *severe* anal pain. Fissures are always visible on examination. Thrombosed hemorrhoids appear as tender firm blue swellings. If a fissure or thrombosed hemorrhoids are not present and there is tenderness in the perirectal tissues, the clinician should consider the diagnosis of perirectal abscess. In these settings, digital rectal and anoscopy examinations are unnecessarily painful and best postponed. Patients with suspected perirectal abscesses should be referred to a surgeon for consideration of examination under anesthesia.

Management. Only symptomatic hemorrhoids require treatment. Sixty-five percent of patients improve over weeks without any treatment, although two thirds experience recurrent disease. Controlled trials document that bulk laxatives such as psyllium decrease bleeding and discomfort over weeks; other sources of dietary fiber (fruits, vegetables, bran, whole grains) may be equally effective. Nonprescription creams/suppositories and sitz baths have not been scientifically tested, although they are safe and effective according to many patients. If symptoms fail to resolve with conservative treatment (bulk laxatives, sitz baths), patients should be referred to a surgeon for any of a number of outpatient procedures designed to repair the anal cushions and prevent prolapse. Rubber-band ligation, injection sclerotherapy, infrared coagulation, bipolar diathermy, and direct-current electrotherapy all are safe (minimal temporary pain and bleeding) and effective (80% response). Fewer than 7% of all patients referred for fixation procedures fail to respond and ultimately require hemorrhoidectomy.

Most patients with thrombosed external hemorrhoids or pain from fissures improve after 2 to 3 days of conservative management (rest, bulk laxatives, sitz baths); the fissure itself may require weeks to heal. Patients with persistent pain or chronic fissures may require surgery (excision for thrombosed hemorrhoids; lateral sphincterotomy for fissures).

Follow-Up. Hemorrhoids and fissures rarely result in hospitalization. Long-term studies demonstrate that fixation procedures reduce hemorrhoidal recurrence rates in the few patients who have unresponsive symptoms. Complications of chronic fissures, which affect less than 10%, are anal fistula and perirectal abscess.

Cross-References: Colorectal Cancer Screening (Chapter 90), Inflammatory Bowel Disease (Chapter 97), Sigmoidoscopy and Colonoscopy (Chapter 104).

REFERENCES

1. Johanson JF, Rimm A. Optimal nonsurgical treatment of hemorrhoids: A comparative analysis of infrared coagulation, rubber band ligation, and injection sclerotherapy. Am J Gastroenterol 1992;87:1601–1606.

   Meta-analysis of five randomized clinical trials showed that the initial response to treatment was equivalent with all three techniques, but patients with rubber-band ligation had the best long-term results (and the most post-procedure pain).

2. Kluiber RM, Wolff BG. Evaluation of anemia caused by hemorrhoidal bleeding. Dis Colon Rectum 1994;37:1006–1007.

   Of 131 patients with concurrent anemia and hemorrhoids, 95% had separate causes for the anemia. In those with anemia due to hemorrhoids, 14% had coagulopathy and 84% described spurting blood or clots during defecation.

3. Mazier WP. Hemorrhoids, fissures, and pruritus ani. Surg Clin North Am 1994;74:1277–1292.

   This is an excellent overview of clinical features and management. Of 500 patients presenting to a colorectal surgeon with a complaint of "hemorrhoids," the final diagnoses were hemorrhoids in 50%, thrombosed hemorrhoids in 19%, fissures in 8%, and miscellaneous in 23%.

4. Moesgaard F, Nielsen ML, Hansen JB, Knudsen JT. High-fiber diet reduces bleeding and pain in patients with hemorrhoids. Dis Colon Rectum 1982;25:454–456.

   In this double-blind randomized placebo trial in 52 patients, 6 weeks of psyllium reduced hemorrhoidal symptoms. The drug was effective whether or not the patient was constipated.

5. Shub HA, Salvati EP, Rubin R. Conservative treatment of anal fissure. Dis Colon Rectum 1978;21:592–593.

   In 317 patients with fissures (mean duration of 24 weeks), over one half responded to conservative nonsurgical treatment.

· ·

104 Sigmoidoscopy and Colonoscopy

Procedure

DAVID C. DUGDALE

SIGMOIDOSCOPY

Indications and Contraindications. Indications for endoscopic evaluation of the anus, rectum, and colon are (1) hematochezia; (2) microscopic intestinal blood loss in asymptomatic patients (colonoscopy preferred but sigmoidoscopy combined with barium enema examination is appropriate when full colonoscopy is not available); (3) suspected antibiotic-associated colitis or inflammatory bowel disease; (4) chronic bloody or inflammatory diarrhea; (5) tenesmus or rectal or perineal pain; (6) fistula in ano, perirectal abscess, and atypical rectal fissures; (7) chronic small-volume diarrhea; and (8) screening for colorectal neoplasia.

The only absolute contraindication to sigmoidoscopy is suspected or impending bowel perforation (e.g., toxic megacolon, acute diverticulitis). Relative contraindications include hemodynamic instability, an uncooperative patient, and colonic distention. Sigmoidoscopy is often performed by primary care physicians, especially for the purpose of screening for neoplasia. Available data indicate that 15 to 25 procedures are required for adequate initial training of practitioners. The number of procedures required to maintain a practitioner's skills is not known.

Rationale. Most pathology responsible for hemodynamically insignificant, recurrent hematochezia is located within the reach of a sigmoidoscope. Direct visualization of the pseudomembranes of antibiotic-associated colitis or the characteristic ulcerations of inflammatory bowel disease, along with histologic confirmation, is often diagnostic of these diseases. Both rigid and flexible sigmoidoscopes are available. Rigid sigmoidoscopes are inexpensive, partly disposable, easy to clean, and easier to use than flexible sigmoidoscopes. Flexible sigmoidoscopy examines more of the colon and is more comfortable for the patient but requires more operator training time. Flexible sigmoidoscopes are relatively expensive ($13,000) and more difficult to clean. In spite of these factors, flexible sigmoidoscopy has replaced rigid sigmoidoscopy for most purposes. The recently developed disposable flexible sigmoidoscope sheath system greatly reduces the need for cleaning but is quite expensive ($60).

Methods

Rigid Sigmoidoscopy. The patient's rectosigmoid may be prepared with a cleansing enema; if proctitis is suspected, a tap water enema is preferred because commercial enemas may induce a mild proctitis and cause diagnostic confusion. Commercial phosphate-containing enemas may also be hazardous in patients with renal insufficiency. Patient acceptance of rigid sigmoidoscopy is increased if a modified left lateral decubitus position is used. In this position, the pelvis and buttocks extend over the operator's side of the table and the shoulders are brought forward over the opposite side of the table for balance and security. The traditional jackknife-prone position (useful when liquid stool or blood is encountered) requires a special table and places the patient in an unusual, psychologically vulnerable position. After a careful digital rectal examination, the lubricated plastic disposable instrument is inserted very slowly through the anal sphincters with the obturator in place. After the sphincter has been traversed (usually after 2 to 3 cm), the instrument must be pointed immediately toward the patient's back to follow the rectum along the sacral curve. Failure to follow this normal anatomy can result in perforation of the anterior rectal wall. The obturator is then removed, the lens cap closed, and the path of the colon is followed, with the instrument advanced only after direct visualization of the judiciously inflated lumen ahead. The instrument is 25 cm long, but the average depth of insertion is 15 to 20 cm. The distal rectal vault just proximal to the anal canal, where low-lying lesions may be missed, must be carefully inspected. A clean suction catheter can be used to stiffen a flexible biopsy forceps to obtain superficial mucosal biopsy specimens. The procedure should take about 5 minutes.

Flexible Sigmoidoscopy. After two cleansing enemas, the flexible sigmoidoscope is introduced under direct vision as far as is comfortably possible (average 50 cm). The mucosa is usually inspected during withdrawal of the instrument. A retroflexed view of the distal rectal vault should be performed. Flexible biopsy forceps are used to obtain superficial mucosal biopsy specimens. Procedure time should be 10 to 15 minutes.

Cost and Complications. The usual charge for rigid sigmoidoscopy is $60 to $100 (physician and facility charges); for flexible sigmoidoscopy it is $200 to $400. The major complication of sigmoidoscopy is perforation (rigid, 0.002% to 0.02% incidence; flexible, 0.01% incidence); the rate of procedure-associated bacteremia is very low, even with biopsy. If a polyp is seen, a grasp biopsy should be performed to determine if the polyp is neoplastic. The use of cautery to remove neoplasms by sigmoidoscopy is contraindicated in the enema-prepared bowel because of the risk of colonic explosion. The high incidence of synchronous neoplasia proximal to the area examined makes fully prepared colonoscopy the procedure of choice for definitive evaluation of and therapy for polyps found by sigmoidoscopy.

COLONOSCOPY

Indications and Contraindications. Indications for endoscopic evaluation of the entire colon include (1) asymptomatic microscopic gastrointestinal blood loss; (2) unexplained iron deficiency anemia; (3) known or suspected neoplasia found on barium enema examination or sigmoidoscopy (remove polyps; screen the entire colon for synchronous neoplasia); (4) ulcerative pancolitis present for longer than 10 years (screening for dysplasia); (5) a history of adenomatous polyps or colon cancer (screening usually recommended every 3 to 5 years after the last colonoscopy that either demonstrated no polyps or removed all lesions); and (6) a strong family history of colon cancer (at least two first-degree relatives or familial cancer syndrome).

The contraindications to colonoscopy are similar to those for sigmoidoscopy. Additional contraindications include the concurrent use of anticoagulants or aspirin or a history of bleeding disorders.

Rationale. Colonoscopy is the most specific and sensitive method for examining the colon for mucosal abnormalities and allows definitive therapy in many patients with localized neoplasia.

Methods. The bowel must be thoroughly prepared for colonoscopy. The patient must adhere to a liquid diet for 2 days before the procedure and ingest a purgative the day before the procedure. This may be 90 mL of a highly concentrated sodium phosphate laxative or 4 to 6 L of an osmotically balanced sodium sulfate solution containing polyethylene glycol (GoLYTELY or Colyte). The former is easier to take but causes more fluid and electrolyte shifts; the latter is preferred for patients with a history of congestive heart failure or severe renal or hepatic disease. Patients should discontinue oral iron intake at least 1 week before the procedure. The procedure typically requires 30 to 60 minutes and is usually an outpatient procedure. Because parenteral sedation is usually provided during colonoscopy to prevent and treat abdominal cramps, the patient should be instructed to have someone drive him or her home. Patients are usually able to resume a regular diet immediately after the procedure.

Cost and Complications. The usual charge for colonoscopy is $1000 to $1500 (physician and facility charges). The most significant complications of bowel preparation with polyethylene glycol–containing solutions are nausea (6%) and vomiting (2%). The incidence of perforation with colonoscopy is 0.2% to 0.4% during diagnostic studies and 0.3% to 1.0% during procedures with polypectomy. The postpolypectomy coagulation syndrome consists of pain, peritoneal irritation, and fever; it probably represents a microperforation but usually does not require surgery. Visible bleeding occurs in 0.03% of diagnostic studies and 0.7% to 2.5% of cases with polypectomy but rarely leads to surgical intervention. Postpolypectomy bleeding may be immediate, but in up to one half of cases, it is delayed by 2 to 7 days. Cardiopulmonary complications related to oxygen desaturation, vagally mediated bradycardia, and sedation do occur but are rarely life threatening. The mortality rate for colonoscopy is 0.03%. The incidence of bacteremia in colonoscopy, even with polypectomy, is low, and recommendations for endocarditis prophylaxis are the same as those for upper endoscopy (1995 American Society for Gastrointestinal Endoscopy recommendations: consider prophylaxis [but not required] for patients with prosthetic heart valves, a history of endocarditis, systemic-pulmonary shunt, or synthetic vascular graft less than 1 year old; prophylaxis is not recommended in all other cases including prosthetic joints).

Cross-References: Periodic Health Assessment (Chapter 8), Colorectal Cancer Screening (Chapter 90), Diarrhea (Chapter 91), Inflammatory Bowel Disease (Chapter 97), Hemorrhoids and Anal Fissures (Chapter 103), Upper Gastrointestinal Endoscopy (Chapter 105).

REFERENCES

1. American Society for Gastrointestinal Endoscopy. Antibiotic prophylaxis for gastrointestinal endoscopy. Gastrointest Endosc 1995;42:630–635.

   This article provides recommendations of the American Society for Gastrointestinal Endoscopy for endocarditis prophylaxis during gastrointestinal procedures.

2. Durack DT. Prevention of infective endocarditis. N Engl J Med 1995;332:38–44.

   A current review of recommendations for endocarditis prophylaxis during gastrointestinal procedures is presented.

3. Katon RM, Keefe EB, Melnyk CS. Flexible Sigmoidoscopy. Orlando, FL, Grune & Stratton, 1985.

   Additional comparative data for rigid sigmoidoscopy, flexible sigmoidoscopy, and colonoscopy are given along with specific techniques for performing flexible sigmoidoscopy.

4. Waye JD, Lewis BS, Yessayan S. Colonoscopy: A prospective report of complications. J Clin Gastroenterol 1992;15:347–351.

   Morbidity data on colonoscopy (n = 2097) include a 5% complication rate, 2% hospitalization rate, and no deaths.

105 Upper Gastrointestinal Endoscopy

Procedure

LONNY M. HECKER

Indications. Upper gastrointestinal endoscopy is commonly known as esophagogastroduodenoscopy (EGD). A fiberoptic or video endoscope is passed through the oral cavity to directly visualize the esophagus, stomach, and proximal duodenum.

DYSPEPSIA. Dyspepsia, broadly defined as upper abdominal discomfort or pain, is a common indication for EGD. Only persons with upper abdominal distress associated with signs or symptoms suggesting serious disease or that persist despite an appropriate trial of therapy should undergo EGD. However, because even the symptoms of upper gastrointestinal cancer may initially respond to acid suppression, the British Society of Gastroenterology reserves empirical therapy for those younger than age 45 and expands the indications for prompt endoscopy to include patients older than age 45 with recent onset of dyspepsia or change in dyspeptic symptoms and all patients with dyspepsia in whom long-term therapy is planned. Several studies have suggested that prompt endoscopy in patients with dyspepsia was cost effective when compared with radiography or empirical therapy.

Helicobacter pylori has been generally accepted as the causative agent for 92% of all duodenal ulcers and most gastric ulcers that are not related to aspirin or nonsteroidal anti-inflammatory drugs (NSAIDs). In light of this, guidelines have included individuals with dyspepsia who are positive for *H. pylori* on noninvasive testing as appropriate for endoscopy. Empirical antibiotic therapy for these individuals is not recommended because the value of treating chronic dyspepsia in the absence of ulcer disease has not been established.

NAUSEA AND VOMITING. Persistent nausea and vomiting is generally considered an appropriate indication for upper endoscopy.

IMMUNOCOMPROMISE. Immunocompromised patients with dyspepsia warrant prompt endoscopy because of the increased frequency of infections (*Candida*, cytomegalovirus, and herpesviruses) and cancer (Kaposi's sarcoma and non-Hodgkin's lymphoma).

DYSPHAGIA OR ODYNOPHAGIA. Difficulty swallowing almost always indicates a significant esophageal pathologic process. Early endoscopy can offer rapid diagnosis of a variety of causes (Schatzki's rings, reflux strictures, or cancers) for which endoscopic therapy may be readily available (e.g., dilation, stent placement, and laser). Barium esophagograms, commonly ordered before endoscopy, may be helpful in severe dysphagia but are unnecessary in most cases.

Odynophagia is most commonly caused by infectious or pill esophagitis for which endoscopy may offer prompt diagnosis and therapeutic guidance.

RADIOGRAPHIC FINDINGS OF ESOPHAGEAL OR GASTRIC ULCERS. Ulcers in the esophagus or stomach always merit endoscopy and biopsy to rule out cancer. A benign radiographic appearance may be misleading, and empirical acid suppression may result in temporary pain relief and even ulcer healing in a small percentage of malignancies. Radiographic findings of mass lesions in the upper gastrointestinal tract are another frequent indication for upper endoscopy with biopsy. Duodenal ulceration without mass effect is rarely neoplastic and does not routinely justify endoscopy. The need for endoscopy with biopsy to document the presence of *H. pylori* will likely diminish when improved noninvasive testing (e.g., breath tests) becomes widely available.

GASTROINTESTINAL BLEEDING. EGD facilitates the diagnosis and treatment of patients with active upper gastrointestinal bleeding and in selected patients with either occult blood loss or iron deficiency anemia when colonoscopy is negative.

SMALL BOWEL BIOPSY. Upper endoscopy can be very helpful in the evaluation of patients with chronic diarrhea when diseases of the small bowel such as celiac sprue are suspected. It may also be used to sample duodenal fluid in cases of suspected bacterial overgrowth or gallbladder microlithiasis.

Contraindications. Absolute contraindications to endoscopy include the following: (1) severe, unstable, or life-threatening cardiac or pulmonary disease; (2) known or suspected perforated viscus; and (3) atlantoaxial instability. Upper endoscopy is also contraindicated in circumstances in which the patient refuses to give informed consent and in those instances in which the patient remains uncooperative despite adequate sedation. Inadequate circulating clotting factors or platelet counts below $60,000/mm^3$ are contraindications to mucosal biopsy. Most authorities recommend stopping aspirin 7 days before and other NSAIDs 2 days before elective endoscopy. Other prescribed medications may be taken up to and including the day of the procedure with small sips of water.

Rationale. The double-contrast upper gastrointestinal series is the main alternative to EGD. Endoscopy is more sensitive and specific than contrast medium–enhanced radiography in the diagnosis of most upper gastrointestinal mucosal disease. Endoscopy for the diagnosis of gastric cancer has published sensitivities of 94% to 100% and specificity of 100%, whereas radiography has a sensitivity of 50% to 89% and a specificity of 95% to 100%. Diagnostic endoscopy is generally quite safe. Patients tolerate endoscopy well, and many prefer it to contrast radiography. The most significant advantage of endoscopy may be the ability to biopsy the mucosa and offer a variety of therapeutic modalities.

The cost of upper endoscopy is decreasing ($789), although it remains relatively expensive when compared with radiography ($312). These figures, based on charges at the University of Washington, include both institutional and professional fees.

Methods. The clinical evaluation before an endoscopy should include a directed history and physical examination. In addition to elucidating the factors prompting the endoscopy one should focus on overall cardiopulmonary status, bleeding disorders, cardiac valvular pathology, swallowing disorders, drug intolerances, signs of unstable dentition, and use of anticoagulants, aspirin, and

NSAIDs. A discussion regarding the nature of the procedure, benefits, alternatives, and risks should occur before scheduling. Patients are generally instructed to avoid oral intake, except for medications, after midnight of the day before the procedure. Patients should be instructed to bring a driver to the procedure because the use of sedation (e.g., meperidine and midazolam) will prohibit operation of a vehicle or heavy machinery or the signing of legal documents until the following day.

Routine diagnostic upper endoscopy should require no more than 15 minutes and usually can be done in the outpatient setting.

Complications. The process of obtaining informed consent dictates that one inform patients that the risks of endoscopy include, but are not limited to, cardiopulmonary complications, perforations, and bleeding. The overall complication rate for diagnostic upper endoscopy is low (0.13%–0.24%), and reports of serious cardiopulmonary complications are fairly uncommon. Continuous monitoring of heart rate and blood pressure, pulse oximetry, and often electrocardiography have become common during endoscopy. Bleeding (0.03%) and perforation are fairly rare occurrences in diagnostic endoscopy. Pharyngeal trauma occurs during intubation in a small but unknown number of patients. The risk of endocarditis is exceedingly low. The American Heart Association recommends antibiotic prophylaxis only during esophageal dilation or sclerotherapy in patients with a history of endocarditis, systemic pulmonary shunts, or prosthetic valves. Most patients who require antibiotics before dental procedures do not need prophylaxis before endoscopy.

Cross-References: Dyspepsia (Chapter 95), Dysphagia and Heartburn (Chapter 96), Peptic Ulcer Disease (Chapter 102).

REFERENCES

1. American Society of Gastrointestinal Endoscopy. Appropriate Use of Gastrointestinal Endoscopy. Manchester, MA, American Society of Gastrointestinal Endoscopy, May 1989.
   Well designed guidelines from the pre–H. pylori era are presented.

2. Axon ATR, et al. Guidelines on appropriate indications for upper gastrointestinal endoscopy. BMJ 1995;310:853–856.
   Several studies show that early endoscopy is cost effective compared with empirical therapy or radiography.

3. Bytzer P, et al. Empirical H2-blocker therapy or prompt endoscopy in management of dyspepsia. Lancet 1994;343:811–816.
   Empirical therapy was associated with higher costs and lower patient satisfaction.

4. Dajani AS, et al. Prevention of bacterial endocarditis: Recommendations by the American Heart Association. JAMA 1990;264:2919–2922.
   Clear and concise guidelines indicate when antibiotic prophylaxis is necessary.

5. Newcomer MK, Brazer SR. Complications of upper gastrointestinal endoscopy and their management. Gastrointest Endosc Clin North Am 1994;4:551–570.
   Therapeutic endoscopy is associated with substantially higher risk, with esophageal dilation, pneumatic dilation for achalasia, and placement of esophageal endoprostheses having the highest risk of perforation.

Musculoskeletal Disorders

106 General Approach to Arthritic Symptoms

Symptom

RICHARD H. WHITE

Epidemiology. Nontraumatic joint pain is a common problem in all age groups. There are more than 200 different causes of arthritis, many with their own unique epidemiology. The prevalence of osteoarthritis varies markedly with age. The radiographic changes of osteoarthritis are noted in less than 5% of individuals younger than age 35 and in over 70% of those aged 65 and older. The annual incidence of rheumatoid arthritis is 2 to 4 per 100,000 adults; the prevalence of definite rheumatoid arthritis is approximately 1%. The prevalence of gout increases with age and with the serum uric acid concentration; in men aged 45 to 64 years, the prevalence is approximately 34 per 1000, and in women it is approximately 14.5 per 1000. The incidence of systemic lupus erythematosus (SLE) is 4 to 6 per 100,000 persons per year, with a prevalence of approximately 50 per 100,000; the disease occurs much more frequently in women and more commonly in blacks.

Synovitis (tender, thickened, palpable synovium, with or without heat and redness) is to be distinguished from traumatic injury, tendinitis (e.g., lateral epicondylitis or heel spur), the myofascial pain syndromes, and fibromyalgia. Synovitis can be classified as monarticular or polyarticular.

MONARTICULAR ARTHRITIS

Epidemiology. The incidence of acute monarticular synovitis increases with advancing age, as crystal-induced arthritides (gout, pseudogout) become more common. Patients with three or fewer affected joints should usually be approached as though they have a monarticular problem.

Etiology. In individuals younger than 40 years old, the most common causes of monarticular synovitis are septic arthritis (particularly gonococcal arthritis), reactive arthritis (Reiter's syndrome), and gout; or it can be a peripheral

Table 106–1. CAUSES OF MONARTICULAR SYNOVITIS

Acute	Chronic
Septic arthritis	Septic arthritis
Neisseria gonorrhoeae	Tuberculosis
Staphylococcus aureus	Fungal arthritis
Streptococci	Lyme disease
Haemophilus influenzae	Chronic gout
Other gram-negative rods	Chronic pseudogout
Gout	Post-traumatic degenerative arthritis
Pseudogout (calcium phosphate	Reactive arthritis
deposition disease)	Loose body, mechanical derangement
Reactive arthritis	Neuropathic arthropathy
Reiter's syndrome	Pigmented villonodular synovitis
Inflammatory bowel disease	Sarcoid arthritis
Acute sarcoidosis	
Acute rheumatic fever	
Spondylitis (HLA-B27 related)	
Psoriatic arthritis	
Aseptic necrosis	
Other: hemarthrosis, mechanical problem,	
initial manifestation of a connective	
tissue disease, metastatic cancer,	
lymphoma	

manifestation of spondylitis or the initial manifestation of a polyarticular disorder (e.g., rheumatoid arthritis) (Table 106–1). After age 40 the most common causes are gout, pseudogout, septic arthritis, and reactive arthritis.

Chronic monarticular arthritis should prompt an evaluation for infection, particularly tuberculous or fungal. Chronic crystal-induced arthritis, primary osteoarthritis, post-traumatic degenerative arthritis, and a persisting reactive arthritis can also lead to chronic monarticular synovitis.

Clinical Approach. The patient should be carefully questioned about sexual activity, history of ocular inflammation (reactive arthritis), pulmonary symptoms (pneumonia, sarcoidosis), bowel symptoms (inflammatory bowel disease, reactive arthritis), genitourinary symptoms (gonococcal disease, reactive arthritis), and previous rash (erythema nodosum with sarcoid and inflammatory bowel disease, erythema chronicum migrans with Lyme disease, psoriasis with psoriatic arthritis). Fever commonly accompanies acute monarticular synovitis associated with septic arthritis, gout, pseudogout, and reactive arthritis. Several days of migratory polyarthralgias may precede the characteristic hemorrhagic skin pustules and synovitis of gonococcal arthritis, which occurs more commonly in women. Acute gout characteristically develops abruptly with striking erythema over the affected joint or joints.

Physical examination of the affected joint or joints may reveal, in addition to an effusion, exquisite pain on motion in any plane (septic arthritis), marked overlying redness (gout), or an adjacent subcutaneous tophus (gout). Other important findings include metastatic lesions (septic arthritis), oral ulcerations (reactive arthritis), ocular inflammation (reactive arthritis, sarcoid), tophi (gout), or signs of skin breakdown (portal of entry for septic arthritis). Although septic arthritis can affect any joint, involvement of certain joints is characteristic of certain diagnoses: the first metatarsophalangeal joint (gout, rarely pseudogout), the isolated small joints of the foot (psoriatic arthritis, reactive arthritis), the midtarsal joints (gout), the ankle (reactive arthritis, gout), the knee (gout, pseudogout, reactive arthritis), and the wrists (pseudogout).

Aspiration of the joint is mandatory to diagnose septic and crystal-induced arthritis. If only a few drops of fluid are available, one drop should be submitted for crystal examination (followed by Gram stain), while the remainder is sent for bacterial and fungal culture. A joint fluid white blood cell count less than 15,000 cells/mm^3 is uncommon in septic arthritis; a count of greater than 100,000 cells/mm^3 is characteristic of infection but is also seen in crystal-induced and reactive arthritis. Polarizing microscopy may reveal intracellular negatively birefringent needle-shaped crystals characteristic of gout, or smaller, rhomboidal, positive birefringent crystals characteristic of pseudogout. Plain radiographs are usually unremarkable but may show findings consistent with gout (erosion with an overhanging lip, tophus), pseudogout (chondrocalcinosis), a neuropathic process (advanced joint destruction), or a loose body. In puzzling cases, a radiograph of the pelvis may reveal bilateral or unilateral sacroiliitis, suggesting that the peripheral arthritis is a manifestation of one of the spondylitides (ankylosing spondylitis, reactive arthritis).

Pending the results of synovial fluid culture and analysis, any patient with fever, severe joint pain, and an elevated synovial fluid white blood cell count should be admitted to the hospital and treated for septic arthritis.

If crystal-induced arthritis is diagnosed, treatment with a nonsteroidal anti-inflammatory drug (NSAID) is usually effective (see Chapter 119, Gout/Hyperuricemia). When NSAID therapy is contraindicated, a tapering dose of prednisone is the treatment of choice. Intra-articular injection of a long-acting corticosteroid preparation is not recommended until a firm diagnosis is established and the arthritis is unresponsive to rest and NSAID therapy.

Follow-Up. Any patient not admitted to the hospital requires close follow-up because the possibility of infection is not excluded until synovial cultures have proved sterile and joint symptoms begin to resolve. The clinician should telephone the patient and schedule a follow-up visit for 2 to 3 days after the initial evaluation. Resolution of crystal-induced arthritis may require several weeks, and in cases of reactive arthritis, it may take weeks to months.

POLYARTICULAR ARTHRITIS

Epidemiology and Etiology. Acute polyarticular synovitis is relatively uncommon in all age groups. Polyarthralgias are common, especially in patients with generalized osteoarthritis.

The most common causes of polyarticular synovitis are (1) postinfectious arthritis (e.g., influenza, coxsackievirus, rubella), (2) rheumatoid arthritis, (3) SLE, (4) reactive arthritis, and (5) psoriatic arthritis (Table 106–2).

Clinical Approach. In patients with physical signs of polyarticular synovitis, the initial diagnostic goal is to exclude life-threatening conditions such as subacute bacterial endocarditis, SLE, and systemic vasculitis. Other useful findings, in

Table 106–2. CAUSES OF ACUTE POLYARTICULAR SYNOVITIS

Causes	Common Features
Common Causes	
Acute viral syndrome	Polyarthralgias, resolution in days to weeks
Rheumatoid arthritis	Metacarpophalangeal joints, wrists, knees, ankles, forefoot, positive rheumatoid factor assay
Systemic lupus erythematosus (SLE)	Hands and large joints, positive antinuclear antibody (ANA) assay, other features of SLE
Reactive arthritis	Oligoarticular, especially joints in the lower extremities
Psoriatic arthritis	Psoriatic rash, oligoarticular or polyarticular disease
Less Common Causes	
Gout	Usually asymmetric, oligoarticular; tophi often present
Pseudogout	Usually oligoarticular, in knees, wrists, elbows
Gonococcal	True synovitis present in only a few joints
Acute rheumatic fever	Lower extremity joints, migratory, elevated antistreptolysin-O titer
Sarcoidosis	Erythema nodosum, hilar adenopathy
Systemic rheumatic diseases	
Sjögren's syndrome	Dry eyes, dry mouth, positive ANA assay
Polymyositis/dermatomyositis	Proximal weakness, characteristic rash, elevated creatine phosphokinase levels
Scleroderma/CREST syndrome	Sclerodactyly, Raynaud's phenomenon, telangiectasia
Mixed connective tissue disease	Raynaud's phenomenon, myositis, positive ANA assay, positive anti-RNP
Still's (adult) disease	Sore throat, fever, evanescent macular rash
Vasculitis	Signs and symptoms of a multisystemic disorder
Polymyalgia rheumatica	Age > 50, high erythrocyte sedimentation rate, shoulder/hip girdle pain
Serum sickness	After exposure to foreign protein
Subacute bacterial endocarditis	Murmur, fever, positive blood cultures
Erosive osteoarthritis	Swelling, heat in interphalangeal joints, radiographic changes

CREST, calcinosis cutis, Raynaud's phenomenon, esophageal dysfunction, sclerodactyly, and telangiectasia.

addition to the pattern of joint involvement, include (1) new onset of severe hypertension (vasculitis), (2) fever (SLE, endocarditis, Still's disease, vasculitis, disseminated gonorrhea, gout), (3) rash (SLE, Still's disease, vasculitis, dermatomyositis, endocarditis, gonococcal arthritis, Behçet's disease), (4) oral ulceration (SLE, viral, Behçet's disease, reactive arthritis), (5) dry eyes and dry mouth (primary Sjögren's syndrome, rheumatoid arthritis, SLE), (6) Raynaud's phenomenon (scleroderma, mixed connective tissue disease, SLE), (7) ocular inflammation (SLE, reactive arthritis, Behçet's disease, sarcoidosis), and (8) serositis (SLE, vasculitis, familial Mediterranean fever). Certain combinations of findings may be diagnostic (e.g., malar rash, serositis, and arthritis for SLE; diarrhea, arthritis, and uveitis for reactive arthritis).

Initial laboratory testing should include a complete blood cell count, platelet count, urinalysis, and serum creatine phosphokinase (CPK), creatinine, and liver function tests. Hemolytic anemia or thrombocytopenia suggests SLE; leukopenia is compatible with SLE or human immunodeficiency virus infection. An elevated CPK level suggests myositis or vasculitis. Proteinuria or urinary casts suggest a systemic immune complex process (subacute bacterial endocarditis, SLE, vasculitis). Radiographs of the involved joints are not usually helpful unless symptoms persist for weeks to months, after which findings typical of rheumatoid arthritis, psoriatic arthritis, or erosive osteoarthritis may appear.

Other tests include the following: (1) blood cultures if there is *any* suspicion of endocarditis; (2) arthrocentesis and synovial fluid analysis, including white blood cell count, crystal examination, and culture; (3) antinuclear antibody assay (see Chapter 123, Interpretation of Serologic Tests); (4) rheumatoid factor assay; (5) chest radiography to look for infiltrates, fibrosis, hilar adenopathy, or pleural effusion; and (6) serum complement levels (C3 and CH_{50}). Low levels of serum complement are consistent with immune complex formation (SLE, serum sickness, endocarditis, hepatitis); high levels indicate an acute phase reactant (reactive arthritis, rheumatoid arthritis, polymyalgia rheumatica).

Other more specific serologic tests should be ordered only when clinical findings indicate an appreciable probability (e.g., pretest probability > 20%) that a particular disease is present (e.g., antineutrophil cytoplasmic antibody in patients with suspected Wegener's granulomatosis).

Management. If the symptoms of the polyarthritis are mild and if endocarditis or sepsis is unlikely, outpatient management is appropriate. If sepsis or endocarditis is suspected or if an acute multisystemic disorder (SLE or vasculitis) is likely, the patient should be admitted to the hospital. Pending the results of initial studies, outpatients can be managed with NSAIDs and bed rest; physical therapy with daily range-of-motion exercises should be ordered as soon as possible to preserve the function of the involved joints. If joint inflammation is profound and does not respond to these measures, referral for rheumatologic evaluation is recommended. Low-dose prednisone (7.5 mg/d) can be given to patients with suspected rheumatoid arthritis who do not respond to nonsteroidal therapy.

Follow-Up. Outpatients started on anti-inflammatory drugs should be followed in 2 to 3 days to monitor the patient's response to therapy.

Cross-References: Psoriasis (Chapter 32), Redness of the Eye (Chapter 37), Dry Eyes and Excessive Tearing (Chapter 38), Pleural Effusion (Chapter 65), Inflammatory Bowel Disease (Chapter 97), Low Back Pain (Chapter 107), Shoulder Pain (Chapter 108), Hip Pain (Chapter 109), Wrist and Hand Pain (Chapter 110), Knee Pain (Chapter 111), Ankle and Foot Pain (Chapter 112), Polymyalgia Rheumatica and Temporal Arteritis (Chapter 117), Osteoarthritis (Chapter 118), Gout/Hyperuricemia (Chapter 119), Interpretation of Serologic Tests (Chapter 123), Physical Therapy Care of Outpatients (Chapter 125), Aspiration/Injection of the Knee (Chapter 129), Sexually Transmitted Diseases (Chapter 176).

REFERENCES

1. Arnett FC. Revised criteria for the classification of rheumatoid arthritis. Bull Rheum Dis 1989;38(5):1–6.

   The diagnostic performance of the 1987 revised criteria for rheumatoid arthritis is reported using both the traditional format and a classification tree. The sensitivity is approximately 92%, and the specificity is approximately 89%.

2. Goldenberg DL, Cohen AS. Acute infectious arthritis. Am J Med 1976;60:369–377.

This is a classic article on the bacteriology of acute infectious arthritis and the response to antibiotic treatment plus needle aspiration.

3. Hochberg MC, ed. Epidemiology of rheumatic diseases. Rheumatol Clin North Am 1990;16:499–781.

The entire volume is devoted to the epidemiology of common rheumatic diseases.

4. McCune WJ. Monarticular arthritis. In Kelly WN, Harris ED, Ruddy S, Sledge CB, eds. Textbook of Rheumatology. Philadelphia, WB Saunders, 1989.

An exhaustive discussion is presented.

5. Resnick D, Williams G, Weisman MH, Slaughter L. Rheumatoid arthritis and pseudorheumatoid arthritis in calcium pyrophosphate dihydrate crystal deposition disease. Radiology 1981;140:615–621.

That calcium pyrophosphate dihydrate deposition can mimic rheumatoid arthritis is emphasized.

6. Sargent JS. Polyarticular arthritis. In Kelly WN, Harris ED, Ruddy S, Sledge CB, eds. Textbook of Rheumatology. Philadelphia, WB Saunders, 1989.

This chapter reviews the fundamental differential diagnosis of polyarthritis.

107 Low Back Pain

Symptom

RICHARD A. DEYO

Epidemiology. Nearly 80% of adults have low back pain at some time during their lives. About 14% have an episode of back pain that persists longer than 2 weeks, but only 2% have back pain associated with sciatica, the symptom associated with most cases of herniated disks or spinal stenosis. Lumbar disk herniation occurs most often in 30- to 50-year-old adults, whereas spinal stenosis is most common after age 50.

Etiology. Pain may result from "mechanical" back problems, systemic diseases that affect the spine, and visceral diseases that cause back pain. At least 95% of all back pain is due to mechanical causes, most commonly muscle sprains and strains, degenerative disk disease, and, in older adults, osteoporosis with compression fractures. Herniated disks and spinal stenosis account for only a small proportion of cases. Less common causes include anatomic abnormalities such as spondylolisthesis, severe scoliosis, and some transitional vertebrae. Because an exact diagnosis is often impossible to establish, as many as 85% of patients with back pain will never receive a definitive diagnosis.

"Systemic" causes, which account for less than 2% of cases, include neoplastic, infectious, and inflammatory diseases. Metastatic breast, lung, and prostate cancer are the most common malignancies. Osteomyelitis and epidural abscesses are occasionally found in patients with risk factors such as urinary tract infection, skin infection, or intravenous drug use. The prototypical inflammatory disorder is ankylosing spondylitis. Visceral diseases that cause low back pain include prostatitis, endometriosis, pyelonephritis, nephrolithiasis, and aortic aneurysms.

Clinical Approach. Because definitive diagnosis is often impossible, the initial evaluation should focus on three basic questions: (1) Is there a systemic or visceral cause of pain? (2) Is there neurologic compromise that may require surgical referral? (3) Are other findings present that influence management decisions, regardless of the precise etiology?

Features that raise the suspicion of systemic causes include age older than 50 years, a previous history of cancer, unexplained weight loss, fever, drug or alcohol abuse, corticosteroid use (predisposing to infection), and pain unresponsive to conservative therapy within a few weeks. Ankylosing spondylitis is rare; it occurs most often in men younger than age 40 and is characterized by morning stiffness, improvement with exercise, and a gradual onset.

The only true surgical emergency is the cauda equina syndrome, characterized by urinary retention, saddle anesthesia, and bilateral leg weakness and numbness.

Sciatica is usually the first clue to nerve root irritation and possible neurologic compromise. Sciatica is a sharp or burning pain, usually associated with numbness, that radiates down the posterior or lateral leg and is often aggravated by coughing or sneezing. Radiation below the knee is a more specific indicator of sciatica than is isolated thigh pain.

The most common cause of sciatica is a herniated disk, 95% of which occur at the L4-5 or L5-S1 levels. L5 nerve root involvement results in weakness of the great toe extensors and other dorsiflexors of the foot and in sensory loss along the medial aspect of the foot and in the web space between the first and second toes. Compromise of the S1 nerve root leads to a diminished ankle reflex, weak plantarflexors of the foot, and sensory deficits of the posterior calf and lateral foot. Almost 90% of patients with a herniated disk will have either weak foot dorsiflexion or diminished ankle reflexes. Abnormal straight-leg raising (less than 60 degrees) is found in approximately 80% of patients with a herniated disk but is nonspecific (i.e., it is found in other conditions as well).

Other factors may also influence the choice of therapy, regardless of specific pathoanatomic derangements. For example, narcotic analgesics, highly appropriate in patients with acute severe sciatica, should generally be avoided in patients with chronic pain syndromes (see Chapter 14, Chronic Nonspecific Pain Syndrome). A neurologic deficit probably mandates longer and stricter bed rest. Frank depression or inconsistent physical findings suggest a need for psychological evaluation. Disability compensation proceedings may strongly influence patient perceptions, expectations, behavior, and prognosis.

Plain radiographs of the spine, often unhelpful or even misleading, are recommended only after trauma or when systemic disease is likely (Fig. 107–1). An erythrocyte sedimentation rate greater than 20 mm/h is relatively sensitive for metastatic cancer (about 80%) or infection (90%) but nonspecific. It may be a useful "screening" test for systemic diseases. Computed tomography or magnetic resonance imaging may be misleading, demonstrating herniated disks in over 20% of normal persons without back pain. These studies are indicated only when systemic disease or surgery is a serious consideration (Table 107–1).

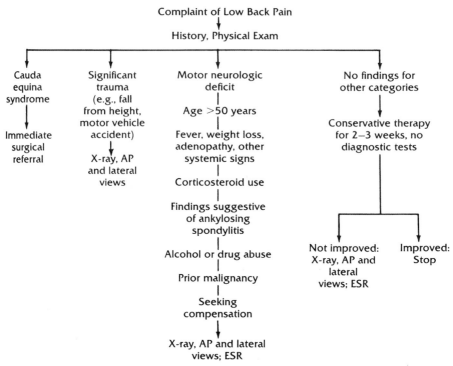

Figure 107–1. Algorithm for the initial approach to a patient with low back pain. Subsequent diagnostic testing is highly individualized, depending on results of the tests shown here, clinical findings, and response to initial therapy. ESR, erythrocyte sedimentation rate. (From Deyo RA. Early diagnostic evaluation of low back pain. J Gen Intern Med 1986;1:328–338. Reproduced by permission.)

Management. The most common error in management is failure to provide patients with strong reassurance and an explanation of their symptoms. The prognosis of acute low back pain is excellent. Discussions with the patient should avoid frightening labels such as "ruptured" disk, "degenerative" spine disease, or even "injury," because these terms imply serious tissue damage that

Table 107–1. INDICATIONS FOR SURGICAL REFERRAL IN THE PATIENT WITH SCIATICA

Cauda equina syndrome (a surgical emergency): characterized by bowel and bladder dysfunction (usually urine retention), saddle anesthesia, bilateral leg weakness, and numbness
Progressive or severe neurologic deficit
Persistent neuromotor deficit after 4 to 6 weeks of conservative therapy
Persistent sciatica, sensory deficit, or reflex loss after 4 to 6 weeks in a patient with positive straight-leg raising sign, consistent clinical findings, and favorable psychosocial circumstances (e.g., realistic expectations; no evidence of depression, substance abuse, or excessive somatization)

From Deyo RA, Loeser JD, Bigos SJ. Herniated lumbar intervertebral disk. Ann Intern Med 1990;112:598–603.

often cannot be documented. Nonthreatening terms such as "muscle strain" or "changes due to wear and tear" are preferable.

For some patients without neurologic deficits, brief bed rest (2 to 3 days) helps reduce pain but does not improve the natural history. Studies suggest that early return to normal activities is usually preferable to either bed rest or early exercise programs. Patients with neurologic deficits may benefit from brief bed rest (e.g., up to 4 days), but with periods of ambulation beginning on day 3. Nonsteroidal anti-inflammatory drugs, including aspirin, relieve pain. Muscle relaxants such as carisoprodol are occasionally beneficial. Use of muscle relaxants and narcotic analgesics should be strictly time limited (e.g., 1 week). Growing evidence suggests that spinal manipulation may be useful for symptom relief in acute back pain.

After the acute phase (about 2 to 4 weeks), patients should be encouraged to begin an exercise program. Strengthening and endurance exercises for the back and lower extremities, as well as general aerobic fitness exercises, improve mobility, reduce fatigue, and decrease the likelihood of recurrences. Weight loss and smoking cessation should be encouraged, because obesity and cigarette smoking have been implicated in epidemiologic studies as causal factors for back pain (nicotine may impair diskal nutrition, raise intradiskal pressure due to coughing, or simply be a marker for anxiety and depression, which prolong pain symptoms).

Complete cure of chronic back pain (more than 3 months) is an unrealistic expectation. Prolonged pain does not warrant surgery in the absence of neurologic and imaging findings that indicate surgically reversible disease. Physical therapy (with emphasis on exercise) and specific pain treatment programs are modalities that may help to restore function. The efficacy of antidepressant drugs in this setting remains uncertain.

Hospitalization is rarely necessary for patients with low back pain unless surgery is scheduled. Indications for surgical referral appear in Table 107–1.

Follow-Up. Patients should be advised to schedule a return visit if they are not improved within 3 weeks. The prognosis of acute low back pain is excellent, with about 80% experiencing substantial improvement within 2 to 3 weeks. Even patients with herniated disks and neurologic deficits usually improve, and most do not require surgery. Most patients will experience recurrence of back pain within 3 to 4 years. Chronic pain carries a less favorable prognosis but may still respond to appropriate management. Other poor prognostic factors include a low educational status, excessive somatization, disability compensation proceedings, and inflexible or unpleasant job circumstances.

Cross-References: Determining Disability: The Primary Physician's Role (Chapter 5), Smoking Cessation (Chapter 12), Chronic Nonspecific Pain Syndrome (Chapter 14), Obesity (Chapter 15), Osteoporosis (Chapter 116), Management of Pain in Patients with Cancer (Chapter 207).

REFERENCES

1. Bigos SJ, Braen G, Bowyer O, et al. Acute low back problems in adults: Assessment and treatment. Clinical Practice Guideline No. 14, AHCPR publication No. 95-0643, Agency for

Health Care Policy and Research, US Department of Health and Human Services, December 1994.

This comprehensive clinical guideline is evidence-based and was produced by a multidisciplinary panel.

2. Deyo RA. Early diagnostic evaluation of low back pain. J Gen Intern Med 1986;1:328–338.

This article focuses on details of the history and physical examination and the value of plain radiography. The algorithm in Figure 107–1 was suggested by this review.

3. Deyo RA, Loeser JD, Bigos SJ. Herniated lumbar intervertebral disc. Ann Intern Med 1990;112:598–603.

The primary care approach to patients with sciatica and suspected disk herniations is reviewed, including indications for surgery.

4. Jensen MC, Brant-Zawadzki MN, Obuchowski N, Modic MT, Malkasian D, Ross JS. Magnetic resonance imaging of the lumbar spine in people without back pain. N Engl J Med 1994;331:69–73.

Over half of "normal" persons had bulging disks, and over one fourth had herniated disks, suggesting that irrelevant and coincidental findings are common with advanced imaging.

5. Malmivaara A, Hakkinen U, Aro T, et al. The treatment of acute low back pain—bed rest, exercises, or ordinary activity? N Engl J Med 1995;332:351–355.

Early return to normal activity was superior to either bed rest or early exercise for patients with acute low back pain.

....

108 Shoulder Pain

Symptom

STEPHAN D. FIHN

Epidemiology and Etiology. Shoulder pain is one of the most common reasons for visiting a primary care provider. It is a frequent problem particularly among the elderly. Probably the most common cause is inflammation of the rotator cuff tendon (especially the supraspinatus) or subacromial bursa, which lies between the deltoid muscle and the rotator cuff tendon (a conjoint tendon of the supraspinatus, infraspinatus, teres minor, and subscapularis muscles). Almost without fail, the reason for inflammation is chronic irritation from impingement of the rotator cuff tendon between the humeral head and the acromion. *Subacromial bursitis,* also known as rotator cuff tendinitis, supraspinatus tendinitis, and painful arc syndrome, usually affects patients older than age 60, often as a result of earlier occupational overuse of the shoulder or, in younger patients, as a result of sports such as swimming.

Much less common are *partial or complete tears of the rotator cuff,* which occur predominantly in patients older than age 50. The supraspinatus is the tendon most often involved. Overuse is often a predisposing factor, although abrupt tears may occur in patients with weakened rotator cuffs who sustain a strain or fall.

Frozen shoulder (adhesive capsulitis) is most common during middle age and is more prevalent in women than in men. It generally follows a period of immobilization that results from trauma to the shoulder, rotator cuff or bicipital tendinitis, rheumatoid arthritis, stroke, myocardial infarction, cervical radiculopathy, herpes zoster infection, distal injuries to the arm, mastectomy, or chest wall surgery. It is also associated with diabetes. Originally thought to be an adhesive bursitis, frozen shoulder is now considered by many experts to be a neuromuscular problem within the spectrum of reflex sympathetic dystrophy (see later).

As described in Chapter 122, *myofascial pain* is a controversial entity of unknown etiology that may involve the shoulder musculature. It typically develops after carrying heavy objects or using the shoulder in an unaccustomed fashion.

It is often erroneously assumed that many cases of shoulder pain are due to *osteoarthritis of the glenohumeral joint*. In fact, in the absence of prior direct trauma, isolated degenerative arthritis of the joint is much less common than periarticular causes of pain and almost always occurs in association with disease of the rotator cuff.

Bicipital tendinitis often occurs in conjunction with rotator cuff tendinitis and is less common as an isolated condition, in which case it typically results from repetitive stress such as overhead painting or ball throwing.

Reflex sympathetic dystrophy (shoulder-hand syndrome, Sudek's atrophy) is an uncommon disorder that manifests with shoulder pain accompanied by signs and symptoms involving the arm, forearm, and hand. These include pain and swelling in the upper extremity, trophic skin changes (atrophy, hyperpigmentation, hypertrichosis, hyperhidrosis, nail changes), and signs of vasomotor instability. The condition is almost always bilateral to some degree, and as with frozen shoulder, there is usually a precipitating event. The etiology is unknown but is postulated to be related to autonomic dysfunction that causes rapidly progressive osteopenia and erosions plus a proliferative synovitis.

Pain from cervical radiculopathy (most often from the C5 region) may radiate to the shoulder. Pain may also be referred to the shoulder in a variety of diseases, including diaphragmatic irritation from gallbladder disease, subphrenic processes, pulmonary infarction, ruptured viscus, Pancoast's tumor, or myocardial infarction. Exceedingly rare causes of shoulder pain include amyloidosis, acromegaly, hemophilia, thoracic outlet syndrome, and brachial neuritis.

Clinical Approach. Most causes of shoulder pain can be identified from the history and physical examination; radiographs are not always necessary. Key elements of the history are acuteness of onset, types of recent activity, a history of distant or recent trauma, stiffness, pain at night, and weakness. Both shoulders should be examined, with the unaffected side used for comparison. The presence of atrophy, swelling, deformity, or tenderness should be noted, with particular attention paid to the area of the supraspinatus tendon (immediately caudal and anterior to the acromion) and to the bicipital groove (points anteriorly with the arm in 10 degrees of internal rotation). Active range of motion should be observed with the patient sitting and moving the arm through forward flexion. External rotation is measured with the arm fully adducted and the elbow flexed to 90 degrees. Internal rotation is checked by having the patient move the thumb up the spine as far as possible, with assistance from the other hand if necessary. Passive range of motion should be performed with the patient supine to eliminate rotation of the thorax and reflex guarding.

There is usually no history of trauma in patients with subacromial bursitis and supraspinatus tendinitis. The pain begins gradually over several days and is more severe at night, particularly when lying on the affected side. Pain may be limited to the subacromial region or may extend around the shoulder girdle or down the arm. Subacromial tenderness is present and occasionally extends into the bicipital groove. A classic finding is a "painful arc" of abduction between 40 and 120 degrees. The patient will limit true abduction by elevating the shoulder. Internal rotation is painful; external rotation is normal. The "impingement sign" may be positive, producing subacromial pain when the arm is forwardly elevated to the maximum while the shoulder girdle is depressed. The diagnosis is confirmed by subacromial injection of 1 to 2 mL of 1% lidocaine, which greatly improves pain and function. In straightforward cases, radiographs are unnecessary, but they may demonstrate calcium in the supraspinatus tendon if they are obtained.

The pain of rotator cuff tears is indistinguishable from that of rotator cuff tendinitis. After acute tears there may be accumulation of fluid in the subacromial bursa, causing swelling. In more long-standing cases, atrophy of the supraspinatus and infraspinatus may be detectable. Passive range of motion is usually normal, but pain and limitation of active range of motion are present. Subacromial instillation of lidocaine relieves the pain but weakness persists, sometimes apparent in the patient's inability to maintain the arm at 90 degrees of abduction (drop arm sign). Plain radiographs of the shoulder may show the humeral head to be osteopenic and to ride high against the acromion. Arthrography shows extravasation of contrast material from the glenohumeral joint into the subacromial bursa. Ultrasound, computed tomography, and magnetic resonance imaging can display tears of the rotator cuff. Ultrasound ($200) and computed tomography (typically $600–$700) are less expensive and more readily available, whereas magnetic resonance imaging may be more accurate, with a sensitivity of 92% and specificity of over 90% for complete tears. Partial tears may not be visible.

Symptoms of frozen shoulder overlap with those of subacromial bursitis and rotator cuff tears. Patients present with mild to moderate shoulder pain or stiffness of subacute onset. Atrophy of the shoulder girdle may be present. There is restricted range of active and passive motion in *all* planes. Typically, abduction is limited to less than 40 degrees and external rotation to no more than 30 degrees. Instillation of lidocaine in the subacromial space does not substantially improve function. Radiographs are not specific, although osteoporosis of the humeral head is common. Not required for diagnosis, arthrography shows a small, tight joint capsule.

Patients with myofascial shoulder pain usually give no history of prior shoulder problems. The pain may be localized around the shoulder or may extend down the arm. Trigger points may be identified in one or more locations, including the supraspinatus, infraspinatus, and teres minor. Radiographs are normal.

In bicipital tendinitis, pain is the predominant symptom and may involve the entire shoulder girdle. Both active and passive range of motion are usually normal, although sometimes performed tentatively. Resisted flexion and supination of the forearm is painful (Yergason's sign). There is tenderness in the bicipital groove, but unless it is extreme, this finding is nonspecific. Calcifications of the biceps tendon are uncommon.

In reflex sympathetic dystrophy there is often burning pain of the shoulder and hand, occasionally with swelling. Radiographs demonstrate osteopenia, and radionuclide bone scans often demonstrate marked uptake on the affected side.

Management. Initial treatment of subacromial bursitis consists of nonsteroidal anti-inflammatory drugs, avoidance of stressful use of the shoulder, and rest for 2 weeks, followed by exercise (Table 108–1). Codman's pendulum exercises are performed by flexing slightly at the waist and gently swinging a 6- to 8-lb weight (e.g., a plastic milk jug filled with water) in a slow circular motion to increase the subacromial space with traction. Isometric exercise should also be performed with a loop of surgical tubing placed over the hands, palms in opposition, and externally rotating at the shoulder. Instillation of an aqueous steroid preparation into the subacromial bursa may help some patients who do not respond to these measures (see Chapter 127, Injection of the Subacromial Bursa). A second injection may be performed in 6 to 8 weeks if the first fails to provide relief. Arthrography, ultrasonography, or computed tomography may be warranted. Small tears of the rotator cuff may heal with conservative treatment similar to that for tendinitis or bursitis. Larger tears require surgical repair.

Physical therapy is the mainstay of treatment for frozen shoulder and consists of daily firm but gentle range-of-motion exercises. The patient may begin by "loosening up" with a warm shower. In the supine position, the contralateral arm is used to move the affected shoulder, using a stick behind the back if necessary to assist with external rotation. Intra-articular corticosteroid injections may be helpful.

Therapy for myofascial pain involves cessation of the aggravating activity, nonsteroidal anti-inflammatory drugs, and heat. If symptoms fail to abate with these measures, stretching exercises plus application of a vapocoolant spray may be helpful, or the trigger point may be injected with 1% lidocaine.

Table 108–1. COMMON SHOULDER SYNDROMES

Problem	Symptoms and Signs	Treatment
Rotator cuff tendinitis and subacromial bursitis	Gradual onset of pain, especially at night; subacromial tenderness; "painful arc"	Initially NSAIDs and rest 2 wk; if no response at 4 to 6 wk, intrabursal corticosteroid injection; then exercises
Rotator cuff tear	Similar to above but weakness that persists after intrabursal lidocaine injection	For partial tears, same as above ± corticosteroid injection; for complete tears, referral to orthopedic surgeon

Treatment of bicipital tendinitis is similar to that for rotator cuff tendinitis. Injection of corticosteroids around the tendon may help in stubborn cases.

Early treatment of reflex sympathetic dystrophy with high-dose corticosteroids (i.e., 60 mg/d of prednisone, tapered over 4–6 weeks) appears beneficial. If this fails, sympathetic blocks and, in refractory cases, sympathectomy may be considered.

Follow-Up. Early follow-up in person or by telephone helps to determine if therapy is effective and helps to reinforce recommended exercises. Referral to a physical therapist for a few visits often helps to speed recovery. Chronic pain or limitation of motion lasting more than 3 to 6 months suggests chronic impingement of the acromion on the rotator cuff or a rotator cuff tear and should prompt orthopedic referral.

Cross-References: Myofascial Pain Syndromes (Chapter 122), Physical Therapy Care of Outpatients (Chapter 125), Trigger Point Injection (Chapter 126), Injection of the Subacromial Bursa (Chapter 127).

REFERENCES

1. Kozin F, McCarty DJ, Sims J, Genant H. The reflex sympathetic dystrophy syndrome: 1. Clinical and histologic studies. Evidence for bilaterality, response to corticosteroids and articular involvement. Am J Med 1976;60:321–338.

   A classic study of 11 patients, delineating clinical and radiologic features and demonstrating improvement with prednisolone, 60 to 80 mg/d for 2 weeks and tapered over 12 weeks. Unfortunately, the evaluation of treatment was uncontrolled.

2. Matsen FA III, Kirby RM. Office evaluation and management of shoulder pain. Orthop Clin North Am 1982;13:453–475.

   An orthopedist's view is presented. Examination of the shoulder is described and shoulder exercises are illustrated.

3. Rogers LF, Hendrix RW. The painful shoulder. Radiol Clin North Am 1988;26:1359–1371.

   The radiographic appearance of common and uncommon problems of the shoulder is described with plain radiographs, arthrograms, and computed tomography scans.

4. Simkin PA. Tendinitis and bursitis of the shoulder: Anatomy and therapy. Postgrad Med 1983;73:177–190.

   The author provides an excellent description of the anatomy, pathophysiology, diagnosis, and management of these problems.

5. Smith DL, Campbell SM. Painful shoulder syndromes: Diagnosis and management. J Gen Intern Med 1992;7:328–339.

   This thorough review includes clear descriptions and illustrations.

109 Hip Pain

Symptom

GREGORY C. GARDNER

Etiology. Hip pain may originate from disease within the joint (articular), from conditions outside the joint (periarticular), or from a more distant source (referred) (Table 109–1). Most patients seen by the primary care physician have bursitis, myofascial conditions, or osteoarthritis.

Clinical Approach. Examination should focus on range of motion of the patient's hip, palpation of surrounding structures, stance, and gait. It is especially important to recognize soft tissue causes of pain. Having the patient point to the area of pain is helpful in sorting out the various diagnostic possibilities.

ARTHRITIS. Arthritis of the hip joint itself usually manifests with groin pain, sometimes radiating to the knee. Although *osteoarthritis* generally causes pain aggravated by weight bearing, advanced disease may cause rest pain that is especially severe at night. Physical examination in early osteoarthritis reveals loss of hip extension and internal rotation. Radiographs may show characteristic changes. The pain of *inflammatory arthritis* is sometimes continuous and is accompanied by morning stiffness that lasts for hours but improves with use. To distinguish rheumatoid arthritis from ankylosing spondylitis, the two most common causes of inflammatory arthritis of the hip, the pattern of other joints affected and radiographs are helpful. Patients with *infectious arthritis* of the hip usually experience fever and intense groin pain. During examination they hold the hip in slight flexion and resist any attempt to move it. The most common responsible organism is *Staphylococcus aureus*.

BURSITIS. Of 18 bursae found around the hip, only 3 typically cause hip pain. Patients with *trochanteric bursitis* usually complain of pain during ambula-

---

Table 109–1. DIFFERENTIAL DIAGNOSIS OF PAIN IN THE HIP REGION

Arthritis	Neuropathy
Osteoarthritis	Lateral femoral cutaneous nerve
Rheumatoid arthritis	Miscellaneous
Ankylosing spondylitis	Femoral/inguinal hernias
Infectious arthritis	Referred pain
Bursitis	Fractures
Trochanteric	Osteonecrosis
Iliopsoas	Tumors
Ischial	
Myofascial syndromes	
Tensor fascia lata fasciitis	
Fibromyalgia	
Muscle/tendon strains	

tion or when lying on the affected side. On examination the trochanteric bursa, located just posterior and superior to the greater trochanter, is tender. The *iliopsoas bursa* lies behind the iliopsoas muscle, lateral to the femoral vessels and just anterior to the hip joint. When it is inflamed, pain may be felt in the thigh, pelvis, or groin. On examination, the bursa is tender and patients hold the hip in flexion to avoid painful extension. Computed tomography is rarely indicated but may help distinguish iliopsoas bursitis from an intra-articular pathologic process in refractory cases. *Ischial bursitis,* or "weaver's bottom," is most often caused by prolonged sitting. Tenderness is found over the ischial tuberosity.

MYOFASCIAL CONDITIONS. The iliotibial band is a wide band of fascia that begins at the lateral ilium and ends at the lateral knee. The taut fascia may slip over the greater tuberosity and cause painless snapping of the hip. In others, the fascia becomes inflamed, causing a dull ache at the lateral hip and thigh. Stretching the fascia reproduces the pain and confirms the diagnosis: the patient lies with the affected side up while the straightened leg is adducted and drawn over the edge of the examining table. *Iliac apophysitis* describes a condition in which maximal tenderness is found over the iliac crest at the insertion of the tensor fascia lata.

Fibromyalgia occurs most often in women and leads to generalized body pain, sleep disturbances, fatigue, headache, and irritable bowel symptoms (see Chapter 121). Of the many tender points present, two near the hip are located at the trochanteric bursa and high gluteal areas.

A variety of muscle strains may produce hip pain, including strains of the hip adductors, abductors, and hamstrings. The patient interview usually uncovers injury or overuse. Maximal tenderness is located in the specific muscles or their insertions, and isometric contraction of the specific muscles reproduces the pain.

ENTRAPMENT NEUROPATHY. Entrapment of the lateral femoral cutaneous nerve at the anterior superior iliac spine (meralgia paresthetica) causes painful paresthesia in the groin and lateral thigh (see Chapter 144, Entrapment Neuropathies).

MISCELLANEOUS. Femoral or inguinal hernias may cause groin pain and are easily found during examination. Pain from sacroiliac joint arthritis, lumbar radiculopathies (especially L3-L4 disk herniations), and renal colic may be referred to the hip region.

Although most hip fractures cause acute pain, stress fractures may be more insidious and may be apparent on bone scans long before radiographs are abnormal.

Risk factors for *osteonecrosis of the femoral head* include corticosteroid use, alcohol abuse, hemoglobinopathies, scuba diving, and systemic lupus erythematosus. Patients note pain with weight bearing and at night. Radiographs, normal in early disease, eventually show progressive collapse of the femoral head. Magnetic resonance imaging is the most sensitive test for early diagnosis, and a limited screening with this modality can be used to reduce costs when evaluating possible osteonecrosis. The more extensive the femoral head involvement, the more the disease will progress.

A variety of *tumors* may metastasize to the acetabulum and femoral head, including those of prostate, breast, thyroid, renal, and lung cancer. Osteoid osteoma, a benign tumor, may involve the femoral head or neck and cause severe pain that sometimes responds dramatically to aspirin. Bone scans are the most sensitive diagnostic tests for osteoid osteoma and metastatic tumors.

Management

ARTHRITIS. Treatment of arthritis of the hip depends on the specific cause (see Chapter 118, Osteoarthritis). Because septic arthritis of the hip can cause rapid destruction of the hip, hospitalization, parenteral antibiotic administration, and urgent consultation with an orthopedic surgeon is mandatory.

BURSITIS. Treatment of bursitis includes local heat and ultrasound, massage, gentle stretching exercises, and anti-inflammatory medication. Local corticosteroid injections are often helpful (see Chapter 128, Injection of the Trochanteric Bursa).

MYOFASCIAL CONDITIONS. The treatment for tensor fascia lata tendinitis includes physical therapy with stretching, massage, local application of heat and ultrasound, and anti-inflammatory medication. Injection of a local anesthetic into particularly tender areas is also helpful (see Chapter 122). Most muscle strains are self-limited. Analgesic medication and local application of ice relieve acute pain. If symptoms persist, physical therapy and anti-inflammatory medications are beneficial.

MISCELLANEOUS. No satisfactory treatment exists for established osteonecrosis of the femoral head. Modification of risk factors may help prevent other joints from being similarly affected. Patients with advanced disease may require joint replacement for pain relief.

The treatment of osteoid osteoma is surgical excision.

Cross-References: Low Back Pain (Chapter 107), Osteoporosis (Chapter 116), Osteoarthritis (Chapter 118), Fibromyalgia (Chapter 121), Myofascial Pain Syndromes (Chapter 122), Physical Therapy Care of Outpatients (Chapter 125), Trigger Point Injection (Chapter 126), Injection of the Trochanteric Bursa (Chapter 128), Entrapment Neuropathies (Chapter 144).

REFERENCES

1. Polisson RP. Sports medicine for the internist. Med Clin North Am 1986;70:469–489.
2. Simkin PA, Gardner GC. Osteonecrosis: pathogenesis and practicalities. Hosp Pract 1994;29(3):73–84.

   Both of these sources discuss various musculoskeletal problems commonly encountered in athletes (including hip pain) and provide otherwise hard-to-find information on iliac apophysitis.

110 Wrist and Hand Pain

Symptom

GREGORY C. GARDNER

Etiology. Table 110–1 is a list of the most common conditions causing wrist and hand pain, organized by anatomic abnormality. Traumatic conditions are not covered in this chapter.

Clinical Approach. Evaluation of the hand and wrist focuses on careful inspection for swelling and deformity, palpation, and range-of-motion testing.

ARTHRITIS. Although it may be difficult to distinguish arthritis from tenosynovitis, passive movement of the affected joint causes pain in arthritis but not in tenosynovitis. Active movement causes pain in both conditions.

The pattern of joint involvement differentiates the various forms of arthritis. Helpful laboratory tests include assays for antinuclear antibodies and rheumatoid factor, determination of erythrocyte sedimentation rate, and synovial fluid crystal analysis and culture. *Osteoarthritis* involves the distal interphalangeal joints and proximal interphalangeal joints, sparing the metacarpophalangeal joints. Heberden's and Bouchard's nodes are often found. *Rheumatoid arthritis* involves the metacarpophalangeal and proximal interphalangeal joints and wrists in a symmetric pattern. Patients with *gout* may have tophaceous deposits about the digits. *Psoriatic arthritis* may involve any joint of the hand or wrist, usually asymmetrically, and is often associated with a characteristic rash and pitting of the nails.

The clinician must have a high degree of suspicion for *infectious arthritis,* especially when monarthritis affects the wrist. Bacterial arthritis rarely affects the small joints of the hand except after puncture wounds (e.g., human bites). Disseminated gonococcal infection may cause an acute arthritis associated with tenosynovitis and vesiculopustular skin lesions.

TENOSYNOVITIS. *Flexor tenosynovitis* may produce a trigger finger, which oc-

Table 110–1. CONDITIONS CAUSING WRIST AND HAND PAIN

Arthritis	Neuropathy
Osteoarthritis	Carpal tunnel syndrome
Rheumatoid arthritis	Ulnar nerve entrapment
Psoriatic arthritis	Cutaneous Inflammation
Systemic lupus erythematosus	Paronychia
Crystal arthropathies	Felon
Infectious arthritis	Cellulitis/lymphangitis
Tenosynovitis	Miscellaneous
Flexor tenosynovitis	Raynaud's phenomenon
de Quervain's tenosynovitis	Reflex sympathetic dystrophy
Ganglions	

curs when the inflamed tendon, often with a palpable nodular thickening, impinges on the flexor pulley located at the base of the finger. Tenosynovitis of the abductor pollicis longus and the extensor pollicis brevis tendons (*de Quervain's*) results in a tender distal radius and positive Finkelstein's test (with the thumb gripped beneath the fingers, ulnar deviation of the wrist reproduces the pain). *Ganglions* are synovial cysts that are typically located on the dorsum of the wrist but may also occur over metacarpophalangeal joints. They are occasionally painful and may interfere with joint motion.

NEUROPATHY. *Carpal tunnel syndrome* (median nerve entrapment) and *ulnar nerve entrapment* cause numbness, tingling, and sometimes weakness in the distribution of the affected nerve (see Chapter 144, Entrapment Neuropathies).

SKIN CONDITIONS. *Paronychia,* a common infection located at the nail fold, is usually due to staphylococci. Examination reveals swelling, erythema, and tenderness at the margins of the nail bed. A *felon* is an infection of the distal finger pulp, usually marked by severe pain and tenderness. *Cellulitis* of the hand, common in injection drug users or after trauma, may cause fever, lymphangitis, or axillary adenopathy.

MISCELLANEOUS. *Raynaud's phenomenon* is relatively common and affects women more often than men. After exposure to cold, patients classically develop pain and blanching of the fingers, followed by cyanosis and redness. *Reflex sympathetic dystrophy* is a condition characterized by burning pain, swelling, and exquisite tenderness of the hand, often with similar involvement of the shoulder (hand-shoulder syndrome). The skin of the affected hand is sweaty and thin, and its temperature may alternate between warm and cold. Patients frequently have a history of diabetes, previous trauma, hand or wrist surgery, or myocardial infarction. Radiographs demonstrate mottled osteopenia; bone scans may show markedly increased radioisotope uptake in the affected extremity.

Management. Specific therapy for arthritis depends on an accurate diagnosis (see Chapter 106, General Approach to Arthritic Symptoms; Chapter 118, Osteoarthritis; and Chapter 119, Gout/Hyperuricemia).

Both flexor tenosynovitis and de Quervain's tenosynovitis may respond to wrist splinting and nonsteroidal anti-inflammatory medication. Refractory cases may require local injections of corticosteroids (10–20 mg of methylprednisolone acetate [Depo-Medrol]). If ganglions become problematic, needle aspiration followed by corticosteroid injection may help temporarily, but recurrence is common. Surgery is usually curative.

The treatment of paronychia or felons includes warm soaks and antibiotics. Incision and drainage may be necessary, especially with felons. Hospital admission and parenteral antibiotic administration are indicated for most patients with cellulitis, especially if lymphangitis, adenopathy, and fever are present. Abscesses require surgical drainage.

The treatment of reflex sympathetic dystrophy is prednisone, 60 mg daily in divided doses, slowly tapered over a month. Patients who experience relapse may require a second course. If corticosteroids are ineffective, patients may experience prolonged relief with a series of sympathetic nerve blocks. If these blocks produce only transient relief, surgical sympathectomy should be considered. To be effective, treatment should begin early and include physical therapy.

Cross-References: Psoriasis (Chapter 32), General Approach to Arthritic Symptoms (Chapter 106), Shoulder Pain (Chapter 108), Osteoarthritis (Chapter 118), Gout/Hyperuricemia (Chapter 119), Interpretation of Serologic Tests (Chapter 123).

REFERENCES

1. Cardelli MB, Kleinsmith DM. Raynaud's phenomenon and disease. Med Clin North Am 1989;73:1127–1141.

   The significance of a positive antinuclear antibody assay associated with Raynaud's phenomenon is presented with an excellent discussion on differential diagnosis and treatment.

2. Dorwart BB. Carpal tunnel syndrome: A review. Semin Arthritis Rheum 1984;14:134–140.

   This concise article contains good sections on differential diagnosis and treatment.

3. Kozin F. Reflex sympathetic dystrophy. Bull Rheum Dis 1986;36:1–8.

   The features and treatment of reflex sympathetic dystrophy are reviewed. The author has done a considerable amount of original work delineating this syndrome.

111 Knee Pain

Symptom

GREGORY C. GARDNER

Etiology. The knee is one of the most frequently injured joints in athletes who participate in weight-bearing sports. It is also a common site for nontraumatic arthritis (Table 111–1).

Table 111–1. COMMON CONDITIONS CAUSING KNEE PAIN

Arthritis	Tendinitis
Chondromalacia patellae	Patellar tendinitis
Meniscal tear	Popliteal region tendinitis
Osteoarthritis	Miscellaneous
Rheumatoid arthritis	Osgood-Schlatter disease
Psoriatic arthritis	Osteonecrosis
Gout	
Pseudogout	
Septic arthritis	
Bursitis	
Prepatellar bursitis	
Pes anserine bursitis	
Baker's cyst	

Clinical Approach. With the patient recumbent, the clinician observes the patient's knees for alignment. The examination, which should include the popliteal fossa, focuses on palpation for warmth, effusions, and joint line tenderness.

ARTHRITIS. *Chondromalacia patellae* is a common condition that affects women more than men. The patella of affected patients is not aligned in its track and moves abnormally (i.e., overpull of the vastus lateralis muscle leads to abnormal lateral pull on the patella), causing excessive compression, softening, and fibrillation of the cartilage. Patients report anterior knee pain especially when using stairs or getting up from a chair. Examination may reveal patellofemoral compartment crepitation, a knee effusion, or abnormal patellar tracking. Pressure placed on the patella while the patient contracts the quadriceps muscles may reproduce the pain. Sunrise and lateral radiographs of the knee show the patellofemoral compartment and may demonstrate joint space narrowing or alignment abnormalities.

Meniscal tears usually occur after trauma, especially a twisting injury. Patients usually complain of acute pain, swelling, locking, or episodic "giving way" of the knee. Depending on the site of the tear, the medial or lateral joint lines may be tender. The McMurray test may be positive (i.e., starting with the knee flexed, slow extension with simultaneous internal or external rotation on the tibia produces pain and clicking). Arthrography, magnetic resonance imaging, or arthroscopy confirms the diagnosis.

Osteoarthritis usually involves the medial compartment, but lateral or patellofemoral disease also occurs (see Chapter 118, Osteoarthritis).

The pattern of joint involvement and the presence of psoriatic skin lesions or a positive rheumatoid factor assay distinguish *rheumatoid* (symmetric polyarthritis) from *psoriatic* arthritis (usually asymmetric). *Gout,* a common cause of knee pain, is discussed in Chapter 119. Calcium pyrophosphate dihydrate crystal–induced synovitis, or *pseudogout,* mimics acute gout of the knee and often affects patients bedridden because of acute medical disease or surgery. A thin line of calcified cartilage (chondrocalcinosis) often appears on anteroposterior knee radiographs in patients with pseudogout, and arthrocentesis reveals characteristic crystals (rhomboid and positively birefringent).

Because the knee is the most common joint to become infected, any acute inflammatory knee monarthritis should be regarded as septic arthritis until examination and culture of the joint fluid prove otherwise. *Staphylococcus aureus* is the usual organism, followed by streptococci, gonococci, and other gramnegative organisms. Patients experience fever and severe pain and often guard against any movement of the knee joint. To diagnose gonococcal arthritis, cultures of both joint fluid and other potentially infected sites (urethra, cervix, rectum) are helpful.

BURSITIS. *Prepatellar bursitis* is covered in Chapter 120.

Inflammation of the pes anserine bursa, which is located at the medial knee, usually affects patients with osteoarthritis. Knee pain with walking and nocturnal pain are common; examination reveals local tenderness. Although *medial collateral ligament strain* resembles anserine bursitis, nocturnal pain is less common.

Baker's cyst occurs when knee effusions from any cause accumulate and distend the gastrocnemius and semimembranosa bursae located in the popliteal fossa. Patients typically complain of fullness and pain in the popliteal fossa, especially with walking. A palpable cyst in the medial popliteal fossa may be the only finding, although some cysts may grow quite large and obstruct venous return or even rupture, causing lower extremity swelling (pseudothrombophlebitis; see Chapter 130, Painful and Swollen Calf). Ultrasonography of the popliteal fossa or arthrography confirms suspected cysts.

TENDINITIS. Suprapatellar and *infrapatellar tendinitis* result from overuse, abnormal patellar tracking, or malrotation of the tibia or femur. Infrapatellar tendinitis may also occur in athletes after repetitive jumping ("jumper's knee"). Pain worsens when the patient climbs stairs, and the involved tendon is tender on examination.

Popliteal pain may reflect strain of the hamstring tendons. In these patients posterior knee pain worsens with the straight leg maneuver (i.e., with the hip and knee flexed, the knee is slowly extended).

MISCELLANEOUS. Osgood-Schlatter disease affects teenage boys who are active in sports. Anterior knee pain is typical and is aggravated by activities such as climbing stairs, kicking, or kneeling. Tenderness and swelling over the tibial tubercle may be present. Radiographs may show avulsion of the tubercle.

Of the two types of *osteonecrosis* of the knee, *osteochondritis dissecans* involves the lateral portion of the medial knee compartment and typically affects young men after an episode of trauma. The inflammation may heal spontaneously or may lead to formation of a loose body and symptoms of locking. The radiographic appearance is diagnostic. The second type of osteonecrosis affects the elderly and those taking corticosteroids and involves the medial and lateral femoral condyles. Both knees are affected in over 50% of patients. Patients experience sudden severe knee pain, especially with weight bearing, and have a small to moderate effusion. Radiographs show abnormal findings only after several months and are not as useful for early diagnosis as bone scans or magnetic resonance imaging are.

Management

ARTHRITIS. Chondromalacia patellae is managed with anti-inflammatory medications and quadriceps strengthening exercises (the patient extends the knee while sitting or lying, gradually adding ankle weights to improve conditioning). Rarely, surgery may be necessary.

Meniscal tears initially require rest and anti-inflammatory medications. Arthroscopic surgery is indicated when patients experience locking of the knee or persistent symptoms.

Therapy for *inflammatory arthritis* (e.g., rheumatoid, psoriatic, and crystal-induced arthritis) includes combinations of anti-inflammatory medications, local corticosteroid injections, and disease-modifying agents. Consultation is advised in difficult cases.

Cases of *infectious arthritis* require hospitalization, high doses of parenteral antibiotics, and frequent joint drainage. Consultation with an orthopedic surgeon is advised.

Therapy for osteoarthritis is covered in Chapter 118.

BURSITIS. Therapy for prepatellar bursitis is covered in Chapter 120.

Pes anserine bursitis responds to physical therapy (gentle stretching, ultrasound, massage) and, in unresponsive cases, to corticosteroid injection.

Corticosteroid injections into the knee joint may benefit patients with Baker's cysts, irrespective of whether the underlying arthritis is inflammatory or noninflammatory. In some patients with noninflammatory conditions (e.g., osteoarthritis), the cyst itself may require aspiration and instillation of a corticosteroid preparation (a large-bore [e.g., 19-gauge] needle is needed to aspirate the thick fluid). Surgical excision is sometimes necessary but is difficult, and recurrence is common. Most cysts, even if recurrent, respond to intermittent aspirations and injections. Some patients with Baker's cysts have internal derangements of the knee (i.e., chronic meniscal tear) that require specific therapy.

TENDINITIS. Most forms of tendinitis respond to rest, physical therapy, and anti-inflammatory medications. Corticosteroid injections into the areas of the large tendons about the knee are not recommended because of the risk of rupture.

MISCELLANEOUS. Osgood-Schlatter disease is treated with rest, discontinuation of athletic activity, and anti-inflammatory medications. Casting is useful in resistant cases.

Treatment of osteochondritis dissecans (usually arthroscopic removal of the loose body) is necessary only in those with persistent symptoms.

Osteonecrosis in the elderly or in those taking corticosteroids is initially treated with rest (to reduce stresses on the joint) and analgesics. Surgical treatment in advanced cases includes bone grafts or total joint replacement.

Cross-References: Psoriasis (Chapter 32), General Approach to Arthritic Symptoms (Chapter 106), Osteoarthritis (Chapter 118), Gout/Hyperuricemia (Chapter 119), Prepatellar and Olecranon Bursitis (Chapter 120), Interpretation of Serologic Tests (Chapter 123), Physical Therapy Care of Outpatients (Chapter 125), Aspiration/Injection of the Knee (Chapter 129), Painful and Swollen Calf (Chapter 130), Sexually Transmitted Diseases (Chapter 176).

REFERENCES

1. Raskas D, Lehman RC. Meniscal injuries in athletes: Pinpointing the diagnosis. J Musculoskel Med 1988;5(5):20–28.

   Normal knee anatomy, mechanism of meniscal injury, physical examination for detection of a tear, and management of these injuries are discussed.

2. Rozing PM, Insall J, Nohne WH. Spontaneous osteonecrosis of the knee. J Bone Joint Surg Am 1980;62:2–7.

   The diagnosis and treatment of spontaneous osteonecrosis is detailed for 90 affected knees, along with a discussion of the diagnostic utility of bone scans.

112 Ankle and Foot Pain

Symptom

GREGORY C. GARDNER

Etiology. The most common causes of ankle and foot pain are listed in Table 112–1. Although trauma is not discussed here, the physician should always consider it in the differential diagnosis.

Clinical Approach. With the patient standing as well as sitting, the examination should focus on the presence of swelling, deformity, or tenderness and on the patient's footwear.

ARTHRITIS. In the foot, osteoarthritis affects either the first metatarsophalangeal joint (*hallux valgus*) or previously injured joints. Hallux valgus, which causes pain with walking, is especially common in women who wear narrow-toed shoes. During examination the first metatarsophalangeal joint is tender and protrudes medially, frequently with an adventitious bursa (bunion). Radiographs show typical osteoarthritic changes. *Hallux rigidus* describes a form of osteoarthritis that markedly limits extension of the great toe. *Rheumatoid arthritis* may produce pain and swelling in the ankle, subtalar, or metatarsophalangeal joint. *Psoriatic arthritis* may cause ankle arthritis, metatarsophalangeal joint arthritis, or "sausage digits" (diffuse phalangeal swelling from interphalangeal joint involvement). Characteristic psoriatic skin and nail changes are often present. *Reiter's disease* mimics psoriatic arthritis, but urethral discharge, conjunctivitis, oral ulcerations, characteristic skin changes, plantar fasciitis, or Achilles tendinitis is also found. *Gout* usually affects the first metatarsophalangeal joint and less often the ankle (see Chapter 119). Because *septic arthritis* may also involve the ankle, any acute arthritis at the ankle joint warrants arthrocentesis and culture of the joint fluid.

TENDINITIS AND FASCIITIS. Conditions causing *Achilles tendinitis* include athletic overuse, the spondyloarthropathies (e.g., ankylosing spondylitis, Reiter's

---

Table 112–1. COMMON CONDITIONS CAUSING ANKLE AND FOOT PAIN

Arthritis	Neuropathy
Osteoarthritis	Tarsal tunnel syndrome
Rheumatoid arthritis	Peroneal neuropathy
Psoriatic arthritis	Morton's neuroma
Reiter's disease	Diabetic neuropathy
Gout	Miscellaneous
Septic arthritis	Pes planus
Tendinitis and fasciitis	Stress fracture
Achilles tendinitis	Metatarsalgia
Posterior tibial tendinitis	
Plantar fasciitis	

disease), rheumatoid arthritis, and, if the tendinitis is recurrent, familial hyper-cholesterolemia. Pain worsens with ankle dorsiflexion, and the tendon is tender and sometimes thickened. Inflammation that is maximal 2 to 6 cm distant from the tendon's insertion into the calcaneum is typical of overuse, whereas inflammation maximal at the insertion, a finding called *enthesopathy,* is charac-teristic of the spondyloarthropathies. Chronic tendinitis may lead to tendon rupture. Laboratory testing for lipid abnormalities is indicated in unexplained cases or if the family history suggests hyperlipidemia.

The posterior tibialis tendon lies posterior to the medial malleolus and may become inflamed after athletic overuse or with Reiter's disease or rheumatoid arthritis. Resisted inversion or passive eversion of the ankle provokes the pain, and localized swelling and tenderness may be present. Tendon rupture may occur, leading to progressive flat foot deformity.

Plantar fasciitis affects obese patients, those with flat feet, and, less often, patients with rheumatoid arthritis, Reiter's disease, or ankylosing spondylitis. Patients complain of painful soles, usually beginning immediately with walking. Dorsiflexion of the toes tenses the plantar fascia and may reveal localized tender points anywhere between the calcaneum and metatarsal heads. Radio-graphs may reveal heel spurs, but their significance is unknown because they are also commonly found in asymptomatic persons.

NEUROPATHY. Posterior tibial nerve entrapment occurs at the tarsal tunnel, which is a space confined by the flexor retinaculum just posterior and inferior to the medial malleolus. Risk factors include valgus heel deformity and ankle fracture; women are more often affected than men. The patient typically complains of burning and numbness that extends from the toes and sole to the medial malleolus. Findings include a positive Tinel's sign (pressure over the nerve reproduces the pain) and diminished two-point discrimination and pinprick sensation. Electrodiagnostic studies are confirmatory.

Peroneal neuropathy, which causes footdrop, may result from local compres-sion or a systemic vasculitis (see Chapter 144, Entrapment Neuropathies).

Morton's neuroma is common in middle-aged women and results from entrapment of the interdigital nerve, usually between the third and fourth toes. Toe numbness and burning worsen with walking on hard surfaces or wearing tight shoes. Tenderness is maximal between, rather than on, the metatarsal heads.

Peripheral neuropathy is discussed in Chapter 147.

MISCELLANEOUS. *Pes planus,* or flatfoot, is usually inherited but may result from trauma, generalized hypermobility, or rupture of the posterior tibial tendon. Although usually asymptomatic, pes planus may cause pain in the soles during prolonged standing or walking. Examination reveals an absent longitudinal arch, valgus heel deviation, and a prominent navicular bone.

Stress fractures usually involve the shafts of the metatarsal bones, especially the second metatarsal neck, but may also occur at the calcaneum. Predisposing conditions include trauma or exercise (e.g., long marches of new military recruits), obesity, and osteoporosis. Localized pain and swelling may be present. Although initial radiographs are normal, films several weeks later may reveal callus formation. Bone scan is the most sensitive test for early diagnosis.

Metatarsalgia (pain at the metatarsals) results from wearing high-heeled shoes, obesity, high-arched feet, rheumatoid arthritis, and trauma. Pain is aggravated by standing, and findings of metatarsal tenderness and calluses are common. Simple metatarsalgia must be distinguished from inflammatory arthritis of the metatarsophalangeal joint. Examination may uncover swelling or synovial hypertrophy in cases of inflammatory arthritis.

Management

ARTHRITIS. The treatment of hallux valgus includes using proper shoes (wide toe box, rigid soles, no high heels—some recommend good running shoes), pads to cushion the bunion, and placement of a rocker bar under the metatarsal portion of the shoe. The best candidates for surgical repair are patients with refractory pain despite conservative treatment, not those with isolated cosmetic deformity.

The treatment of inflammatory arthritis includes combinations of anti-inflammatory medication, corticosteroid injections, and specific disease-modifying agents (see Chapter 106, General Approach to Arthritic Symptoms). Patients with septic arthritis require hospitalization, appropriate antibiotics, and consideration of surgical drainage.

The treatment of gout is described in Chapter 119.

TENDINITIS AND FASCIITIS. Achilles tendinitis is managed by rest, gentle stretching, and, especially with spondyloarthropathies, anti-inflammatory medication. Corticosteroid injections are not recommended. Overuse Achilles tendinitis may require casting or splinting to rest the tendon. Refractory overuse tendinitis may improve after surgical stripping of the tendon.

Posterior tibialis tendinitis responds to rest, anti-inflammatory medications, and, in certain cases, splinting or local corticosteroid injection.

Plantar fasciitis usually responds to arch supports, soft-soled shoes, anti-inflammatory medications, and, in some patients, heel cup orthoses and local corticosteroid injection. Less than 2% of patients require surgery.

NEUROPATHY. Tarsal tunnel syndrome may resolve with corticosteroid injections and, if there is a valgus ankle deformity, shoe modifications or orthoses. Most patients, however, require surgical release. Management of peroneal neuropathy appears in Chapter 144.

Morton's neuroma may respond to shoes with a wide toe box and metatarsal rocker bar and to local corticosteroid injections or, if pain persists, to surgical excision.

MISCELLANEOUS. Symptoms of pes planus may improve with the Thomas heel (a device that aligns the heel), firm shoes, and toe-grasping exercises that strengthen the intrinsic muscles. Some patients require rigid-molded inserts, which can be expensive.

Stress fractures are treated with rest, decreased weight bearing, weight loss if appropriate, and analgesic medication. Most fractures resolve within 6 to 8 weeks.

Metatarsalgia responds to metatarsal pads or rocker bars placed behind the metatarsal heads, well-fitting shoes with a wide toe box, weight reduction, softening of the calluses, and toe-grasping exercises.

Cross-References: Corns and Calluses (Chapter 24), Psoriasis (Chapter 32), General Approach to Arthritic Symptoms (Chapter 106), Osteoarthritis (Chapter 118), Gout/Hyperuricemia (Chapter 119), Diabetic Foot Care Education

(Chapter 124), Local Care of Diabetic Foot Lesions (Chapter 134), Entrapment Neuropathies (Chapter 144), Peripheral Neuropathy (Chapter 147), Hyperlipidemia (Chapter 152).

REFERENCES

1. Gerber L. Foot and ankle problems in the arthritides. J Musculoskel Med 1989;6(12):13–28.

   An excellent review article details the anatomy of the ankle and foot region, arthritides that affect this area, and treatment.

2. Mann R. Acquired flatfoot in adults. Clin Orthop 1983;181:46–51.

   The major causes of flatfoot are reviewed, including posterior tibial rupture.

3. Nelen G, Martens M, Burssens A. Surgical treatment of chronic Achilles tendonitis. Am J Sports Med 1989;17:754–759.

   In a large series of patients with chronic idiopathic or overuse Achilles tendinitis, if conservative treatment failed, 90% had an excellent or good response to surgery.

4. Sheon RP, Moskowitz RW, Goldberg VM. Ankle and foot. In Soft Tissue Rheumatic Pain. Philadelphia, Lea & Febiger, 1982.

   This is a useful discussion of common soft tissue foot and ankle problems, with an emphasis on treatment.

113 Restless Legs Syndrome

Symptom

STEVEN R. McGEE

Epidemiology. Patients with restless legs syndrome experience creeping, aching, or writhing sensations in their lower extremities that appear only during rest (usually at night) and subside immediately after movement of the legs. Estimates of prevalence are 2% to 5%.

Etiology. The cause of restless legs syndrome is unknown, although many investigators attribute it to an underactive dopaminergic system. Strong associations occur with iron deficiency anemia, pregnancy, rheumatoid arthritis, and uremia.

Clinical Approach. The clinician should exclude anemia, confirm that the neurologic examination is normal, and consider withdrawing any medication that has been associated with development of restless legs syndrome (i.e., neuroleptics, phenytoin, methsuximide, and antidepressants).

Management. Carbamazepine, levodopa plus benserazide (a peripheral decarboxylase inhibitor), bromocriptine, oxycodone, and clonazepam all are superior to placebo in randomized double-blind trials of patients with restless legs syndrome. The risk of abuse or of side effects with these medications, however, limits their clinical utility (e.g., 40% of patients treated with carbamazepine had side effects despite less than 5 weeks of treatment).

The clinician should reassure patients with restless legs syndrome that the condition spontaneously waxes and wanes over years and may remit for long periods. In the very few patients with severe and refractory symptoms, clonazepam or levodopa preparations may be the treatments with the fewest side effects.

Cross-References: Chronic Renal Failure (Chapter 179), Anemia (Chapter 199), Diagnosis of Pregnancy (Chapter 210).

REFERENCES

1. Gibb WRG, Lees AJ. The restless legs syndrome. Postgrad Med J 1986;62:329–333.

   Clinical features, differential diagnosis, and treatment are reviewed.

2. McGee SR. Restless legs syndrome. JAMA 1991;265:3014.

   A concise up-to-date review is presented.

3. O'Keeffe ST, Noel J, Lavan JN. Restless legs in the elderly. Postgrad Med J 1993;69:701–703.

   Of consecutive geriatric patients with the restless legs syndrome (4.9% of entire series), one fourth had iron deficiency anemia and dramatic relief of symptoms after iron supplementation.

4. Von Scheele C. Levodopa in restless legs. Lancet 1986;2:426–427.

   Seventeen of 20 patients preferred levodopa plus benserazide to placebo.

· ·

114   Muscle Cramps

Symptom

STEVEN R. McGEE

Epidemiology. In surveys of elderly outpatients, the prevalence of nocturnal leg cramps varies between 37% and 56%. Among cramp sufferers, 6% to 24% have symptoms daily.

Etiology. Painful skeletal muscle contractions, or cramps, result from several distinct clinical entities: true cramp, contracture, tetany, and dystonia (Table 114–1).

Isolated bursts of motoneuron action potentials characterize true cramps. The most common example, the ordinary cramp or "charley-horse," develops while resting at night, may be accompanied by fasciculations, affects unilateral calf and ventral foot muscles, and is relieved by muscle stretching. Lower motor

Table 114–1. ETIOLOGY OF MUSCLE CRAMPS

True cramp—motor unit hyperactivity
    Ordinary cramps
    Lower motor neuron disease
    Hemodialysis
    Saline depletion (e.g., heat cramps)
    Drug-induced
        Nifedipine
        β-Agonists (terbutaline, salbutamol)
        β-Blockers with intrinsic sympathomimetic activity
Contracture—electrically silent
    Metabolic myopathy (e.g., McArdle's disease)
    Thyroid disease
Tetany—motor unit and sensory hyperactivity
    Hypocalcemia
    Hypomagnesemia
    Respiratory alkalosis
    Hypokalemia, hyperkalemia
Dystonia
    Occupational cramp
    Phenothiazines, butyrophenones, metoclopramide

Adapted from McGee SR. Muscle cramps. Arch Intern Med 1990;150:511–518. Copyright 1990, American Medical Association.

neuron diseases may cause weakness, atrophy, and fasciculations, as well as true cramps in the affected muscles. Dehydration also produces true cramps, usually associated with hyponatremia; examples include overdiuresis, hemodialysis (excessive ultrafiltration), or heavy muscular activity in high environmental temperatures (heat cramps).

Contractures, in contrast to true cramps, are uncommon, develop not at rest but during exercise, and are characterized by electromyographic silence during the muscle spasm. In metabolic myopathies such as McArdle's disease, exercise depletes available energy stores more rapidly than normal. Because muscle requires energy to relax, contracture occurs. Hypothyroid and hyperthyroid patients may experience either contractures or true cramps.

Tetany consists of characteristic distal extremity muscle cramps (carpopedal spasm) associated with paresthesias and positive Trousseau's and Chvostek's signs. Causes are listed in Table 114–1.

Dystonia produces sustained postures, not always painful, that result from simultaneous contraction of agonist and antagonistic muscles. After years of practice, musicians, writers, and typists, among others, may develop muscle spasms and incoordination during attempts to perform their occupation-specific fine motor tasks. These focal dystonias ("occupational cramps") may ruin careers. Focal dystonias also occur during treatment with antipsychotic and antidopaminergic medications.

Clinical Approach. Symptoms confused with cramps are myotonia, which is a painless disorder marked by percussion myotonia on examination, and claudication, which although described by patients as cramps does not produce palpable hardening of the muscle. Diagnosis of cramps depends largely on the patient interview: the nocturnal calf cramp relieved by stretching of the muscle (ordinary cramp), the steelworker's arm cramp (heat cramps), the asthmatic's cramps provoked by inhalant treatments (β-agonist cramps), or the exercise-induced cramp associated with dark urine (metabolic myopathy). Physical examination emphasizes the search for dehydration, thyroid disease, tetany (Trousseau's and Chvostek's signs), and neurologic disease. If the condition is still undiagnosed, appropriate laboratory tests include assessment of levels of electrolytes, calcium, and magnesium, and, if suggested by signs and symptoms, thyroid function tests.

Management. The physician should withdraw responsible medications, if possible, and treat underlying fluid, electrolyte, or endocrine abnormalities. Patients with newly suspected lower motor neuron disease (weakness and atrophy), dystonia unrelated to medication, or suspected contracture should be referred to a neurologist.

Muscle stretching exercises performed periodically during the day may reduce ordinary nocturnal cramps. Measures that stretch the calf and ventral foot muscles during the night, such as a footboard placed at the end of the bed, also effectively prevent cramps in many patients, although this method has never been scientifically studied. In double-blind placebo-controlled trials, quinine effectively reduced the frequency but not the severity of ordinary cramps. Because the data supporting quinine use are meager, however, and because significant adverse reactions occur (nausea, tinnitus, hypoglycemia, and immune thrombocytopenia), the Food and Drug Administration announced in February 1995 that quinine can no longer be labeled for use in nocturnal cramps. At the time of this writing, the generic form of quinine is still available for treatment of malaria.

Simple writing aids may benefit patients with writer's cramps.

Cross-References: Muscular Weakness (Chapter 137), Common Thyroid Disorders (Chapter 153), Chronic Renal Failure (Chapter 179), Electrolyte Abnormalities (Chapter 182).

REFERENCES

1. Daniell HW. Simple cure for nocturnal leg cramps. N Engl J Med 1979;301:216.

   Forty-four patients with nocturnal calf cramps were cured after 1 week of calf stretching exercises performed three times per day.

2. Layzer RB. Motor unit hyperactivity states. In Vinken PF, Bruyn GW, eds. Handbook of Clinical Neurology. Amsterdam, North-Holland, 1980:295–316.

   This encyclopedic review includes descriptions of exotic cause of cramps, such as tetanus, strychnine poisoning, stiff-man syndrome, and black widow spider bite.

3. Man-Son-Hing M, Wells G. Meta-analysis of efficacy of quinine for treatment of nocturnal leg cramps in elderly people. BMJ 1995:310:13–17.

   A meta-analysis was done of six randomized, double-blind trials (total of 107 patients); compared with placebo, quinine reduced the number of cramps and the number of nights with cramps, but not the severity or duration of individual nocturnal cramps.

4. McGee SR. Muscle cramps. Arch Intern Med 1990;150:511–518.

   This is a thorough overview of cramping conditions; use of quinine and other treatments is presented.

115 Paget's Disease

Problem

DENNIS L. ANDRESS

Epidemiology and Etiology. Paget's disease is characterized by localized areas of enhanced bone turnover, which lead to enlargement and vascularization of compact bone and increased susceptibility to deformity and fracture. Although the etiology is unknown, a viral infection of the bone-resorbing cells (osteoclasts) is suspected. It is more commonly observed in Europe, North America, and Australia, with clinical manifestations usually beginning by the fifth decade. In the United States, Paget's disease is present in 4% of those older than 45 years of age and in 8% of those older than 80 years of age. There is a slight male predominance.

Symptoms and Signs. Most patients are asymptomatic, especially with early disease. The most common symptom is localized pain over affected bone. Bowing deformities of the femur or tibia cause pain from either secondary arthritis or abnormal gait and consequent mechanical stresses. Back pain may be due to vertebral compression fractures, lumbar spinal stenosis, or degenerative changes of the spine. Motor and sensory changes may occur with spinal involvement, whereas cranial nerve palsies or headache occurs in 33% with skull involvement. Long bone involvement produces localized tenderness and warmth. Vertebral disease may cause kyphosis. Extreme skull involvement may produce bone softening and basal flattening that rarely leads to brain stem compression.

Clinical Approach. In asymptomatic patients the only clue to Paget's disease may be the incidental finding of an elevated serum alkaline phosphatase level. When suspected, pagetic bone is most easily identified with scintigraphy. Because bone scans are nonspecific, it is necessary to obtain a radiograph of areas positive on bone scan to identify the characteristic changes. Occasionally, metastatic bone disease becomes a consideration and can be ruled out only by biopsy.

Management. An indication for treatment in asymptomatic patients is a serum alkaline phosphatase level more than three times the upper normal limit. Treatment at this stage prevents severe and prolonged bone resorption and symptoms. In the United States, approved agents for treatment include etidronate and calcitonin. Both are effective, but etidronate is usually preferred because of oral administration and few side effects; the recommended dose is 5 mg/kg/d for 6 months, followed by no treatment for 6 months to prevent osteomalacia. Alendronate will likely be the diphosphonate of choice now that it has been approved in the United States. Calcitonin requires self-injection subcutaneously and causes nausea in 15% of patients but is the preferred choice in severe disease of weight-bearing bones. In 20% of patients, resistance to calcitonin develops. A combination of calcitonin and etidronate may be required in resistant cases.

Follow-Up. An acceptable biochemical response is a 50% reduction in the serum alkaline phosphatase level. Declines in urinary hydroxyproline excretion precede the change in the alkaline phosphatase level. Etidronate has a more long-lasting effect; calcitonin's effect is usually lost within 1 year. Both forms of therapy ameliorate bone pain in the majority of patients but do not correct bone deformities or improve pain from secondary arthritis. Potential long-term problems include fractures, which usually heal normally, and neoplastic degeneration of pagetic bone (< 1% incidence).

Cross-References: Low Back Pain (Chapter 107), Hip Pain (Chapter 109).

REFERENCES

1. Harinck HIJ, Bijvoet OLM, Vellenga CR, et al. Relation between signs and symptoms in Paget's disease of bone. Q J Med 1986;58:133–151.
   The authors present a good review of this disorder.

2. Harinck HIJ, Papapoulos SE, Blanksma HJ, et al. Paget's disease of bone: Early and late responses to three different modes of treatment with aminohydroxypropylidene bisphosphonate (APD). BMJ 1987;295:1301–1305.
   Short-term (10-day) intravenous APD appears to be as effective as long-term oral treatment.

. . . .

116 Osteoporosis

Problem

DENNIS L. ANDRESS

Epidemiology and Etiology. Osteoporosis is defined as reduced bone mass that results in bone fragility and fractures. Approximately 30% of women have one or more fractures after menopause; 25% of these fractures involve the distal radius (Colles' fracture), 50% involve the vertebrae, and 25% involve the hip. One third of all women and 17% of all men suffer a hip fracture before age 90, and 20% of those who sustain a fracture die within 3 months of the event. The major cause of osteoporosis in women is estrogen deficiency (postmenopausal, oophorectomy, prolonged amenorrhea). In men, testosterone deficiency accounts for 30% of spinal osteoporosis. In women and men, osteoporosis also results from age-related declines in bone formation, which lead to reduced bone mass. Risk factors for osteoporosis include white or Asian race, family history of osteoporosis, small body frame, chronic low calcium intake, excessive alcohol intake, and cigarette smoking. Clearly defined secondary causes of osteoporosis include hyperparathyroidism, hyperthyroidism, Cushing's syndrome, multiple myeloma, thyroid replacement therapy, corticosteroid therapy, and chronic heparin treatment.

Symptoms and Signs. Before the occurrence of a fracture, osteoporosis is asymptomatic. Although most fractures are painful, 35% of vertebral fractures are asymptomatic and are manifested only by loss of height or kyphosis (dowager's hump).

Clinical Approach. General screening of all asymptomatic women with measurements of bone density is not appropriate. Such measurements are advocated, however, for the following groups of patients: (1) estrogen-deficient women, (2) testosterone-deficient men, (3) patients with vertebral abnormalities or radiographic osteopenia, (4) patients receiving glucocorticoids, and (5) patients with asymptomatic primary hyperparathyroidism. Spinal bone density measurements are also appropriate for patients with a vertebral fracture. Dual-photon absorptiometry, computed tomography, and dual-energy radiography all measure the bone mineral density of the spine or hip and can be used to diagnose osteoporosis (i.e., > 1 standard deviation [SD] below the mean for young normal subjects that represents peak bone mass). Dual-energy radiograph absorptiometry (cost: $75–$150) is superior because of its precision, accuracy, and low radiation exposure.

In patients with documented osteoporosis, routine laboratory tests include determinations of serum calcium (for hyperparathyroidism), serum thyroid hormone, serum and urine protein electrophoresis (for multiple myeloma), free testosterone (to document male hypogonadism), and alkaline phosphatase (to rule out osteomalacia). A normal serum 25-hydroxyvitamin D level excludes the most common form of osteomalacia. Bone biopsy (after tetracycline labeling) is necessary whenever osteomalacia is suspected (e.g., in subjects with skeletal pain and elevated alkaline phosphatase levels, with or without hypocalcemia).

Management. The initial management of vertebral fractures consists of analgesic therapy and bed rest. Prolonged bed rest increases bone resorption and is discouraged. A back brace may help reduce pain in some patients.

The recommended daily calcium intake for all patients is 1000 to 1200 mg with 400 IU of vitamin D per day. If calcium supplements are required, calcium citrate provides optimal gastrointestinal absorption. Other preventive measures include regular weight-bearing exercise (30 minutes of walking three times per week) and avoidance of medications that may precipitate falling.

In mild to moderate osteoporosis, also sometimes called osteopenia (bone mineral density 1–2 SD below that of young normal subjects), antiresorptive agents such as estrogens and calcitonin prevent further declines in bone mass. Oral estrogen, 0.625 mg/d, is recommended soon after menopause for an 8- to 10-year minimum duration, with appropriate monitoring for the development of neoplasia (see Chapter 161, Menopausal Symptoms, and Chapter 159, Abnormal Uterine Bleeding). The addition of cyclical progesterone produces menstrual cycles and appears to decrease the risk of estrogen-induced endometrial cancer. Calcitonin, though effective, has not been widely accepted because of the need for frequent subcutaneous injections. The future availability of nasally administered calcitonin may make it the preferred choice when estrogen therapy is contraindicated (e.g., in subjects with a history of estrogen-dependent tumor or endometrial cancer, venous embolic disease, or abnormal liver function). Ongoing studies with the bisphosphonate alendronate will determine whether fractures can be prevented in asymptomatic patients with mild to moderate reductions in bone mass.

For patients with severe osteoporosis (bone mineral density > 2 SD below that of young normal subjects), alendronate has been shown to be effective. An additional agent, sodium fluoride, has shown promise for treatment of severe osteoporosis by its effect of increased bone formation and, consequently, bone mass. The slow-release form, which is expected to gain approval from the Food and Drug Administration soon, is well tolerated.

Follow-Up. Yearly bone density measurements are recommended for assessing treatment efficacy.

Cross-References: Periodic Health Assessment (Chapter 8), Low Back Pain (Chapter 107), Hip Pain (Chapter 109), Common Thyroid Disorders (Chapter 153), Menopausal Symptoms (Chapter 161).

REFERENCES

1. Kiel DP, Felson DT, Anderson JJ, et al. Hip fracture and the use of estrogens in postmenopausal women: The Framingham Study. N Engl J Med 1987;317:1169–1174.

   Women who began taking estrogens within 4 years of menopause were protected against subsequent hip fracture.

2. Liberman UA, Weiss SR, Broll J, et al. Effect of oral alendronate on bone mineral density and the incidence of fractures in postmenopausal osteoporosis. N Engl J Med 1995;333:1437.

   This 3-year multidose study demonstrates that, at all doses, bone mineral density increased in the spine and hip. The optimal dose is probably 10 mg/d.

3. Melton LJ, Eddy DM, Johnston CC Jr. Screening for osteoporosis. Ann Intern Med 1990;112:516–528.

   Extensive review of the clinical utility of bone mass measurements as a screening method found that mass screening is not recommended because treatment guidelines have not been generally accepted.

4. Pak CYC, Sakhaee K, Adams-Huet B, et al. Treatment of postmenopausal osteoporosis with slow-release sodium fluoride. Ann Intern Med 1995;123:401–408.

   This is the final report of a randomized trial of slow-release sodium fluoride plus calcium citrate (500 mg) given in cycles of 12 months on, 2 months off, for 3 to 4 years. Bone mineral density increased 4% to 5% per year in the spine and 2% to 4% per year in the femoral neck. These changes were associated with a significant reduction in fracture rate.

5. Seeman E. The dilemma of osteoporosis in men. Am J Med 1995;98:76S–88S.

   A good recent review of male osteoporosis is presented.

117 Polymyalgia Rheumatica and Temporal Arteritis

Problem

GREGORY C. GARDNER

POLYMYALGIA RHEUMATICA

Epidemiology. Both polymyalgia rheumatica and temporal arteritis primarily affect elderly patients, with a mean age at onset of 70 years. These conditions are rare before the age of 50, affect women more than men, and, although data are incomplete, are rare in blacks. The reported annual incidence of polymyalgia rheumatica is 30 to 50 cases per 100,000 per year; the prevalence in predominantly white populations is 500 per 100,000.

Symptoms and Signs. Patients with polymyalgia rheumatica complain of pain and stiffness (often profound and worse in the morning) of the neck, shoulders, thighs, and hips. Fatigue, weight loss, and lassitude may accompany the pain and stiffness, rendering simple tasks such as getting out of bed extremely difficult. Patients often recall the exact day that symptoms began.

Physical examination is usually unremarkable; muscle weakness is *not* found. As many as 20% of patients have synovitis (usually transient) of the shoulders, wrists, or knees.

Clinical Approach. Because other causes of proximal muscle symptoms include hypothyroidism, polymyositis, early rheumatoid arthritis in the elderly, and fibromyalgia, important initial laboratory tests are erythrocyte sedimentation rate (ESR), rheumatoid factor, and creatine phosphokinase determinations and thyroid function tests. In polymyalgia rheumatica, the ESR is very high, often exceeding 100 mm/h, although rare cases with a normal ESR exist. Other laboratory abnormalities seen in polymyalgia rheumatica are anemia, thrombocytosis, and elevated liver alkaline phosphatase levels. Clinicians should question all patients with suspected polymyalgia rheumatica about symptoms suggestive of temporal arteritis.

Management. Most patients with polymyalgia rheumatica respond dramatically in 1 to 2 days to 10 to 20 mg/d of prednisone, although some cases require up to 1 week of treatment before improvement becomes noticeable. The diagnosis should be questioned if there is no response after 1 week. After 1 month of treatment, the prednisone dose is gradually reduced to a maintenance dose of 5 to 7.5 mg/d. Most patients need 2 years of treatment, although some relapse even after as long as 10 years of prednisone.

Any patient who takes more than 7.5 mg/d of prednisone for 6 months or more is at increased risk for corticosteroid-induced osteoporosis. Such patients should take calcium supplements (800–1500 mg/d). Many authorities also prescribe vitamin D supplements if the 24-hour urinary excretion of calcium remains low despite calcium supplementation. Patients who receive vitamin D supplementation should be carefully monitored for hypercalcemia and hypercalciuria.

Follow-Up. Patients who fail to respond to corticosteroids or who become corticosteroid dependent should be referred to a rheumatologist. Corticosteroid-dependent patients may be candidates for methotrexate.

TEMPORAL ARTERITIS

Epidemiology. Temporal arteritis, a giant cell arteritis of the medium to large arteries, is less common than polymyalgia rheumatica, with an incidence of 2 to 18 cases per 100,000 and a prevalence of 234 per 100,000. Although the specific relationship is unclear, most authorities regard temporal arteritis and polymyalgia rheumatica as different manifestations of the same disease process.

Symptoms and Signs. Inflammation of the extracranial arteries causes headache, scalp tenderness, jaw claudication, and visual symptoms (diplopia, ptosis, and transient or permanent visual loss). Inflammation of the vessels of the aortic arch, although infrequent, leads to upper extremity claudication, transient ischemic attacks, or strokes. Polymyalgia rheumatica accompanies temporal arteritis in 40% to 60% of cases.

Physical findings may include prominent temporal arteries, absent temporal artery pulsations, or bruits over large vessels, especially of the upper extremities. Brushing the temporal scalp may elicit tenderness. Eye examination is usually normal unless ischemia has occurred.

Clinical Approach. The ESR in temporal arteritis is frequently very high (often 100 mm/h), although cases with less impressive elevations exist. The clinician should suspect temporal arteritis in any person older than 50 years of age with an unexplained elevation of the ESR and a new headache or transient visual changes. When temporal arteritis is suspected, the best diagnostic test is temporal artery biopsy, an outpatient procedure in which a specimen 2 to 4 cm long is removed from the symptomatic side. Multiple pathologic sections are necessary because the inflammation may involve only small isolated portions of the vessel. If the biopsy results are normal but temporal arteritis is still likely, the other side should be sampled.

Management. When temporal arteritis is strongly suspected, immediate treatment with prednisone while awaiting biopsy is appropriate. Treatment for as long as 1 week does not alter the biopsy results. High doses of prednisone (60 mg/d in divided doses) are initially used to prevent blindness, a complication that may affect patients suddenly and without warning. Some authorities believe that 1 month of high-dose prednisone precludes relapses.

After 1 month of treatment, the prednisone dosage is slowly reduced over 6 months to 5 to 7.5 mg/d and is continued at this level as recommended earlier for patients with polymyalgia rheumatica. Once the daily dose has been reduced to 30 mg, it can be consolidated to a single daily dose. With both polymyalgia rheumatica and temporal arteritis, the best clinical guide to corticosteroid dosing is the patient's symptoms and signs, not the ESR. Although patients without visual symptoms may respond to lower doses of prednisone, this regimen is under investigation and not yet generally recommended.

Recommendations for calcium and vitamin D supplementation are the same as for patients with polymyalgia rheumatica. Other potential complications of large doses of corticosteroids include cataracts, infection, and hyperglycemia.

Cross-References: General Approach to Arthritic Symptoms (Chapter 106), Interpretation of Serologic Tests (Chapter 123), Muscular Weakness (Chapter 137), Headache (Chapter 138).

REFERENCES

1. Delecoeuillerie G, Joly P, Cohen De Lara A, Paolaggi JB. Polymyalgia rheumatica and temporal arteritis: A retrospective analysis of prognostic features and different corticosteroid regimens. Ann Rheum Dis 1988;47:733–739.

   In a large retrospective study, patients with symptoms of polymyalgia rheumatica but without symptoms of temporal arteritis responded to low-dose prednisone even when the temporal biopsy results were positive. The authors suggest that biopsy is unnecessary in this setting and that temporal arteritis without visual symptoms may respond to lower doses of corticosteroids (see text).

2. Healey LA. Rheumatoid arthritis in the elderly. Clin Rheum Dis 1986;12:173–179.

   The clinical presentation of elderly patients with seronegative rheumatoid arthritis was similar to that of patients with polymyalgia rheumatica. They responded well to low doses of corticosteroids.

3. Lauter SA, Reece D, Avioli LV. Polymyalgia rheumatica. Arch Intern Med 1985;145:1273–1275.

   This is a concise and well-written summary of polymyalgia rheumatica and temporal arteritis.

4. Sonnenblick M, Nesher G, Rosin A. Nonclassical organ involvement in temporal arteritis. Semin Arthritis Rheum 1989;19:183–190.

   In this article involvement of unusual organ systems is reviewed. The hepatic alkaline phosphatase level was elevated in up to 60% of patients with temporal arteritis/polymyalgia rheumatica.

• •

118 Osteoarthritis

Problem

GREGORY C. GARDNER

Epidemiology. In the United States, approximately 60 million persons have osteoarthritis. The prevalence rises sharply after the age of 50; by age 60, 50% of persons have clinical osteoarthritis and 80% have some radiographic evidence of osteoarthritis. Not all radiographic changes are symptomatic, however; some studies suggest that only 9% of men and 25% of women with moderate

Table 118–1. CLASSIFICATION OF OSTEOARTHRITIS

Primary

Localized
Generalized (three or more joint areas affected)
Erosive (inflammatory osteoarthritis of the hands)

Secondary

Trauma
Congenital anomaly
    Perthes' disease
    Congenital hip dysplasia
Metabolic
    Calcium pyrophosphate dihydrate deposition
      disease
    Ochronosis
    Hemachromatosis
    Acromegaly
    Gout
Postinflammatory arthritis
    Rheumatoid arthritis
    Infection
Other
    Avascular necrosis
    Charcot joint

to severe radiographic osteoarthritis of the distal interphalangeal joints report symptoms, whereas 56% and 80% of men and women, respectively, with radiographically demonstrated knee involvement have symptoms.

Risk factors depend on the joint affected and include a family history of hand osteoarthritis (especially in women); prior congenital or acquired hip abnormalities (hip arthritis); and obesity and previous trauma (knee arthritis).

A simple classification of osteoarthritis appears in Table 118–1.

Symptoms and Signs. Primary osteoarthritis most commonly affects the hands (distal interphalangeal joints, proximal interphalangeal joints, first carpometacarpal joints), followed by the cervical spine, lumbar spine, hips, knees, and first metatarsophalangeal joints. Pain occurs with use of the joint and is associated with mild morning stiffness (lasting less than 15 minutes) that is most pronounced after rest ("gelling"). Advanced disease may lead to rest pain or nocturnal pain. Loose bodies or degenerative meniscal tears in the knee may cause symptoms of locking or catching.

Many patients may initially notice pain and swelling in the distal and proximal interphalangeal joints, but when deformity of these joints occurs often there is a disappearance of discomfort. Deformities at the distal interphalangeal joints are called Heberden's nodes, whereas the changes at the proximal interphalangeal joints are known as Bouchard's nodes. "Erosive" osteoarthritis, so called because of more severe clinical and radiographic changes, may cause symptoms in the affected hand joints. Osteoarthritis of the spine may cause compression of the spinal cord or nerve roots, leading to spinal stenosis.

Clinical Approach. The diagnosis of primary osteoarthritis depends on (1) involvement of characteristic joints, (2) morning stiffness that is brief (prolonged stiffness suggests other active inflammatory forms of joint disease), (3) laboratory data that are normal (normal erythrocyte sedimentation rate, negative rheumatoid factor assay), and (4) radiographs that are characteristic for osteoarthritis (nonuniform joint space narrowing, osteophytes, bone sclerosis, and subchondral cysts).

Rheumatoid arthritis, psoriatic arthritis, and tophaceous gout may all affect the proximal and distal interphalangeal joints. Calcium pyrophosphate deposition (CPPD) disease, a secondary form of osteoarthritis, should be considered when osteoarthritis affects joints not typically involved by primary osteoarthritis. Radiographs of joints with CPPD often reveal chondrocalcinosis (linear calcification of the cartilage parallel to the underlying bone); aspirated joint fluid shows positively birefringent crystals as viewed with compensated polarized microscopy.

Management. The most effective medications for osteoarthritis are the nonsteroidal anti-inflammatory agents (NSAIDs) (Table 118–2). All NSAIDs except for the nonacetylated salicylates have potential gastrointestinal toxicity (dyspepsia, gastric ulceration or perforation) and renal toxicity (fluid retention, renal insufficiency, renal failure). Low-dose tricyclic antidepressants such as amitriptyline may benefit patients with nocturnal pain.

Topical capsaicin is an attractive alternative for treating digital osteoarthri-

Table 118–2. NONSTEROIDAL ANTI-INFLAMMATORY DRUGS

Drug	Dose Range (mg/d)	Divided Doses (No./d)	Comments	Cost* ($ per Month)
Salicylates				
Aspirin	2400–6000	2–4	Tinnitus	4.80–10.80
Salicylsalicylic acid (salsalate)	2000–5000	2–4	Tinnitus	23.90–59.70
Diflunisal	500–1000	2	Use reduced dose in elderly; longer half-life with higher doses	25.41–50.82
Propionic acids				
Ibuprofen	600–3200	3–4		3.45–24.98
Naproxen	500–1500	2–3		40.42–75.77
Fenoprofen (600-mg tabs)	1200–3200	3–4	Interstitial nephritis	27.50–81.65
Ketoprofen	100–400	3–4		78.80–211.20
Flurbiprofen	200–300	2–3		62.34–95.51
Indoleacetic acids				
Indomethacin	50–200	3–4	Headache	10.07–35.90
Sulindac	300–400	2	Relative renal sparing?	49.77–50.76
Tolmetin	800–1600	3–4	Rare anaphylaxis	45.30–90.60
Fenamates				
Meclofenamate	200–400	4	Diarrhea in up to 15%	43.50–44.58
Diclofenac (Voltaren)	100–200	2–4		60.46–118.85
Oxicams				
Piroxicam	10–20	1	Rash	38.59–64.66

*Generic prices used if available; average wholesale price, 1996 *Drug Topics Red Book.*

tis. At least one controlled study found that a 0.075% capsaicin cream applied to the hand joints may reduce pain by up to 40%. It has to be applied three to four times per day and the effect may be delayed by 1 to 2 weeks. The only side effect appears to be local burning.

Intra-articular corticosteroids, especially when injected in the first carpometacarpal joint, knee, or ankle joints, may result in prolonged benefit. Injections more frequent than every 3 to 4 months, however, should be avoided because they may hasten joint destruction. The usual dose of triamcinolone or equivalent is 30 to 40 mg in the knee, 20 to 30 mg in an ankle, and 10 mg in the small joints of the hand. There is presently no role for oral corticosteroids in the treatment of osteoarthritis.

Physical therapy maintains range of motion and muscle strength around affected joints. In addition, physical therapy manages the painful surrounding bursae and tendons, especially the pes anserine bursae at the medial knee, that are affected by the altered joint mechanics of osteoarthritis. Use of a cane in the hand opposite the affected hip or knee can improve walking.

Joint replacement surgery should be considered in those with refractory pain or markedly altered joint mechanics. In the knee, arthroscopy can remove loose bodies or trim degenerative menisci that may be limiting motion.

Cross-References: General Approach to Arthritic Symptoms (Chapter 106), Low Back Pain (Chapter 107), Shoulder Pain (Chapter 108), Hip Pain (Chapter 109), Wrist and Hand Pain (Chapter 110), Knee Pain (Chapter 111), Ankle and Foot Pain (Chapter 112), Gout/Hyperuricemia (Chapter 119), Physical Therapy Care of Outpatients (Chapter 125), Aspiration/Injection of the Knee (Chapter 129).

REFERENCES

1. Bradley JD, Brandt KD, Katz BP, Kalasinski LA. Comparison of an anti-inflammatory dose of ibuprofen, an analgesic dose of ibuprofen, and acetaminophen in the treatment of patients with osteoarthritis of the knee. N Engl J Med 1991;325:87–91.

   Controlled trial of ibuprofen in two doses was compared to acetaminophen for knee osteoarthritis with no difference of significance noted, although several trends favored the ibuprofen. The authors suggest that acetaminophen is more appropriate therapy in most patients with osteoarthritis owing to its favorable safety profile.

2. Brandt KD. Osteoarthritis. Clin Geriatr Med 1988;4:279–293.

   The most important theories concerning the pathogenesis of osteoarthritis are presented.

3. Davis MA. Epidemiology of osteoarthritis. Clin Geriatr Med 1988;4:241–255.

   Risk factors for and the natural history of osteoarthritis are discussed.

4. Furst DE, Paulus HE. Aspirin and other nonsteroidal anti-inflammatory drugs. In McCarty D, ed. Arthritis and Allied Conditions, 12th ed. Philadelphia, Lea & Febiger, 1993:507–543.

   The mechanism of action of NSAIDs is outlined and each NSAID is discussed individually, detailing its reported adverse reactions.

5. McCarthy GM, McCarty DJ. Effect of topical capsaicin in the therapy of painful osteoarthritis of the hands. J Rheumatol 1992;19:604–607.

   A controlled trial of capsaicin cream was done for osteoarthritis of the hand.

119 Gout/Hyperuricemia

Problem

DOUGLAS S. PAAUW

Epidemiology. Approximately 1.5% of the population experiences an attack of gout. Gout is far more common in men (90% of cases). The average age at onset for men is 48. Women usually do not develop gout until after menopause (average, age 54). Most patients (94%) who develop gout have elevated uric acid levels (hyperuricemia). Patients who are not taking drugs that raise serum uric acid and have a uric acid level between 7 and 8 mg/dL have a 20% risk of developing gout, whereas those with levels over 9 mg/dL have a 90% risk.

Of the many drugs that elevate uric acid, diuretics and alcohol are the most common (Table 119–1). Uncommonly, lead exposure due to drinking "moonshine" produces arthritis (saturnine gout).

Symptoms and Signs. In 90% of cases, the initial attack of gout is acute, is extremely painful, and affects a single joint. Polyarticular involvement is more common in women. An attack frequently follows minor trauma, with symptoms often beginning at night as bedsheets pull against the toe and produce the first awareness of pain. More than 50% of initial attacks affect the first metatarsophalangeal joint (podagra). Other sites commonly involved are the knees, metatarsophalangeal joints, tarsal joints, arch of the foot, and ankles. In patients with osteoarthritis, gout can occur in Heberden's nodes.

Periarticular erythema and edema is common. Dramatic erythema and warmth as well as low-grade fever and chills may accompany the attack and lead to a mistaken diagnosis of cellulitis or septic arthritis. Desquamation of periarticular skin frequently occurs as the attack resolves.

Clinical Approach. Before instituting therapy, especially long-term preventive therapy, the clinician should establish the diagnosis of gout by finding monosodium urate crystals in tophi or synovial fluid leukocytes. Urate crystals are found in 85% of patients with acute gout. The crystals appear yellow under a polarized light microscope with a red compensator when oriented parallel to the axis of the compensator (negatively birefringent).

Table 119–1. DRUGS THAT INCREASE SERUM URIC ACID

Ethanol	Cyclosporine
Nicotinic acid	Ethambutol
Diuretics	Pyrazinamide
Thiazides	Salicylates (low dose, e.g.,
Furosemide	< 600 mg/d)
Chlorthalidone	
Amiloride	
Triamterene	

Table 119–2. TREATMENT OF GOUT: ACUTE ATTACKS AND PROPHYLAXIS

Drug	Dose and Administration	Cost ($ per Week)*†
Acute Gout		
Indomethacin (Indocin)	25–50 mg tid PO	4.94 (23.86)
Ibuprofen (Motrin)	800 mg tid PO	4.18 (7.75)
Naproxen (Naprosyn)	750 mg followed by 250 mg tid PO	14.74 (18.24)
Sulindac (Clinoril)	200 mg bid	13.95 (17.40)
Colchicine	0.6 mg PO qh up to 12 doses until relief or diarrhea/nausea	1.35
Prednisone	30–50 mg qd with rapid taper (over 10 days)	1.52
Triamcinolone hexacetonide	5–20 mg injected into joint	8.18
		Cost ($ per Month)
Prophylaxis		
Probenecid (Benemid)	begin 250 mg bid; increase to 1–3 g/d	9.90 (18.36)
Sulfinpyrazone (Anturane)	100 mg bid	8.79 (21.44)
Allopurinol (Zyloprim)	300 mg qd	6.97 (16.76)
Colchicine	0.6 mg bid	2.90

*Average wholesale price, 1996 *Drug Topics Red Book.*
†Prices in parentheses are for trade drugs.

Because it may be technically difficult to tap a small joint such as the metatarsophalangeal or tarsal joint, a presumptive diagnosis of gout may be made if these joints are affected and the patient is hyperuricemic.

Management. Nonsteroidal anti-inflammatory drugs (NSAIDs) are effective for acute gouty arthritis (Table 119–2). Indomethacin is the most widely used. These medications should be avoided in patients with congestive heart failure, cirrhosis, or renal disease. Colchicine is effective but produces adverse gastrointestinal effects in 70% to 80% of patients taking the drug for acute gout and should be avoided in patients with renal or hepatic insufficiency. Prednisone is an effective alternative for many patients with monarticular gout and contraindications to NSAIDs and colchicine, as are intra-articular corticosteroid injections (e.g., triamcinolone hexacetonide, 5–20 mg). Drugs that lower uric acid should not be started until 4 to 6 weeks after an initial attack, because they may prolong or worsen the attack or precipitate a relapse.

Treatment of elevated uric acid should not be considered unless the patient has tophi, nephrolithiasis, or recurrent gouty arthritis. The cause of hyperuricemia should be sought, and any drugs that elevate the uric acid level should be eliminated if possible (see Table 119–1). A 24-hour urine collection measures uric acid production (normal 24-hour urate excretion is 600 mg). Another option for measuring uric acid excretion is to calculate from a spot mid-morning urine uric acid collection:

$$\frac{\text{urine uric acid} \times \text{serum creatinine}}{\text{urine creatinine}}$$

Normal values are 0.4 mg/dL or less; an acid excretion rate over 0.7 mg/dL indicates an overproducer of uric acid. The vast majority of hyperuricemic patients are underexcretors of uric acid who respond well to the uricosuric agents probenecid and sulfinpyrazone. These drugs should not be used in overproducers (indicated by the presence of tophi or a 24-hour urate excretion > 600 mg), in the presence of impaired renal function (creatinine > 1.5), or in patients with nephrolithiasis. Allopurinol effectively treats both overproducers and underexcretors of uric acid by decreasing uric acid production, but it can cause an exfoliative dermatitis that is occasionally life threatening. Uric acid–lowering drugs should be started while the patient is still taking colchicine or an NSAID, and the anti-inflammatory agent should be continued for an additional 2 to 4 weeks to prevent a gouty flare. Treatment of asymptomatic hyperuricemia is rarely indicated.

Occasionally the clinician will encounter a patient who has been started on a uric acid–lowering drug without having had uric acid crystals demonstrated in joint aspirates. It is reasonable to continue the drug if the patient has a history of hyperuricemia and recurrent monarticular arthritis affecting typical joints and if the arthritis has responded to colchicine or NSAIDs. Otherwise, the patient should be given a trial off therapy to determine whether gouty arthritis recurs.

Follow-Up. A single gout attack requires no follow-up as long as the patient remains asymptomatic. Patients with recurrent attacks should consider treatment of the hyperuricemia, with the goal of reducing the serum acid level below 6 mg/dL. Patients with hyperuricemia and hypertension should avoid diuretics if at all possible.

Cross-References. General Approach to Arthritic Symptoms (Chapter 106), Wrist and Hand Pain (Chapter 110), Knee Pain (Chapter 111), Ankle and Foot Pain (Chapter 112), Aspiration/Injection of the Knee (Chapter 129), Nephrolithiasis (Chapter 174).

REFERENCES

1. Groff GD, Frank WA, Raddatz DA. Systemic steroid therapy for acute gout: A clinical trial and review of the literature. Semin Arthritis Rheum 1990;19:329–336.
   These authors address the issue of corticosteroid use for acute gout. A 10-day taper of prednisone resulted in clinical resolution without rebound arthropathy.

2. Lin HY, Rocher LL, et al. Cyclosporine-induced hyperuricemia and gout. N Engl J Med 1989;3201:287–292.
   Hyperuricemia is a common complication of cyclosporine therapy. Gouty arthritis occurred in 7% of the patients in this study.

3. Roberts WN, Liang MH, Stern SH. Colchicine in acute gout: reassessment of risks and benefits. JAMA 1987;257:1920–1922.
   The dangers of intravenous colchicine are discussed, including reports of two deaths related to neutropenia.

4. Simkin PA, Hoover PL, Paxon CS, Wilson WF. Uric acid excretion: Quantitative assessment from spot, midmorning serum and urine samples. Ann Intern Med 1979;91:44–47.
   This article gives a useful formula for calculating from a midmorning urine sample whether the patient is an overproducer or underexcretor of uric acid.

5. Wallace SL, Singer JZ. Therapy in gout. Rheum Dis Clin North Am 1988;14:441–457.
   The standard therapies for gout are reviewed.

120 Prepatellar and Olecranon Bursitis

Problem

DAVID L. SMITH

Epidemiology and Etiology. The olecranon bursa is situated over the extensor tissue of the elbow; the prepatellar bursa (including the infrapatellar bursa) is located anterior to the knee. These bursae facilitate motion of adjacent tendons but are subject to injury from trauma or infection. Repetitive trauma of the elbow or knee, incurred by laborers such as carpenters or mechanics and through recreation, predisposes to both septic and nonseptic bursitis. Alcoholic patients and patients with neurologic disorders (e.g., seizures, ataxia) or impaired host defense mechanisms and those with bursal involvement from rheumatoid nodules or gouty tophi are also at risk for bursitis. Dermatitis overlying the bursa increases the risk of infection. The incidence of olecranon or prepatellar bursitis is between 0.03% and 0.1% of hospital admissions and outpatient or urgent clinic visits. The ratio of nonseptic to septic cases is 3:1; the ratio of olecranon to prepatellar bursitis is 8:1.

Pathogens that typically cause septic bursitis are *Staphylococcus aureus, S. epidermidis,* and several streptococcal species. Rarely, fungal organisms are implicated. The etiology of nonseptic cases is idiopathic in 60% of patients, traumatic in 35%, and crystal induced in 5%. Crystal-induced cases, secondary to monosodium urate or calcium pyrophosphate deposition, may be precipitated by trauma.

Symptoms, Signs, and Laboratory Findings

SEPTIC BURSITIS. Except for immunocompromised patients, bursal warmth and a surface temperature difference of 2.2°C or greater compared with the contralateral side is observed (Table 120–1). Peribursal edema or cellulitis is noted in about 60% of cases. Spontaneous drainage occurs in 36%. The fluid aspirated from the bursa ranges from purulent to serous. The mean white blood cell count in the aspirated fluid varies between 2000 and 60,000 cells/mm^3, with polymorphonuclear leukocytes predominating. The Gram stain is positive in only 60% of culture-positive cases.

NONSEPTIC BURSITIS. Bursal warmth is found in 50%, tenderness in 20%, and an overlying skin lesion (e.g., dry or cracked skin) in 17% of cases. Aspirated bursal fluid ranges from clear to bloody. The mean leukocyte count in the aspirated fluid is 2500 cells/mm^3 but ranges from 200 to 27,000 cells/mm^3, with mononuclear cells predominating. An olecranon bone spur is radiographically present in 30% of nonseptic olecranon bursitis cases.

Table 120–1. UTILITY OF SELECTED CHARACTERISTICS IN DISTINGUISHING SEPTIC FROM NONSEPTIC BURSITIS*

Characteristic	Sensitivity (%)	Specificity (%)	Positive Predictive Value (%)	Negative Predictive Value (%)	Positive Likelihood Ratio
History of trauma	54	60	30	80	1.4
Warmth on palpation	100	50	38	100	2.0
Surface temperature difference between involved and control sides ($\geq 2.2°C$)	100	94	85	100	16.7
Tenderness	80	63	60	93	1.7
Skin lesion	64	80	54	90	3.2
White blood cell count > 2000/mm³	78	75	53	90	3.1
$\geq$ 50% of white blood cells are polymorphonuclear leukocytes	82	77	53	93	3.6
Positive Gram stain	54	100	100	88	∞

*These features appear to have similar utility in prepatellar bursitis (unpublished observation, DL Smith).

From Smith DL, McAfee JH, Lucas LM, Kumar KL, Romney DM. Septic and nonseptic bursitis: Utility of the surface temperature probe in the early differentiation of septic and nonseptic cases. Arch Intern Med 1989;149:1581–1585. Copyright 1989, American Medical Association.

Clinical Approach. In all cases of newly diagnosed olecranon and prepatellar bursitis, the bursa should be aspirated. A 20-gauge 1-inch needle attached to a 10-ml syringe is adequate to aspirate the bursal contents after skin cleansing. A lateral approach helps to avoid bursal bacterial inoculation through the skin when these areas are exposed to pressure after aspiration.

In some cases the history, examination, and bursal fluid aspirate do not distinguish between septic and nonseptic bursitis. The individual clinical features listed in Table 120–1 assist in determining whether infection is present before culture results are available. When there is uncertainty, antibiotic treatment is usually prudent.

Management

SEPTIC BURSITIS. In cases of localized infection, an antistaphylococcal penicillin (e.g., dicloxacillin, 500 mg every 6 hours) or cephalosporin should be given for 14 days. Clindamycin, 300 mg every 6 hours, is an effective alternative for patients who are allergic to penicillin. Sterilization of the bursa may require prolonged therapy in patients with impaired host defenses. Warm soaks, arm elevation, daily dressing changes, and repeated bursal irrigation and aspiration are also of value. The patient should receive intravenous antibiotics (e.g., nafcillin, 1 g every 4 hours) when extensive arm or leg cellulitis, lymphadenitis, or chills and fever are present. Intravenous antibiotic therapy is administered for 1 to 2 weeks, followed by 10 to 14 days of oral antibiotic therapy.

NONSEPTIC BURSITIS. Idiopathic or traumatic bursitis usually responds to complete evacuation of the sterile bursal sac contents, use of a compression dressing, and an injection of an intrabursal corticosteroid preparation (e.g., 20 mg of methylprednisolone acetate). Bursal sterility must be ensured by culture.

In olecranon bursitis, the corticosteroid injection shortens the course and minimizes recurrences. A 10-day course of an oral nonsteroidal anti-inflammatory agent is effective for crystal-induced cases. Treatment of underlying gout is essential. When rheumatoid nodules involve the bursa, appropriate systemic treatment is required.

Follow-Up. Patients with septic bursitis should be reevaluated within several days. Repeat aspiration may be required to evacuate a recurrent or persistent effusion. Normally, complete resolution occurs within 4 weeks. In protracted septic cases, referral to an orthopedic surgeon for incision and drainage is indicated if parenteral antibiotic use is unsuccessful. Patients with nonseptic bursitis should be reevaluated in 7 to 10 days. Recurrent cases may respond to temporary splinting of the affected joint. Extensor area pads help protect these bursae from further trauma, especially in high-risk patients. Resection of the bursa or underlying bone spur is reserved for chronic cases.

Cross-References: General Approach to Arthritic Symptoms (Chapter 106), Knee Pain (Chapter 111), Gout/Hyperuricemia (Chapter 119).

REFERENCES

1. Ho G, Tice AD. Comparison of nonseptic and septic bursitis: Further observations on the treatment of septic bursitis. Arch Intern Med 1979;139:1269–1273.

   A helpful analysis of bursal fluid findings is provided.

2. McAfee JH, Smith DL. Olecranon and prepatellar bursitis: Diagnosis and treatment. West J Med 1988;149:607–610.

   The authors review the anatomy, clinical features, and management of olecranon and prepatellar bursitis.

3. Pien FD, Ching D, Kim E. Septic bursitis in a community practice. Orthopedics 1991;14:981–984.

   This is a useful descriptive analysis of septic bursitis in a private setting.

4. Smith DL, McAfee JH, Lucas LM, Kumar KL, Romney DM. Septic and nonseptic bursitis: Utility of the surface temperature probe in the early differentiation of septic and nonseptic cases. Arch Intern Med 1989;149:1581–1585.

   A surface temperature probe reading helps distinguish septic from nonseptic cases.

5. Smith DL, McAfee JH, Lucas LM, Kumar KL, Romney DM. Treatment of nonseptic olecranon bursitis. Arch Intern Med 1989;149:2527–2530.

   A controlled prospective clinical trial demonstrated efficacy of intrabursal methylprednisolone acetate compared with an oral anti-inflammatory agent.

121 Fibromyalgia

Problem

JOHN B. STIMSON

Epidemiology. Fibromyalgia is a clinical syndrome of generalized aching and stiffness that is associated with the finding of numerous tender points in characteristic locations (Table 121–1). The terms *fibrositis* and *primary* or *secondary fibromyalgia* have been abandoned. In contrast to myofascial pain syndrome, patients with fibromyalgia experience generalized instead of focal discomfort, have no trigger points on examination, and respond less well to treatment (see Chapter 122, Myofascial Pain Syndromes). Although no cause or characteristic laboratory abnormality has been identified, the clinical syndrome of fibromyalgia is characteristic enough that most physicians accept it as a real entity. The prevalence of fibromyalgia among over 3000 randomly selected residents of Wichita, Kansas, was 2.0%. Five percent of unselected patients in a general medical clinic satisfy criteria for fibromyalgia. Seventy percent to 90% of affected patients are women.

Symptoms and Signs. The most common symptom is prolonged (i.e., > 3 months) multifocal pain, accompanied by fatigue, morning stiffness, and nonrestorative sleep. Patients may report prolonged morning stiffness similar to that seen in rheumatoid arthritis. The pain typically worsens with acute stress, exposure to cold, inactivity or overactivity, and changes in barometric pressure. Less common complaints are headaches, irritable bowel symptoms, sensations

---

Table 121–1. AMERICAN COLLEGE OF RHEUMATOLOGY 1990 CRITERIA FOR THE CLASSIFICATION OF FIBROMYALGIA

1. Widespread pain for more than 3 months.
   "Widespread" requires both right- and left-sided pain, pain above and below the waist, and axial skeletal pain. Low back pain is regarded as being below the waist.
2. Pain on palpation in at least 11 of 18 of the following tender point sites:
   Occiput: bilateral, at the suboccipital muscle insertions.
   Low cervical: bilateral, at the anterior aspects of the intertransverse spaces at C5-C7.
   Trapezius: bilateral, at the midpoint of the upper border.
   Supraspinatus: bilateral, at origins, above the scapula spine near the medial border.
   Second rib: bilateral, at the second costochondral junctions, just lateral to the junctions on upper surfaces.
   Lateral epicondyle: bilateral, 2 cm distal to the epicondyles.
   Gluteal: bilateral, in upper outer quadrants of buttocks in anterior fold of muscle.
   Greater trochanter: bilateral, posterior to the trochanteric prominence.
   Knee: bilateral, at the medial fat pad proximal to the joint line.

Wolfe F, Smythe HA, Yunus MB, et al. The American College of Rheumatology 1990 criteria for the classification of fibromyalgia: Report of the Multicenter Criteria Committee. Arthritis Rheum 1990;33:160–172.

of numbness or swelling, reactive hyperemia of the skin, and Raynaud's phenomenon.

Tender points, the hallmark of fibromyalgia, are discrete areas over muscle, ligaments, or fat pads that produce local pain when moderately firm pressure is applied with a single finger or thumb. The appropriate technique uses pressure insufficient to produce pain in normal individuals or uninvolved sites in affected individuals. In contrast to the trigger points seen in myofascial pain syndromes, palpation of tender points generally does not cause referred pain, and tender points are not confined to muscle.

Depression is no more common than among patients with rheumatoid arthritis, although patients with fibromyalgia do report high stress levels.

Clinical Approach. The patient interview does not reliably differentiate fibromyalgia, rheumatoid arthritis, and osteoarthritis. Chronic generalized pain refractory to anti-inflammatory medications suggests fibromyalgia. Low back pain is common and hand involvement is rare in fibromyalgia, in contrast to rheumatoid arthritis. Physical examination in patients with fibromyalgia, however, is remarkable for the absence of joint abnormalities (unless a coincidental arthritic disorder is present) and the presence of characteristic tender points. Control areas not expected to be tender in fibromyalgia (e.g., middle of the forehead, fingertips) should be examined to exclude psychogenic pain or malingering.

Diagnostic criteria for fibromyalgia are listed in Table 121–1. Laboratory evaluation is unnecessary unless a coexisting condition is suspected. A normal erythrocyte sedimentation rate helps exclude most inflammatory conditions, such as rheumatoid arthritis, polymyalgia rheumatica, ankylosing spondylitis, myositis, lupus erythematosus, and vasculitis. Although hypothyroidism can cause generalized aching, tender points are unusual on examination.

Management. Therapy for fibromyalgia is generally disappointing. Far greater benefit is achieved by reassurance than by any pharmacologic therapy currently available. Patients benefit from learning they have a recognizable condition that does not progress or cripple and that does not warrant further diagnostic testing. Various medications produce minor benefit in some patients. Cyclobenzaprine (10–40 mg/d) or low-dose amitriptyline (10–50 mg at bedtime) may improve sleep and slightly lessen daytime fatigue and aching. Nonsteroidal anti-inflammatory medications can help some patients, but the small benefit may not justify the risks. A controlled trial of prednisone, 15 mg/d, showed no benefit. Low-impact cardiovascular conditioning (e.g., stationary cycling) helps some patients, although initial worsening for 2 weeks is the rule. Use of narcotics for pain management is to be avoided.

Cross-References: Chronic Nonspecific Pain Syndrome (Chapter 14), General Approach to Arthritic Symptoms (Chapter 106), Myofascial Pain Syndromes (Chapter 122), Common Thyroid Disorders (Chapter 153).

REFERENCES

1. Carett S, Lefrancois L. Fibrositis and primary hypothyroidism. J Rheumatol 1988;15:1418–1421.
   Hypothyroid patients frequently have diffuse aching, but multiple tender points were no more frequent than in the general medical clinic population.

2. McCain GA, Bell DA, Mai FM, Halliday PD. A controlled study of the effects of a supervised cardiovascular fitness training program on the manifestations of primary fibromyalgia. Arthritis Rheum 1988;31:1135–1141.

Some 50% of patients with fibromyalgia who underwent a 5-month cardiovascular fitness training program significantly improved, compared with 10% of patients who underwent a simple stretching program.

3. Wolfe F, Smythe HA, Yunus MB, et al. The American College of Rheumatology 1990 criteria for the classification of fibromyalgia: Report of the Multicenter Criteria Committee. Arthritis Rheum 1990;33:160–172.

The authors report a study in which 293 patients considered to have fibromyalgia and 265 controls with rheumatic conditions most likely to be confused with fibromyalgia were examined in a standardized and blinded fashion. The information was used to develop the 1990 criteria for the diagnosis of fibromyalgia.

● ●

122 Myofascial Pain Syndromes

Problem

JOHN B. STIMSON

Epidemiology. Myofascial pain syndromes usually affect overused or injured muscles, may persist long after the actual muscle injury, and are associated with discrete, tender areas within muscle called trigger points. The pathophysiology is unknown. A given trigger point, which may be further stimulated by moderate pressure or needle insertion, causes referred pain in characteristic patterns, just as ischemic foci in cardiac muscle cause referred neck, jaw, or arm pain. The overall prevalence of myofascial pain syndrome is unknown but is reportedly as high as 55% to 85% in patients attending pain clinics.

Symptoms and Signs. Myofascial pain is poorly localized and can include sensations of tingling, numbness, or skin hyperalgesia. In the involved muscle, trigger points are often found within palpable firm bands, which may visibly twitch during palpation or needle puncture. Because stretching of affected muscles causes pain, patients often keep muscles in a shortened position and restrict motion of nearby joints.

Common clinical syndromes and associated trigger points include (1) temporomandibular joint syndrome from masseter muscle trigger points; (2) arm or shoulder pain from scapular muscle trigger points; (3) occipital headache and neck pain from trapezius or posterior neck muscle trigger points; (4) anterior chest pain from sternal, pectoral, sternocleidomastoid, or serratus anterior muscle trigger points (at times misdiagnosed as ischemic cardiac pain); (5) low back pain from lumbar spinal muscle trigger points; and (6) sciatica from gluteal muscle trigger points.

Table 122–1. CAUSES OF SOFT TISSUE PAIN

Trigger points in muscle	Reflex dystrophies
Bursitis, tendinitis, tenosynovitis, arthritis	Referred pain syndromes from viscera
Phlebitis or deep venous thrombosis	Mononeuritis multiplex
Hematoma in muscle	Central nervous system pain syndromes
Nerve entrapment syndromes	

Clinical Approach. Familiarity with common trigger points and their referred pain patterns is essential to the diagnosis. The examiner strokes his or her fingers perpendicular to the affected muscle fibers and searches for palpable bands. Moderately firm pressure over these bands may identify the actual trigger point. If the examination fails to elicit discrete tenderness and produce referred pain, a true trigger point and a myofascial cause for pain are unlikely.

Other causes of soft tissue pain appear in Table 122–1. Joint or tendon crepitation, tenderness over bony structures, reflex loss, and muscle wasting are not features of myofascial pain syndromes and generally point to the correct diagnosis.

Management. Established myofascial pain responds poorly to conventional therapy for musculoskeletal pain, such as heat and anti-inflammatory agents. Instead, measures directed at the responsible trigger point are most effective: vapocoolant spray (chlorofluoromethane) or trigger point injection with a local anesthetic, followed by stretch of the involved muscle (see Chapter 126, Trigger Point Injection). A single treatment may be effective, but often treatments repeated every 2 to 4 days are necessary until sustained improvement is achieved. Correction of postural abnormalities or occupational overuse may prevent relapses.

Cross-References: Acute Chest Pain (Chapter 73), Recurrent Chest Pain (Chapter 74), General Approach to Arthritic Symptoms (Chapter 106), Low Back Pain (Chapter 107), Shoulder Pain (Chapter 108), Hip Pain (Chapter 109), Fibromyalgia (Chapter 121), Trigger Point Injection (Chapter 126), Headache (Chapter 138).

REFERENCES

1. Simons DG, Travell JG. Myofascial pain syndromes. In Wall PD, Melzack R, eds. Textbook of Pain. New York, Churchill Livingstone, 1984:263–276.

   Excellent maps of referred pain patterns for common trigger points are included.

2. Travell J, Rinzler SH. Pain syndromes of the anterior chest muscles: Resemblance to effort angina and myocardial infarction, and relief by local block. Can Med Assoc J 1948;59:333–338.

   Case reports illustrate that myofascial pain can mimic pain from ischemic cardiac muscle, resulting in hospital admission.

3. Travell JG, Simons DG. Myofascial Pain and Dysfunction: The Trigger Point Manual. Baltimore, Williams & Wilkins, 1983.

   Comprehensive review of location and treatment techniques for trigger points in the most important muscles in the upper (volume 1) and lower (volume 2) body includes otherwise difficult-to-find techniques for stretching each muscle.

123 Interpretation of Serologic Tests

Procedure

RICHARD H. WHITE

Indications and Contraindications. Numerous serologic tests are available that may aid in the diagnosis of specific rheumatic diseases. Those serologic tests with high *specificity* should be ordered to verify suspected diagnoses. For example, a high level of antibody to double-stranded DNA or to the Smith (Sm) antigen is specific for systemic lupus erythematosus (SLE), and an elevated level of antibody to neutrophil cytoplasmic antigens is specific for Wegener's granulomatosis and related disorders (polyarteritis nodosa and crescentic glomerular nephritis). Tests with high *sensitivity* should be ordered to help exclude a diagnosis when clinical findings are equivocal. For example, a negative antinuclear antibody assay essentially excludes the diagnosis of SLE.

Methods. The serologic tests most frequently ordered are listed in Table 123–1, together with the sensitivity, specificity, and clinical utility of each test. Each laboratory has a different range for normal and abnormal values.

Test Interpretation. Results of a fluorescent antinuclear antibody test are usually reported as a titer, together with a pattern. A *rim* pattern is rare and is specific for SLE. A *speckled* pattern is common, nonspecific, and frequently present in high titer in patients who have no manifestations of a rheumatic disease. A *nucleolar* pattern is less common and is nonspecific. A *centromere* pattern is rare and is not the same as a positive test for anticentromere antibody. A *homogeneous* pattern is common, nonspecific, usually present in low titer (less than 1:640), and characteristic for drug-induced antinuclear antibody.

In the absence of signs and symptoms of the rheumatic disease under consideration, a positive serologic test is not diagnostic. For example, in patients with isolated chronic fatigue, a positive Lyme titer (enzyme-linked immunosorbent assay for IgG) is not diagnostic for Lyme disease. A positive antinuclear antibody assay without findings of lupus is meaningless and sometimes occurs with subclinical autoimmune disease or with certain medications.

Cross-References: Principles of Screening (Chapter 7), General Approach to Arthritic Symptoms (Chapter 106).

Table 123–1. INTERPRETATION OF SEROLOGIC TESTS

Serologic Tests	Sensitivity	Specificity	Clinical Utility
ANA	SLE (95%), MCTD (99%), drug-induced SLE (99%)	Low; associated with many disorders	A negative test helps to exclude SLE, MCTD, and drug-induced SLE
RF	RA (85%–90%)	Low; associated with many disorders	A positive test helps classify patients with polyarthritis for greater than 3 mo
Anti-dsDNA	SLE (50%–60%) (with active disease)	High, > 95% for SLE	A positive test helps to diagnose SLE
Anti-Sm (Smith)	SLE (30%–40%)	High, > 98% for SLE	A positive test helps to diagnose SLE
Anti-(U1) RNP	MCTD (100%)	Low, seen in SLE, PSS, RA, discoid lupus	A negative test excludes MCTD
Antihistone	Drug-induced SLE (100%)	Low, seen in SLE, RA	Not helpful
Anti-Ro (SSA)	Sjögren's (60%–70%)	Low, seen in SLE, RA	Associated with aggressive Sjögren's neonatal SLE, neonatal heart block
Anti-La (SSB)	Sjögren's (50%–60%)	Low, seen in SLE	Not useful
Anticentromere	CREST syndrome (50%–90%)	High for CREST, PSS, or Raynaud's	Minimal value over clinical findings alone
Anti-SCL$_{70}$ (Anti-Topo 1)	Scleroderma (20%)	High, > 95% for scleroderma	Positive test is helpful in the diagnosis of scleroderma
Anti-JO$_1$	Polymyositis (30%)	?	Associated with myositis and interstitial fibrosis
ANCA	Wegener's granulomatosis: Generalized (95%) Limited (67%)	High, > 99% for Wegener's granulomatosis	A positive test helps diagnose Wegener's granulomatosis and related disorders (e.g., polyarteritis)
Lyme titer	High for subacute and chronic Lyme disease	Low, < 90%	Helpful when there is a high titer *and* clinical manifestations of Lyme disease

ANA, antinuclear antibody; ANCA, antineutrophil cytoplasmic antibody; CREST, calcinosis cutis, Raynaud's phenomenon, esophageal dysfunction, sclerodactyly, and telangiectasia; MCTD, mixed connective tissue disease; PSS, progressive systemic sclerosis; RA, rheumatoid arthritis; RF, rheumatoid factor; RNP, ribonucleoprotein; SLE, systemic lupus erythematosus.

REFERENCES

1. Barbour AG. The diagnosis of Lyme disease: Rewards and perils. Ann Intern Med 1989;110:501–502.

   This article is a summary of the current status regarding the role of serologic testing in the diagnosis of Lyme disease. The test should be ordered solely to confirm a diagnosis based on epidemiologic and clinical evidence.

2. Falk RJ, Hogan S, Carey TS, Jennette C, Glomerular Disease Collaborative Network. Clinical course of anti-neutrophil cytoplasmic autoantibody–associated glomerulonephritis and systemic vasculitis. Ann Intern Med 1990;113:656–663.

   Prospective study of 70 patients with anti-neutrophil cytoplasmic autoantibody documented its specificity for Wegener's granulomatosis and the related disorders crescentic glomerulonephritis and polyarteritis nodosa.

3. Slater CA, Davis RB, Shmerling RH. Antinuclear antibody testing. A study of clinical utility. Arch Intern Med 1996;56:1421–1425.

   This study demonstrates that the sensitivity of the antinuclear antibody test is high while the positive predictive value for SLE and other rheumatic diseases is low.

4. Tsokos GC, Pillemer SR, Klippel JH. Rheumatic disease syndromes associated with antibodies to the Ro (SS-A) ribonuclear protein. Semin Arthritis Rheum 1987;16:237–244.

   Associations between anti-Ro antibody and (1) antinuclear antibody–negative SLE, (2) subacute cutaneous SLE, (3) neonatal SLE, and (4) extraglandular Sjögren's syndrome are reviewed.

5. Wade JP, Sack B, Schur PH. Anticentromere antibodies: Clinical correlates. J Rheumatol 1988;15:1759–1763.

   The presence of anticentromere antibody is less specific than previously thought in the screening of unselected patients with rheumatic disease.

6. White RH, Robbins DL. Clinical significance and interpretation of antinuclear antibodies. West J Med 1987;147:210–213.

   The diagnostic utility of the antinuclear antibody test is reviewed.

. . . .

124 Diabetic Foot Care Education

Procedure

JESSIE H. AHRONI

Indications and Contraindications. All patients with diabetes should be taught the basic principles of foot care, although there is no evidence that young persons with healthy feet require detailed advice. Those with neuropathy, vascular disease, or a history of foot ulceration or amputation should receive periodic intensive, comprehensive foot care education.

Rationale. For the patient with neuropathy, vascular disease, orthopedic deformity, or a history of foot infection or ulceration, an education program can reduce the incidence of recurrent ulceration and limb amputation. Insensitivity to a 5.07 monofilament can identify patients at high risk for foot ulceration and lower extremity amputation. In one study the odds ratio of subsequent ulceration was 9.9 (95% CI 4.8–21.0) and of amputation was 17 (95% CI 4.5–95.0) compared with those who retained sensation.

Methods. The clinician should review the principles of foot care with high-risk diabetic patients at every visit and with low-risk patients at least once a year. The essentials of self-care for persons with diabetes are listed below:

1. Inspect the feet and interdigital areas daily (e.g., whenever putting on or taking off socks). A mirror may be helpful. If the patient is unable, a family member should perform the inspection.

2. Wash and dry the feet thoroughly, especially between the toes. A thin layer of lamb's wool can be used to separate overlapping or contacting toes and help prevent maceration. The clinician should caution the patient about avoiding hot-water burns by checking the bath water temperature with the forearm or elbow. Routine soaking is not recommended.

3. Moisturize dry skin (except between the toes) with an emollient such as lanolin or hand lotion.

4. Cut or file toenails straight across the contour of the toe, being sure all sharp edges are filed smooth. If the patient does not see well or has difficulty reaching his or her feet, this may be done by a family member, nurse, or podiatrist.

5. Avoid self-treatment of corns, calluses, or ingrown toenails. Chemicals, sharp instruments, or razor blades should never be used on the feet by a patient. A patient with good judgment can use a pumice stone to gently buff away minor calluses or rough skin. Flaky fungal debris can be loosened and removed with a soft nail brush during regular bathing.

6. Wear well-fitting soft cotton or wool socks. The patient should not use hot-water bottles or heating pads for cold feet.

7. Avoid walking barefoot to avoid puncture wounds and burns from hot sand or pavement.

8. Examine the shoes daily for internal cracks, loose linings, pebbles, and other irregularities that may irritate the skin. Soft leather or canvas shoes that have cushioned insoles and fit well at the time of purchase are best. Changing shoes during the day can limit repetitive local pressure.

9. Seek prompt medical attention for any problems (e.g., cuts, blisters, calluses, and any wounds that do not heal or any signs of infection such as redness, swelling, pus, drainage, or fever). Fungal infections should be promptly treated with antifungal cream, spray, or powder and behavioral or footwear changes to keep the area between the toes clean and dry.

Cost and Complications. Although the actual costs of diabetic foot problems and amputations are unknown, these conditions are undoubtedly expensive and disabling. Greater use of preventive services has the potential to lessen this burden.

Cross-References: Diabetic Retinopathy (Chapter 44), Local Care of Diabetic Foot Lesions (Chapter 134), Diabetes Mellitus (Chapter 154).

REFERENCES

1. Ahroni JA. Teaching foot care creatively and successfully. Diabetes Educator 1993;19:320–325.
   This article describes comprehensive diabetic foot screening and includes practical suggestions for teaching foot self-care skills and knowledge.

2. Davidson JK, Algona M, Goldsmith M, Borden J. Assessment of program effectiveness at Grady Memorial Hospital, Atlanta. In Steiner G, Lawrence OA, eds. Educating Diabetic Patients. New York, Springer, 1981;329–348.

   A comprehensive diabetes evaluation, education, and treatment center decreased severe hypoglycemia, ketoacidosis, hospital days, and amputations and improved patient and professional satisfaction.

3. Edmonds ME, Blundell MP, Morris ME, Thomas EM, Cotton LT, Watkins PJ. Improved survival of the diabetic foot: The role of a specialized foot clinic. Q J Med 1986;60:763–771.

   A comprehensive, multidisciplinary foot clinic achieved a high rate of ulcer healing and reduced the number of amputations in diabetic patients.

4. Reiber GE, Boyko EJ, Smith DG. Lower extremity foot ulcers and amputations in diabetes. In National Diabetes Data Group, ed. Diabetes in America, 2nd ed. Washington, DC, National Institutes of Health, 1995.

   Current population-based analytic and experimental studies demonstrate that diabetic foot ulcers and amputations are important and costly problems.

5. Rith-Najarian SJ, Stolusky TS, Gohdes DM. Identifying diabetic patients at high risk for lower-extremity amputation in a primary health care setting: A prospective evaluation of simple screening criteria. Diabetes Care 1992;15:1386–1389.

   A few medical history questions and a simple clinical examination can stratify patients with diabetes into risk categories for subsequent foot ulceration or lower extremity amputation.

• •

125 Physical Therapy Care of Outpatients

Procedure

SARAH JACKINS

Indications and Contraindications. Physical therapy offers a variety of treatments that assist in the management of many medical conditions.

There are three routes to follow in considering a referral to physical therapy (Table 125–1): (1) no referral—the primary care provider provides early measures that in and of themselves provide all the needed treatment; (2) late referral—the provider's early measures are not sufficient and the patient is referred to a physical therapy program; and (3) early referral—cases in which the patient will do best when physical therapy referral is initiated early on.

Rationale. In the outpatient setting, physical therapy is primarily aimed at aiding recovery from an injury and preventing secondary complications during that recovery process. Physical therapists educate patients with regard to how they can participate in their recovery and prevent future injuries.

The trend these days is for patients to take on more responsibility for their health, and that includes their rehabilitation for a particular condition. The

Table 125–1. INDICATIONS FOR REFERRAL FOR PHYSICAL THERAPY

Patient has a decrease in function secondary to musculoskeletal limitation of pain
Examples of musculoskeletal conditions that respond to physical therapy include
    Recurrent ankle sprains
    Persistent anterior knee pain
    Frozen shoulder or other joint restrictions
    Low back pain
    Whiplash
    Persistent tendinitis at any joint
    Repetitive stress injuries such as carpal tunnel syndrome
    Fractures
    Following orthopedic surgery
    Reflex sympathetic dystrophy

Table 125–2. COMMON PHYSICAL THERAPY PROCEDURES

Procedure	Indications	Contraindications
Exercise		
Flexibility/stretching	Stiffness	Unstable joint
Assisted		
Passive		
Strengthening	Weakness	
	Instability	
Isometric	Inflamed joint	
Isotonic/isokinetic		Inflamed joint
Modalities		
Heat	Aches, pains	Acute injury
Superficial (hot packs,		Decreased sensation
infrared, fluidotherapy,		Malignancy
whirlpool)		Impaired circulation
Deep	Contracture	Inflamed joint
Ultrasound		
Cold	Muscle spasm	Decreased sensation
	Acute injury	Raynaud's syndrome
		Cold urticaria
		Impaired circulation
Hydrotherapy	Wound cleansing/débridement	Acute injury
Massage	Myofascial syndrome/	Acute injury
	fibromyalgia	Open wound
		Hemorrhage
Posture/body mechanics	Back pain	None
training	Work-related injuries	
Splint	Joint requiring immobilization	
	secondary to inflammatory	
	process; contractures	
	Protection after orthopedic	
	repair	

physical therapist becomes more and more of an instructor and coach. As a part of this, the trend is away from the use of many passive modalities and toward more active exercise.

Methods. When making a referral for physical therapy, it is very helpful for the physician to include the diagnosis and pertinent medical history: presence of any cardiac limitations, any infectious disease that is not handled by universal precautions (e.g., tuberculosis), and precautions regarding weight bearing (as in the case of a fracture) or against resisted exercise (as in the time immediately after a rotator cuff tear repair).

Ideally, the physician and the physical therapist should agree on the general treatment philosophy of therapy. Given the physician's general recommendations, the therapist provides a specific treatment plan (Table 125–2). The physician also communicates any known insurance guidelines that limit the number of treatment sessions the therapist can offer; the therapist can present these limits as supporting the idea that the patient will get better and will not be dependent on therapy for an especially long time.

Cost and Complications. Most third-party payers cover physical therapy services, but these may be capped by dollar amounts or number of treatment sessions. Charges vary depending on various factors, including location. Typical charges for an hour of therapy are between $75 and $150.

Cross-References: General Approach to Arthritic Symptoms (Chapter 106), Low Back Pain (Chapter 107), Shoulder Pain (Chapter 108), Hip Pain (Chapter 109), Knee Pain (Chapter 111), Ankle and Foot Pain (Chapter 112), Fibromyalgia (Chapter 121), Myofascial Pain Syndromes (Chapter 122).

REFERENCES

1. American College of Sports Medicine. Resource Manual for Guidelines for Exercise Testing and Prescription, 2nd ed. Philadelphia, Lea & Febiger, 1993.

   This is an authoritative reference for exercise measurement and guidelines

2. Lehmann JF. Therapeutic Heat and Cold, 4th ed. Baltimore, Williams & Wilkins, 1990.

   This reference provides a thorough explanation of physical agents, scientific rationales, and applications.

3. Malone TR, McFoil TG. Orthopedic and Sports Physical Therapy, 3rd ed. St. Louis, CV Mosby, 1996.

   This presents a comprehensive review of indications for physical therapy techniques for a variety of musculoskeletal conditions.

4. Michlovitz SL. Thermal Agents in Rehabilitation. Philadelphia, FA Davis, 1986.

   The author provides descriptions of physical therapy modalities and uses.

126 Trigger Point Injection

Procedure

JOHN B. STIMSON

Indications and Contraindications. Prolonged myofascial pain syndromes with reproducible trigger points (see Chapter 122, Myofascial Pain Syndromes) justify trigger point injection. Soft tissue pain or tender muscles without trigger points are unlikely to respond to injection and should not be treated in this manner. Tender points seen in fibromyalgia also respond poorly to injection. True allergy or a previous idiosyncratic reaction to local anesthetics are the only contraindications to trigger point injection. Coagulopathy or anticoagulant therapy render patients more likely to develop small hematomas at injection sites and are relative contraindications.

Rationale. Whether abnormalities of muscle, nerves, or both cause trigger points is unknown. Nonspecific therapy with analgesics, rest, and heat is generally ineffective. Empirical treatment of trigger points with local anesthetic injections or chlorofluoromethane spray, however, reduces pain and restores normal muscle length and function. Interestingly, needle insertion without injection or saline injection alone is also sometimes effective, although local anesthetic injections are probably superior.

Methods. A reproducible discrete trigger point is a prerequisite to trigger point injection. After palpation, a 22- to 25-gauge needle is inserted into the muscle to locate the exact spot that reproduces the patient's pain. Once the trigger point is located, 1 to 2 mL of anesthetic is injected. If the trigger point cannot be located with the needle, a larger amount of anesthetic should be infiltrated in the general area. When the site is anesthetic, the muscle is passively stretched to restore full range of motion. Short-acting anesthetics without epinephrine, such as 1% procaine or lidocaine, are preferred because they produce less muscle necrosis at the injection site than long-acting anesthetics (e.g., bupivacaine) or those containing epinephrine. A 1½-inch needle is sufficient to reach essentially all trigger points in the upper body. Lumbar and gluteal trigger points may require longer needles and more expertise to locate. Repeated treatments every few days are sometimes necessary to achieve sustained improvement, though no specific guidelines exist.

Complications. Trigger point injection is quite safe if simple precautions are observed. If not properly performed, intravascular or intraneural injections can occur. Pneumothorax is an uncommon complication of injections in the thorax. Up to 50 mL of 1% procaine or lidocaine can be safely infiltrated into soft tissues before concerns about neurologic or cardiac toxicity arise. These volumes far exceed those required for multiple trigger point injections.

Cross-References: Low Back Pain (Chapter 107), Shoulder Pain (Chapter 108), Myofascial Pain Syndromes (Chapter 122).

127 Injection of the Subacromial Bursa

Procedure

STEPHAN D. FIHN

Indications and Contraindications. For the primary care provider, injection of the shoulder usually refers to injection of the subacromial bursa. Injection of the glenohumeral joint should be performed only by those with training and substantial experience. The response to injection of the subacromial bursa with 1% lidocaine is useful in differentiating subacromial bursitis from other causes of shoulder pain, particularly rotator cuff tears and frozen shoulder. Randomized trials have shown that patients with subacromial bursitis who fail to respond to treatment with nonsteroidal agents, heat, and exercise often respond favorably to injection of a long-acting corticosteroid preparation into the bursa.

Contraindications to injection include suspected infection of the shoulder joint, surrounding structures, or overlying skin and the presence of a prosthetic shoulder joint. Contraindications to corticosteroid injection are a suspected rotator cuff tear and a history of repeated corticosteroid injections.

Rationale. Injection of lidocaine into the subacromial bursa can be helpful in deciding which patients with significant shoulder pain should have an early referral to an orthopedic surgeon or for imaging tests such as magnetic resonance imaging or arthrography. Injection of a corticosteroid into an inflamed bursa can provide substantial relief of pain and improvement in range of motion to patients with otherwise stubborn symptoms.

Methods. The patient should be seated comfortably with the hands folded in the lap. After thorough hand washing, the clinician should locate the acromion. The area immediately anterior and inferior to the acromion should be palpated with the index finger of the same hand as the side of the patient being examined (e.g., right index finger on right shoulder). The area of maximal tenderness should be pressed firmly with the examining finger while the clinician holds the patient's elbow with his or her other hand and passively abducts and adducts the arm. At the point of maximal tenderness or in the immediate vicinity, the clinician should feel his or her finger enter the space between the lower border of the acromion and the humeral head. This spot should be marked using gentle pressure with a retracted ball-point pen or the open end of a pen cap. The location marked is usually 1 to 2 cm below the acromion and 1 to 2 cm anterior to it. If there is marked disparity between the point of maximal tenderness and the spot marked, the shoulder should be reexamined to confirm the diagnosis. Otherwise, the shoulder should be scrubbed with a povidone-iodine solution and allowed to dry.

Meanwhile, the examiner should place 2 to 4 mL of 1% lidocaine (without epinephrine) into a 10-mL syringe. If a corticosteroid is also to be injected, it should be mixed with the lidocaine in the syringe. Aqueous methylprednisolone acetate suspension, 20 to 40 mg, is the corticosteroid preparation of choice, although aqueous dexamethasone phosphate, 2 to 6 mg, and triamcinolone hexacetonide, 20 to 40 mg, are acceptable alternatives.

Wearing sterile gloves, the physician may then raise a skin wheal with 1 to 2 mL of 1% lidocaine at the previously marked location, although in most cases this is unnecessary. If a corticosteroid is being injected, the physician should then briskly shake the syringe to disperse the corticosteroid suspension in the lidocaine. A 23- to 27-gauge, 1½-inch needle should be placed on the syringe. The physician then places the tip of the needle on the previously marked spot and advances it directly in the horizontal plane. The needle is slowly passed through the deltoid muscle so that it passes beneath the acromion until it reaches a hard surface, which is the rotator cuff tendon overlying the humerus. The needle is then withdrawn slightly to avoid injecting directly into the tendon. After gentle aspiration, the contents of the syringe are slowly instilled. Only minimal resistance should be felt. If resistance is encountered, injection is reattempted after backing the needle out 2 or 3 mm. When the contents of the syringe have been dispensed, the needle is withdrawn and placed in an appropriate disposal container and an adhesive bandage is placed over the injection site.

After injection, the patient should be asked to move the shoulder gently to distribute the injected materials and to determine whether the pain is diminished. If the purpose of the injection was solely diagnostic (i.e., no corticosteroids were given), the examiner should passively abduct the shoulder. If pain is still present, the injection may have been performed improperly or the differential diagnosis was inaccurate. If there is full range of motion without pain, a frozen shoulder is excluded. In this case, strength of the shoulder girdle should be tested. If strength is normal, the diagnosis is most likely subacromial bursitis, although a partial rotator cuff tear could be present. If there is weakness in abduction and external rotation, rupture of the rotator cuff is probable.

If corticosteroids have been instilled, the same maneuvers should be performed. Patients should be forewarned that when the effect of the lidocaine wears off, in several hours, the pain may recur for a day or so before the full effect of the corticosteroid is felt. If no relief is obtained, the patient should be reexamined and the diagnosis reconsidered. If pain disappears but recurs in several weeks or months, the injection may be repeated. Thereafter, corticosteroid injections should not be given more than once every 6 months (and less often if possible).

Costs and Complications. Injection of the subacromial bursa is generally a very safe procedure with few adverse effects. Occasional patients may find their pain made worse by injection. Injection directly into the rotator cuff tendon, especially the supraspinatus tendon, may cause rupture. Repeated injections may contribute to thinning of the rotator cuff. Infection or hematomas after injection are exceedingly rare. The cost of injection varies widely, depending on physician fees, although an average charge is $70 to $100.

Cross-Reference: Shoulder Pain (Chapter 108).

REFERENCES

1. Adebajo AO, Nash P, Hazleman BL. A prospective double-blind dummy placebo controlled study comparing triamcinolone hexacetonide injection with oral diclofenac 50 mg TDS in patients with rotator cuff tendinitis. J Rheumatol 1990;17:1207–1210.

   In a prospective double-blind, placebo-controlled study, both treatments were superior to placebo but triamcinolone injection was somewhat more effective than the nonsteroidal agent.

2. Bulgen DY, Binder AI, Hazleman BL, Dutton J, Roberts S. Frozen shoulder: Prospective clinical study with an evaluation of three treatment regimens. Ann Rheum Dis 1984;43:353–360.

   A small randomized trial compared intra-articular corticosteroids, physical therapy, ice therapy, and no therapy in 42 patients. Shortly after entry, the corticosteroid-treated group showed more improvement in pain and function, although at 6 months the groups were all equally improved.

3. Dacre JE, Beeney N, Scott DL. Injections and physiotherapy for the painful stiff shoulder. Ann Rheum Dis 1989;48:322–325.

   In a randomized single-blind trial comparing injection with triamcinolone, 6-week physical therapy, or both, all patients showed significant improvements by 6 weeks with further improvement at 6 months. Injection provided the fastest relief and was less expensive than physical therapy.

4. Petri M, Dobrow R, Neiman R, Whiting O'Keefe Q, Seaman WE. Randomized, double-blind, placebo-controlled study of the treatment of the painful shoulder. Arthritis Rheum 1987;30:1040–1045.

   In a randomized, double-blind, placebo-controlled study of 100 patients with painful shoulders, both subacromial bursa injection with triamcinolone and naproxen therapy were more effective than placebo, whereas injection was superior to naproxen in relieving pain and promoting overall clinical improvement.

5. White RH, Paull DM, Fleming KW. Rotator cuff tendinitis: Comparison of subacromial injection of a long acting corticosteroid versus oral indomethacin therapy. J Rheumatol 1986;13:608–613.

   A small controlled trial involving 40 patients failed to demonstrate a benefit beyond that provided by indomethacin.

128 Injection of the Trochanteric Bursa

Procedure

RICHARD H. WHITE

Indication. The only indication for injection of the trochanteric bursa is to diagnose and treat suspected trochanteric bursitis.

Rationale. When hip pain is associated with exquisite tenderness over the lateral and posterior aspect of the greater trochanter, inflammation of one or more of the bursae that lie between the gluteus maximus, gluteus medius, and the greater trochanter is likely. The best way to confirm the diagnosis of trochanteric bursitis is to inject 8 to 10 mL of lidocaine 1% into the region of the bursa, which should ameliorate most of the pain in 5 to 10 minutes.

The cause of bursal inflammation is unknown but is thought to be mechanical. It is not due to infection or a crystal-induced process but instead is associated with low back pain and osteoarthritis of the hip. Injection is necessary for diagnosis, because tenderness over the greater trochanter is nonspecific and is sometimes seen in degenerative or inflammatory arthritis of the hip and with aseptic necrosis of the femoral head.

Methods. Choosing the exact location for the injection is critical. With the patient lying on the opposite hip and with underwear removed, the clinician should palpate the femur, working from the mid thigh upward. The upper extent of the femur (trochanter) should be identified and a small mark made on the skin. The iliac crest should also be identified 4 or 5 inches cephalad. The area of maximal tenderness should be over the *posterior* aspect of the trochanter and may extend caudad 10 to 14 cm.

In obese patients, the trochanter may be difficult to palpate. In addition, the bursa is usually located more than 1½ inches beneath the surface of the skin, making use of a spinal needle (usually 21 gauge) necessary. In many instances, even the tip of the spinal needle may not reach the trochanter until the hub of the spinal needle touches the skin.

After locating and marking the area of greatest tenderness, the clinician cleanses the overlying skin with alcohol and anesthetizes the epidermis and dermis with 1 mL of lidocaine 1%. The patient should be approached from the back, so that he or she does not see the long spinal needle. Sterile gloves are required because insertion of the spinal needle requires two hands. After the skin is prepared with an iodine solution, the needle is inserted directly perpendicular to the trochanter. Numerous points of resistance and sudden "pops" or giving-way sensations are felt as the needle passes through fascial planes. Once the bone has been touched, the clinician may be confident that the basic direction of the injection is correct. Failure of the spinal needle to touch the bone by the time the needle hub reaches the skin suggests that the angle of the search was incorrect. The needle should be withdrawn and reinserted until the needle tip touches the femur.

Injections of lidocaine should be "fanned out," with 3 mL placed right over the trochanter, 3 mL placed several centimeters superiorly, and the final 3 mL placed several centimeters caudad.

Only patients who respond to the initial lidocaine injection will benefit from additional injection of 40 mg of a long-acting form of methylprednisolone or its equivalent. Corticosteroids should be injected at the time of the initial visit. Most patients with trochanteric bursitis experience marked relief of pain for many months; return of the pain in several days suggests either that the injection was not made in the correct location or that there is another cause for the pain.

Costs and Complications. The complications associated with injection of the trochanteric bursa are local pain and bacterial infection. If proper technique is employed, the risk of introducing infection is very low.

Cross-Reference: Hip Pain (Chapter 109).

REFERENCES

1. Gordon ET. Trochanteric bursitis and tendinitis. Clin Orthop 1961;20:193–202.

   The author reviews the clinical manifestations of trochanteric bursitis.

2. Larsson L-G, Baum J. The syndromes of bursitis. Bull Rheum Dis 1986;36:1–8.

   Common bursitis syndromes and their treatment are reviewed.

3. Ramon D, Haslock I. Trochanteric bursitis: A frequent cause of "hip" pain in rheumatoid arthritis. Ann Rheum Dis 1982;41:602–603.

   Trochanteric bursitis was present in 15% of an unselected group of 100 patients with rheumatoid arthritis.

4. Schapira D, Nahir M, Scharf Y. Trochanteric bursitis: A common clinical problem. Arch Phys Med Rehabil 1986;67:815–817.

   Most patients also had lumbar spine arthrosis or ipsilateral hip damage.

129 Aspiration/Injection of the Knee

Procedure

RICHARD H. WHITE

Indications and Contraindications. The principal indications for arthrocentesis are (1) to obtain joint fluid for analysis in the setting of monarticular or polyarticular arthritis of unknown etiology, (2) to remove joint fluid as a therapeutic maneuver, and (3) to inject a therapeutic agent, usually a corticosteroid preparation, to treat an inflammatory arthritis. The only contraindication is suspected hemarthrosis due to an uncorrectable coagulopathy, such as acquired antibody to von Willebrand's factor, because bleeding may be impossible to control. Overlying cellulitis is not a contraindication to aspiration of the knee, which should be performed if there is any suspicion of septic arthritis; antibiotics should be administered intravenously to treat the cellulitis as soon as arthrocentesis is completed.

Rationale. Analysis and culture of synovial fluid can aid in the diagnosis of a number of causes of arthritis, including (1) septic arthritis, based on Gram stain and culture results; (2) gout, based on the finding of negatively birefringent crystals; (3) pseudogout, based on the presence of small, positively birefringent crystals; (4) inflammatory arthritis, based on a joint fluid white blood cell count greater than 2000 cells/mm^3, with no crystals and a negative culture; (5) noninflammatory arthritis, based on a synovial white blood cell count less than 2000 cells/mm^3; and (6) hemarthrosis. Synovial fluid should be aspirated whenever there is an unexplained arthropathy leading to an effusion, particularly if infection is suspected.

Although a large number of joint fluid tests are available (e.g., protein level, glucose, quality of the mucin clot), only a microbiologic culture, examination for crystals, and determination of the synovial white and red blood cell counts provide useful information. Even these tests, however, are imperfect: culture results may be falsely positive (contamination) or falsely negative; crystals may be seen in cases of septic arthritis; crystals, especially calcium pyrophosphate, may be difficult to see; or the synovial fluid white blood cell count may lead to inaccurate classification. The entire clinical picture, only one part of which is synovial fluid analysis, forms the basis for diagnosis.

Methods. Before aspirating a knee joint, the clinician cleans the point of entry with alcohol and anesthetizes the skin with 0.5 to 1 mL of lidocaine 1%. An injection of lidocaine into deep subcutaneous tissues is unnecessary. The skin is then cleansed with an iodine-containing solution. Because joint fluid can be very viscous, a No. 18 or No. 19 needle is needed for aspiration. Appropriate collection tubes should be available, including a tube for cell count and differential, a tube to save fluid for synovial crystal analysis, and an appropriate container for microbiologic culture. A 5-ml syringe is adequate for small effusions; larger collections should be removed with a 50-mL syringe.

To obtain joint fluid from the knee, the easiest and safest site to insert a needle is the medial or lateral suprapatellar recess. The joint fluid is forced into the suprapatellar recess by the clinician's applying pressure with the nondominant hand, positioning the palm just below the patella, with the thumb running along one edge of the patella and the fingers along the opposite edge. With the syringe in the dominant hand, the clinician inserts the needle above the superior edge of the patella, aimed to pass just beneath the cartilaginous surface of the patella. Often there is a popping sensation when the joint space has been entered. The dominant hand withdraws the plunger to remove the joint fluid. If an assistant is available to compress the joint fluid, the physician is freed to operate the syringe with both hands.

Joint fluid may be difficult to aspirate, particularly in patients with rheumatoid arthritis. Hypertrophied synovium, which may be mistaken for joint fluid, consists of thousands of microvilli that can occlude the lumen of a needle when too much negative pressure is applied. If no joint fluid is retrieved, reducing the negative pressure being applied to the syringe and rotating the needle often results in a successful tap.

Occasionally, one may want to inject a therapeutic agent into the joint after removing the joint fluid (e.g., 20–40 mg triamcinolone hexacetonide). This requires either using a three-way stopcock or removing the syringe from the needle hub while the needle tip remains in the joint space. Any exchange of syringes must be performed using sterile technique; the first syringe should be only gently tightened on the needle, allowing easy removal during the procedure.

After aspiration, the iodine solution should be wiped off the skin with alcohol to prevent skin sensitization.

Costs and Complications. The complications associated with aspiration of the knee are pain and bacterial contamination. Avoiding needle contact with the patella minimizes pain. If aseptic technique is followed, the likelihood of introducing bacteria into the joint space is less than 1 in 2000 aspirations.

Cross-References: General Approach to Arthritic Symptoms (Chapter 106), Knee Pain (Chapter 111), Osteoarthritis (Chapter 118), Gout/Hyperuricemia (Chapter 119).

REFERENCES

1. Bomalaski JS, Lluberas G, Schumacher HR Jr. Monosodium urate crystals in the knees of patients with asymptomatic nontophaceous gout. Arthritis Rheum 1986;29:1480–1484.

   In 50 patients with a prior diagnosis of gout, aspiration of noninflammatory joint fluid revealed monosodium urate crystals in 29 (58%).

2. Moll JMH. Management of Rheumatic Diseases. London, Chapman & Hale, 1983:213–238.

This chapter includes a description of local injection/aspiration techniques.

3. Schmerling RH, Delbanco TL, Tosteson ANA, Trentham DE. Synovial fluid tests: What should be ordered? JAMA 1990;264:1009–1014.

Chemistry studies, including glucose, protein, and lactic dehydrogenase levels, provided misleading or redundant information in classifying inflammatory versus noninflammatory joint fluid.

4. Schumacher HR Jr. Synovial fluid analysis and synovial biopsy. In Kelly WN, Harris ED Jr, Ruddy S, Sledge CB, eds. Textbook of Rheumatology. Philadelphia, WB Saunders, 1989:637–664.

A thorough overview of synovial fluid analysis is presented.

SECTION XI
Vascular Disorders

∙∙∙

130 Painful and Swollen Calf

Symptom

STEVEN R. McGEE

Epidemiology. Acute deep venous thrombosis (DVT) occurs with an annual incidence of 1 per 1000 in the general population. The mean age of affected patients is 60 years, with men affected as often as women. The left leg is involved more often than the right. Fewer than one half of outpatients with DVT have the conventional risk factors, such as prolonged immobility, recent surgery, trauma, malignancy, congestive heart failure, pregnancy, or deficiencies of antithrombin III, protein C, or protein S. Of the remaining cases, some may be due to two recently identified risk factors, genetic resistance to activated protein C and hyperhomocysteinemia.

Etiology. The most important causes of the acutely painful and swollen calf are cellulitis, deep venous thrombosis, Baker's cyst, and muscle hematoma. When outpatients with acute calf swelling are studied with both venograms and arthrograms (cellulitis is clinically excluded), Baker's cysts are found in about 30%, acute DVT in 25%, both Baker's cyst and DVT in 10%, and neither diagnosis in 35%.

Acute DVT usually originates in the venous sinuses of the soleus muscle. When it is confined to the calf (i.e., "distal" DVT), clinically significant pulmonary emboli are unlikely. DVTs that propagate from the calf to involve at least the popliteal vein ("proximal" DVT) cause (symptomatic) pulmonary emboli in as many as 50% of untreated patients, sometimes with a fatal outcome. *Baker's cysts* are distended gastrocnemiosemimembranosus bursae that usually communicate with the knee joint and may enlarge from any cause of knee arthritis (e.g., rheumatoid arthritis, osteoarthritis, loose body). Baker's cysts may cause acute swelling that is indistinguishable from DVT (pseudothrombophlebitis), either because of dissection or rupture of the cyst into the calf or because of pressure of the enlarging cyst on the popliteal vein. *Muscle hematomas* may result from calf muscle tears, often after trauma or excessive exercise. *Cellulitis* is a spreading infection of the skin and subcutaneous tissues, usually caused by group A streptococcus or *Staphylococcus aureus*.

Clinical Approach. The most important diagnosis to address is acute DVT, not only because untreated patients may die, but because empirical anticoagulation without a firm diagnosis may promote bleeding in patients with unsuspected Baker's cysts or muscle hematomas.

Some patients with muscle hematomas or ruptured Baker's cysts have small ecchymotic crescents near the medial or lateral malleoli as the only clue. Muscle hematomas otherwise cause little leg discoloration because the blood lies beneath deep muscle fascia. Cellulitis may cause shaking chills and high fever, with the findings of a hot extremity, bright well-demarcated redness, lymphangitis, and tender local lymph nodes.

Certain combinations of patient risk factors (e.g., presence or absence of active cancer, recent immobilization, strong family history) and physical signs (e.g., > 3 cm difference in calf circumference) do allow the clinician to assign to their patients a low, intermediate, or high probability of DVT, but because no combination of findings is absolutely diagnostic, further objective testing is necessary.

Although contrast venography is the gold standard test for DVT, it has several disadvantages, including expense, radiation exposure, invasiveness, and tendency to induce DVT (1% to 2%). Furthermore, as many as 10% of studies are inadequate for interpretation, and in another 10% radiologists differ on the test's interpretation.

Most clinicians now use *real-time compression ultrasonography* or *Duplex ultrasonography* to diagnose DVT. In symptomatic outpatients, these techniques are more sensitive (0.97) and specific (0.97) than *impedance plethysmography* (sensitivity = 0.92, specificity = 0.95). Real-time ultrasonography directly visualizes the vein and its compressibility (clots render veins incompressible). One additional advantage to real-time ultrasonography is that 5% to 10% of studies reveal other diagnoses such as Baker's cysts or muscle hematomas. Duplex ultrasonography combines real-time ultrasonography with Doppler measurements of flow in the vein.

If the ultrasound test is positive for proximal DVT, no further tests are necessary and anticoagulation should be initiated. If the initial ultrasound test is negative, the test should be repeated within 1 week because up to 7% of all DVTs are first identified only during serial testing (suggesting that some distal DVTs, missed on the first test, propagate over time into the popliteal vein). Serial testing is especially important if symptoms persist in patients with moderate or high probability of DVT; serial testing is probably unnecessary in those with low probability or if symptoms resolve. If both ultrasound tests are negative, anticoagulation can be safely withheld (the incidence of documented venous thromboembolism in these patients during 6-month follow-up is only 1.5%). Contrast venography still may have a limited role in (1) the diagnosis of DVT in patients with high probability of DVT (e.g., a patient with recent cancer, > 3 cm asymmetric swelling, recent immobilization, and no alternative diagnosis) but persistently negative ultrasound tests and (2) the diagnosis of suspected recurrent DVT when there are no previous ultrasound results available for comparison.

To diagnose a Baker's cyst, real-time ultrasonography is equivalent to arthrography in most studies. Patients with obvious knee effusions on examination require arthrocentesis (see Chapter 129, Aspiration/Injection of the Knee).

Management. Patients with proximal DVTs require at least 5 days of heparin anticoagulation (continuous intravenous heparin, adjusted twice-daily subcutaneous heparin, or daily subcutaneous low-molecular-weight heparin) and warfarin anticoagulation (the warfarin is usually started on day 1). Low-molecular-weight heparin offers the opportunity to manage these patients strictly as outpatients, although daily clinic or nurse visits are necessary to monitor the warfarin dose and International Normalized Ratio (INR). Thrombolysis is no longer recommended for most DVTs because the reduction in postphlebitic syndrome (40% vs. 90%) is far outweighed by the increased risk of central nervous system bleeding (0.9% vs. 0.2%) and death (0.5% vs. 0.1%).

Those patients with cellulitis, especially when fever or lymphangitis is present, are best managed in the hospital with parenteral antibiotics. The remaining patients with an acutely swollen leg usually respond to leg elevation and nonsteroidal anti-inflammatory agents over 1 to 2 weeks.

Follow-Up. A common reason for recurrent cellulitis is untreated tinea pedis.

Chapter 201 reviews chronic anticoagulation, which is usually recommended for 3 to 6 months after the first DVT, and for longer periods if the DVT is recurrent. In patients with DVT, the clinician should not routinely screen for the "hypercoagulable state" (i.e., activated protein C resistance or deficiencies of protein C, protein S, antithrombin III, or plasminogen) until studies demonstrate that a positive finding would change the current recommendations on chronic anticoagulation outlined earlier.

Cross-References: Pleuritic Chest Pain (Chapter 61), Knee Pain (Chapter 111), Aspiration/Injection of the Knee (Chapter 129), Chronic Anticoagulation (Chapter 201).

REFERENCES

1. Heijboer H, Buller HR, Lensing AWA, Turpie AGG, Colly LP, Cate JWT. A comparison of real-time compression ultrasonography with impedance plethysmography for the diagnosis of deep-vein thrombosis in symptomatic outpatients. N Engl J Med 1993;329:1365–1369.

   In a randomized trial of 985 consecutive outpatients with suspected DVT, serial compression ultrasonography was the superior test.

2. Hillner BE, Philbrick JR, Becker DM. Optimal management of suspected lower-extremity deep vein thrombosis. Arch Intern Med 1992;152:165–175.

   This article presents a decision analysis of 24 management strategies for patients with suspected deep venous thrombosis, written before the study by Heijboer and colleagues. The optimal approach was to perform a single real-time ultrasonogram; serial testing saved more lives but at a cost of $390,000 per each additional life saved.

3. Weinmann EE, Salzman EW. Deep-vein thrombosis. N Engl J Med 1994;331:1630–1641.

   The authors present a well-referenced and comprehensive review of the diagnosis, clinical epidemiology, prevention, and management of deep venous thrombosis.

4. Wells PS, Hirsh J, Anderson DR, et al. Accuracy of clinical assessment of deep-vein thrombosis. Lancet 1995;345:1326–1330.

   A complicated point system (with major and minor criteria) allowed accurate stratification of 529 outpatients with suspected deep venous thrombosis into high (16% of patients), moderate (27%), and low (57%) probability groups. With contrast venography, thromboses were found in 85%, 33%, and 5%, respectively.

5. Wigley RD. Popliteal cysts: Variations on a theme of Baker. Semin Arthritis Rheum 1982;12:1–10.

   An excellent review of Baker's cysts is provided.

131 Raynaud's Syndrome

Symptom

STEVEN R. McGEE

Epidemiology. Raynaud's syndrome (intermittent vasospasm of the fingertips) affects up to 5% of the population. The mean age at onset is 30 years. The disease is more common in women (70%–90% of cases), in northern climates, during colder months, and in users of hand-held vibratory tools (e.g., jackhammers, grinders, chain saws).

Etiology. Raynaud's syndrome is either *primary* (vasospastic, formerly termed *Raynaud's disease*) or *secondary* to systemic disease that affects the small arteries of the hand (obstructive, formerly termed *Raynaud's phenomenon*). Large surveys from vascular surgery clinics suggest that 40% of cases are primary and 60% are secondary, with two thirds of the secondary cases resulting from connective tissue disease, most commonly systemic sclerosis, the CREST syndrome (calcinosis, Raynaud's phenomenon, esophageal hypomotility, sclerodactyly, telangiectasia), or systemic lupus erythematosus (SLE). Other secondary causes, among many, include arterial diseases (atherosclerosis, Buerger's disease), cryoglobulinemia, multiple myeloma, myxedema, and frostbite. However, because of the high prevalence of Raynaud's syndrome (5%) and the low incidence of systemic sclerosis (5 to 10 new cases per 1 million population per year), these data probably reflect referral bias and overestimate the prevalence of secondary cases seen in general practice settings.

Medications associated with an increased incidence of Raynaud's syndrome include β-blockers, sympathomimetics, ergotamine, vinblastine, and bleomycin.

Clinical Approach. The diagnosis depends entirely on a characteristic history: after emotional upset or exposure to cold, patients experience attacks of discrete pallor that extend at least to the distal interphalangeal joint. Cyanosis and rubor may sequentially follow the pallor, although only 20% of patients have the full triphasic color response. The syndrome usually affects both hands and sometimes involves the toes, ears, and cheeks but typically spares the thumbs. Numbness, tingling, or burning frequently accompanies the attack, which usually lasts 30 to 60 minutes; severe pain is rare. The differential diagnosis includes cyanotic diseases of the central (hypoxemia, hemoglobin abnormalities) or peripheral (low cardiac output, peripheral vascular disease) type. These diseases differ because they lack discrete attacks of pallor; furthermore, central cyanosis may worsen with warming of the extremity and involves the tongue and buccal mucosa.

The patient interview focuses on the patient's medications (including over-the-counter cold remedies), occupation, and symptoms suggestive of connective tissue disease (arthralgia, rash, dysphagia, tight skin, sicca syndrome symptoms of dry eyes and mouth). The clinician should closely examine the patient's pulses and skin (ulcers, sclerodactyly, telangiectasia). Routine laboratory tests include a complete blood cell count, erythrocyte sedimentation rate, chemistry profile, urinalysis, and antinuclear antibody assay. Because vasospasm alone never causes digital ulcers or gangrene, patients with these findings, as well as those with absent pulses on examination, should be referred to a vascular surgeon for consideration of arteriography.

Management. About 90% of patients respond to (1) discontinuing offending medications and cigarette smoking, (2) limiting occupational exposure to vibratory tools, and (3) using mittens and insulated fabrics to minimize exposure to cold.

Pharmacologic therapy for Raynaud's syndrome, given during the colder months, is appropriate for the few patients who have frequent disabling symptoms despite the measures listed earlier. Double-blind placebo-controlled trials document the efficacy of nifedipine (10 mg orally three times a day), diltiazem (30 to 120 mg three times a day), and prazosin (slowly advanced to 1 mg orally three times a day). In one study, nifedipine was found superior to prazosin.

Surgery is indicated only for documented proximal arterial stenosis. Upper extremity sympathectomy has been abandoned because relapses were common.

Follow-Up. The frequency of attacks waxes and wanes over years. The course of primary Raynaud's syndrome, present at least 2 years, is benign: 9 years later, fewer than 5% of patients have signs of connective tissue disease.

Cross-References: Smoking Cessation (Chapter 12), General Approach to Arthritic Symptoms (Chapter 106), Wrist and Hand Pain (Chapter 110), Interpretation of Serologic Tests (Chapter 123).

REFERENCES

1. Cardelli MB, Kleinsmith DM. Raynaud's phenomenon and disease. Med Clin North Am 1989;73:1127–1141.

   The author presents an overview of etiology, pathophysiology, and management.

2. Gerbracht DD, Steen VD, Ziegler GL, Medsger TA, Rodnan GP. Evolution of primary Raynaud's phenomenon (Raynaud's disease) to connective tissue disease. Arthritis Rheum 1985;28:87–92.

   Only 4 of 87 patients with primary Raynaud's syndrome had developed signs of connective tissue disease a decade later. Antinuclear antibody and anticentromere antibody assays did not help predict who would develop connective tissue disease.

3. Houtman PM, Kallenberg CGM, Fidler V, Wouda AA. Diagnostic significance of nailfold capillary patterns in patients with Raynaud's phenomenon. J Rheumatol 1986;13:556–563.

   Although a decrease in nail fold capillary loops helped distinguish primary from secondary Raynaud's syndrome (sensitivity = 46%, specificity = 92%), the diagnosis of connective tissue disease was obvious from other clinical findings.

4. Jobe JB, Sampson JB, Roberts DE, Beetham WP. Induced vasodilation as treatment for Raynaud's disease. Ann Intern Med 1982;97:706–709.

   A controlled study demonstrated the efficacy of Pavlovian conditioning: simultaneous exposure of the body to cold and the hands to warm, repeated over 3 weeks, resulted in lasting benefit.

5. Rodeheffer RJ, Rommer JA, Wigley F, Smith CR. Controlled double-blind trial of nifedipine in the treatment of Raynaud's phenomenon. N Engl J Med 1983;308:880–883.

   Moderate or marked improvement occurred in 60% of patients.

132 Peripheral Arterial Disease

Problem

KAJ JOHANSEN

Epidemiology and Etiology. Most patients with symptoms and signs of peripheral arterial disease have atherosclerosis. The age-adjusted prevalence of claudication is 0.3% in men and 0.1% in women. Claudication is five times more common in patients with diabetes. Patients with peripheral arterial disease are generally older than 50 years, and almost all have smoked extensively. Many are hypertensive, and hyperlipidemia is more common in this patient population. Although only a minority have diabetes, over half of the lower extremity amputations in the United States are performed in diabetics.

Abdominal aortic aneurysm (AAA) is found in 2% of unselected autopsy series and in at least 10% of patients attending a vascular surgery clinic. AAA rarely occurs before the age of 60; it is predominantly a disease of elderly men with a past or current history of smoking. Hypertension is common in AAA patients, and first-degree relatives of AAA patients have at least an eightfold higher likelihood of developing AAA themselves, in comparison with an age-matched control population.

Symptoms and Signs. Claudication is exercise-related muscle discomfort. Classically, patients are asymptomatic at rest and begin walking without difficulty, but at distances of from as little as a few feet to four to six blocks they note the onset of calf muscle distress characterized as "aching," "tiredness," or "burning." Symptoms appear sooner with uphill walking or walking up stairs, because such activity makes use of the gastrocnemius and soleus muscles obligatory.

Claudication is usually diagnostic of a high-grade atherosclerotic stenosis or occlusion of the superficial femoral artery in the thigh. Less common distributions of atherosclerotic arterial occlusive disease may cause claudication in the gluteal or thigh muscles, which when associated with absent femoral pulses, impotence in men, and thigh muscle atrophy (the Leriche syndrome) suggests aortoiliac occlusive disease.

Very rarely, instep claudication is noted in patients with diffuse tibial artery occlusive disease. This almost always occurs in young male patients addicted to cigarette smoking and is virtually pathognomonic for thromboangiitis obliterans (Buerger's disease).

Much less commonly, patients with peripheral arterial disease present with nocturnal rest pain or tissue loss (heel or toe gangrene or a nonhealing ischemic ulcer of the foot). Virtually all such patients have a prior history of claudication, and examination of their lower extremities typically shows retarded capillary refill, loss of hair growth, and thickened nails. Advanced cases manifest dependent rubor, pallor with elevation, and coolness.

The absence of diabetes or a smoking history should suggest another diagnosis (e.g., lumbar spinal stenosis, trauma, myositis, or another nonvascular cause). Neurogenic or pseudoclaudication may occur in individuals with lumbar spinal stenosis or osteophytic impingement on lumbosacral nerve roots. Such patients may have few or no symptoms at rest but may develop calf pain after walking or even standing for a period of time. These individuals' pain is characteristically sharper and more burning. Such individuals usually have normal pulses on physical examination, normal Doppler pressure indices (see later), and history, physical examination findings, and spinal imaging studies consistent with chronic back disease (e.g., degenerative disk disease, healed fractures, or prior back operations).

AAA is rarely symptomatic before rupture. Up to 50% of patients with AAA ultimately die of aneurysmal rupture. Hospital mortality rates from AAA rupture vary from 30% to 70%; overall, the mortality (including those who die at home or en route to the hospital) exceeds 90%. On the other hand, the operative mortality associated with elective repair of AAAs discovered before rupture is less than 5%, even in octogenarians.

Clinical Approach. The diagnosis of peripheral arterial disease in the patient with claudication is implied by absent popliteal and pedal pulses on physical examination and by diminished Doppler pressures at the ankle. Ankle/brachial indices (ABIs) (see Chapter 135) are diminished in direct proportion to the walking distance. A normal ABI is about 1.0; one- to two-block claudication is generally associated with an ABI of 0.6 to 0.8; whereas patients with severe (less than one-block) claudication have an ABI of 0.4 to 0.6. Patients with rest pain, arterial ulcers, or gangrene have an ABI below 0.4.

Although claudication is diagnostic of significant arterial occlusive disease, patients with claudication are at greater risk of subsequent cardiovascular mortality than of limb loss. In one study, limb loss after onset of claudication occurred in only 7% of claudicants during the next 5 years, and in only 12% by 10 years, whereas cardiovascular mortality was 27% during the first 5 years and 63% at 10 years. Accordingly, close attention to the cardiac status of patients with claudication is warranted.

A single abdominal ultrasound examination performed after age 60 in men or women with a history of smoking, peripheral vascular disease, or a relative with a known AAA should detect more than 90% of all AAAs. Individuals with a normal abdominal aortic ultrasound study at the age of 60 need be evaluated no further. Those with a small AAA, less than 4 cm in diameter, should undergo repeat abdominal ultrasonography every 6 months and should be referred to a vascular surgeon when the size of the AAA exceeds 5 cm. Patients with an AAA of any size should be instructed to seek medical attention immediately should new abdominal, flank, or back pain occur.

Management. Claudication in most patients stabilizes or improves with simple measures such as weight loss, daily aerobic exercise, and, most important, cessation of cigarette smoking. Treatment of hyperlipidemia and hypertension may be beneficial. In compliant patients, pentoxifylline (Trental) may be useful: a prospective multicenter trial showed a small but significant improvement in walking distance. Gastrointestinal upset accompanies the administration of pentoxifylline in 5% to 10% of patients. A 3-month supply (400 mg orally three times a day) costs approximately $144.

A very small number of patients with severe claudication may be considered for arterial reconstruction. Because such operative or endovascular procedures are only moderately successful, they should be proposed only if nonoperative means, including smoking cessation, have failed and the patient's employability or quality of life is significantly affected. Arteriography is warranted only when a therapeutic intervention—balloon dilation, stenting, or surgical reconstruction—is contemplated.

By contrast, *all* individuals with rest pain, arterial ulcers, or gangrene require an intervention, either arterial reconstruction or amputation. Lower extremity arteriography always shows atherosclerotic occlusions at two or more levels. Because such patients' coronary or cerebrovascular occlusive disease is proportionately more advanced as well, the 5-year survival rate after the onset of rest pain or lower extremity gangrene in the nondiabetic patient is substantially less than 50%.

No nonoperative therapy exists for AAA. All AAAs larger than 5 cm should be repaired, and AAAs with diameters between 4.5 and 5 cm should be repaired in younger or healthy patients and those living in remote locales. Few contraindications to AAA surgery exist, other than rapidly terminal conditions such as metastatic cancer or severe chronic pulmonary disease. Occasional long-term survivors develop graft complications, such as anastomotic pseudoaneurysm.

Follow-Up. The clinician should monitor the patient's symptoms and ankle pressures or ABIs every 3 to 6 months. Any improvement in ankle pressures and symptoms can be appropriately ascribed to exercise or smoking cessation programs; such positive feedback is often very encouraging to the patient. After an arterial reconstructive procedure, regular follow-up (usually by the vascular surgeon) is important to detect vessel or graft occlusion (from arterial neointimal hyperplasia or progression of atherosclerosis).

Because aneurysmal arterial degeneration is a systemic disorder, follow-up of patients with AAAs should include ultrasound surveillance of femoral and popliteal arteries for asymptomatic dilation.

Cross-References: Smoking Cessation (Chapter 12), Ankle and Foot Pain (Chapter 112), Diabetic Foot Care Education (Chapter 124), Leg Ulcers (Chapter 133), Doppler Measurement of Ankle Pressures (Chapter 135), Hyperlipidemia (Chapter 152), Diabetes Mellitus (Chapter 154), Preoperative Cardiovascular Problems (Chapter 218).

REFERENCES

1. Boyd AM. Natural course of arteriosclerosis of lower extremities. Proc R Soc Med 1962;55:591–599.

   A classic study from the prevascular surgery era documents that lower extremity claudication is a relatively insensitive predictor of limb loss but a very good indicator of an early coronary demise.

2. Collin J. Screening for abdominal aortic aneurysms. Br J Surg 1985;72:851–852.

   Because abdominal aortic aneurysms are usually asymptomatic and are diagnosed on physical examination in fewer than half of cases, screening of populations at risk seems warranted. Such an approach, however, requires consideration of the resource expenditures necessary to manage the large number of asymptomatic lesions thus discovered.

3. Criqui MH, Langer RD, Fronek A, et al. Mortality over a period of 10 years in patients with peripheral arterial disease. N Engl J Med 1992;326:381–386.

In this prospective study, subjects with peripheral arterial disease had a relative risk of death varying from 3 (all causes) to 15 (severe symptomatic peripheral arterial disease).

4. Johansen K, Kohler TR, Nicholls S, Zierler RE, Clowes AW, Kazmers A. Ruptured abdominal aortic aneurysm: The Harborview experience. J Vasc Surg 1991;13:240–247.

Despite (or perhaps because of) skilled prehospital paramedic care, rapid diagnosis, timely operation, and expert postoperative care, 70% of patients with ruptured abdominal aortic aneurysms died. This toll, and the extraordinary utilization of health care resources used to try to salvage patients with ruptured aneurysms, underscores the importance of abdominal aortic aneurysm screening programs.

5. Porter JM, Cutler BS, Lee BY, et al. Pentoxifylline efficacy in the treatment of intermittent claudication: Multicenter controlled double-blind trial with objective assessment of chronic arterial occlusive disease patients. Am Heart J 1982;104:66–72.

A multicenter trial found a small but significant benefit of pentoxifylline in increasing walking distance, probably by altering whole blood viscosity and red cell deformability, when administered to patients with claudication.

. . . .

133 Leg Ulcers

Problem

STEVEN R. McGEE

Epidemiology. Venous ulcers, which account for up to 90% of all leg ulcers, affect 0.2% to 0.4% of the population. The prevalence of venous ulcers increases with age, and the female-to-male ratio is approximately 2:1.

Etiology. Table 133–1 is a list of the most important causes of leg ulceration. Fifty percent to 75% of patients with sickle cell disease have leg ulcers.

Venous ulcers result from venous valvular incompetence and chronic venous hypertension, sometimes because of previous deep venous thrombophlebitis. Although the exact cause is debatable, many authorities attribute the actual ulceration to capillary leakage of fibrin (which may impair oxygen diffusion) or to stasis of white blood cells (which may release toxic metabolites).

Table 133–1. LEG ULCERS: ETIOLOGY*

Venous†	Pyoderma gangrenosum
Arterial†	Tumors
Neuropathic†	Squamous cell carcinoma
Vasculitis	Mycosis fungoides
Hemoglobinopathy	
Sickle cell disease	
Infectious	
Sporothrix schenckii	
Mycobacterium marinum	

*A more complete differential diagnosis appears in reference 4.
†Most common causes.

Clinical Approach. The clinician should ask the patient how rapidly the ulcer developed and whether there is associated trauma, claudication, edema, or symptoms of systemic disease (e.g., fever, weight loss). Pain is common from all causes except neuropathic ulcers. The examination focuses on the ulcer's location, appearance (base and edge), and associated skin, vascular, and neurologic findings.

Venous ulcers, which may appear abruptly, are classically located over the medial malleolus but may be over the lateral malleolus, distal leg, or dorsal surface of the foot. Affected patients have findings of underlying venous insufficiency, such as edema or venous (stasis) dermatitis (pruritic erythematous rash on the distal third of the calf with scaling and weeping and skin hyperpigmentation from hemosiderin and melanin). The ulcer base consists of granulation tissue (red pebbly tissue reflecting new capillary tufts of wound healing) and frequently contains abundant yellow-green exudate. *Arterial ulcers* develop gradually, affect the foot distal to the ankle (tips of toes, "kissing ulcers" between toes, heel, plantar metatarsal heads), and have a necrotic base without granulation tissue. Affected patients have claudication; some also experience rest pain that improves with dangling of the leg. Associated findings include absent pulses, delayed capillary refill, thin hairless skin, and dependent rubor. When arterial ulcers occur in male smokers younger than 40 years of age, especially if associated with superficial thrombophlebitis and instep claudication, the diagnosis of thromboangiitis obliterans (Buerger's disease) should be considered. *Neuropathic ulcers* occur from pressure against bony prominences (metatarsal heads, heel, toes) and affect patients with peripheral sensory neuropathy.

Vasculitic ulcers, which resemble arterial ulcers, may be associated with a blue nonpalpable lacelike discoloration of the extremity (livedo reticularis). Sometimes there may be the associated findings of subcutaneous nodules and systemic disease (fever, weight loss, and abnormalities of kidneys, joints, nerves, or gastrointestinal system). Ulcers in patients with *sickle cell disease* resemble venous ulcers. The ulcer of *pyoderma gangrenosum* appears abruptly (over days), is very painful, and is diagnosed clinically (not by biopsy) by its characteristic violet undermined edge, ragged heaped-up border, and surrounding red halo.

Management. The treatment of venous ulcers should reduce the patient's venous hypertension and leg edema, using measures such as leg elevation, elastic bandages, elastic support stockings, or Unna's boot. For most patients, over-the-counter support hose are probably as effective as the more expensive custom-made stockings. Patients should put on the stockings before arising in the morning and wear them the entire day. When patients have arthritis or other debilities that make dressing with these stockings difficult, elastic bandage wraps are an alternative. *Unna's boot* is a generic term for bandages impregnated with glycerin, sorbitol, gelatin, zinc oxide, and calamine that are wrapped around the leg (Dome-Paste, GeluCast). One advantage of Unna's boot is that it is left in place and removed 1 week later in the doctor's office, allowing the physician to follow closely the progress of the ulcer and preventing the patient from manipulating or scratching the ulcer during the week.

Synthetic occlusive dressings (e.g., DuoDerm) help débride the ulcer, significantly reduce pain, promote healing, and, because patients often learn to change them themselves, facilitate outpatient management. The dressing should cover the ulcer and at least a 3-cm margin of surrounding skin, and it should be changed only after it starts to leak exudate at the edges (an average of every 5 days, range 1 to 10 days). The patient should learn that this accumulation of exudate (which is sometimes foul smelling) is normal, that infection is rare, and that premature removal of the dressing may pull off the new epithelium and retard healing. Because some form of compression therapy must accompany occlusive dressings in patients with significant edema, many clinicians combine Unna's boot with occlusive dressings. The only major contraindication to occlusive dressings is an established infection.

No study clearly demonstrates the superiority of any of these treatments over the others, with most ulcers healing over 6 to 12 weeks. Despite the typical yellow-green exudate that often is colonized with bacteria, randomized controlled trials demonstrate that *routine* administration of antibiotics (topical or systemic) does not promote healing of venous ulcers. When the patient has signs of infection (fever, lymphangitis, rapidly spreading erythema, and tenderness), antibiotics are clearly indicated.

Patients with arterial ulcers should be referred to a vascular surgeon for consideration of a revascularization procedure. Care of diabetic foot ulcers appears in Chapter 134. Patients with suspected pyoderma gangrenosum should be seen by a dermatologist; if the diagnosis is confirmed, corticosteroids are the preferred treatment.

Follow-Up. The patient should be seen every 1 to 2 weeks, until the ulcer is clearly healing and the patient understands the treatment regimen, at which time the follow-up intervals may be increased. At each visit, the clinician should measure the size of the ulcer (product of the two maximum perpendicular diameters). Any ulcer that is failing to improve or develops a nodular or heaped-up edge should be sampled to exclude cancer, vasculitis, or infection. Large ulcers may require skin grafting. Because venous ulcers have the tendency to recur, the clinician should counsel the patient to avoid trauma and to seek treatment for edema or dermatitis.

Cross-References: Principles of Dermatologic Diagnosis and Therapy (Chapter 22), Eczema (Chapter 28), Edema (Chapter 77), Inflammatory Bowel Disease (Chapter 97), Diabetic Foot Care Education (Chapter 124), Peripheral Arterial Disease (Chapter 132), Local Care of Diabetic Foot Lesions (Chapter 134), Doppler Measurement of Ankle Pressures (Chapter 135), Diabetes Mellitus (Chapter 154), Sickle Cell Disease (Chapter 200).

REFERENCES

1. Douglas WS, Simpson NB. Guidelines for the management of chronic venous leg ulceration: Report of a multidisciplinary workshop. Br J Dermatol 1995;132:446–452.

   This is a scientific, concise, and well-referenced review.

2. Falanga V. Occlusive wound dressings: Why, when, which? Arch Dermatol 1988;124:872–877.

   The author presents a practical review of the various available occlusive dressing materials.

3. Rijswijk L, Brown D, Friedman S, Degreef H, Roed-Petersen J, et al: Multicenter clinical evaluation of a hydrocolloid dressing for leg ulcers. Cutis 1985;35:173–176.

In an uncontrolled study of DuoDerm in 152 leg ulcers that were refractory to other measures, including Unna's boot, 62% healed over a mean of 51 days and 80% had significant pain relief. No patient developed infection.

4. Young JR. Differential diagnosis of leg ulcers. Cardiovasc Clin 1983;13:171–193.

The author provides an encyclopedic review with many clinical points.

134   Local Care of Diabetic Foot Lesions

Procedure

JESSIE H. AHRONI

Indications and Contraindications. Foot lesions are common in patients with diabetes, particularly the elderly and those with sensory neuropathy. In one study, 86% of amputations followed potentially preventable minor trauma and cutaneous injury. To prevent progression to chronic nonhealing wounds, gangrene, or refractory infections, all diabetic foot lesions—discrete ulcers, blisters, calluses, abscesses, or fissures—require prompt and aggressive care.

Rationale. Healing requires a bed of clean granulation tissue, treatment and drainage of infections, dressings for protection, and control of edema.

Methods. Thorough débridement with a sharp instrument should remove superficial debris, fibrin, and remnants of necrotic or nonviable tissue, including eschar. Callus around an ulcer, especially in the plantar area, should be carefully pared with a scalpel to create a flat, saucerized area. Topical débriding and cleansing applications cannot replace proper surgical débridement. If a sinus tract, abscess, or deep infection is discovered, it must be incised to provide drainage. Clinicians are sometimes hesitant to incise lesions on diabetic feet for fear of creating a nonhealing wound. However, undrained pus and devitalized, infected tissue represent a greater hazard; early complete drainage of deep infections affords the best chance of saving the foot.

Virtually all open wounds will become colonized with various microorganisms, but uninfected lesions do not require antibiotic treatment. Determining which lesions are infected is a clinical task that is sometimes difficult. The presence of purulent secretions or two or more of the classic signs and symptoms of inflammation (induration, redness, warmth, tenderness) usually indicates infection. Mild infections, in patients not previously treated with antibiotics, are usually caused by aerobic gram-positive cocci, especially *Staphylococcus aureus,* and generally respond well to outpatient management with oral antibiotics.

Despite differences of opinion and the lack of good data on the details of local care, wound dressings should be applied according to accepted principles for such care. Dressings are used to protect the area from trauma, to protect the wound from contamination, and to contain wound drainage. They should not contain materials that harm growing cells or predispose to sensitization, and they should be easy to apply, comfortable, and nonadherent. Occlusive dressings (e.g., Duoderm) are not recommended for diabetic foot lesions.

For most lesions, cleansing with normal saline is sufficient. Harsh antiseptics, including hydrogen peroxide and iodine solutions, are best avoided. Topical antibiotics have no place in the treatment of diabetic foot infections.

A single layer of nonadherent dry sterile fine-mesh gauze dressing (Owens Non-Adherent Dressing or equivalent) is cut to the size of the ulcer with sterile scissors and placed evenly over the wound with forceps. The gauze should touch the entire wound surface. This fine-mesh gauze is then covered with a plain gauze pad and gauze wrap (Kerlix or equivalent) and taped in place.

When necessary, damp-to-dry dressings can be used to provide additional gentle débridement of lesions and remove wound debris that remains after instrument débridement. A saline-moistened gauze pad opened to two-ply thickness can be laid over the wound and air dried for 1 to 2 hours once or twice a day, for 2 or 3 days. Removing the dried dressing débrides necrotic tissue; but because it can also damage newly forming epithelium, damp-to-dry dressings should be discontinued as soon as exudation is minimal. Soaking should be avoided because it macerates the skin, damages granulation tissue, opens small fissures that are portals to infection, and may result in hot-water burns.

Leg edema, whether from local infection or systemic causes, can adversely affect local cutaneous circulation and wound healing. Elevating the affected extremity may be sufficient to control local edema, but in some cases diuretics are required. When arterial flow is severely compromised, the leg should be elevated only to the level of the heart. Elastic wraps or compression hose, fitted so as not to restrict arterial flow, may also be useful.

Pressure from walking can increase edema, prevent a wound from healing, or cause further foot problems. Patients should be instructed to avoid walking, even around the house, except as absolutely necessary until skin closure occurs. When ambulation is essential, appropriate footwear is crucial. Optimal footwear should provide the following: (1) correct width sizing, (2) even weight distribution over the plantar surface of the foot, (3) a rounded, fairly high toe box, (4) a removable padded insole with energy-absorbing properties under which accommodative pads may be placed, (5) soft upper materials, (6) relatively low cost, (7) aesthetic acceptability, and (8) comfort. Protective temporary shoes with moldable insoles should be used when the patient's usual footwear is inappropriate for necessary ambulation. After healing, patients without major foot deformities may use good-quality running shoes. In some cases, specially constructed shoes, molded insoles, metatarsal bars, or rocker bottoms may be needed.

The basic principles of diabetic foot care that all patients must be taught are described in Chapter 124, Diabetic Foot Care Education.

Complications. Patients who cannot perform or obtain good outpatient local care, who have signs of systemic toxicity (e.g., high fever, hypotension, severe hyperglycemia, acidosis), or who have an infection that is immediately threatening to life or limb (i.e., accompanied by extensive cellulitis, lymphangitis, deep space infection, gangrene, crepitus, gas in the tissues, or osteomyelitis) should be admitted to the hospital for treatment.

Cost. The actual cost of diabetic foot problems in the United States is unknown. Comprehensive diabetic foot care programs have reported high ulcer healing rates and reductions in amputations and hospital stays.

Cross-References: Edema (Chapter 77), Diabetic Foot Care Education (Chapter 124), Peripheral Arterial Disease (Chapter 132), Leg Ulcers (Chapter 133), Doppler Measurement of Ankle Pressures (Chapter 135), Diabetes Mellitus (Chapter 154).

REFERENCES

1. Katz S, McGinley K, Leyden JJ. Semipermeable occlusive dressings: Effects on growth of pathogenic bacteria and reepithelialization of superficial wounds. Arch Dermatol 1986;122:58–62.

   Six commercially available semiocclusive dressings used on experimentally induced wounds in humans all provided microenvironments conducive to the growth of resident and pathogenic bacteria; there were no differences in the rates of reepithelialization.

2. Lipsky BA, Pecoraro RE, Larson SA, Hanley ME, Ahroni JH. Outpatient management of uncomplicated lower-extremity infections in diabetic patients. Arch Intern Med 1990;150:790–797.

   Previously untreated infections are usually caused by aerobic gram-positive cocci and generally respond well to outpatient management with oral antibiotics.

3. Pecoraro RE, Ahroni JH, Boyko EJ, Stensel VL. Chronology and determinants of tissue repair in diabetic lower extremity ulcers. Diabetes 1991;40:1305–1313.

   The authors identify and quantify important factors affecting impaired wound healing in 46 diabetic outpatients receiving comprehensive local wound care.

4. Pecoraro RE, Reiber GE, Burgess E. Pathways to diabetic limb amputation: A basis for prevention. Diabetes Care 1990;13:513–521.

   The causal pathways to diabetic limb amputation are defined in 80 patients, emphasizing minor trauma.

5. Rith-Najarian SJ, Stolusky TS, Gohdes DM. Identifying diabetic patients at high risk for lower-extremity amputation in a primary health care setting: A prospective evaluation of simple screening criteria. Diabetes Care 1992;15:1386–1389.

   This report provides a few medical history questions and a simple clinical examination that can stratify patients with diabetes into risk categories for subsequent foot ulcerations or lower-extremity amputation.

135 Doppler Measurement of Ankle Pressures

Procedure

KAJ JOHANSEN

Indications and Contraindications. The hand-held Doppler ultrasonic probe allows rapid, accurate, and noninvasive measurement of lower extremity arterial pressure, which is a reasonable indicator of tissue perfusion. Use of this technique is indicated to confirm suspected peripheral arterial disease, to exclude the diagnosis in other cases, and to evaluate patients serially during exercise programs or after arterial reconstructive surgery.

Contraindications include a recent limb operation or other conditions that make use of a pneumatic pressure cuff painful. Doppler pressures cannot, of course, be measured when the limb has been amputated and may be unreliable in diabetics, in whom calcification of the arterial media renders the calf arteries noncompressible.

Rationale. In the normal adult, systolic arterial pressure at the ankle equals brachial artery pressure, and pedal pulses should be palpable. Because it is difficult to palpate a pedal pulse with a pressure of less than 70 or 80 mm Hg, a simple noninvasive means of measuring pressure in arteries with atherosclerotic stenoses or occlusions is necessary. Individuals with symptoms (e.g., claudication) suggesting arterial occlusive disease but whose ankle pressures are normal may have another cause for the pain, such as lumbar spinal stenosis.

Ankle pressure measurement and calculation of the ankle/brachial index (ABI) reliably indicate perfusion to the level of the muscular arteries of the ankle in patients with atherosclerosis (excluding diabetics).

Methods. The technique is simple and rapid. A standard arm blood pressure cuff is placed on the calf just above the ankle. A dollop of ultrasound gel is placed over the posterior tibial artery (just behind the medial malleolus) and over the dorsalis pedis artery (one to three fingerbreadths lateral to the meridian of the foot on its dorsal surface), and the arterial signal is located with the hand-held Doppler device. The cuff is then inflated to suprasystolic levels, and the higher of the two systolic pressures (either the dorsalis pedis or the posterior tibial artery) is recorded just as for measuring arm blood pressure (i.e., by the first sounds of arterial flow as the blood pressure cuff is "bled" down toward zero). The higher of the two brachial artery pressures is then measured in the same fashion. The ABI equals the higher pedal systolic pressure divided by the higher of the two brachial systolic pressures.

The normal ABI should be approximately 1.0 (range, 0.90–1.2). Patients with one-block claudication generally have an ABI of 0.6 to 0.8, those with severe (less than one-block) claudication have an ABI of 0.4 to 0.6, and those with limb-threatening ischemia (rest pain, gangrene, nonhealing ulcers) have an ABI of less than 0.4.

Cost and Complications. No significant complications have been reported with this technique. This method is highly reliable in standard lower extremity arterial occlusive disease but may be unreliable in diabetics (in whom measurement of toe blood pressure by strain-gauge plethysmography in the vascular laboratory appears to be much more dependable). A hand-held ultrasonic flow detector can be purchased for $300 to $600 and should last at least 5 years. Because costs of measuring the ABI in a vascular laboratory setting may range from $60 to $200, measurement of Doppler pressures and ABI calculation in the office setting can be both clinically useful and cost-effective.

Cross-References: Peripheral Arterial Disease (Chapter 132), Leg Ulcers (Chapter 133).

SECTION XII
Neurologic Disorders

. . . .

136 Tremor

Symptom

THOMAS D. BIRD

Epidemiology. The prevalence of tremor in the general population or in the outpatient clinical setting has never been precisely determined. However, it is a relatively common sign. Approximately 500,000 Americans suffer from Parkinson's disease, and this represents only one of several relatively common causes of tremor.

Etiology. The most common cause of a *resting tremor* is Parkinson's disease. Phenothiazines and other dopaminergic blocking agents may also produce a resting tremor. The most common causes of a *postural tremor* are anxiety, benign essential tremor, toxins, medication (e.g., alcohol, caffeine, lithium, β-adrenergic agonists, phenytoin, and mercury), and metabolic disorders (e.g., hyperthyroidism). An *intention* or *action tremor* is usually associated with benign essential tremor or diseases of the cerebellar system such as multiple sclerosis, alcoholic cerebellar degeneration, primary or metastatic tumors of the cerebellum, postanoxic syndrome, and paraneoplastic cerebellar degeneration (usually seen with carcinoma of the lung or ovary).

Clinical Approach. Postural tremor is a fine regular movement of the fingers or hands when the arms are outstretched. It is usually not present at complete rest. Anxiety, the side effects of medication, or an underlying metabolic disturbance are the most common explanations. The major problem in the differential diagnosis of tremor is distinguishing the tremor of Parkinson's disease from essential tremor or disorders of the cerebellum. The tremor of Parkinson's disease is rapid, rhythmic, most evident in the fingers ("pill rolling"), present at rest, and often improved with intention or action. Most important, the tremor of Parkinson's disease rarely occurs in isolation but rather is associated with other characteristics of the parkinsonian syndrome. These include bradykinesia, cogwheel rigidity, masked facies, stooped posture, a festinating gait, a tendency toward retropulsion when standing, micrographia, and decreased voice volume. Parkinsonian tremor may be asymmetric and may involve the head and lower extremities. Note that a parkinsonian syndrome may be caused by neuroleptic dopaminergic blocking agents used to treat psychosis.

Benign *essential tremor* is rarely present at rest, is present with the arms

431

outstretched, and is much worse with action or intention. Essential tremor may also produce a horizontal or vertical head tremor and a "quivering voice" and is often familial. It is usually bilateral but may be worse on one side. It does not usually involve the lower extremities or produce gait ataxia. The handwriting of patients with essential tremor is large and irregular compared with the micrographia of Parkinson's disease. Patients with essential tremor may have considerable difficulty with handwriting, drinking from a cup or glass, or any activity involving hand movement. In fact, a useful clinical test is to observe the patient with tremor drinking from a full cup of water. The patient with essential tremor often has great difficulty and spills the liquid, whereas the patient with Parkinson's disease is slow but successful in the maneuver, except in the late stages of the disease. Furthermore, the patient with essential tremor does not have the other associated clinical signs of Parkinson's disease.

Both Parkinson's disease and essential tremor are slowly progressive over many years. Parkinson's disease generally becomes much more handicapping because of rigidity, bradykinesia, and an approximately 20% incidence of dementia.

As an isolated finding, the hand tremor of essential tremor is indistinguishable from the hand tremor of other cerebellar disorders. However, other disorders of the cerebellum are much more likely to also be associated with nystagmus, dysarthria, and gait ataxia, none of which is expected with benign essential tremor.

The assessment of tremor may also involve the question of the presence of asterixis, myoclonus, or chorea. *Asterixis* refers to brief recurring lapses in muscle contraction, best demonstrated with the arms outstretched and the hands dorsiflexed at the wrist. This is commonly seen in metabolic disorders such as azotemia and early hepatic encephalopathy. *Myoclonus* usually refers to brief, lightning-like contractions or jerks of an isolated limb or the entire trunk. *Chorea* refers to sudden, irregular, sometimes "semi-purposeful" jerking of the limbs that may also involve the face or trunk. Chorea may be a side effect of levodopa medications used to treat Parkinson's disease.

Management. The tremor of Parkinson's disease may improve with levodopa preparations or anticholinergic agents (such as trihexyphenidyl or benztropine) or a combination of the two. Selegiline (a monoamine oxidase-B inhibitor) may also be of value early in the course of Parkinson's disease; detailed clinical trials are in progress. Mild (truly benign) essential tremor often requires no treatment. However, essential tremor may not be "benign" and may interfere with daily activities. The observation that essential tremor often improves with a small amount of alcohol is a useful point in the history but usually is not an appropriate basis of therapy. No medication completely eliminates the tremor, and side effects often prevent increases in dosage. However, several drugs ameliorate essential tremor, including low doses of phenobarbital (30–90 mg/d), benzodiazepines (chlordiazepoxide, 20–50 mg/d), and β-blocking agents (propranolol, 40–160 mg/d). Patients with tremor should avoid caffeine.

Cross-References: Parkinsonism (Chapter 145), Generalized Anxiety (Chapter 186).

REFERENCES

1. Anouti A, Koller WC. Tremor disorders: Diagnosis and management. West J Med 1995;162:510–513.

   A focused review of the differential diagnosis and treatment of various causes of tremor is presented.

2. Bain PG, Findley LJ, Thompson PD, Gresty MA, Rothwell JC, Harding AE, Marsden CD. A study of hereditary essential tremor. Brain 1994;117:805–824.

   This article is a detailed description of the relatively common condition of inherited essential tremor.

3. Cleeves L, Findley LJ, Koller W. Lack of association between essential tremor and Parkinson's disease. Ann Neurol 1988:24:23–26.

   The authors provide a useful comparison of the features of Parkinson's disease and essential tremor.

4. Elble RJ, Koller WC. Tremor. Baltimore, Johns Hopkins University Press, 1990.

   This is an extensive review of the causes and treatment of tremor.

5. Koller WC, Busenbark K, Miner K, et al. The relationship of essential tremor to other movement disorders: Report on 678 patients. Ann Neurol 1994;35:717–723.

   Essential tremor is contrasted to other causes of tremor and movement disorders.

■ ■

137 Muscular Weakness

Symptom

JOHN RAVITS

Etiology and Symptoms and Signs. Weakness, an objective loss of muscle strength, is a frequent problem seen by primary care clinicians and by neurologists. It is often confused with *lassitude,* a feeling of weariness without actual weakness, or with other kinds of neurologic dysfunction such as pain, incoordination, rigidity, and apraxia. *Paresis* refers to incomplete loss of strength, and *plegia* or *paralysis* refers to complete loss of strength. *Upper motor neuron weakness* is caused by lesions in the central nervous system (CNS) and is characterized by weakness affecting groups of muscles (usually extensor muscles in the arms and flexor muscles in the legs), loss of fine-skilled movements, increased muscle tone (spasticity), increased reflexes, and extensor plantar responses. *Lower motor neuron weakness* is caused by lesions in the peripheral nervous system and is characterized by weakness in specific distributions (such as a ventral root or a peripheral nerve), fasciculations, muscle atrophy, decreased muscle tone (flaccidity), and decreased reflexes.

Lassitude and fatigue (distinct from true muscular weakness) may result from a variety of metabolic diseases (e.g., thyroid disease, Addison's disease, diabetes), systemic inflammatory conditions (e.g., polymyalgia rheumatica), anemia, hepatic disease, renal disease, infections (e.g., subacute bacterial endo-

carditis, urosepsis, flulike illnesses, mononucleosis, tuberculosis, human immunodeficiency virus infection), malignancy, chronic fatigue syndrome, and psychiatric problems (previously called neurasthenia) (see Chapter 21, Fatigue).

The distribution of true muscle weakness provides clues to its cause.
Monoparesis refers to a weakness in a single limb and is usually of the lower
motor neuron type. It is caused by radiculopathy, plexopathy, or mononeuropathy. Monoparesis of an upper motor neuron type indicates a discrete lesion in
the CNS, usually from strokes, neoplasms, or multiple sclerosis. *Hemiparesis*
refers to weakness on one side of the body and usually indicates a CNS lesion
contralateral to the weak side. The more typical causes are stroke, neoplasms,
infections, trauma, or perinatal injury. *Quadriparesis* refers to weakness in the
arms and legs. If it is of the lower motor neuron type, it indicates peripheral
nervous system dysfunction. *Distal weakness* with relative sparing of proximal
muscles is the hallmark of polyneuropathy. It is usually caused by toxic-metabolic neuropathies such as diabetes, vitamin B_{12} deficiencies, demyelinating
neuropathies such as Guillain-Barré syndrome, paraproteinemic neuropathies,
and hereditary neuropathies. *Proximal muscle weakness* with relative sparing of
distal muscles is the hallmark of myopathy. The usual causes of myopathy
are polymyositis, toxic-metabolic myopathy (e.g., thyroid disease, Cushing's
syndrome), and muscular dystrophy. Also, defective neuromuscular transmission such as myasthenia gravis or myasthenic syndrome may simulate myopathy.
If quadriparesis has the features of upper motor neuron weakness, it indicates
spinal cord disease (myelopathy) at or above the cervical level. The most
common causes of myelopathy include compression from spondylosis or disk
disease, trauma, tumors (either primary tumors or metastatic disease), myelitis,
and multiple sclerosis.

Paraparesis refers to weakness of the legs. If it is of the lower motor neuron
type, it indicates polyneuropathy, Guillain-Barré syndrome, myopathy, multiple
mononeuropathies, or abnormalities of the cauda equina (usually from neoplasms, lumbar stenosis, or lumbar disk disease). If paraparesis is of the upper
motor neuron type, it indicates myelopathy at the thoracic or upper lumbar
levels; the usual causes are compression from spondylosis or disk disease,
trauma, tumors (either primary or metastatic), myelitis, and multiple sclerosis.

Diffuse weakness may indicate, in addition to any of the above conditions,
multiple sclerosis, multiple strokes, posterior circulation strokes, and degenerative conditions such as motor neuron disease. *Episodic weakness* may indicate
transient ischemic attacks, multiple sclerosis, myasthenia gravis, and periodic
paralysis.

Clinical Approach. In addition to the character and pattern of weakness, the
patient interview should identify associated symptoms and signs. In particular,
the presence or absence of ocular bulbar symptoms, sensory disturbance, pain,
sphincter dysfunction, and autonomic dysfunction must be noted. One must
know the clinical context, such as the patient's general medical health, age,
other systemic diseases such as diabetes, malignancy, arthritis, vascular disease,
alcoholism, and medications. The family history may shed light on some
patients' weakness. The physician should identify associated orthopedic problems (e.g., kyphoscoliosis) and cutaneous markings (e.g., café-au-lait spots) and
examine the axial, shoulder, hip girdle, and appendicular muscles for atrophy,

fasciculations, muscle tone, and weakness. "Give-way weakness" is ratchety rather than smooth and is often seen in the patient who is co-contracting muscles other than those being examined. Although this usually represents functional overlay or malingering, it may be evident in a frightened patient with an underlying organic problem. Patients in pain often do not make a full effort, especially if the muscle contraction puts the body part into a position of greater pain; these patients are best examined isometrically, because contraction of the muscle does not produce movement about a joint. Reflexes must be carefully tested and compared for symmetry; Jendrassik's maneuver (i.e., the patient contracts a muscle group other than that being tested) may help elicit an otherwise absent reflex.

Laboratory testing includes a complete blood cell count, erythrocyte sedimentation rate, chemistry panel, muscle enzyme evaluation, and acetylcholine receptor antibody determination (when myasthenia gravis is suggested). Radiographs of the chest and spine may be particularly important. Magnetic resonance imaging of the head or relevant regions of the spinal axis may ultimately be necessary to define the cause of weakness, but because of its expense there should be a clear definition of the weakness and its differential diagnosis and the need for magnetic resonance imaging. Electromyography, nerve conduction studies, muscle biopsies, and nerve biopsies may identify neuromuscular abnormalities in selected cases. Examination of the cerebrospinal fluid may demonstrate a cytoalbuminologic dissociation in Guillain-Barré syndrome, abnormal immunoglobin findings in multiple sclerosis or myelitis, or abnormal cytologic findings in carcinomatous infiltration of the meninges.

One of the most dreaded and treatable complications of weakness is respiratory weakness. In rapidly evolving weakness or weakness in which respiratory compromise is apparent or possible, hospitalization and mechanical ventilation may be appropriate.

Cross-References: Fatigue (Chapter 21), Low Back Pain (Chapter 107), Multiple Sclerosis (Chapter 141), Entrapment Neuropathies (Chapter 144), Peripheral Neuropathy (Chapter 147), Electromyography and Nerve Conduction Studies (Chapter 149).

REFERENCES

1. Adams RD, Victor M, eds. Principles of Neurology, 6th ed. New York, McGraw-Hill Information Services, 1997.

   The first half of this standard textbook of neurology is a discussion of cardinal manifestations of disease and differential diagnosis; in the second half the various disease processes are detailed.

2. Rowland LP, ed. Merritt's Textbook of Neurology, 8th ed. Philadelphia, Lea & Febiger, 1989.

   This is another very good standard neurology textbook.

138 Headache

Symptom

JOYCE E. WIPF

Epidemiology. Headaches affect 90% of the population, accounting for about 2% of all visits to emergency departments or primary care physicians. About 50% of adults experience a severe or disabling headache at some time, and 1% have daily headaches. Migraine headaches affect nearly 10% of adults, accounting for frequent missed workdays (averaging more than 2 workdays missed per month in one survey). Headaches in patients older than 65 are less common, affecting only 40%, and are more likely to be due to a serious pathologic process.

Etiology. Over 80% of headaches are idiopathic and benign. It is believed that all of these represent a similar neurogenic disorder involving serotonin. In the most recent (1988) International Headache Society classification, terms such as *vascular headache, muscle contraction,* and *classic* and *common migraine* were eliminated. The current major categories are (1) tension-type headaches (e.g., psychogenic, nonspecific daily headaches), (2) migraine headaches (e.g., migraine with or without aura), (3) cluster headache, and (4) mixed headaches with features of more than one type.

Migraine and tension-type headaches may be indistinguishable and have overlapping features; they probably represent a continuum of the same process. *Tension-type headaches* are usually bilateral (90%) and located at the vertex, temporal, or frontal area; less than 20% are occipital. They may be episodic or chronic, often feature prominent fatigue, and usually respond within hours to analgesics. A typical *migraine* consists of unilateral throbbing discomfort that lasts 1 to 3 days. Associated mood changes and gastrointestinal symptoms may precede the headache by minutes to hours. Reversible neurologic auras (most commonly visual scotomas or flashing lights and less commonly focal weakness, numbness, tingling, mild aphasia, or confusion) may precede, accompany, or even follow the pain phase of the headache. Migraines rarely occur more often than once or twice a week. *Cluster headaches,* usually seen in middle-aged men, are characterized by paroxysms of severe unilateral pain, usually of the orbit, and associated ipsilateral autonomic changes, such as lacrimation, erythema of the eye, nasal congestion, and Horner's syndrome. Cluster headaches often recur in groups over consecutive days or weeks. Another headache type is *carotidynia,* which is characterized by unilateral anterior neck pain with tenderness of the ipsilateral carotid artery and floor of the mouth.

Factors that may precipitate headaches include ingestion of certain dietary items (strong or aged cheeses containing tyramine, alcohol, chocolate, canned figs, cured meats containing nitrate, monosodium glutamate, caffeine), sleep deprivation or excess, stress, menstruation, and various medications (e.g., oral contraceptives; vasodilators such as hydralazine, minoxidil, prazosin, and nifedipine; or β-blockers with sympathomimetic or partial agonist activity such as acebutolol and pindolol).

Organic causes of headache include *mass lesions* (e.g., brain tumor, abscess, subdural hematoma, subarachnoid or intracerebral hemorrhage), *meningitis*, *sinusitis*, *vascular causes* (carotid or basilar artery stenosis, aneurysm, temporal arteritis), *intracranial hypertension* (hydrocephalus, pseudotumor cerebri), *medical conditions* (malignant hypertension, pheochromocytoma, carbon monoxide poisoning, hypoxia, hypercapnia, anemia, glaucoma), *neuralgia*, and miscellaneous diseases of the bones, joints, and teeth.

Clinical Approach. The clinician's goal is to distinguish the common idiopathic headaches from the uncommon organic causes. The interview (with open-ended questions) identifies the pattern and location of headache and determines previous treatments for headaches, associated symptoms, and precipitating factors. Symptoms traditionally associated with migraine, such as throbbing, photophobia, and gastrointestinal distress, may be seen in a severe headache of any type.

Features that suggest a possible organic cause include the patient's complaint of "worst headache ever"; a headache that is "different" from before; a headache precipitated by position change, cough, or exertion; a history of trauma or fever; and abnormal mentation or other neurologic findings. Features that suggest benign headaches include young age (< 35), a history of a previous identical headache, normal vital signs, normal neurologic findings, and pain relieved by oral analgesics.

Routine laboratory tests include a complete blood cell count, chemistry screen, and, in patients older than 40, an erythrocyte sedimentation rate (to exclude temporal arteritis) and screening for glaucoma. Computed tomography of the head is indicated in patients with trauma, worrisome historical features, or focal neurologic findings. Magnetic resonance imaging may better evaluate those patients with suspected posterior fossa lesions. Lumbar puncture is indicated in patients with acute fever and headache. If bacterial meningitis is strongly suspected, antibiotics should be administered without delay, even before completion of the diagnostic workup.

Management. The clinician should initially clarify the patient's specific concerns. Although physicians often assume that relief of headache is the patient's primary concern, studies suggest that patients more often seek medical attention for reassurance that no serious pathologic process exists. Therapy for headache encompasses (1) avoidance of precipitating factors, (2) treatment of acute attacks, and (3) prophylaxis for migraine headaches (Table 138–1).

Nondrug therapies, including behavioral modification and relaxation training to help patients cope with stress, may benefit patients with recurrent headaches.

Patients with headaches that persist beyond 72 hours (status migrainosus) are frequently volume depleted and should receive intravenous fluids before drug treatment. Ergotamines, which are available in oral, sublingual, aerosolized, rectal, and parenteral forms, are most effective when given early during a migraine headache, are contraindicated in patients with atherosclerotic cardiovascular disease, and may actually promote headaches if used more than 2 days per week. Other effective medications include nonsteroidal anti-inflammatory

Table 138-1. THERAPY FOR HEADACHES—ACUTE ATTACK

Drug	Dose	Side Effects	Cost ($)*
Oral			
Nonsteroidal anti-inflammatory		Gastrointestinal distress, ulceration and bleeding, rash, renal effects, tinnitus, edema	
Aspirin	650 mg q4h		0.01 (325 mg)
Naproxen	250–375 mg tid		0.66 (250 mg)
Acetaminophen	650 mg q4h	Overdose: nausea, vomiting, hepatotoxicity	0.01 (325 mg)
Barbiturates			
Fiorinal (50 mg butalbital, caffeine, and aspirin)	1–2 tabs q4h (max. 6 tabs/d)	Nausea and vomiting, constipation, sedation, dizziness, drug dependency	0.48 (tab)
Ergotamines			
Cafergot (1 mg ergotamine and caffeine)	2 tablets PO at start of attack, 1 additional tablet every 30 min (max. 6/d or 10/wk)	Vasoconstriction,† nausea, vomiting, transient bradycardia or tachycardia	0.56–1.05 (tab)
Ergostat (2 mg ergotamine)	1 sublingual tablet at first symptoms, then repeat q1/2h × 2, prn (max. 3/24 h or 5/wk)		0.74 (tab)
Sumatriptan (Imitrex)	25–100 mg PO; may repeat × 1 in 2 h	Coronary vasospasm,‡ mild increase in blood pressure, dysesthesias	8.95 (25 mg) 10.15 (50 mg)
Parenteral			
Sumatriptan (Imitrex)	6 mg SQ; may repeat × 1 in 1 h	Same as in oral administration; erythema and stinging at injection site	35.11 (6 mg)
Ketorolac (Toradol)	30–60 mg IM	Gastrointestinal distress, dizziness, insomnia, renal effects	8.05 (60 mg)
Dihydroergotamine	1 mg IM or IV (preceded by 10 min with 10 mg IM or IV metoclopramide)	Coronary vasospasm,‡ nausea and vomiting, flushing, drowsiness, anxiety	9.69 (1 mg)
Prochlorperazine	10 mg slow IV × 1 (max. 5 mg/min), used alone or with other therapies	Drowsiness, orthostatic hypotension (extrapyramidal symptoms are rare)	1.81–6.81 (10 mg)
Chlorpromazine	7.5 mg IV over 3 min, may repeat × 3 at 7-min intervals	Hypotension	1.05–6.91 (25 mg)
Meperidine	25–75 mg IM with 25–50 mg hydroxyzine	Hypotension, drug dependency	0.70–1.28 (100 mg)

*Average wholesale price, 1996 *Drug Topics Red Book*.
†Ergotamines are contraindicated in patients with coronary artery disease, peripheral vascular disease, hypertension, and impaired renal/hepatic function.
‡Sumatriptan is contraindicated in coronary artery disease or uncontrolled hypertension.
Note: Avoid joint use of ergotamines and sumatriptan within 24 h.

Table 138–2. PROPHYLAXIS OF MIGRAINES

Drug	Dose	Side Effects	Cost ($)*
β-blocker			
Propranolol	80–320 mg/d	Bronchospasm, hypotension, fatigue, impotence	0.12–0.88 (80 mg)
Tricyclic antidepressant			
Amitriptyline	50–175 mg/d	Anticholinergic symptoms, orthostatic hypotension	0.04–0.74 (50 mg)
Anticonvulsant			
Divalproex sodium (Depakote)	250–1000 mg/d	Nausea, diarrhea, sedation, decreased libido	0.31 (250 mg)
Calcium channel blockers			
Verapamil	80–120 mg tid	Postural hypotension, edema, constipation, facial flushing	0.28–0.62 (120 mg)
Cyproheptadine (Periactin)	6–12 mg bid	Sedation, weight gain, appetite stimulation	0.04 (4 mg, generic) 0.39 (4 mg, Periactin)
Methysergide (Sansert)	2 mg bid	Vivid dreams, hallucinations; pericardial, cardiac, pulmonary, and retroperitoneal fibrosis with long-term use	1.64 (2 mg)

*Average wholesale price, 1996 *Drug Topics Red Book.*

agents, which are underutilized. Ketorolac, an injectable nonsteroidal medication, is effective as a single dose in the emergency department setting or administered by the patient at home. Antiemetics such as prochlorperazine and metoclopramide have been shown in controlled trials to relieve acute headache in addition to relieving nausea and vomiting associated with severe headaches.

Sumatriptan, a serotonin-receptor agonist, has proven effective for both migraine and cluster headaches and is available in subcutaneous injection and oral preparations. Sumatriptan and ergotamines should not be given within 24 hours of one another because both can produce vasospasm. Narcotic medications are best avoided in both acute and chronic headaches.

Drug-induced headache should be considered in any patient with daily headaches. Analgesic medications including acetaminophen, nonsteroidal antiinflammatory agents, barbiturates, ergotamines, and narcotics have been shown to precipitate daily headaches when used frequently. Such medications can also nullify the benefits of prophylactic medications. One should consider discontinuing daily symptomatic medications in any patient with frequent headaches and monitoring headache frequency by means of a headache diary.

A 3- to 6-month trial of prophylactic medications (Table 138–2) is reasonable when migraines are frequent, complicated (associated reversible neurologic deficits), or refractory to abortive treatments. β-blockers are useful prophylactic agents but do not alleviate prodromes and may actually aggravate them. Pindolol and acebutolol should not be used because of their sympathomimetic effects. Patients with refractory migraines should be referred to a headache specialist. Treatment with the lysergic acid derivative methysergide is rarely necessary and should be limited to 4 months, followed by a 1-month period without the medication because of its potentially severe side effects.

Medications for cluster headaches include ergotamines, divalproex, lithium, tricyclic antidepressants, and methysergide; 100% oxygen may rapidly relieve cluster headache and associated autonomic symptoms.

Follow-Up. Within a few weeks of starting a new drug, a follow-up appointment should be scheduled to monitor the patient's response and side effects. Those with frequent severe migraines should be given prophylaxis for a limited period of 3 to 6 months. Headaches refractory to therapy deserve further evaluation for an intracranial lesion, despite a normal neurologic examination, because occasional mass lesions present without localizing findings and respond temporarily to drug therapies. Although controversial, current evidence does not conclusively demonstrate that migraine is a risk factor for stroke.

Cross-References: Screening for Glaucoma (Chapter 35), Polymyalgia Rheumatica and Temporal Arteritis (Chapter 117), Myofascial Pain Syndromes (Chapter 122).

REFERENCES

1. Frishberg BM. The utility of neuroimaging in the evaluation of headache in patients with normal neurologic examinations. Neurology 1994;44:1191–1197.

   The author concluded from data in several studies that scans are not beneficial in patients with headache and normal neurologic examination. Most patients studied were younger than age 60, and abnormalities found on scans were generally incidental findings.

2. International Headache Society. The classification and diagnosis criteria for headache disorders, cranial neuralgia and facial pain. Cephalalgia 1988;8(suppl 7):1–96.

This lists the 1988 changes in classification of headaches. The previously used term muscle contraction type is now included under tension headache. Migraines are no longer categorized as "classic" or "common" types but as migraine with or without aura.

3. Kumar KL. Recent advances in the acute management of migraine and cluster headaches. J Gen Intern Med 1994;9:339–348.

Tables of the International Headache Society's migraine diagnostic criteria are presented, along with an excellent discussion of drug efficacy data, including newer agents such as sumatriptan and ketorolac.

4. Matthew NT, Kurman R, Perez F. Drug induced refractory headache—clinical features and management. Headache 1990;30:634–638.

Drug-induced headache and patterns of analgesic use are defined. Concomitant use of symptomatic medications can precipitate daily headaches and also nullify the effects of prophylactic medications. Discontinuing daily symptomatic medications results in improvement of headache and improved response to prophylactic therapy.

5. Matthew NT, Saper JR, Silberstein SD, et al. Migraine prophylaxis with divalproex. Arch Neurol 1995;52:281–286.

A double-blind, randomized trial showed that 48% of divalproex-treated patients and 14% of placebo-treated patients had a 50% or greater reduction in migraine frequency from baseline.

139 Seizures

Symptom

JAMES J. COATSWORTH and LAIRD G. PATTERSON

Epidemiology and Etiology. Between 0.5% and 1% of the population suffer from epilepsy, and up to 5% have a single seizure. The incidence is 20 to 50 per 100,000 population per year, increasing after age 60. Seizures result from a wide variety of primary central nervous system diseases (e.g., brain tumors, infection, and degenerative diseases) or systemic disturbances (e.g., drug withdrawal, electrolyte imbalance, renal or hepatic failure, or hypoxia). In patients with a known seizure disorder, certain factors increase susceptibility to seizures (e.g., sleep deprivation, stress, menstruation, drugs). The term *epilepsy* refers to chronic recurrent seizures, whether or not the cause is known.

Symptoms and Signs. Seizures are classified as either focal (partial) or generalized; focal seizures may or may not impair consciousness (Table 139–1). A detailed history relying on witnesses is important to characterize events immedi-

Table 139–1. CLASSIFICATION OF SEIZURES

Generalized seizures (no focal onset)	Partial seizures (focal onset)
Absence (petit mal)	Simple (consciousness not impaired)
Tonic-clonic (grand mal)	Motor
Myoclonic	Sensory
	Autonomic
	Psychic
	Complex (consciousness impaired)

ately preceding and following a suspected seizure. For example, focal motor or sensory manifestations before or after the seizure suggest a seizure caused by a localized cerebral structural lesion. Additional historical points of importance include evidence of head trauma, use of drugs or alcohol, and compliance with seizure medications.

A careful neurologic examination may yield clues that the episode was a seizure (tongue biting, incontinence) or that a structural problem is present (mild hemiparesis, reflex asymmetry, extensor plantar response). Careful physical examination may help identify skin lesions of tuberous sclerosis (adenoma sebaceum) or neurofibromas, suggesting associated von Recklinghausen's disease.

Clinical Approach. The practitioner should classify the type of seizure and define any underlying pathologic process that may require specific treatment. An electroencephalogram (EEG) may assist in confirming the clinical diagnosis and help differentiate partial from generalized seizures. Videotape monitoring in combination with an EEG may help differentiate true seizures from pseudoseizures.

Patients with seizures related to alcohol or drug withdrawal who have normal neurologic findings and no head trauma need not undergo EEG, computed tomography, or magnetic resonance imaging, because these studies almost always show no abnormality. Patients with partial seizures, focal abnormalities on the EEG, or other unexplained neurologic signs should undergo head computed tomography or magnetic resonance imaging to evaluate potential pathologic causes.

Laboratory testing is rarely useful but should exclude hypoglycemia, hypocalcemia, and hyponatremia. Hospitalization is indicated in patients with electrolyte abnormalities or those who have multiple seizures that recur within a short period of time.

Management. A single seizure does not constitute a diagnosis of epilepsy and does not necessarily require treatment. Because 40% of adults will experience recurrent seizures within 2 or 3 years of their first seizure, those with a progressive cerebral disorder or clearly abnormal EEGs should usually receive medication after the initial event. Patients with postconcussion seizures, alcohol withdrawal seizures, or drug-related seizures do not require antiepileptic treatment.

Therapy should begin with the least toxic drug at a relatively low dose that is increased gradually if seizures recur. Primary generalized seizures respond best to phenytoin, carbamazepine, or valproic acid. Partial seizures should be treated with the same drugs, starting with carbamazepine and moving to phenytoin or valproic acid as required.

Primidone and phenobarbital are less frequently used because of their sedating side effects. Patients who experience recurrent seizures despite an adequate serum level of an initial antiepileptic medication sometimes require the addition of a second antiepileptic medication. Phenobarbital is a commonly used second drug, especially in patients with partial seizures. Patients requiring two or more drugs require careful monitoring of symptoms and drug levels to prevent toxicity (Table 139–2).

Two new antiepileptic drugs are now available and provide greater flexibility of drug choice. Gabapentin is an add-on drug with few side effects or drug interactions. Lamotrigine is useful as an add-on drug but can also be used for monotherapy.

Sophisticated epilepsy centers and neurosurgical procedures have been developed for properly selected patients. This represents a major advance in the management of complex or pharmacologically refractory seizure disorders.

Pregnant epileptic women seem to have more obstetric complications, and their children seem to have more fetal abnormalities. Seizure medications are likely responsible for some of these complications. Although withdrawal of antiepileptic agents before pregnancy is advisable in women with prolonged remissions from epilepsy, most patients require medication despite the risks. Treatment with phenytoin, valproic acid, and combinations of agents should be avoided if possible. Serum drug levels should be monitored monthly during the last trimester and again after delivery.

Follow-Up. During the first few weeks of therapy, toxic effects and compliance should be carefully monitored. Once the condition has been stabilized, the patient should return to the clinic every 6 to 12 months. It must be remembered that symptoms may be satisfactorily controlled with lower-than-therapeutic serum levels, and, conversely, many patients tolerate high serum levels without complications. Therapeutic drug levels are therefore an adjunct to drug evaluation rather than an absolute guide.

Discontinuing medications is best done in consultation with an experienced neurologist. Most authorities recommend a repeat EEG before discontinuing medications. Up to 40% of patients who are seizure free on medication for 2 or more years will experience relapse with discontinuation. The chance of relapse decreases with the passage of time after withdrawal. Other factors favoring successful withdrawal include a normal EEG at the time of withdrawal, generalized epilepsy, and an epileptic history of short duration. Drugs should be discontinued gradually over 4 to 6 weeks to avoid precipitating seizures. Patients with structural brain diseases as a cause of seizures are best continued on treatment.

Patients with well-controlled epilepsy do not need repeated imaging studies or EEGs. Those who fail treatment or show progressive neurologic abnormalities require reevaluation.

Cross-References: Compliance (Chapter 4), Syncope (Chapter 75), Alcohol Withdrawal (Chapter 142), Electroencephalography (Chapter 148).

Table 139-2. COMMONLY USED ANTIEPILEPTIC MEDICATIONS IN ADULTS

Drug	Usual Daily Dose (mg)	Plasma Half-life Plasma (h)	Therapeutic Range (μg/mL)	Adverse Effects	Cost ($) per Day*
Phenytoin	300–400	24	10–20	Ataxia, diplopia, gingival hyperplasia, hirsutism, low folate level	0.51
Carbamazepine	600–1200	12–17	4–12	Dizziness, leukopenia	1.05
Primidone	750–1250	12	5–15	Drowsiness	0.45
Valproic acid	1000–1500	5–20	50–100	Nausea, vomiting, sedation	1.00
Phenobarbital	90–120	48–144	20–40	Sedation	0.15

*Average wholesale price, 1995 *Drug Topics Red Book*, for lower range of common daily dose.

REFERENCES

1. Berg AT, Shinnar S. Relapse following discontinuation of antiepileptic drugs. A meta-analysis. Neurology 1994;44:601–608.

   Relapse rates after drug withdrawal are reviewed and analyzed with recommendations and criteria for discontinuing antiepileptic drug therapy.

2. Brodie MJ, Dichter MA. Antiepileptic drugs. N Engl J Med 1996;334:168–175.

   A thorough review of the diagnosis and appropriate treatment of seizures is provided.

3. Dichter MA, Brodie MJ. New antiepileptic drugs. N Engl J Med 1996;334:1583–1590.

   The authors present an excellent summary of the pharmacology and indications for using the most recently introduced antiepileptic drugs.

4. Engel J Jr. Surgery for seizures. N Engl J Med 1996;334:647–652.

   A concise overview is given of the role of surgery in the treatment of refractory seizure disorders.

5. Wilder BJ, ed. Rational polypharmacy in the treatment of epilepsy. Neurology 1995;45(suppl 2):S1–S38.

   Guidelines are presented for the classification, evaluation, and treatment of seizures.

■ ■

140 Dementia

Symptom

DAVID G. FRYER and LAIRD G. PATTERSON

Epidemiology. *Dementia* refers to the gradual loss of cognitive function that occurs over many months or years, eventually resulting in total dependency. It is most common in older patients. About 15% of patients older than 75 years of age suffer from some degree of dementia; in 5% of cases, the dementia is severe.

Etiology. Alzheimer's disease is the most common cause of dementia, followed by multi-infarct dementia. Less common causes include the acquired immunodeficiency syndrome (30% to 65% of patients with advanced disease), head injury, alcohol-related cerebral degeneration, and Parkinson's disease. Communicating hydrocephalus, hypothyroidism, hyperparathyroidism, central nervous system vasculitis, brain tumor, vitamin B_{12} deficiency, Creutzfeldt-Jakob disease, neurosyphilis, and Pick's disease are rare causes.

Clinical Approach. Only the demonstration at autopsy of excessive numbers of neurofibrillary tangles and senile plaques containing amyloid beta protein confirms the diagnosis of Alzheimer's disease. Because brain biopsy is almost never justified or helpful, and because no laboratory test for Alzheimer's disease exists, the diagnosis during life depends on demonstration by the patient of (1) impaired short- and long-term memory; (2) altered abstract thinking, judgment, or personality sufficient to interfere with social activity or work; and (3) exclusion of factors that cause delirium.

Although older patients have more difficulty with memory and tasks requiring spatial organization, this normal deterioration differs from dementia because it preserves vocabulary and spelling and improves with offered cues. The abnormal memory of Alzheimer's disease, in contrast, is always associated with some degree of dysphasia and does not improve by use of association. For example, unlike normal elderly persons, patients with Alzheimer's disease can recall a list of related words no better than they can a list of random words.

The clinician should inquire about cardiovascular disease, head trauma, alcohol consumption, human immunodeficiency virus exposure, and current medications. There may be a family history of dementia.

The Folstein Mini-Mental State Examination (Table 140–1) can gauge the degree of dementia but may be normal in very intelligent, educated patients with some mild cognitive impairment. More detailed neuropsychological testing may be needed to assess vocational abilities, establish legal competency, or distinguish dementia from depression.

The neurologic examination is otherwise normal in patients with Alzheimer's disease until late in its course. Headache, seizures, or focal neurologic deficits (e.g., hemiparesis) suggest a different cause, such as tumor or

Table 140–1. THE MINI-MENTAL STATE EXAMINATION

	Score*
Orientation	
What is the year, season, month, day of month, and day of week?	5
Where are we (i.e., state, county, town, building floor)?	5
Registration	
Examiner names three objects, then asks patient to repeat them.	3
Attention and Calculation	
Serial sevens (five successive subtractions from 100), or spell "world" backward.	5
Recall	
What were the three objects learned earlier? (One point for each correct answer)	3
Language and Praxis	
Examiner points to a pencil and a watch and asks patient to name them.	2
Patient is asked to:	
Repeat "no ifs, ands, or buts."	1
Follow the three-stage verbal command, "Take this piece of paper in your right hand, fold it in half, and put it on the floor."	3
Follow the written command, "Close your eyes."	1
Make up and write a sentence.	1
Copy a simple figure (e.g., intersecting pentagons).	1
Maximum Total Score:	30

*Scores less than 24 generally signify dementia or delirium.
Adapted from Folstein M, et al. J Psychiatr Res 1975;12:189–198.

subdural hematoma, whereas gait disturbance and urinary incontinence suggest communicating normal-pressure hydrocephalus.

Routine laboratory tests include a complete blood cell count, erythrocyte sedimentation rate, chemistry profile, and determination of thyroid-stimulating hormone and vitamin B_{12} levels. Lumbar puncture, electroencephalography, and computed tomography or magnetic resonance imaging are not helpful as routine tests. These tests are appropriate in cases with (1) abrupt onset of dementia, (2) onset before age 60 years, (3) focal neurologic signs, (4) recent seizures or new-onset headache, or (5) immunosuppression. Single-photon emission computed tomography (SPECT) often shows decreased blood flow in the parietal cortex in Alzheimer's disease, but its place in the evaluation of dementia has not been established. In the future, biologic markers may contribute to the diagnosis of Alzheimer's disease. Some individuals at risk carry alleles for apolipoprotein E. Others may have amyloid precursor protein or tau protein in the cerebrospinal fluid.

Clues to the diagnosis of multi-infarct dementia are (1) a stepwise progression of dementia, (2) associated hypertension or diabetes, (3) findings of peripheral vascular disease or previous cerebrovascular accidents, (4) pseudobulbar palsy with exaggerated laughing or crying, and (5) pyramidal or extrapyramidal signs due to deep white matter and brain stem ischemia.

The differential diagnosis of dementia includes delirium and depression ("pseudodementia"). *Delirium* also involves defective memory and cognitive function but, unlike dementia, is characterized by clouding of consciousness, disordered sleep pattern, and more abrupt development over hours or days. Types of delirium include the agitated type, where patients are excited and distractible, often with hallucinations that provoke unpredictable or violent behavior (followed by amnesia for such episodes), and the retarded type, where patients are lethargic and apathetic, with depressed mood and motor activity. The evaluation of patients with delirium emphasizes the search for medication intoxication (especially anticholinergic, antiparkinsonian, antidepressant, nonsteroidal anti-inflammatory, antihistamine, and narcotic medications) and acute physical illnesses (such as urinary tract infection, pneumonia, uremia, volume depletion, hypokalemia, hypoxia, hypoglycemia, and hepatic failure).

Pseudodementia refers to a memory disturbance that results from depression and responds to antidepressive drug therapy. In pseudodementia, the depression usually precedes the abnormal memory, the onset may be abrupt, the severity may plateau rather than progress, and the mental status examination is often characterized by profound apathy. Depression may also occur in true dementia.

Management. Although most causes of dementia are untreatable, many patients improve after treatment of associated conditions, such as adverse drug reactions, depression, and malnutrition.

Treatable causes of dementia are hydrocephalus, subdural hematoma, hyperparathyroidism, vitamin B_{12} deficiency, hypothyroidism, and chronic central nervous system infection. Sedatives, neuroleptic drugs (e.g., haloperidol), and antidepressants (e.g., amitriptyline) may provide some relief of symptoms for agitated, paranoid, or depressed patients but require careful dosage adjustment to avoid accentuating confusion and disorientation.

Demented patients benefit from repeated explanations that reinforce orientation, for example, reminders of what has been done, what is going to happen, what building they are in, and other points of reference. In those with dysphasia, the clinician and family should emphasize nonverbal aspects of communication (e.g., gestures). Patients with dementia are often inclined to wander and should wear an identification bracelet or necklace. Other helpful measures include attaching neck chains to eyeglasses, illuminating the bedroom at all times, labeling drawers and appliances at home, and establishing a toileting program in which the person is reminded to go to the bathroom at regular intervals. Patients and their families should be made aware of the risk of driving, and driving skills may require formal assessment. Family members often benefit from community support groups and, as they are burdened by the responsibilities of caring for the patient, by short respites during which the patient is temporarily admitted to a nursing home. Although no highly effective treatment is available for Alzheimer's disease, some patients with mild or moderate dementia may demonstrate mild improvement in cognition temporarily with tacrine. Psychoactive drugs such as haloperidol or anticonvulsants are occasionally used to control disruptive behavior. These drugs should be used cautiously with treatment begun with small doses because the risk of toxicity is substantial.

Follow-Up. Patients should be reevaluated at 6- to 12-month intervals if the diagnosis of dementia is uncertain or not convincingly established after the initial workup. Other patients need reassessment if there is sudden or more rapid than expected decline. Superimposed illness or depression may aggravate the dementia. Follow-up for purposes of behavior management and family/caregiver support is often necessary.

Cross-References: Parkinsonism (Chapter 145), Cerebrovascular Disease (Chapter 146), Common Thyroid Disorders (Chapter 153), Screening for Depression (Chapter 185), Management of Depression (Chapter 189), HIV Infection: Evaluation of Common Symptoms (Chapter 205).

REFERENCES

1. Clarfield AM. The reversible dementias: Do they reverse? Ann Intern Med 1988;109:476–486.
   In this excellent review of dementia, emphasis is placed on treatable causes and guidelines for evaluating dementia; useful tables are included.

2. Corey-Bloom J, et al. Diagnosis and evaluation of dementia. Neurology 1995;45:211–218.
   This is a concise review of the approach to investigating the demented patient. This background paper for practice parameter issued by the American Academy of Neurology contains an excellent algorithm for dementia diagnosis and workup.

3. Friedland RP. Alzheimer's disease: Clinical features and differential diagnosis. Neurology 1993;43(suppl 4):45–51.
   The author provides a review of dementia with emphasis on Alzheimer's disease.

4. Román GC, et al. Vascular dementia: Diagnostic criteria for research studies. Neurology 1993;43:250–259.
   An attempt is made to clarify the diagnosis of vascular dementia by establishing criteria that have both clinical and research applications.

5. Winkler MA. Tacrine for Alzheimer's disease. JAMA 1994;271:1023–1024.
   This is an editorial discussing the rational use and limitations of tacrine.

141 Multiple Sclerosis

Problem

JAMES B. MACLEAN

Epidemiology. The etiology of multiple sclerosis is unknown, but the disease may result from immunologic alterations triggered by a viral infection in genetically susceptible individuals. The incidence is greater in northern latitudes, particularly in individuals who resided in these regions during the early years of life. Family members of patients with multiple sclerosis have a nearly five times higher incidence of developing the disease than the general population.

Symptoms and Signs. Multiple sclerosis is classically defined by the appearance of central nervous system lesions, identified clinically, that are separated in both time and location. There is an enormous variety in the presenting symptoms and signs of multiple sclerosis because the pathologic lesions, plaques in the white matter, may appear anywhere in the central nervous system or even in the peripheral nervous system. The more common symptoms include monocular visual loss, focal numbness with clumsiness, imbalance, bilateral leg weakness with sensory distortion, double vision, and autonomic symptoms (particularly bowel and bladder dysfunction). Less frequent symptoms include trigeminal neuralgia, vertigo, hearing loss, peripheral neuropathic patterns, and hypothermia. Helpful diagnostic signs include internuclear ophthalmoplegia, monocular optic atrophy, incomplete myelopathy (particularly Brown-Séquard patterns), bilateral horizontal and vertical nystagmus, an evolving spastic hemiparesis, focal ataxia, and midline ataxia with various gait abnormalities.

Seventy-two percent of patients present with a single symptom, with attacks recurring about once per year. Some 20% to 40% of patients have a benign course without progression, whereas the remainder develop progressive disease, usually within 6 or 7 years after onset. About 10% to 15% of patients have a malignant course. Symptoms lasting more than 1 year are usually permanent.

Clinical Approach. Because there is no definitive diagnostic test, the diagnosis of multiple sclerosis is based on clinical findings. Although its role in diagnosis is not truly defined, magnetic resonance imaging (MRI) is used to display patchy lesions of demyelination in the paraventricular white matter. MRI with gadolinium enhancement may differentiate active disease from more chronic disease. MRI is less useful for identification of plaques in the optic nerve or spinal cord. About 95% of patients with definite clinical multiple sclerosis have abnormal MR images after 2 years of symptoms. MRI changes, however, are not specific and may be caused by tumor nodules or vascular lesions. This lack of specificity, combined with wide use of MRI in patients who lack definite symptoms and signs of multiple sclerosis, has led to overdiagnosis, particularly in the elderly.

In 90% of patients with definite multiple sclerosis, cerebrospinal fluid studies demonstrate an increase in immunoglobulin G. Evoked potentials (visual, somatosensory, and auditory) may identify definite sites of abnormalities and help meet the criteria of lesions separated in space. At present, MRI is the most useful diagnostic test, with cerebrospinal fluid changes the second most useful in confirming a clinical suspicion of multiple sclerosis.

Management. There is no cure for multiple sclerosis, and management involves symptomatic therapy only.

Several medications have been introduced that lessen the frequency and severity of exacerbations in patients with remitting exacerbating disease and also seem to lessen the disability compared with controls at 2 to 3 years. Interferon beta-1b (Betaseron) is being used to lessen the frequency and severity of exacerbations. The medication is given subcutaneously on alternate days and is well tolerated, although there continues to be considerable discussion as to the quality of the original data regarding its short- and long-term effects. This medicine should be used only after appropriate neurologic referral. Copolymer 1 (Copaxone) has been studied at 20 mg subcutaneously once a day, and it, too, has been shown to decrease frequency and severity of exacerbations and to lessen disability at 2 to 3 years. Interferon beta-1b has been shown to decrease the plaque burden on follow-up MR images during treatment. This has not been shown or studied with copolymer 1. Whether combination therapy with copolymer 1 and type 1 interferons will be additive needs further study. High-dose intravenous methylprednisolone, 1 g/d for 3 days, followed by a rapid oral prednisone taper, has been used in acute exacerbations of multiple sclerosis and has been found useful in reversing deterioration and accelerating recovery, at least in the short term. The overall impact on disability is yet to be determined. None of these therapeutic regimens has been shown to be effective in patients with chronic progressive multiple sclerosis.

The management of individuals with multiple sclerosis can be divided into prophylactic, curative, symptomatic, and restorative management. Some symptomatic therapies can be exceedingly useful in managing patients with multiple sclerosis and need to be understood for maximal care of these patients. Self-catheterization has been useful to prevent urosepsis, recurrent urinary tract infections, and problems with bladder spasm. Baclofen (Lioresal) can be used for spasticity, but sufficient amounts need to be given, up to 60 or 80 mg/d, before deciding that the medication is not useful. There is always a tradeoff with increasing weakness. Dantrolene as well as diazepam can be useful in this regard. Clonazepam (Klonopin) is helpful for nocturnal extensor spasms, as is carbamazepine (Tegretol). Botulinum toxin (Botox) injection can help decrease muscle tone in patients with spasticity. Intrathecal baclofen with a pump has proven very useful in mobilizing multiple sclerosis patients with severe extensor and flexor leg spasms out of wheelchairs. Paroxysmal muscle spasm (tic douloureux) is treatable with carbamazepine, divalproex (Depakote), phenytoin (Dilantin), or corticosteroids. Some patients with multiple sclerosis have action tremor, and propranolol (Inderal), primidone (Mysoline), or clonazepam can be useful to control it. Vasopressin nasal spray has been used to decrease nocturnal urination and to allow better sleep. Bowel regimens obviously are exceedingly important. Fatigue can be treated with amantadine (Symmetrel), pemoline (Cylert), methylphenidate (Ritalin), or even fluoxetine (Prozac). Pain is a common problem in patients with multiple sclerosis, and carbamazepine, amitriptyline (Elavil), or phenytoin may be useful. Vertigo can be responsive to dimenhydrinate (Dramamine), meclizine (Antivert), clonazepam, or tranylcypromine patches. Patients with severe double vision from intranuclear ophthalmoplegia do better with alternate eye patching.

Interferon alfa, cyclosporine, colchicine, azathioprine, and plasmapheresis are ineffective and may be harmful. The efficacy of total lymphoid irradiation and monoclonal antibodies is under investigation.

Follow-Up. Regular follow-up is essential to confirm the diagnosis and to assist families and patients with the numerous psychosocial problems that arise. Indicators of a favorable prognosis include an intermittent course with asymptomatic intervals, early onset (before the age of 40), isolated optic neuritis or sensory symptoms, a long first remission time, and lack of malignant progression within 5 years. Poor prognostic indicators include a rapidly progressive course, late onset, and an initial presentation with motor, cerebellar, or sphincter impairment. Prognosis is unrelated to sex, number of attacks, psychological symptoms, or any laboratory or imaging findings.

Cross-References: Constipation (Chapter 93), Muscular Weakness (Chapter 137), Urinary Incontinence (Chapter 172).

REFERENCES

1. Papadopoulos FM, McFarlin DE, Pationas NJ, et al. A comparison between chemical analysis and MRI with the clinical diagnosis of multiple sclerosis. Am J Clin Pathol 1987;88:365–368.

   MRI revealed findings suggestive of multiple sclerosis in 48 of 51 patients with definite multiple sclerosis (as determined by clinical examination), 4 of 4 with possible multiple sclerosis, and 1 of 6 without multiple sclerosis.

2. Rolak L. Multiple sclerosis. In Appel SH, ed. Current Neurology, vol 9. Chicago, Year Book Medical Publishers, 1989.

   Excellent current information on multiple sclerosis is provided.

3. Scheinberg L, Smith CR. Rehabilitation of patients with multiple sclerosis. Neurol Clin 1987;5:585–600.

   Important suggestions, often forgotten, that help in the management of chronic multiple sclerosis are presented.

4. Shapiro RT. Symptom management. In Multiple Sclerosis. New York, Demos Publications,1987.

   The author presents helpful clinical suggestions in the care of multiple sclerosis patients.

5. Thompson AJ, Hutchinson M, Brazil J, et al. A clinical and laboratory study of benign multiple sclerosis. Q J Med 1986;58:69–80.

   In a study of 400 patients, 42% of those with disease for more than 10 years had a benign course. Early onset of disease and long first remission correlated with a favorable prognosis.

142 Alcohol Withdrawal

Problem

STEVEN R. McGEE

Epidemiology. The abrupt interruption of sustained exposure to alcohol may produce the alcohol withdrawal syndrome. Risk factors for major withdrawal (or delirium tremens) include prior history of major withdrawal, infection, and prolonged exposure to alcohol.

Symptoms and Signs. Alcohol withdrawal consists of minor and major syndromes (Table 142–1). Three or more weeks of consistent drinking may precede major withdrawal.

Most patients experience minor symptoms such as irritability, tremor (six to eight cycles per second, an exaggeration of the physiologic tremor), anorexia, and insomnia. These symptoms usually last days and are easy to treat. In a few patients, minor symptoms blend over days into major withdrawal.

Hallucinations (more commonly visual than auditory) occur early after the last drink (< 48 hours) and appear in 25% of those with minor withdrawal. Withdrawal seizures are generalized seizures that also appear early (< 48 hours). Although 50% of seizures are single, multiple seizures (e.g., two to six seizures over several hours) may occur. In minor withdrawal, fever is unusual (< 25% of cases) and indicates infection (usually pneumonia). In major withdrawal, fever is common (> 80%), although infections are found in only 50% (in the remainder, the fever presumably occurs because of autonomic and motor hyperactivity).

Clinical Approach. Outpatient management is most appropriate for patients who voluntarily decide to stop drinking. Table 142–2 lists the indications for patient hospitalization. Detoxification centers in some communities provide alternatives to inpatient care when, for example, a patient manifests only minor symptoms without associated illness (favoring outpatient treatment) but is unknown to the physician and has no stable residence (favoring inpatient treatment).

The history and physical examination should focus on the search for

Table 142–1. MINOR VS. MAJOR WITHDRAWAL

	Minor	Major
Onset (hours from last drink)	Early (6–48 h)	Late (> 48 h)
Frequency	Common	Uncommon
Disorientation?	No	Yes
Autonomic hyperactivity?*	Mild	Marked

*Tachycardia, hypertension, fever, mydriasis, diaphoresis.

Table 142–2. OUTPATIENT VS. INPATIENT CARE

Inpatient Care Indicated

Associated illness (infection, fever, liver disease, pancreatitis,
    gastrointestinal bleeding, dehydration, ataxia, head trauma)
Major withdrawal present
Hallucinations
Previous history of major withdrawal
Social factors (isolation)
Abuse of other drugs—barbiturates, cocaine
First seizure

Outpatient Care Appropriate

Minor symptoms only
Absence of significant associated illness
Availability of physician daily during withdrawal
Commitment to abstinence
Adequate social support (friends/family)

associated illnesses that require treatment and increase the risk of major withdrawal (see Table 142–2). Wernicke's encephalopathy—ophthalmoplegia (usually lateral rectus palsies), ataxia, and/or encephalopathy (somnolence, confusion)—responds to thiamine, although 80% of patients ultimately develop Korsakoff's psychosis. Computed tomography of the head adds little to the evaluation of withdrawal seizures, unless (1) the seizure is atypical for withdrawal (multiple seizures over days, focal seizure), (2) the neurologic examination reveals asymmetric findings, or (3) there is evidence of head trauma.

Management. Patients should receive thiamine (100 mg orally per day for three doses) and a loading dose of a sedating medication that is subsequently slowly withdrawn. In several placebo-controlled trials, benzodiazepines were superior to other sedating medications in calming the patient and reducing the progression to seizures and delirium. The doses of benzodiazepine listed in Table 142–3 apply only to minor withdrawal; treatment of major withdrawal requires hospital admission and parenteral administration of benzodiazepines.

Long-acting benzodiazepines (e.g., chlordiazepoxide, diazepam) are preferred for the outpatient management of alcohol withdrawal because they are the least expensive benzodiazepines and because the drug and active metabolites have very long elimination half-lives (50 hours or more), which allows the clinician to prescribe just a loading dose (see Table 142–3). Further doses are unnecessary because the drug self-tapers over days. In one study, such front-loading schedules resulted in a smaller benzodiazepine requirement and shorter treatment duration as compared with fixed-dose schedules. In patients with liver disease, however, the long-acting agents are not recommended because significant drug accumulation and oversedation may occur. Short-acting benzodiazepines (e.g., lorazepam, oxazepam) are safe in these patients, but their doses must be tapered (fixed-dose schedule) over several days.

Atenolol (50–100 mg/d, based on pulse and blood pressure), when given *with* benzodiazepines, results in more rapid normalization of vital signs and may reduce alcohol craving. Clonidine also restores normal vital signs more quickly but, like atenolol, does not prevent seizures or delirium and should not

Table 142–3. DRUG TREATMENT OF MINOR WITHDRAWAL

Drug	Dose (mg)*
Long-acting†	
Chlordiazepoxide	50 mg PO q3–4h until calm, then stop (maximum, six doses)
Diazepam	10 mg PO q3–4h until calm, then stop (maximum, six doses)
Short-acting‡	
Lorazepam	2 mg PO tid (+2 mg)‡
Oxazepam	30 mg PO tid (+30 mg)‡

*Average doses listed. Physicians should monitor the patient's course carefully to determine whether more or less sedation is necessary.

†Loading dose alone is adequate (usual requirement varies between two and six doses). Drug self-tapers over several days.

‡Short-acting drugs must be tapered over 4 days. For example, patient receives 18 1-mg lorazepam tablets: day 1 dose is 2 mg q8h plus an additional 2 mg as needed (e.g., at bedtime), day 2 dose is 2 mg in morning, 1 mg at afternoon, 2 mg at evening; day 3 dose is 1 mg q8h; day 4 dose is 1 mg in morning, 1 mg in evening.

be used alone. Drugs to avoid during withdrawal include propranolol (which increases hallucinations) and phenothiazines (which increase seizures). Seizure prophylaxis with phenytoin is unnecessary.

Follow-Up. All patients should enter alcohol rehabilitation treatment. Frequent visits with the primary physician during subsequent months provide important emotional support to the patient.

Cross-References: Alcohol Problems (Chapter 10), Tremor (Chapter 136), Seizures (Chapter 139).

REFERENCES

1. Hayashida M, Alterman AI, McLellan AT, et al. Comparative effectiveness and costs of inpatient and outpatient detoxification of patients with mild-to-moderate alcohol withdrawal syndrome. N Engl J Med 1989;320:358–365.

   Outpatient detoxification (daily clinic visits) was as effective and safe as inpatient treatment in patients with mild-to-moderate withdrawal, with similar 6-month rehabilitation rates and significantly less cost.

2. Horwitz RI, Gottlieb LD, Kraus ML. The efficacy of atenolol in the outpatient management of the alcohol withdrawal syndrome. Arch Intern Med 1989;149:1089–1093.

   Although all received benzodiazepines, atenolol resulted in more rapid normalization of vital signs, less craving for alcohol, and fewer treatment failures. Atenolol did not affect seizures, delirium, or tremor.

3. Naik P, Lawton J. Pharmacologic management of alcohol withdrawal. Br J Hosp Med 1993;50:265–269.

   An excellent, concise review of recent advances is presented.

4. Saitz R, Mayo-Smith MF, Roberts MS, Redmond HA, Bernard DR, Calkins DR. Individualized

treatment for alcohol withdrawal; a randomized double-blind controlled trial. JAMA 1994;272:519–523.

Patients were randomized to fixed-schedule benzodiazepine (four times a day and as needed) versus symptom-triggered therapy (as needed only, every hour). Symptom-triggered therapy resulted in significantly less total drug, fewer days of treatment, and no difference in seizures or delirium.

5. Turner R, Lichstein P, Peden J, Busher J, Waivers L. Alcohol withdrawal syndromes: A review of pathophysiology, clinical presentation, and treatment. J Gen Intern Med 1989;4:432–444.
   This is an outstanding review.

· ·

143 Idiopathic Facial Palsy

Problem

STEVEN R. McGEE

Epidemiology. Bell's palsy, the acute onset of facial weakness, occurs with an annual incidence of 25 per 100,000. Age incidence increases until age 30, after which it levels off. The palsy occurs equally in men and women, on both sides of the face, and during each season of the year. The term refers only to those facial palsies of unknown cause.

Symptoms and Signs. Unilateral facial weakness usually appears abruptly, although symptoms in some individuals may progress over 1 or 2 days. Associated symptoms include facial pain (33%–62%), increased (34%–68%) or decreased (2%–17%) tearing, facial numbness (26%–32%), hyperacusis (21%–29%), and alterations of taste (19%–57%). The pain centers around the ear and usually lasts 3 days, rarely longer than 1 week. Increased tearing occurs because the weak orbicularis oculi muscle cannot contain and direct tears down the nasolacrimal duct. Decreased tearing reflects damage to the greater superficial petrosal nerve, which accompanies the facial nerve through the skull. Hyperacusis, the perception of sounds as louder and brasher in the ipsilateral ear, results from involvement of the stapedius branch of the facial nerve. Abnormal taste is variably found and probably reflects the examiner's diligence; in other settings after surgical section of the chorda tympani, most patients do not notice alterations of taste.

Physical examination reveals a decreased nasolabial fold, a widened palpebral fissure, and weakness of the eyebrow, eyelid, and mouth muscles. One third of patients experience only incomplete paralysis, a harbinger of quick and complete recovery. Upward rotation of the eyeball during attempted bilateral eye closure (Bell's phenomenon) has dual significance: it convinces the examiner that the patient is indeed trying to close the eye, and it helps protect the cornea during sleep even when the eyelid muscles are weak. Hypoesthesia of the trigeminal nerve (facial sensation) and glossopharyngeal nerve (degree of gag reflex) may occur on either side of the face.

Clinical Approach. Topographic testing of lacrimation, hearing, and taste to pinpoint the site of discrete facial nerve lesions has limited value in Bell's palsy, probably because the lesion is patchy and incomplete. All patients with eye pain should have a slit lamp examination to search for corneal abrasions and ulcers.

The differential diagnosis of facial paralysis includes trauma, infections or tumors of the ear or parotid gland, Lyme disease, Ramsay Hunt syndrome, sarcoidosis, and central facial palsy. Gradual development of weakness over several days or weeks suggests infection or tumor. Ramsay Hunt syndrome, a *herpes zoster* infection of the geniculate ganglion, produces facial paralysis with vesicles in the auricle. In Lyme disease, 10% of patients develop facial palsies, usually weeks to months after the tick bite. These palsies may be bilateral, may be associated with other cranial nerve abnormalities, and may remit without treatment. Serology provides the diagnosis.

Any disease of the central nervous system that interrupts the supranuclear fibers to the facial nucleus produces central facial palsy. In contrast to Bell's palsy, central facial palsy preserves voluntary movements of the upper face. Furthermore, emotional movements of the mouth, such as during laughter or crying, are paradoxically unaffected by central palsies.

Management. The physician should reassure the patient that facial paralysis does not represent a stroke. Eye protection includes the use of artificial tears during the day (one to two drops four times a day) and ophthalmic ointments at night. Massage and facial nerve electrical stimulation do not hasten recovery. Although corticosteroids may decrease facial pain and have few complications in Bell's palsy, two double-blind placebo-controlled studies failed to document a beneficial effect on recovery of muscle strength. Surgical decompression of the facial nerve is not helpful and may be harmful.

Follow-Up. Fifty percent of patients begin to recover within 2 weeks and return to normal within 2 months. The remaining half improve slowly over months. Predictors of incomplete recovery include complete facial paralysis, age older than 40, pain other than ear pain, and the Ramsay Hunt syndrome. Although minor degrees of weakness may persist, 90% of patients are satisfied that their face has returned to normal. Careful examination after recovery may reveal two complications: contracture (increased muscle tone) and associated movements (e.g., the ipsilateral eye may wink when the patient smiles or the corner of the mouth may curl when the patient closes the eye). Abnormal reinnervation of the lacrimal gland with regenerating salivary gland nerves occurs in 5% and causes crocodile tears (tearing during eating).

Cross-References: Herpes Zoster (Chapter 30), Redness of the Eye (Chapter 37), Foreign Bodies and Corneal Abrasions (Chapter 42).

REFERENCES

1. Adour KK. Diagnosis and management of facial paralysis. N Engl J Med 1982;307:348–351.
   In one of the largest series of facial palsy cases, 80% of patients had associated dysesthesia or hypesthesia of the trigeminal or glossopharyngeal nerve or both.

2. Caruso VG. Facial paralysis from Lyme disease. Otolaryngol Head Neck Surg 1985;93:550–553.

   Lyme disease should be suspected when there is bilateral paralysis.

3. Gates GA. Facial paralysis. Otolaryngol Clin North Am 1987;20:113–131.

   Outstanding review of anatomy, pathophysiology, clinical evaluation, and treatment of facial paralysis.

4. May M, Klein SR, Taylor FH. Idiopathic (Bell's) palsy: Natural history defies steroid or surgical treatment. Laryngoscope 1985;95:406–409.

   Written by an authority who previously advocated decompression of the facial nerve for selected patients, this study demonstrated no difference in outcome between the surgically treated group and those receiving conservative management.

5. Wolf SM, Wagner JH, Davidson S, Forsythe A. Treatment of Bell palsy with prednisone: A prospective randomized study. Neurology 1978;28:158–161.

   Eighty-eight percent of treated patients and 80% of control patients completely recovered, an insignificant difference.

■ ■

144 Entrapment Neuropathies

Problem

LAIRD G. PATTERSON

MEDIAN NERVE ENTRAPMENT NEUROPATHY

Epidemiology and Etiology. Carpal tunnel syndrome is the most common nerve entrapment syndrome, affecting 0.1% of the general population. It is found in 15% of workers in high-risk industries and is more frequent in middle-aged women. Associated conditions include congenitally small carpal tunnels, wrist trauma, tenosynovitis, collagen vascular disease, diabetes, hypothyroidism, pregnancy, paraproteinemias, and Raynaud's syndrome. Other median nerve entrapment syndromes are rare.

Symptoms and Signs. The median nerve arises from the C6–T1 nerve roots and innervates the flexor muscles of the wrist and fingers. Sensory symptoms are classically confined to the thumb, index finger, and middle finger, although paresthesias may affect the entire hand, forearm, or even upper arm. Nocturnal dysesthesias may awaken the patient, and activities such as sewing, kneading dough, washing dishes, writing, or driving may precipitate or aggravate symptoms. Actual weakness is often minimal because the abductor pollicis brevis is the only primary muscle involved; however, complaints of diminished grip strength and poor dexterity are often voiced. Symptoms are commonly unilateral and affect the dominant hand, but they may be bilateral.

In severe carpal tunnel syndrome, the abductor pollicis brevis muscle is weak and the thenar eminence appears atrophic. Altered sensation may be detected in all median nerve–innervated fingers, especially the index and middle fingers. Phalen's maneuver (hyperflexion of the wrist) for 1 minute may reproduce symptoms. Tinel's sign (tingling or pain produced by gentle percussion of the median nerve at the wrist) may be elicited. Both tests have a sensitivity of approximately 50% and a specificity of approximately 80%. These tests do not prove the diagnosis of carpal tunnel syndrome but provide additional confirmatory clinical information.

Conditions that resemble carpal tunnel syndrome include cervical radiculopathy (C6 or C7), middle brachial plexus lesions, and median nerve lesions at or above the elbow. Rarely, cervical cord abnormalities such as demyelinating disease, syringomyelia, or mass lesions may mimic carpal tunnel syndrome. Findings that suggest other sources of hand numbness include sensory or motor abnormalities proximal to the wrist, asymmetric deep tendon reflexes, or neck pain.

Clinical Approach. The patient interview and physical examination will identify most patients with carpal tunnel syndrome. Electrodiagnostic studies are positive in 90% of cases if both sensory and motor conduction are tested. Electromyography rarely contributes to the diagnosis. In selected cases, laboratory tests should include erythrocyte sedimentation rate, antinuclear antibody and rheumatoid factor assays, fasting glucose level determinations, thyroid function studies, and serum protein electrophoresis.

Management. Symptoms respond to rest, application of a wrist splint, and use of anti-inflammatory medications. Some patients, particularly those who continue to have pain as a major symptom, may benefit from corticosteroids injected under the flexor retinaculum.

About one third of patients fail conservative management and should be considered for surgery. Ninety percent of these patients, if they have persistent pain or weakness as well as classic neurologic findings and abnormal electrophysiologic tests, will benefit from surgery performed by experienced surgeons. Patients with thenar atrophy are less likely to recover. If both hands are affected, the more symptomatic hand should be treated first.

Follow-Up. If surgery is recommended, neurologic consultation is recommended to confirm the diagnosis and obtain necessary electrophysiologic tests. The physician should assess the patient's symptoms, weakness, and atrophy at monthly intervals so that a timely decision regarding surgical therapy can be made if conservative treatment fails.

ULNAR NERVE ENTRAPMENT NEUROPATHY

Epidemiology and Etiology. Ulnar entrapment, the second most common entrapment syndrome, may result from elbow trauma, chronic subluxation of the nerve at the ulnar groove, arthritis, or osteophyte formation at the elbow. Other risk factors are diabetes and chronic confinement to bed. Thirty percent to 50% of cases are idiopathic.

Symptoms and Signs. The ulnar nerve arises from the C8–T1 nerve roots, passes behind the elbow through the ulnar groove into the cubital tunnel (formed by the two heads of the flexor carpi ulnaris), and then enters the hand by way of Guyon's canal (except for the abductor pollicis brevis, part of the opponens pollicis, and the first and second lumbricals) and supplies sensation to the fifth finger and the ulnar aspect of the fourth finger and hand.

The nerve is most susceptible to trauma at the ulnar groove, cubital tunnel, wrist, and palm. The usual initial symptoms are nocturnal paresthesias in the ulnar distribution or numbness accompanying repetitive elbow flexion. Grip strength may be gradually and subtly affected. Sensory symptoms usually reflect entrapment at the elbow, whereas pure motor involvement usually represents injury to the deep palmar branch but may occur with injury at the elbow or wrist as well.

Entrapment of the ulnar nerve at the elbow causes weakness of the intrinsic muscles of the hand (abduction of the index finger and of the little finger against resistance are simple tests) and classic sensory loss in the ulnar distribution. Palm or wrist entrapment does not affect sensation because the sensory branches bifurcate before the ulnar nerve passes into the hand. Percussion at the ulnar groove or wrist as well as elbow or wrist flexion may provoke symptoms and help localize the ulnar entrapment.

Clinical Approach. Other conditions mimic ulnar entrapment, such as infiltration or compression of the inferior brachial plexus by tumor, motor neuron disease, syringomyelia, lesions of the cervical roots or cords, or, rarely, thoracic outlet syndrome. The presence of Horner's syndrome (unilateral ptosis, myosis, and anhidrosis of the face), sensory abnormalities proximal to the wrist, weakness outside the ulnar nerve distribution, or asymmetric reflexes suggests causes other than ulnar nerve entrapment.

Electrophysiologic studies (nerve conduction studies and electromyography) help to distinguish the various causes of weakness and numbness in the hand. Chest radiography or imaging studies of the cervical cord and brachial plexus are indicated when more proximal lesions are suspected. The clinician should also consider generalized polyneuropathy due to diabetes or alcohol abuse, which may be superimposed on ulnar neuropathy.

Management. Conservative measures, such as elbow splinting or padding, and avoidance of aggravating positions or activity often reverse symptoms. If the condition progresses despite conservative treatment, it may be necessary to refer the patient to an experienced orthopedic or neurologic surgeon for nerve decompression or transposition.

Follow-Up. Monthly follow-up during the early phases of the condition is advisable. Weakness may progress without symptoms, and any decision regarding surgery should be made within 6 months of the onset of symptoms to ensure a good outcome. Ulnar neuropathy due to a single traumatic event will usually resolve without surgery, although it may take 6 to 12 months. Neurologic consultation to confirm the diagnosis of ulnar neuropathy is recommended. Neurologic follow-up is also recommended, because progressive ulnar nerve dysfunction can be relatively silent and may result in a useless hand if surgical intervention is delayed.

RADIAL NERVE ENTRAPMENT NEUROPATHY

Epidemiology and Etiology. Radial entrapment is uncommon, representing only 1% of upper extremity entrapment neuropathies. Most lesions are proximal to the elbow and usually result from trauma to the axilla or humerus. Ten percent to 15% of fractures of the humerus result in radial neuropathy. Most cases result from the use of crutches, hyperextension of the arm during surgery, or pressure in the axilla or upper arm during sleep or coma.

Symptoms and Signs. The radial nerve arises from the C5–T1 nerve roots and innervates the triceps, brachioradialis, and extensor muscles of the wrist and fingers. Patients note weakness but rarely have sensory complaints. Pain is uncommon, although trauma to the nerve as it passes through the supinator muscle may be accompanied by severe pain and tenderness, resembling "tennis elbow."

Weakness is generally limited to wrist and finger extensor muscles, although proximal entrapment weakens the triceps and brachioradialis. Sensory loss is usually confined to the dorsal web space between the thumb and forefinger.

Clinical Approach. Because of the technical difficulties, electrophysiologic studies are less helpful in radial entrapment than in other entrapment neuropathies. Lesions of the brachial plexus, nerve roots, cervical cord, or cerebral cortex may mimic the distal extensor weakness of a radial neuropathy.

Management. Most radial entrapment neuropathies, whether proximal or distal, will recover with time and avoidance of aggravating positions or activity. In cases of severe wristdrop and finger extensor weakness, a cock-up wrist splint provides comfort and improves function. Although it is rarely necessary, some patients with persistent pain require exploration and decompression of the radial nerve as it passes through the supinator muscle.

Follow-Up. Recovery from the radial lesions takes 6 to 24 weeks. Follow-up appointments every 1 or 2 months are adequate. The use of nerve conduction studies or electromyography for prognostic purposes is rarely necessary.

LATERAL FEMORAL CUTANEOUS NERVE ENTRAPMENT NEUROPATHY (MERALGIA PARESTHETICA)

Epidemiology and Etiology. Entrapment of the lateral femoral cutaneous nerve occurs as the nerve passes through the lateral portion of the inguinal ligament at the anterior superior iliac spine. Entrapment may be idiopathic or the result of chronic injury from tight clothing, obesity, pregnancy, or frequent leaning against a bench or cupboard at waist height.

Symptoms and Signs. The lateral femoral cutaneous nerve is a purely sensory nerve and is composed of fibers from the L1–L3 nerve roots. Entrapment causes burning, stinging, itching, tingling, or numbness in an ovoid area of the anterolateral thigh. The pain is often aggravated by standing, hyperextending the leg, or lying flat. Hyperpathia may occur, causing discomfort when clothing or bedclothes lightly touch the affected area. Dysesthesias gradually subside, often to be replaced by painless anesthesia.

Examination demonstrates sensory loss confined to the anterolateral thigh.

Testing temperature or light touch sensation often identifies the sensory loss more easily than testing with a pin.

Clinical Approach. The typical history and examination are usually sufficient to make the diagnosis of lateral femoral cutaneous nerve entrapment. Electrophysiologic studies can confirm the diagnosis but are difficult to perform and usually unnecessary.

Other common conditions may mimic lateral femoral cutaneous nerve entrapment, such as intrapelvic or retroperitoneal processes that infiltrate the lateral femoral cutaneous nerve or a high lumbar root lesion that manifests with purely sensory symptoms. Computed tomography and magnetic resonance imaging are useful in selected cases.

Treatment. Initial treatment includes weight loss, if appropriate, and avoidance of tight clothing and positions that exacerbate symptoms. If pain is severe, it may be relieved by a nerve block at the inguinal ligament with methylprednisolone (Depo-Medrol), 60 to 80 mg, and a local anesthetic. Although it is rarely necessary, patients with persistent pain may require surgical decompression.

PERONEAL NERVE ENTRAPMENT NEUROPATHY

Epidemiology and Etiology. Injury to the peroneal nerve usually occurs at the fibular head and results from direct trauma, fracture of the fibula, compression with casts or tight stockings, or prolonged pressure on the nerve that occurs in bedridden patients or those who repeatedly cross their legs, squat, or kneel. Occasionally a fibrous band or mass in the fibular tunnel entraps the nerve. It is the most common mononeuropathy in the leg.

Symptoms and Signs. The most common presentation is painless weakness of foot dorsiflexion and eversion, although pain may occur early in the course of entrapment or compression. Although the common peroneal nerve is affected in most cases, isolated deep branch involvement produces weakness and only minimal sensory loss in the dorsal web space between the first and second toes, and isolated peripheral branch involvement results in weak foot eversion and extensive sensory loss of the lower calf, dorsal foot, and medial toes. Reflexes are not affected in peroneal entrapment.

Clinical Approach. The typical sensory loss and weakness of peroneal entrapment may be mimicked by sciatic nerve pathology, L5 root, or even upper motor neuron lesions. The findings of absent ankle or patellar reflexes or of weak foot inversion, plantarflexion, or knee or hip movements suggest conditions other than peroneal entrapment. Electromyography and nerve conduction testing help identify the lesion.

Management. Removal of the identified risk factor usually allows recovery. An ankle-foot orthosis prevents ankle injury if the footdrop is severe. Conservative care almost invariably leads to recovery, although rare patients have persistent weakness and may require exploration of the nerve at the fibular head. Electrophysiologic studies are useful to follow and predict recovery.

Follow-Up. The clinician should examine patients monthly until clear-cut recovery is documented, because a decision regarding surgery should be made within 3 to 6 months of the onset of symptoms.

Cross-References: Alcohol Problems (Chapter 10), Low Back Pain (Chapter 107), Hip Pain (Chapter 109), Wrist and Hand Pain (Chapter 110), Ankle and Foot Pain (Chapter 112), Myofascial Pain Syndromes (Chapter 122), Raynaud's Syndrome (Chapter 131), Peripheral Neuropathy (Chapter 147), Electromyography and Nerve Conduction Studies (Chapter 149), Common Thyroid Disorders (Chapter 153), Diabetes Mellitus (Chapter 154).

REFERENCES

1. Dawson DM, Hallett M, Millender LH. Entrapment Neuropathies, 2nd ed. Boston, Little, Brown & Co, 1990.

   The authors provide an excellent comprehensive discussion of entrapment neuropathies.

2. Nakano KK. The entrapment neuropathies. Muscle Nerve 1978;1:264–279.

   This is a compact review of the important entrapment syndromes.

3. Pelmear PL, Taylor W. Carpal tunnel syndrome and hand–arm vibration syndrome. Arch Neurol 1994;51:416–420.

   This article reviews the commonly encountered difficulty of distinguishing carpal tunnel syndrome from symptoms due to repetitive strain and arm–hand vibration.

4. Quality Standards Subcommittee of the American Academy of Neurology. Practice parameters for carpal tunnel syndrome (summary statement). Neurology 1993;43:2406–2409.

   This is an excellent summary of diagnostic criteria with an algorithm.

5. Spinner RJ, Bachman JW, Amadio PC. The many faces of carpal tunnel syndrome. Mayo Clin Proc 1989;64:829–836.

   A detailed clinical review of the most common entrapment neuropathy is presented.

. . . .

145 Parkinsonism

Problem

LAIRD G. PATTERSON

Epidemiology and Etiology. Parkinson's disease affects approximately 1% of the population older than the age of 50. The peak incidence occurs in the fifth and sixth decades, with men more likely to be affected than women in a ratio of 3:2. The disease is distributed worldwide and affects all ethnic groups, and the prevalence has been stable for at least 100 years. A single genetic cause is unlikely, and definite environmental causes have not been identified. Mortality was two to three times higher before levodopa was available but is now similar to that in age-related cohort groups.

Extrapyramidal signs appear when dopamine levels in the putamen and caudate are reduced by 80% or more.

Symptoms and Signs. The onset is insidious and often unrecognized by the patient or family for several years. Many symptoms are nonspecific and include arthralgias, depression, vague sensory or balance complaints, stiffness, fatigue, and generalized slowing, all of which may be attributed to arthritis or aging.

Tremor is the first symptom in about 50% of patients but often appears late or not at all. Unilateral stiffness or clumsiness, diminished arm swing, dragging a leg, difficulty getting out of low seats or out of a car, poor postural reflexes, slowed gait, sialorrhea (excessive saliva), decreased facial expression, restless legs, or a dystonic foot may be presenting symptoms. Patients often report symptoms of seborrhea, micrographia, or flexed posture. Patients with unilateral tremor as a predominant initial feature of the disease at onset fare better as a group in both response to treatment and overall prognosis.

The signs of early Parkinson's disease may be subtle. A 4- to 6-Hz tremor is usually not present at rest but can occur with activity. Rigidity is often minimal but can be elicited by reinforcement techniques such as making a fist with the hand contralateral to the limb being tested. Decreased blink rate (normal, 12–15 blinks per minute), infrequent postural adjustment, slowness in dressing or adjusting glasses, and difficulty getting out of a chair are all manifestations of bradykinesia. Gait is often shuffling or difficult to initiate. Festination, a tendency to chase the center of gravity when walking, and loss of postural reflexes appear as the disease progresses. Rapid alternating movements that progressively diminish in amplitude, micrographia, mumbling, and stammering may also be present. Deep tendon reflexes are generally normal but may become hyperactive in affected extremities. The plantar reflex is usually normal. Eye movement abnormalities include restricted upward gaze and diminished saccadic movements. Other findings such as orthostatic hypotension, dementia, and ataxic gait may be seen but if encountered early may signify other conditions. Despite sensory symptoms, the sensory examination is usually normal.

Clinical Approach. A clinical diagnosis of Parkinson's disease is possible in at least 80% to 90% of cases, although patients with atypical features may need further studies. Conditions that mimic Parkinson's disease include frontal and midline tumors, chronic subdural hemorrhage, multiple infarcts, normal-pressure hydrocephalus, and Wilson's disease. Other degenerative diseases such as Huntington's chorea, multisystem atrophy, Shy-Drager syndrome, progressive supranuclear palsy, olivopontocerebellar atrophy, Creutzfeldt-Jakob disease, and even Alzheimer's disease can produce parkinsonian features. Neuroleptic medications, metoclopramide, and sedative/hypnotic drugs may produce extrapyramidal side effects. Intoxication with methyl-phenyl-tetrahydropyridine (MPTP), a toxic byproduct produced during illicit manufacture of a meperidine analog, causes a striking parkinsonian syndrome.

Although the diagnosis of Parkinson's disease is based on clinical criteria, patients who are younger than the age of 50 or who have atypical features may require further studies. Magnetic resonance imaging or computed tomography can exclude most structural causes of extrapyramidal dysfunction. A normal ceruloplasmin level and eye examination make Wilson's disease unlikely. A careful family history may reveal relatives with Huntington's chorea or olivopontocerebellar atrophy. Creutzfeldt-Jakob disease is suggested if the electroencephalogram shows myoclonic activity.

Management. The initial management of Parkinson's disease is straightforward, but management becomes quite complex as the disease progresses. Neurologic consultation is usually necessary to confirm the diagnosis and to aid in management. Patients are usually not treated until their symptoms begin to affect their lifestyle, job, or relationships. Education of the patient and family is an important aspect of treatment. Stretching and aerobic exercises should be done by all patients, including those on pharmacologic therapy. Vitamin E (800 units/d) is generally started at the time of diagnosis because of its theoretic neuroprotective effect as a free radical scavenger, although evidence confirming its benefit is lacking.

Pharmacologic therapy begins with levodopa and carbidopa, a decarboxylase inhibitor (Table 145–1). A 1:4 ratio of carbidopa to levodopa is preferred, to minimize systemic dopaminergic side effects. An initial dose of carbidopa/levodopa, 25/100 mg two or three times daily, is usually well tolerated and may provide symptom relief for several years in early disease. If wearing-off of the medication effect occurs or motor fluctuations appear as the disease progresses, a more frequent dosage schedule or switching to the long-acting carbidopa/levodopa (Sinemet CR) preparation may improve the response. As the total dose of levodopa is increased up to 500 or 600 mg/d, dopamine agonists such as bromocriptine (Parlodel) or pergolide (Permax) may be added. The pergolide dose is generally 10% of the bromocriptine dose. The combination of low-dose levodopa and a dopamine agonist seems to prolong the period of effective therapy. After 3 to 5 years, however, most patients begin to have treatment complications, such as early wearing-off of the medication effect, rapidly fluctuating motor symptoms ("on-off phenomenon"), (i.e., still posture) dyskinesias, and hallucinations, which require changing the frequency or size of the dose. The addition of selegiline (Eldepryl), 5 mg twice daily, a monoamine oxidase (type B) inhibitor, may be warranted because it often improves the effectiveness of levodopa. Controversy exists regarding whether it delays progression of the disease as well. Restricting protein in the diet may improve the response to levodopa.

Other medications that are used in Parkinson's disease are generally less effective but may contribute to further improvement in selected cases. These include amantadine or various anticholinergic medications such as trihexyphenidyl (Artane), which may partially alleviate symptoms but may cause some memory difficulty. Antidepressant therapy not only treats depression but also may enhance the effectiveness of levodopa by decreasing synaptic dopamine reuptake.

A variety of stereotactic surgical procedures such as thalamotomy, thalamic stimulation, pallidotomy, and transplantation of fetal and genetically engineered cells have been shown to have benefit in appropriately selected cases.

Follow-Up. Patients with early disease should be seen every 4 to 6 months. As the disease progresses and complications occur, closer follow-up becomes necessary. Disease complications in addition to those related to therapy include autonomic dysfunction, depression, inanition, sleep disturbances, dementia, delirium, and the dangers of immobility such as pneumonia and thrombophlebitis. Intercurrent illness or surgery often exacerbates the symptoms and signs of Parkinson's disease. Most patients with moderate to advanced disease will need to be managed with the help of a neurologist.

Table 145–1. ANTIPARKINSON MEDICATIONS

Agent	Daily Dose (mg)	Major Side Effects	Cost ($) per Tablet*
Carbidopa/levodopa (regular) (Sinemet)	10/100–150/1500	Dyskinesias, nausea, anorexia, orthostatic hypotension, cardiac arrhythmias, confusion, hallucinations	
10/100 mg			0.42
25/100 mg			0.43
25/250 mg			0.60
Sinemet (long-acting)	25/100–250/1000	Dyskinesias, nausea, anorexia, orthostatic hypotension, cardiac arrhythmias, confusion, hallucinations	
25/100 mg			0.68
50/200 mg			1.47
Trihexyphenidyl (Artane) 2 mg	1–20	Drowsiness, urine retention, constipation, confusion, hallucinations, tachycardia	0.02
Benztropine (Cogentin) 2 mg	1–6	Drowsiness, urine retention, constipation, confusion, hallucinations, tachycardia	0.02
Bromocriptine (Parlodel)	5–20	Nausea, dyskinesias, confusion, hallucinations, dizziness, syncope	
2.5 mg			1.52
5.0 mg			2.42
Pergolide (Permax)	1–5	Nausea, dyskinesias, confusion, hallucinations, dizziness, syncope	
0.05 mg			0.36
0.25 mg			0.92
1.00 mg			2.54
Amantadine (Symmetrel) 100 mg	200	Confusion, hallucinations, psychosis, hypotension, livedo reticularis, edema	0.31
Selegiline (Eldepryl) 5 mg	5–10	Exacerbates levodopa side effects, headache, insomnia, fainting	2.16

*Average wholesale price, 1995 *Drug Topics Red Book*.

Cross-References: Tremor (Chapter 136), Dementia (Chapter 140), Electroencephalography (Chapter 148).

REFERENCES

1. An algorithm for the management of Parkinson's disease. Neurology 1994;44(suppl 10):5–50.

   This is an up-to-date comprehensive review of the management of all aspects of Parkinson's disease.

2. Dogali M, et al. Stereotactic ventral pallidotomy for Parkinson's disease. Neurology 1995;45:753–761.

   This is a discussion of the rationale and outcome of surgical therapy.

3. Fahn S, ed. Therapy of Parkinson's disease: Four critical issues. Neurology 1994;44(suppl 1):5–20.

   This article highlights several of the major problems encountered in the treatment of Parkinson's disease.

4. Jenner P. The rationale for the use of dopamine agonists in Parkinson's disease. Neurology 1995;45(suppl 3):6–12.

   The author provides a concise review of dopamine agonist physiology and pharmacology.

5. Tolosa ES, et al. New and emerging strategies for improving levodopa treatment. Neurology 1994;44(suppl 6):35–44.

   Novel approaches for the management of levodopa-related complications are presented.

146 Cerebrovascular Disease

Problem

LYNNE P. TAYLOR

Epidemiology and Etiology. Stroke refers to the sudden appearance of a focal neurologic deficit, caused by thrombotic (65%–80%) or embolic (5%–15%) arterial occlusion or cerebral hemorrhage (15%–20%). Stroke ranks third as a cause for death in the United States, where there are over 2 million stroke survivors and 500,000 new strokes each year.

The treatment of risk factors for stroke has reduced this incidence in recent years. Hypertension, cardiac disease, diabetes, polycythemia, and a history of transient ischemic attacks (TIAs—episodes of focal neurologic dysfunction lasting less than 24 hours) all increase the risk of stroke. Cigarette smoking, excessive alcohol use, recreational drug use (cocaine), sedentary lifestyle, obesity, and hyperlipidemia also increase the risk, although it is uncertain whether interventions for these factors reduce the risk of stroke. Isolated systolic hypertension is a particularly important risk factor in the elderly, and decreasing the systolic blood pressure toward a target of 140 mm Hg produces a decreasing incidence of cerebrovascular events.

Atherothrombotic disease includes both extracranial (carotid and vertebrobasilar atherosclerosis) and intracranial occlusive disease (lacunar strokes). Lacunar strokes are small (1–20 mm in diameter), usually affect the deep hemispheric white matter or brain stem, and are associated with hypertension and diabetes. The pathologic process is distinct and thought to be related to lipohyalinosis of tiny penetrating blood vessels.

Emboli originate from arterial, aortic arch, or cardiac thrombi. It is important to identify cardiogenic embolic disease, because these patients have a high risk of recurrent stroke (6 to 12 times higher than stroke patients without a cardiac source), and 10% to 20% of recurrent emboli recur within the subsequent 2 weeks. Sources of cardioembolism are atrial fibrillation (45%), myocardial infarction or ventricular aneurysms (25%), rheumatic heart disease (10%), prosthetic heart valves (10%), and other sources such as bacterial endocarditis (10%).

Intracerebral hemorrhage may result from severe hypertension, amyloid angiopathy, or bleeding into a bland infarct.

Symptoms and Signs. It is useful to divide strokes into small vessel (lacunar infarcts) and large vessel occlusive disease, which can be further subdivided into anterior (carotid, middle cerebral, anterior cerebral arteries) or posterior (posterior cerebral, vertebrobasilar arteries) circulation.

Because *lacunar* infarcts involve a small, dense area of a white matter tract, deficits tend to be subtle and often either pure motor or pure sensory. The face, arm, and leg are often equally affected. Common patterns include dysarthria–clumsy hand, ataxic hemiparesis, and pure motor stroke. Large vessel strokes usually destroy a much larger portion of brain than the tiny lacunes and, therefore, more commonly involve cortical structures.

Amaurosis fugax, a brief, stereotypical, monocular visual loss described by patients as a curtain descending over an eye, is typical of carotid artery disease. Stroke involving the middle cerebral artery distribution generally produces a mixed motor and sensory disturbance that maximally involves the face and arm, with relative sparing of the leg. Expressive or receptive aphasia may occur in left (dominant) hemisphere strokes, and confusion and cortical neglect in right hemispheric (nondominant) strokes. Strokes in the region of the anterior cerebral artery produce hemianesthesia and hemiparesis that is more pronounced in the leg.

Posterior cerebral artery strokes classically cause a contralateral homonymous visual field deficit, generally without other neurologic findings, and are frequently clinically silent or produce only vague visual complaints. Vertebrobasilar system symptoms include vertigo, headache, nausea, vomiting, or hiccoughs in association with a hemiparesis that may be unilateral, bilateral, or alternating. Typical neurologic findings, in addition to hemiparesis, include nystagmus, ocular motor palsies, and other cranial nerve findings.

Embolic strokes classically produce maximal deficit at onset and are noticed by the patient on arising in the morning. A seizure occurs at the time of the embolic event in 5% to 10% of cases. *Thrombotic strokes* tend to pursue a more stuttering course, with symptoms that wax and wane before the deficit becomes maximal. Cerebral hemorrhage produces symptoms abruptly at any time of the day, usually accompanied by headache.

Clinical Approach. A proper diagnostic and therapeutic approach to stroke and TIA depends heavily on the correct identification of (1) the neuroanatomic location of the lesion, (2) the likely cause, and (3) risk factors for stroke. The general physical examination focuses on peripheral blood vessels; hypertensive retinal changes and Hollenhorst plaques on ophthalmoscopic examination, blood pressure in both arms, pulse contour, bruits of the carotid and other arteries, and the heart (irregular rhythm, murmur).

The neurologic examination should detail the degree and distribution of motor and sensory findings as well as such "cortical" findings as apraxia, aphasia, neglect, or hemianopsia. After the examination, the clinician should attempt to localize the lesion within the neuraxis, define its vascular distribution, and then exclude other diseases that mimic stroke (Table 146–1). Because stroke, by definition, occurs suddenly, *slowly progressive* symptoms that worsen over days or weeks should be considered to be due to a tumor (or subdural hematoma) until proven otherwise.

Routine laboratory tests include electrocardiography; chest radiography; blood glucose testing; a complete blood cell count; and determination of prothrombin time, activated partial thromboplastin time, platelet count, and cholesterol level. In most cases, computed tomography (CT) of the head is needed to exclude other abnormalities (see Table 146–1), confirm the size and site of the infarct, and evaluate for areas of previous silent ischemia in other vascular distributions that may suggest cardiogenic embolic disease. As a tool to exclude hemorrhage, CT is usually done without contrast medium enhancement on an emergent basis only in those patients under consideration for immediate anticoagulation. Magnetic resonance imaging is more expensive and less available than CT and should be reserved for identification of lacunar infarcts too small to be seen on CT or when lesions in the posterior fossa are suspected. When cardiogenic embolic disease is suspected (suspicious history and abnormal heart examination, electrocardiogram, or chest radiograph), echocardiography is necessary to look for left atrial enlargement, valvular disease, left ventricular dysfunction, and intracardiac clot. In unexplained cases of embolic stroke, echocardiography with bubble contrast may identify a right-to-left shunt, or blood cultures may identify the bacteremia of endocarditis. Transesophageal echocardiography is the preferred technique when possible because it increases the detection of potential cardioembolic sources and allows imaging of the aortic arch, a newly recognized source of atheroemboli. Echocardiographic abnormalities associated with increased risk are spontaneous echo contrast in the atrium and atrial septal aneurysms.

Duplex ultrasonography, which uses pulsed echo imaging to visualize the carotid artery and a Doppler signal to measure blood flow, is indicated for patients with symptoms in the anterior circulation. Depending on the laboratory, it has a sensitivity of 85% to 100% and a specificity close to 90%. Patients

Table 146–1. DIFFERENTIAL DIAGNOSIS OF STROKE

Tumor	Inner ear disturbance
Subdural hematoma	Multiple sclerosis
Seizures	Hypoglycemia
Migraine	

with a history of TIA or stroke, if they have stenosis greater than 70% on noninvasive testing and are surgical candidates, should be further evaluated with carotid angiography. Intra-arterial digital subtraction technique is preferred to conventional angiography because a smaller catheter and a lower dose of contrast material are used. The morbidity from angiography should be less than 2% (stroke, wound hematoma, infection). In many centers, magnetic resonance angiography and spiral CT are producing images comparable in vascular detail to standard angiography, without the risk, and will likely replace this test over the next few years.

In young patients (< 50 years old) with unexplained ischemic strokes, the physician should consider hematologic causes such as antithrombin III deficiency, polycythemia vera, lupus anticoagulant, and anticardiolipin antibodies. The prevalence of stroke attributed to hematologic disorders is 0% to 7%.

Management. Proper medical treatment depends on whether patients are (1) asymptomatic with normal neurologic findings, (2) previously symptomatic but now with normal neurologic findings, or (3) currently symptomatic.

Asymptomatic patients should be helped to modify risk factors such as smoking, excessive alcohol use, hypertension, poorly controlled diabetes, and perhaps hypercholesterolemia. Young (< 79 years) patients with more than 60% carotid artery stenosis should be considered for *prophylactic* surgery if an experienced surgeon (< 2% morbidity) is available.

Unless contraindicated, patients should be placed on long-term oral anticoagulant therapy, as outlined in Chapter 82, Atrial Fibrillation, and Chapter 201, Chronic Anticoagulation. Asymptomatic patients with carotid bruits should learn about the symptoms of TIAs and modify their risk factors. The role of carotic duplex testing in these patients will remain unclear until studies are available on the economics of screening large number of asymptomatic patients.

Previously symptomatic but currently neurologically normal patients may have been having TIAs. Patients with crescendo TIAs (TIAs that occurred within the previous week and are increasing in frequency) should be admitted to the hospital for evaluation and possible anticoagulation. A patient with a more remote single neurologic event can be evaluated as an outpatient and managed with risk factor modification and initiation of aspirin therapy, 325 mg orally every morning (Table 146–2). All of these patients should also be referred to a neurologist to ensure that vascular pathology is correlated carefully with symptoms.

Patients with crescendo TIAs thought to be of cardiogenic origin (e.g., atrial fibrillation, after myocardial infarction) should be immediately anticoagulated with heparin, as long as the CT scan excludes hemorrhagic stroke, the systolic blood pressure is less than 170 mm Hg, and there is no large cerebral infarct that could increase the risk of an intraparenchymal hemorrhage. Data on anticoagulation of patients with TIAs in other settings are lacking.

There is rarely a role for anticoagulation in completed stroke if the deficit is profound. Management in these patients emphasizes supportive care and measures to prevent aspiration, deep venous thrombosis, and contracture. To avoid enlarging the ischemic area, hypertension should not be treated in an acute stroke unless the systolic pressure consistently exceeds 180 to 190 mm Hg and the diastolic pressure exceeds 100 mm Hg.

Table 146–2. ORAL ANTIPLATELET/ANTICOAGULANT DRUGS

Clinical Setting	Drug	Dose	Cost ($) per Day*
Atherothrombotic disease	Aspirin (enteric coated)	300–1200 mg/d	0.01–0.05
Cardiogenic emboli	Warfarin	See Chapter 201 (Chronic Anticoagulation)	0.44†
Transient ischemic attacks resistant to aspirin	Warfarin‡	See Chapter 201 (Chronic Anticoagulation)	0.44†

*Average wholesale price, 1996 *Drug Topics Red Book.*
†Individual doses vary; price listed is for 5 mg/d.
‡Data are lacking; treatment is empirical.

Symptomatic patients with hemodynamically significant carotid stenosis (70% or greater) and possibly those with an ulcerated plaque require carotic endarterectomy if it is ipsilateral to the site of TIA, as demonstrated in the North American Symptomatic Carotid Endarterectomy Trial. Carotid endarterectomy is also appropriate for patients who have had a small completed stroke with good remaining functional abilities, although in this situation surgery is often delayed for 6 weeks.

Lacunar strokes are generally treated with control of hypertension. There is no role for anticoagulation, although a single aspirin a day is often prescribed empirically.

More experimental means of treatment for stroke include the use of tissue plasminogen activator, which if given intravenously in the first 6 hours after the onset of symptoms is purported to limit the extent of the neurologic deficit. Complications, including parenchymal hemorrhage, have been described, and it is not yet clear if this therapy will have a role outside of stroke study centers.

Follow-Up. In the course of evaluation, patients are often discovered to have high-grade asymptomatic stenoses in the nonsymptomatic carotid artery. These patients should be followed closely for evidence of neurologic symptoms and with repeat studies as clinically indicated. The value of endarterectomy in asymptomatic carotid stenosis is controversial; this procedure may be found to benefit younger patients, men, and those with high-grade critical stenoses (> 80%).

Patients should be followed at 6-month intervals to monitor symptoms and reinforce risk factor modification.

Cross-References: Smoking Cessation (Chapter 12), Dizziness (Chapter 20), Visual Impairment (Chapter 36), Ophthalmoscopy (Chapter 46), Syncope (Chapter 75), Atrial Fibrillation (Chapter 82), Essential Hypertension (Chapter 85), Echocardiography (Chapter 89), Peripheral Arterial Disease (Chapter 132), Muscular Weakness (Chapter 137), Polycythemia (Chapter 198), Chronic Anticoagulation (Chapter 201).

REFERENCES

1. Barnett HJ, Eliasziw M, Meldrum HE. Drug therapy: Drugs and surgery in the prevention of ischemic stroke. N Engl J Med 1995;332:238–248.

The authors present a thoughtful review examining the benefits of aspirin and warfarin in atrial fibrillation and following MI, as well as approaches to prevent stroke in patients with carotid stenosis.

2. Executive committee for ACAS study. Endarterectomy for asymptomatic carotid artery stenosis. JAMA 1995;273:1421–1428.

This multicenter randomized trial involving 1662 patients with a 60% or greater asymptomatic stenosis showed an overall reduction in death or stroke over 5 years from 11% to 5.1% among those undergoing endarterectomy.

3. Mohr JP. Lacunes. Stroke 1982;13:3–10.

This is an excellent clinical description of lacunar infarcts.

4. North American Symptomatic Carotid Endarterectomy Trial. N Engl J Med 1991;325:445–453.

This trial demonstrated benefit of endarterectomy over medical treatment for symptomatic patients with 70% to 99% carotid stenosis by angiography.

5. Stroke prevention in atrial fibrillation study. Circulation. 1991;84:527–539.

Stroke decreased 42% per year in a patient with nonrheumatic atrial fibrillation treated with acetylsalicylic acid and 67% when treated with warfarin (Coumadin).

147 Peripheral Neuropathy

Problem

JOYCE E. WIPF

Epidemiology. Peripheral neuropathy is a disease of neural structures outside the brain and spinal cord, which may involve abnormalities of axons (axonopathy) or myelin sheaths (demyelination) and may affect any combination of motor, sensory, or autonomic nerves. Although peripheral neuropathy may be congenital (e.g., the peroneal muscle atrophy of Charcot-Marie-Tooth disease), acquired neuropathy is much more common, occurring in a wide variety of medical disorders, including half of patients with long-standing diabetes and up to 15% with newly diagnosed diabetes. The incidence of lower extremity amputation in the diabetic population is 15 times greater than in individuals without diabetes; most are in the setting of neuropathy and peripheral vascular disease. An estimated 50% of these amputations can be prevented with appropriate foot care and prevention of minor trauma.

Etiology and Symptoms and Signs. Because the causes are so diverse, peripheral neuropathy may be acute, subacute, or chronic, and symptoms may fluctuate or remain constant.

Common motor symptoms are weakness, muscle twitching, and cramps. Sensory symptoms include numbness, dysesthesia (painful sensations), cold feet, stumbling, and unsteady gait. Involvement of autonomic nerves may result in impotence, retrograde ejaculation, diaphoresis or loss of sweating, incontinence, urine retention, constipation, diarrhea, orthostatic dizziness, or flushing. Diabetics with autonomic neuropathy may become unaware of episodes of hypoglycemia or may develop symptoms of gastroparesis (postprandial nausea, vomiting, bloating, and early satiety).

Neurologic examination may reveal weakness, fasciculation, atrophy, ataxia, wide-based gait, abnormal sweating, diminished or absent reflexes, and orthostatic hypotension. Sensory findings include areas of hypoesthesia (sometimes surrounded by a zone of hyperesthesia) or complete loss of sensation, with vibratory and position sensation usually disappearing before loss of pinprick and temperature sensation. Patients with neuropathic arthropathy may have diminished pulses and various foot abnormalities, including flat longitudinal arches, a tendency to evert and externally rotate the ankle, a shorter and wider foot, swelling, and painless punched-out ulcers. Signs of autonomic neuropathy include small dark-adapted pupil size, delayed pupillary response to light, resting tachycardia, and loss of sinus arrhythmia. The electrocardiogram may reveal evidence of silent myocardial ischemia.

It is helpful to classify the patient's peripheral neuropathy as polyneuropathy (the most common type), radiculopathy (compression of nerve roots), mononeuropathy, entrapment neuropathy, or mononeuropathy multiplex.

Polyneuropathy usually affects both legs in a symmetric "stocking-glove" distribution with varying combinations of motor, sensory, or autonomic findings. Progressive disease may involve the thighs, trunk, and shoulders. Although diabetes is the most common cause, polyneuropathy may occur in many different systemic disorders. Sixty-five percent of patients with renal failure who are starting dialysis have a mixed sensorimotor polyneuropathy, often associated with the restless legs syndrome. Alcoholism and nutritional deficiencies (thiamine, pyridoxine, vitamin B_{12}, and pantothenic acid) cause a subacute polyneuropathy that may progress to severe weakness and atrophy. In vitamin B_{12} deficiency, the neuropathy may precede anemia.

Some 2% to 5% of all patients with malignancy have polyneuropathy, usually a mixed sensorimotor type, although other specific paraneoplastic syndromes occur (e.g., Lambert-Eaton syndrome with myasthenia-type weakness). Common associated tumors are small cell carcinoma of the lung (accounting for more than 50% of paraneoplastic neuropathy in some series) and those producing a paraproteinemia (e.g., plasmacytoma, multiple myeloma).

Although the neuropathy of rheumatologic diseases (e.g., vasculitis) is usually a mononeuropathy, 5% of patients with long-standing rheumatoid arthritis and 10% with systemic lupus erythematosus have polyneuropathy. Other important causes of polyneuropathy are medications and environmental toxins (Table 147–1), metabolic conditions (amyloidosis, hypothyroidism, and chronic liver failure), and human immunodeficiency virus infection. Rapidly progressive sensorimotor polyneuropathy occurs in the Guillain-Barré syndrome.

Common *mononeuropathies*, which affect single nerves, are cranial nerve palsies, especially those of nerves III, IV, VI, and VII, and entrapment neuropathies, especially of the median nerve at the carpal tunnel, the ulnar nerve at the elbow or wrist, the lateral femoral cutaneous nerve at the inguinal ligament, and the posterior tibial nerve at the tarsal tunnel (see Chapter 144, Entrapment Neuropathies).

Mononeuropathy multiplex (asymmetric proximal motor neuropathy) involves

Table 147-1. DRUGS AND TOXINS CAUSING PERIPHERAL NEUROPATHY*

Drugs	Toxins
Antibiotics	*Metals*
Nitrofurantoin	Lead (adults)
Chloramphenicol	Arsenic
Metronidazole	Lithium
Sulfonamides	Mercury
	Gold
Antituberculous	Platinum
Isoniazid	? Copper, zinc, bismuth
Ethambutol	
Ethionamide	*Occupational*
	Methyl-*n*-butyl ketone (solvent)
Antineoplastic	*n*-Hexane (contact cements)
Vincristine	Dimethylaminopropionitrile
Vinblastine	(manufacture of polyurethane foam)
Cisplatin	Carbon disulfide
Procarbazine	Allyl chloride (manufacture of epoxy
Etoposide (VP-16)	resin, pesticides)
Teniposide (VM-26)	Organophosphates (pesticides)
Aramycin	Thallium (rat poison)
Nitrogen mustard	Methyl and ethyl alcohol
Other	
Zidovudine	
Hydralazine	
Glutethimide	
Phenytoin	
Amiodarone	
Amitriptyline	
Imipramine	
Disulfiram	
Dapsone	

*Most cause axonal degeneration.

several noncontiguous nerve trunks and is characterized by severe unilateral pain, followed by weakness and muscle atrophy, in the low back or hips, sometimes extending to the thigh and knee. Sensory loss, if any, is mild. Symptoms usually progress over days, but most patients experience gradual recovery. This neuropathy results from multifocal ischemic infarcts of the lumbar plexus and other regional nerve trunks and is associated with diabetes, leprosy, sarcoidosis, polyarteritis nodosa, and cryoglobulinemia.

Diabetic amyotrophy (symmetric proximal motor neuropathy), which is frequently associated with other neuropathies, features profound weight loss, wasting, and progressive weakness of the hip and thigh muscles bilaterally, often with proximal shoulder girdle involvement. It is often very painful, although sensory loss is unusual. Symptoms may progress rapidly over several weeks and then slowly improve over months. *Diabetic neuropathic cachexia* is usually seen in middle-aged men and mimics metastatic cancer, with profound weight loss, severe diffuse pain, and absence of focal neurologic abnormalities. Recovery occurs after months to a year.

Clinical Approach. The patient interview should focus on systemic diseases, medications, and exposure to toxins or chemicals. Genetic neuropathies are diagnosed from a careful family history and examination of blood relatives. The clinician's major diagnostic goals are to identify treatable diseases and potential environmental causes. Even individuals with diabetes or alcohol abuse may have other reasons for neuropathy and deserve careful evaluation. Routine laboratory tests should include a complete blood cell count; urinalysis; a VDRL test; evaluation of glucose, creatinine, thyroid-stimulating hormone, and vitamin B_{12} levels; and a recent chest radiograph. In patients with bone pain or elevated serum total proteins, an erythrocyte sedimentation rate should be obtained along with serum and urine protein electrophoresis.

Electrodiagnostic studies (see Chapter 149, Electromyography and Nerve Conduction Studies) distinguish demyelinating from axonal degeneration (e.g., most metabolic and toxic etiologies cause axonal degeneration) and are most useful in patients with unilateral neuropathies to confirm radiculopathy, entrapment, or mononeuropathy multiplex. Nerve biopsies are indicated in patients with unexplained asymmetric or multifocal neuropathies or when nerves are enlarged on examination.

Management. The clinician should treat the underlying disease and eliminate any causative agents. Tight control of insulin-dependent diabetes has been shown to reduce the risk of neuropathy and other microvascular complications. There is preliminary evidence in non–insulin-dependent diabetes that peripheral neuropathy is more likely with poor glycemic control. Aldose-reductase inhibitors (e.g., sorbinil) may transiently improve nerve function in diabetic neuropathy but with the potential of significant toxicity. Diabetic gastroparesis may respond to metoclopramide, 10 mg orally four times a day, or cisapride, 10–20 mg orally four times a day. If evaluation of the patient's chronic diarrhea or constipation does not reveal a treatable cause, a bowel program may be beneficial.

The major concern for most patients with polyneuropathy is discomfort from dysesthesia. Non-narcotic analgesics are most useful and include nonsteroidal anti-inflammatory agents, acetaminophen, and tricyclic antidepressants (amitriptyline, 50–150 mg/d orally; desipramine, 25–250 mg/d). Alternative antidepressants, such as paroxetine, 40 mg/d, may benefit patients with side effects to tricyclic agents. Paroxetine was superior to placebo but less effective than imipramine in one randomized trial of diabetic neuropathy. If severe pain persists, a 3-month trial of anticonvulsant medication (e.g., phenytoin or carbamazepine) may be beneficial, following the same therapeutic drug levels used for patients with seizures. Topical capsaicin cream, derived from hot capsicum peppers, will diminish neuropathic pain, although up to 10% of patients have intolerable side effects, such as site burning, cough, rash, and skin irritation.

Symptomatic orthostatic hypotension resulting from autonomic neuropathy may respond to the use of support hose, withdrawal of exacerbating drugs (e.g., tricyclic antidepressants, diuretics), and counseling the patient to rise slowly from a seated or supine position. Mineralocorticoid therapy (fludrocortisone, 0.1–0.2 mg twice daily) is helpful in refractory cases.

Many patients benefit from a referral to a physical therapist, who may recommend splints, specific exercise programs, or aids for ambulation. Nerve blocks for intractable focal pain are rarely required. Management of specific entrapment neuropathies is discussed in Chapter 144.

Follow-Up. During regular follow-up visits, the clinician should carefully examine the skin for signs of infection or ulceration and should monitor for any progression of the neuropathy. All patients with polyneuropathy should inspect their feet daily, always wear shoes, and avoid testing water temperature with their feet. Any patient with new or persistent focal foot pain should undergo radiographic evaluation to exclude osteomyelitis, fracture, or dislocation.

Cross-References: Alcohol Problems (Chapter 10), Diarrhea (Chapter 91), Constipation (Chapter 93), Abdominal Pain (Chapter 94), Ankle and Foot Pain (Chapter 112), Restless Legs Syndrome (Chapter 113), Diabetic Foot Care Education (Chapter 124), Physical Therapy Care of Outpatients (Chapter 125), Leg Ulcers (Chapter 133), Local Care of Diabetic Foot Lesions (Chapter 134), Muscular Weakness (Chapter 137), Entrapment Neuropathies (Chapter 144), Electromyography and Nerve Conduction Studies (Chapter 149), Diabetes Mellitus (Chapter 154), Erectile Dysfunction (Chapter 169), Urinary Incontinence (Chapter 172).

REFERENCES

1. The Diabetes Control and Complications Trial Research Group. The effect of intensive diabetes therapy on the development and progression of neuropathy. Ann Intern Med 1995;122:561–568.

   This multicenter North American trial randomized type 1 insulin-dependent diabetics to intensive therapy versus conventional insulin injections once or twice daily and found that intensive therapy reduced the development of neuropathy by 64% after 5 years of follow-up.

2. He F. Occupational toxic neuropathies: An update. Scand J Work Environ Health 1985;11:321–330.

   An extensive review is presented of environmental and work-related chemicals and toxins associated with peripheral neuropathy.

3. Monforte R, Estruch R, Valls-Solé J, et al. Autonomic and peripheral neuropathies in patients with chronic alcoholism: A dose-related toxic effect of alcohol. Arch Neurol 1995;52:45–51.

   This study of hospitalized patients with alcoholism found that 24% had evidence of autonomic neuropathy and 32% had peripheral neuropathy, unrelated to nutritional status.

4. Partanen J, Niskanen L, Lehtinen J, Mervaala E, Siitonen O, Uusitupa M. Natural history of peripheral neuropathy in patients with non-insulin-dependent diabetes mellitus. N Engl J Med 1995;333:89–94.

   Patients with newly diagnosed NIDDM and control subjects were observed at baseline and 5 and 10 years later. At baseline, the prevalence of polyneuropathy was 8% in those with NIDDM compared with 2% of controls; at 10 years, 42% of NIDDM patients and 6% of controls had neuropathy. Higher mean fasting glucose and glycoglobin levels were risk factors for development of neuropathy.

5. Wright J. Review of the symptomatic treatment of diabetic neuropathy. Pharmacotherapy 1994;14:689–697.

   The author covers the pathophysiology of pain in diabetic peripheral neuropathy and drug therapy efficacy in prospective randomized studies. Antidepressants are first-line agents, with benefit also demonstrated by phenytoin and carbamazepine. Topical capsaicin cream 0.075% applied four times a day was shown to be more effective than placebo cream, but 11% of capsaicin-treated patients withdrew from the study because of adverse effects.

148 Electroencephalography

Procedure

JAMES J. COATSWORTH

Indications and Contraindications. Electroencephalography (EEG) is useful in evaluating patients with seizures or suspected seizures, recurrent loss of consciousness, metabolic disorders (delirium), sleep disorders, and brain injury. Computed tomography and magnetic resonance imaging are superior to EEG in evaluating suspected brain tumors, stroke, multiple sclerosis, and arteriovenous malformations. There are no contraindications to EEG, although tracings from uncooperative patients may include artifacts and be uninterpretable.

Rationale. The EEG records the cortical electrical activity of the brain. Two important types of EEG abnormalities are slowing (slow waves) and epileptiform activity (spike waves), either focal or generalized.

Even between actual seizures, patients with generalized epilepsy may exhibit generalized spike and slow-wave discharges; those with focal (partial) epilepsy may have focal spikes or slow waves. Anterior temporal spikes are characteristic of patients with complex partial seizures. An accompanying slow-wave focus suggests structural lesions such as tumor or infarct. Metabolic encephalopathy may cause generalized slow waves, a helpful finding in the assessment of the comatose patient.

Although a positive EEG confirms the diagnosis of epilepsy, some patients with documented epilepsy have normal EEGs between seizures.

All results require clinical correlation because minor abnormalities, although nonspecific, may be subtle indications of serious disease.

Methods. By using 16 separate amplifying units, the EEG is very sensitive to artifacts produced by eye blinking, movement, perspiring, and swallowing. A routine EEG takes 60 to 90 minutes to complete and is painless.

Certain procedures that are used to activate latent seizure foci are hyperventilation (to produce alkalosis-induced cerebral vasoconstriction), stroboscopic stimulation, and sleep (with or without sedatives).

EEG by telemetry or with videotape monitoring may be useful in evaluating patients who have frequent seizures unresponsive to medications and in patients with pseudoseizures. Such patients should be referred to epilepsy centers where such monitoring is performed.

Cost. The cost of EEG is about $340.

Cross-References: Sleep Apnea Syndromes (Chapter 64), Syncope (Chapter 75), Seizures (Chapter 139), Dementia (Chapter 140).

REFERENCES

1. Kiloh LG, et al. Clinical Electroencephalography, 4th ed. London, Butterworths, 1981.
   This comprehensive textbook on electroencephalography is an excellent source of information.
2. Kooi KA, et al. Fundamentals of Electroencephalography, 2nd ed. Hagerstown, MD, Harper & Row, 1978.
   The usefulness of EEG in various settings is discussed.

149 Electromyography and Nerve Conduction Studies

Procedure

JOHN RAVITS

Indications and Contraindications. Electromyography (EMG) and nerve conduction studies are specialized tests of neuromuscular function. These tests are often used to evaluate muscular weakness, sensory change (either hyperfunctioning, such as paresthesia, or hypofunctioning, such as anesthesia), or pain (especially when focal). There are no absolute contraindications to the test, although anticoagulated patients are at increased risk for hematomas.

Rationale. EMG and nerve conduction studies are often invaluable in the diagnosis of anterior horn cell disorders (e.g., amyotrophic lateral sclerosis and polio), radiculopathies, plexopathies, mononeuropathies (including nerve injuries and entrapment syndromes), polyneuropathies, myopathies, and disorders of neuromuscular junction transmission. These studies (1) help confirm and measure abnormalities of the peripheral nervous system, especially when symptoms exist without signs; (2) help localize lesions (e.g., differentiate radiculopathy from plexopathy or myopathy from neuromuscular junction disorders); (3) assess the extent of disease when there are widespread abnormalities, not all of which are clinically apparent (e.g., anterior horn cell disease); (4) provide useful prognostic information (e.g., nerve injury and Guillain-Barré syndrome); and (5) monitor the course of a disease (e.g., nerve injuries, entrapment syndromes, and polyneuropathies).

Nerve conduction studies are extremely sensitive in detecting carpal tunnel syndrome, polyneuropathy, and entrapment syndromes but are less sensitive for radiculopathy or myopathy. False-negative results may occur because the abnormalities are not continuously present, the techniques used are insensitive, the referral occurred early in the course of a disease (before diagnostic abnormalities appeared), or the electromyographer is inexperienced.

Methods. EMG and nerve conduction studies are often referred to as "EMG," but they are two separate procedures. *Nerve conduction studies* evaluate nerve function and use an electrical impulse to depolarize nerves; electrodes placed over the skin record sensory or motor potentials. *EMG* evaluates muscle function and uses needle electrodes that are inserted into muscle to record muscle action potentials. Spontaneous activity, which refers to muscle potentials appearing while the muscle is inactive, is normally absent; abnormalities include fibrillations, fasciculations, and myotonic discharges. Voluntary activity refers to muscle potentials appearing during voluntary muscle activation. Voluntary activity is evaluated for size of the potentials (amplitude and duration), morphology of the potentials, and recruitment (as muscle is activated from minimal to maximal effort). Newer computerized techniques include a single-fiber EMG and quantitative EMG.

The neurophysiologist usually performs a combination of nerve conduction studies and EMG, depending on the particular clinical problem. For example, a patient with upper extremity radiculopathy may undergo nerve conduction studies to exclude peripheral nerve entrapments, followed by EMG to search for muscle denervated in a myotomal pattern.

Cost and Complications. EMG and nerve conduction studies are expensive: an EMG of two extremities costs approximately $350, and nerve conduction studies of two nerves (motor and sensory) costs about $390. Because this expense far exceeds that of a neurologic consultation, these studies should be obtained judiciously, often in consultation with a neurologist. Although the test may be uncomfortable, complications of local infection and local hematoma are extremely rare.

Cross-References: Low Back Pain (Chapter 107), Ankle and Foot Pain (Chapter 112), Muscular Weakness (Chapter 137), Entrapment Neuropathies (Chapter 144), Peripheral Neuropathy (Chapter 147).

REFERENCES

1. Kimura J. Electrodiagnosis in Diseases of Nerve and Muscle: Principles and Practice, 2nd ed. Philadelphia, FA Davis, 1989.

   This is a standard textbook on technical and clinical aspects of EMG and nerve conduction studies.

2. Warmolts JR. Electrodiagnosis in neuromuscular disorders. Ann Intern Med 1981;95:599–608.

   The author reviews neuromuscular physiology and electrodiagnosis.

SECTION XIII
Endocrine Disorders

· ·

150 Cholesterol Screening

Screening

LINDA E. PINSKY

Epidemiology. Epidemiologic, observational, and interventional studies clearly demonstrate a causal role of hypercholesterolemia in coronary artery disease, a condition that affects approximately 7 million Americans and is the most common cause of death in both men and women in the United States. The risk of coronary artery disease rises 2% to 3% for every 1% increase in total serum cholesterol. Twenty percent of adult Americans have a cholesterol level of greater than 240 mg/dL, which, in a middle-aged man, indicates a 9% to 12% risk of his developing symptomatic coronary artery disease within 7 to 9 years.

Age is the best predictor of death from coronary artery disease, with a 100-fold increase between ages 40 and 80. Other established risk factors for coronary artery disease include elevated cholesterol level, hypertension, and cigarette smoking (Table 150–1). For a nonsmoking, normotensive 55-year-old man with a total cholesterol level less than 200 mg/dL, the probability of having a heart attack within 8 years is 31/1000. If he smokes, the risk is 46/1000; if he has high cholesterol (> 260 mg/dL) and smokes, it is 64/1000. With the addition of hypertension (systolic greater than 150 mm Hg) to smoking and hypercholesterolemia, his risk of myocardial infarction within 8 years is 95/1000.

Rationale. In some individuals coronary artery disease may present with anginal pain, but in many its initial presentation is sudden death or myocardial infarction. In 1995, one third of the 1.5 million Americans who had myocardial infarctions did not survive. Resting and exercise electrocardiograms lack sensitivity and specificity for asymptomatic coronary artery disease and are not cost effective. Even if coronary artery disease is detected early, the only intervention shown to improve outcome is modification of risk factors. Thus, it is important to detect and reduce risk factors. Reduction of low density lipoprotein (LDL)-cholesterol below 100 mg/dL leads to regression of atherosclerotic plaques and decreases the incidence of myocardial infarction in individuals with known cardiac disease.

Lowering cholesterol in individuals with known coronary artery disease

Table 150–1. ESTABLISHED RISK FACTORS FOR CORONARY HEART DISEASE

Positive Factors

Nonmodifiable

Age: men ≥ 45 years, women ≥ 55 years or premature menopause without estrogen replacement
Family history of premature coronary heart disease
  Myocardial infarction/sudden death in first-degree female relative < 65 years or in first-degree
  male relative < 55 years

Modifiable

Increased total or low density lipoprotein
Cigarette smoking (current)
Hypertension: ≥ 140/90 mm Hg or treated
High density lipoprotein (HDL) < 35 mg/dL
Diabetes mellitus
Obesity*: especially visceral (central) obesity
Physical inactivity*

Negative Factor

High HDL ≥ 60 mg/dL†

Bold type indicates risk factors NCEP II uses with total cholesterol to determine need for lipoprotein analysis.

*Obesity and inactivity, although not considered risk factors in NCEP classification, are seen as areas of intervention.

†If present, negates one positive risk factor in above determination.

decreases both cardiac and noncardiac mortality. Primary prevention studies have shown decreased cardiac mortality, although some studies have also found short-term increases in all causes of mortality, raising concerns about the risk-benefit ratio of medically treating hypercholesterolemia in lower-risk populations.

Routine screening of adults is recommended by many advisory groups (Tables 150–2 through 150–4). The US Preventive Services Task Force and the American College of Physicians recommendations reflect concern about the potential risks of lipid-lowering medication and suggest delaying the age at onset of laboratory cholesterol screening to focus screening on higher-risk groups in whom the risk-benefit ratio and cost-effectiveness is greater. The National Cholesterol Education Program (NCEP) Adult Treatment Panel II guidelines take a more aggressive approach to screening while recognizing the different risk-benefit ratios in primary and secondary prevention.

The applicability of guidelines to any specific patient must always be considered. The applicability of findings from studies in middle-aged men, a higher-risk population, to women and young men, lower-risk populations, has been questioned. Clinical manifestations of coronary artery disease and myocardial infarction occur, respectively, 10 and 20 years later on average in women than in men. Data from primary prevention trials on the effects of treatment on all-cause and cardiovascular mortality in women are limited and inconclusive. While awaiting more conclusive studies, extrapolations from studies in men suggest that the approach to primary prevention for premenopausal women should resemble that used for younger men, given the similarities in epidemiology and pathophysiology. Data from secondary prevention trials, while still limited, favor treatment.

Table 150–2. AMERICAN COLLEGE OF PHYSICIANS— 1996 CHOLESTEROL SCREENING GUIDELINES

Target Population

Middle-aged adults*
  Men: age 35–65 years
  Women: age 45–65 years

Frequency

Variable, depending on test results
  If results are normal, test once.
  If results are near treatment threshold, repeat at least every 5 years.

Primary Prevention

Screening of total cholesterol appropriate but not mandatory (confirm
  abnormal results with repeat test)

Secondary Prevention

Do lipoprotein analysis.

*Selective screening of young adults with history or physical examination suggesting a familial lipoprotein disorder or at least two other risk factors for coronary heart disease.

Studies of cholesterol screening in the elderly suggest that a low high density lipoprotein (HDL)-cholesterol is an independent predictor of coronary artery disease events for all groups. The predictive value of a mild to moderately elevated total or LDL-cholesterol is uncertain in individuals older than 70 without cardiac disease. Screening and treatment is indicated in those with known coronary artery disease, regardless of age. In both primary and secondary prevention, screening should not be done in individuals whose life expectancy, quality of life, or personal wishes would prohibit interventions based on the results.

Table 150–3. US PREVENTIVE SERVICES TASK FORCE CHOLESTEROL SCREENING GUIDELINES—1995

Target Population

Middle-aged adults*
  Men: age 35–65 years
  Women: age 45–65 years

Frequency

Variable, depending on test results
  If results are normal, test at least once.
  Periodic screening is most important during times of cholesterol increase (middle-
  aged men, perimenopausal women, weight gain).

Primary Prevention

Screening of total cholesterol recommended (confirm abnormal results with repeat test)

Secondary Prevention

Do lipoprotein analysis.

*Selective screening of young adults with history of very high cholesterol or premature coronary artery disease; or with other major risk factors for coronary heart disease.

Table 150–4. NATIONAL CHOLESTEROL EDUCATION PROGRAM ADULT TREATMENT PANEL II CHOLESTEROL SCREENING GUIDELINES

Target Population

Adults ≥ 20 years old

Frequency

Once every 5 years if results are normal (total cholesterol ≤ 200 mg/dL and high density lipoprotein (HDL) cholesterol ≥ 35 mg/dL)

Primary Prevention

Check total cholesterol and HDL-cholesterol (confirm abnormal results with repeat test). Do lipoprotein analysis if the mean of two test results show any of the following:
   (HDL)-cholesterol < 35 mg/dL
   Total cholesterol > 200 mg/dL and two or more risk factors*
   Total cholesterol > 240 mg/dL

Secondary Prevention

Do lipoprotein analysis.

*See Table 150–1.

Screening in the younger population is reasonable if interventions involve dietary and lifestyle modifications, rather than medication, thus decreasing both the cost and associated risks (there are no reports of increased mortality with diet-associated low cholesterol). Additionally, earlier screening may allow healthy adults to recognize the relationship between health risk and their behavior. As a result, these individuals can begin to establish dietary and lifestyle habits that may make the use of potent lipid-lowering medications when they are older unnecessary. Whether measuring blood cholesterol increases compliance with recommendations for lowering coronary artery disease risk through lifestyle modifications is not known, so the decision to screen cholesterol levels solely for this purpose should be individualized.

Strategy. All individuals should be assessed for risk factors for coronary artery disease and the presence or absence of atherosclerotic disease at approximately age 20. Routine initial screening of blood cholesterol levels should be done beginning in middle age; screening may be done at a younger age, based on individualized assessment of risk factors or potential benefits for lifestyle interventions. Laboratory screening should not be done if it will have no bearing (immediate or long term) on the patient's risk stratification, education and counseling, or management plan. Interpretation of cholesterol levels in terms of the need for fasting lipoprotein analysis should follow the NCEP Adult Treatment Panel II guidelines shown in Table 150–4.

On average, individuals with desirable cholesterol levels should have repeat testing approximately every 5 years. Variations in frequency should be made on a case-by-case basis. Screening of cholesterol levels is especially appropriate during periods when levels may be changing, as in middle-aged men and perimenopausal women, after initial prescription of oral contraception, or with weight gain. Screening less frequently than every 5 years is appropriate for a younger individual without risk factors for coronary artery disease whose lifestyle already incorporates all the interventions that might result from the screening.

Cholesterol evaluation should continue after the age of 65 to 70 in individuals with known coronary artery disease. Asymptomatic individuals older than 70 generally do not require testing. Other factors, such as life expectancy related to concurrent illness and personal preference, are pivotal in the decision to screen.

Action. All individuals should receive advice on modification of the risk factors associated with coronary artery disease, including diet, exercise, obesity, and smoking cessation.

Individuals with borderline cholesterol levels without other risk factors for coronary artery disease should be followed yearly. Individuals with increased cholesterol levels (a total cholesterol greater than 240 mg/dL or an HDL-cholesterol level less than 35 mg/dL or a total cholesterol value of 200 to 240 mg/dL in the presence of two or more risk factors) require further evaluation and possible treatment, as discussed in Chapter 152.

Cross-References: Principles of Screening (Chapter 7), Periodic Health Assessment (Chapter 8), Angina (Chapter 78), Hyperlipidemia (Chapter 152).

REFERENCES

1. American College of Physicians. Guidelines for using serum cholesterol, high-density lipoprotein cholesterol and triglycerides as screening tests for preventing coronary heart disease in adults. Ann Intern Med 1996;124:515–531.

   These guidelines are revised from a previous ACP guideline to focus screening on high-risk groups in whom the benefit-risk ratio of treatment is significantly increased.

2. Corti MC, Guralnik JM, Salive ME, Harris T, Field TS, Wallace RB, Berkman LF, Seeman TE, Glynn RJ, Hennekens CH, et al. HDL cholesterol predicts coronary heart disease mortality in older persons. JAMA 1995;274:539–544.

   These researchers found HDL-C predictive of coronary artery disease in the elderly, in contrast to the lack of association found in a subset population of this study reported earlier by Krumholz.

3. Grover SA, Coupal L, Hu X. Identifying adults at increased risk of coronary disease. How well do the current cholesterol guidelines work? JAMA 1995;274:801–806.

   NCEP II guidelines designate 15% of population as high risk, with 45% of eventual deaths from coronary artery disease occurring in this group. These are the best results of any expert guidelines studied. The superiority of a computer risk model is proposed. Other studies advocate use of total cholesterol/HDL-cholesterol ratio as the most accurate measure.

4. Summary of the second report of the National Cholesterol Education Program (NCEP) Expert Panel on Detection, Evaluation, and Treatment of High Blood Cholesterol in Adults (Adult Treatment Panel II). JAMA 1993;269:3015–3023.

   This widely used guideline advocates aggressive screening; it is modified from Adult Treatment Panel I to reflect different approaches to primary and secondary prevention and the growing recognition of the importance of HDL-cholesterol.

5. Verschuren WMM, Jacobs DR, Bioemberg B, et al. Serum total cholesterol and long term coronary heart disease mortality in different cultures. JAMA 1995;264:131–136.

   The 25-year follow-up of the Seven Countries Study found cholesterol level linearly related to coronary heart disease mortality across cultures, with the same relative increase in mortality rates with a given cholesterol increase. Of note, absolute coronary artery disease mortality rates at a given cholesterol level are vastly different, indicating "other factors such as diet that are typical for cultures with a low CHD risk are also important with respect to primary prevention."

151 Gynecomastia

Symptom

DOUGLAS S. PAAUW

Epidemiology. Gynecomastia (enlargement of the male breast) is a common problem, affecting 30% to 40% of men. The prevalence of gynecomastia increases with advancing age, probably because of testicular failure.

Etiology. Gynecomastia usually results from an increased ratio of estrogens to androgens, although in many cases the precise cause is unknown. Transient gynecomastia is common during puberty (40% to 70% of normal boys), probably because of a short-lived increase in plasma estrogen-to-androgen ratio.

The broad range of recognized causes is given in Tables 151–1 and 151–2. Drug-induced gynecomastia is common and may occur because of the drug's intrinsic estrogen activity (digitalis, marijuana), inhibition of testosterone synthesis (spironolactone, ketoconazole), or direct damage to the testes (cytotoxic agents) (see Table 151–2). The cause of gynecomastia due to cimetidine is unclear, but males receiving a dose of greater than 1 g/d have a 40-fold increased risk of gynecomastia compared with nonusers. Regular ingestion of milk or meat from estrogen-treated animals can cause gynecomastia.

Clinical Approach. The history should emphasize the patient's present medications, use of alcohol, and reproductive history. The physical examination focuses on the breasts (size and consistency), the testes (size, nodules, and symmetry), and any evidence of hyperthyroidism or chronic liver disease. A cushingoid appearance or recent onset of hypertension suggests adrenal disease. Gynecomastia may be asymmetric. Almost all breast carcinomas present as a unilateral, usually painless mass. Although breast cancer in males is rare (1% of all breast cancer cases), patients with signs suggestive of cancer (bleed-

Table 151–1. CAUSES OF GYNECOMASTIA

Physiologic	Increased estrogen production
Pubertal gynecomastia	Hermaphroditism
Gynecomastia of aging	Testicular tumors
Decreased androgen production or	Bronchogenic carcinoma
androgen resistance	Increased peripheral conversion to estrogen
Congenital	Congenital adrenal hyperplasia/adrenal
Congenital anorchia	tumors
Klinefelter's syndrome	Liver disease
Testicular feminization	Malnutrition
Acquired	Thyrotoxicosis
Alcoholism	Drugs
Myotonic dystrophy	Idiopathic gynecomastia
Orchitis	
Renal failure	

Table 151–2. MEDICATIONS ASSOCIATED WITH GYNECOMASTIA

Amiodarone	Finasteride
Amphetamines	Isoniazid
Calcium channel blockers	Ketoconazole*
Human chorionic gonadotropin	Marijuana
Cimetidine*	Methyldopa
Clomiphene	Phenothiazines
Cytotoxic agents	Reserpine
Digitalis	Spironolactone*
Diazepam	Tricyclic antidepressants
Estrogen*	

*Most common.

ing, fixation, regional adenopathy, eccentric breast mass) should have an immediate biopsy. Risk factors for breast carcinoma in males include family history of breast cancer as well as Klinefelter's syndrome (20-fold increased risk).

If the cause remains unknown despite a thorough history and physical examination, laboratory tests should include liver function tests, human chorionic gonadotropin determination (to exclude ectopic hCG from testicular and nontesticular tumors), thyroid function tests (30% of men with hyperthyroidism have gynecomastia), and measurement of testosterone levels (to exclude hypogonadism). If examination suggests Klinefelter's syndrome (small firm testes, eunuchoid habitus, and long limbs), karyotyping is indicated.

Management. If gynecomastia is drug induced, removal of the offending drug usually results in a decrease in breast size within several months. Reassurance and explanation are frequently all that is required in most cases of gynecomastia. Breast carcinoma is no more likely in patients with gynecomastia than in other males (except patients with Klinefelter's syndrome).

Cross-References: Alcohol Problems (Chapter 10), Cirrhosis and Chronic Liver Failure (Chapter 99), Common Thyroid Disorders (Chapter 153), Male Infertility (Chapter 156), Erectile Dysfunction (Chapter 169), Scrotal Mass (Chapter 183).

REFERENCES

1. Carlson HE. Gynecomastia. N Engl J Med 1980;303:795–799.

   This article is an excellent overall review of gynecomastia.

2. Dolsky RL. Gynecomastia: Treatment by liposuction subcutaneous mastectomy. Dermatol Clin 1990;8:469–478.

   Liposuction is described as a cosmetic treatment for gynecomastia. The operative complication rate is very low.

3. O'Hanlon D, Kent P, Kerin MJ, Given F. Unilateral breast masses in men over 40: A diagnostic dilemma. Am J Surg 1995;170:24–26.

   Most breast carcinomas present as a painless unilateral mass. In this series, 18% of the masses were malignant. Risk factors for breast carcinoma included family history of breast cancer or a previous history of carcinoma.

4. Rodriquez LA, Jick H. Risk of gynecomastia associated with cimetidine, omeprazole, and other antiulcer drugs. BMJ 1994;308:503–506.

   Use of cimetidine but not ranitidine or omeprazole was associated with increased risk of developing gynecomastia (relative risk 7.2). The risk increases with increased dose.

5. Tanner LA, Bosco LA. Gynecomastia associated with calcium channel blocker therapy. Arch Intern Med 1988;148:379–380.

   Thirty-one cases of gynecomastia with calcium channel blocker use were reported to the Food and Drug Administration. The underlying mechanism is unknown.

152 Hyperlipidemia

Problem

LINDA E. PINSKY

Epidemiology and Etiology. Hyperlipidemia is one of several modifiable risk factors, along with cigarette smoking, hypertension, diabetes, physical inactivity, and obesity, associated with increased risk of coronary artery disease. The association of increasing coronary artery disease risk with increasing cholesterol levels is continuous, and the demarcation between normal and abnormal levels is somewhat arbitrary. Fifty percent of adult Americans have a cholesterol level of greater than 200 mg/dL, and 20% have a level greater than 240 mg/dL.

Individuals with familial hypercholesterolemia and familial combined hyperlipidemia, which are autosomal dominant traits, are at markedly increased risk of heart disease, with the first myocardial infarction occurring at a mean age of 40 years in affected men and 10 years later in affected women. In familial hypercholesterolemia, a low density lipoprotein (LDL) receptor defect often results in cholesterol levels above 300 mg/dL. Familial hypercholesterolemia (seen in 1 in 500 persons in its heterozygous state) causes 5% of myocardial infarctions occurring before age 60. In familial combined hyperlipidemia, estimated to occur in 1 in 100 persons, increased production of apoprotein B causes elevated triglyceride (TG) or cholesterol levels or both. Approximately 15% of individuals with myocardial infarction before age 60 have familial combined hyperlipidemia. In contrast, persons with elevated triglyceride levels due to familial hypertriglyceridemia are not thought to be at increased risk for coronary artery disease.

Several studies have demonstrated that reductions in cholesterol among high-risk men, especially those with documented coronary disease, can substantially reduce the risk of myocardial infarction and cardiovascular death. On average, a 1% reduction in cholesterol results in a 2% decrease in coronary artery disease events, attributable to stabilization and, in some cases, regression of atherosclerotic plaques.

Signs and Symptoms. Clinical evaluation centers on determining the presence of hyperlipidemia and, if present, whether it is due to a genetic syndrome or due to a diet, disease, or drug that can be altered. Symptoms of hyperlipidemia result from associated diseases (e.g., angina with hypercholesterolemia, pancreatitis with chylomicron syndrome). In the absence of definitive signs or symptoms, the risk of coronary artery disease is determined based on the presence of existing coronary heart disease as well as assessment of nonlipid risk factors for coronary artery disease, such as cigarette smoking, diabetes, hypertension, obesity, and inactivity. Elevated cholesterol levels should be suspected in anyone with a strong family history of premature coronary artery disease (i.e., a family history of a myocardial infarction or sudden death occurring in a female relative younger than 65 or a male relative younger than 55). Signs and symptoms of secondary causes of hyperlipidemia should also be sought, particularly those of hypothyroidism, diabetes, nephrotic syndrome, and liver or biliary disease.

On physical examination, central obesity (increased intra-abdominal fat assessed by a waist-hip ratio of 0.95) may indicate syndrome X, a condition associated with insulin resistance and dyslipidemia. Lipid abnormalities in this condition include increased triglyceride levels, low levels of high density lipoprotein (HDL)-cholesterol, and an increased fraction of small dense LDL-cholesterol, a subclass of LDL-cholesterol that is protein rich. Arcus corneae occurring in patients in their 20s or 30s suggests hypercholesterolemia but is not specific for this condition. Increased β-lipoproteins and associated increased LDL-cholesterol may be manifested by visible cutaneous and subcutaneous deposits of cholesterol: xanthelasmas or tendinous xanthomas. Xanthelasmas (yellowish plaques on the eyelids) may also be a sign of hypothyroidism or aging. Tendinous xanthomas, commonly found on the extensor tendons of the hand or as thickening (7 mm) of the Achilles tendon, are diagnostic of familial hypercholesterolemia. Remnant removal disease (sometimes referred to as type III disease) may result in palmar and tuberous xanthomas appearing in the palmar creases and on the elbows and knees, respectively. In chylomicron syndrome, acute elevations in triglyceride levels (e.g., caused by medications) precipitate the appearance of eruptive xanthomas on the buttocks and extensor surfaces of the elbows and knees. Pancreatitis (with symptoms of nausea, vomiting, and epigastric pain radiating to the back) can occur when triglyceride levels reach 1000–2000 mg/dL.

Clinical Approach. Evaluation for hyperlipidemia should include a nonfasting measurement of total and HDL-cholesterol in individuals without known atherosclerotic disease and a fasting lipoprotein analysis in those with disease. A total cholesterol level greater than 240 mg/dL or an HDL-cholesterol level less than 35 mg/dL is abnormal and should be followed by a fasting lipoprotein analysis. A borderline cholesterol level of 200 to 240 mg/dL in an individual with two or more risk factors requires further evaluation. Because of individual and laboratory variations in cholesterol measurements, abnormal results should be confirmed with repeat testing and the mean results of two or three tests used. (Risk factor assessment and screening criteria are discussed in Chapter 150.)

LDL-cholesterol is calculated using the following formula:

$$LDL\text{-}C = Total\text{-}C - HDL\text{-}C - TG/5.$$

Secondary causes of hyperlipidemia should be sought in individuals with coronary heart disease with LDL-cholesterol greater than 100 mg/dL and in individuals without known coronary heart disease with either LDL-cholesterol greater than 160 mg/dL or two or more risk factors and LDL-cholesterol of 130 to 159 mg/dL. Secondary causes include type II diabetes mellitus, hypothyroidism, obstructive liver disease, and nephrotic syndrome. Medications that raise lipids include cyclosporine (cholesterol); estrogen, alcohol, or β-blockers (triglycerides); and diuretics, anabolic steroids, and sometimes glucocorticoids (cholesterol and triglycerides).

Lipid factors such as lipoprotein (a), apoprotein B, and apoprotein A-II play a role in the genesis of coronary heart disease. Although not cost-effective for general evaluation, measurement of these factors may help define level of risk in certain individuals with an exceptionally strong family history.

In patients with pancreatitis due to hypertriglyceridemia, the plasma may be milky white. Evaluation of fasting triglycerides and lipoprotein analysis can confirm and classify the hypertriglyceridemia.

Management. Multiple studies have demonstrated that decreasing cholesterol levels with diet or medications results in a decreased risk of coronary artery disease. Decreasing saturated fat and cholesterol intake reduces total and LDL-cholesterol levels up to 30% in controlled situations and about 10% on average in outpatient settings. The Oslo Study Diet and Antismoking Trial (primary prevention) found a 47% lower incidence of myocardial infarction (fatal and nonfatal) and sudden death in the group given dietary treatment and instruction in smoking cessation as compared with controls. The Lifestyle Heart Trial demonstrated angiographic regression of coronary atherosclerotic lesions in individuals given therapy with diet and exercise but without lipid-lowering medications. Recommendations from the National Cholesterol Education Panel (NCEP) Adult Treatment Panel II emphasize lifestyle modification, especially dietary changes, as the initial therapy for hyperlipidemia (Table 152–1). For elevated LDL-cholesterol levels, the first stage of treatment involves a step I diet in which the amount total fat consumed should not exceed 30% of the total calories, with saturated fat limited to 8% to 10% of the total calories and cholesterol intake less than 300 mg/d. For a person on a 2000-kcal step I diet, total daily fat intake should not exceed 67 g and daily saturated fat intake should be 22 g. (The average American diet has 36 to 40 g of saturated fat.) If this diet is unsuccessful, or if the individual is already consuming a step I diet at the time of diagnosis, a step II diet is suggested. This diet differs in that saturated fat is limited to less than 7% of the total calories. Referral to a nutritionist improves compliance rates, especially for adopting a step II diet. Weight loss and physical activity should also be stressed. Smoking cessation and reduction of other nonlipid risk factors are equally or more important for lowering the patient's risk of coronary heart disease.

For most individuals, dietary therapy should be tried for 6 months before beginning drug therapy. Exceptions to this in primary prevention are rare and may include middle-aged and older individuals (men older than age 45 and postmenopausal women) with cholesterol levels well above 220 mg/dL in whom drug therapy may be recommended after intensive dietary therapy has begun.

Table 152-1. NATIONAL CHOLESTEROL EDUCATION PANEL ADULT TREATMENT PANEL II GUIDELINES FOR INITIATION OF DIETARY AND DRUG THERAPY

Primary Prevention

Begin dietary therapy (step I* or step II† diet) if
LDL >130 mg/dL and two or more risk factors	Goal <130 mg/dL
LDL >160 mg/dL	Goal <160 mg/dL

Begin drug therapy if man >35 years or postmenopausal woman‡ and §
LDL >160 mg/dL and two or more risk factors	Goal <130 mg/dL
LDL >190 mg/dL	Goal <160 mg/dL

Secondary Prevention

Begin dietary therapy (step II diet)† if LDL >100 mg/dL	Goal <100 mg/dL
Begin drug therapy if LDL >130 mg/dL§	Goal <100 mg/dL

*Step I diet: total fat ≤ 30% of total calories; saturated fat 8%–10% of total calories; cholesterol 300 mg/d.

†Step II diet: total fat ≤ 30% of total calories; saturated fat < 7% of total calories; cholesterol 300 mg/d.

‡Consider estrogen replacement therapy first.

§Unless the LDL-cholesterol is extremely high, dietary therapy should be tried for 6 months before beginning drug therapy.

Individuals at markedly increased risk for coronary artery disease, such as those with severe forms of primary hypercholesterolemia (e.g., familial hypercholesterolemia) or severe secondary dyslipidemias (e.g., diabetes mellitus), also may require early drug therapy, regardless of age.

If LDL-cholesterol goals are not achieved after 6 months of dietary therapy, adjunct therapy with medications may be considered for men older than age 35, postmenopausal women, and anyone with known coronary artery disease (see Table 152–1). Although effects of diet and drug therapy are additive, medications have a substantially greater effect. The decision to begin medications, especially in primary prevention, must be made carefully, with the patient's participation, weighing the benefits versus the risks, because it may mean lifelong drug therapy. Age, gender, other risk factors, the etiology and duration of the dyslipidemia, past compliance, co-morbid conditions, and individual preferences should be taken into account. The initial medication choice is made on the basis of the specific lipoprotein abnormality (see Table 152–2 for suggested therapy by condition and Table 152–3 for therapy by drug action). If after a sufficient trial the desired effect is not achieved, adding a second agent is generally more effective and has fewer side effects than increasing the dose of the first agent. Good combinations are low doses of bile acid–binding resins added to niacin or to 3-hydroxy-3-methylglutaryl-coenzyme A (HMG-CoA) reductase inhibitors. Referral to a specialist is indicated for the use of other medication combinations.

A low HDL-cholesterol level is a risk factor for coronary artery disease; however, there are no studies demonstrating that increasing HDL-cholesterol decreases the risk. Smoking cessation, increased activity, and weight loss raise the HDL level and should be suggested, but medication (e.g., nicotinic acid) should not be used if a low HDL-cholesterol is the only indication. Similarly, elevated levels of lipoprotein (a) are associated with an increased risk of

Table 152–2. PATTERNS OF HYPERLIPIDEMIA

Lipid Testing Results	Plasma Lipoproteins Elevated/ Phenotype	Causes of Primary Hyperlipidemia	Causes of Secondary Hyperlipidemia	Drug Therapy First Choice
Increased cholesterol, and normal triglyceride levels	LDL/IIA	Familial hypercholesterolemia Familial combined hyperlipidemia Familial defective apo-B-100 Undefined	Acute intermittent porphyria Anorexia nervosa Cushing's syndrome Dysglobulinemia Hyperparathyroidism Hypothyroidism Nephrotic syndrome Obesity Glucocorticoid use	HMG-CoA reductase inhibitor Nicotinic acid Bile acid binding resins
Combined elevation of cholesterol and triglyceride levels (triglycerides 1 to 3 times cholesterol)	LDL and VLDL/ IIB	Familial hypercholesterolemia Familial combined hyperlipidemia Undefined	Same as in phenotype IIA above	Nicotinic acid HMG-CoA reductase inhibitors
	Chylomicrons and VLDL remnant/III	Remnant removal disease	Diabetes mellitus Dysglobulinemia Hypothyroidism Systemic lupus erythematosus Obesity	Fibrates Nicotinic acid HMG-CoA reductase inhibitor (Postmenopausal estrogen therapy may be helpful.)
Primary elevation of triglycerides		Familial hypertriglyceridemia Familial combined hyperlipidemia	Acute intermittent porphyria Alcoholism Diabetes mellitus Dysglobulinemia Hypothyroidism Nephrotic syndrome Obesity Pregnancy Renal failure Use of diuretics, β-blockers, estrogens, glucocorticoids	Nicotinic acid (except in type II diabetics)
Moderate to marked increases of cholesterol levels and more marked increases of triglyceride levels	Chylomicrons present and elevated/I	Lipoprotein lipase or apoprotein C II deficiency	Diabetes mellitus Dysglobulinemia Systemic lupus erythematosus Pancreatitis	Gemfibrozil
	Chylomicrons present and VLDL elevated/V	Familial hypertriglyceridemia (Lipoprotein lipase or apoprotein C II deficiency)	As in phenotype IV above	

HMG-CoA, 3-hydroxy-3-methyglutaryl-coenzyme A.

Table 152-3. DRUG THERAPY FOR DYSLIPIDEMIA

Category	Indications for Use	Effects on Serum Lipids		Contraindications	Generic Name	Brand Name	Usual Daily Doses	Cost ($ per Month)* (range = dose)
Nicotinic acid	Increased TG, Lp(a), or small dense LDL Decreased HDL	↓ LDL ↑ HDL ↓ TG ↓ Lp(a)	20–25% 10–20% 20–40% 35%	Chronic liver disease ? Gout non-insulin-dependent diabetes mellitus	Niacin	Generic	500–2000 mg tid	2.57–6.90
Fibrates	Increased TG Chylomicron syndrome, remnant removal disease	↓ LDL ↑ HDL ↓ TG	5–10% 6% 30%	Gallstones	Gemfibrozil	Generic Lopid	600 mg bid	55.66 65.74
HMG-CoA reductase inhibitor	Increased LDL	↓ LDL ↑ HDL ↓ TG	20–25% 2–15% 10–30%	Active or chronic liver disease ? Cyclosporine, gemfibrozil, niacin	Lovastatin Pravastatin Simvastatin Fluvastatin	Mevacor Pravachol Zocor Lescol	20–80 mg 10–40 mg 5–40 mg 20–40 mg	62.53–225.09 50.64–92.17 53.42–103.13 31.92–35.70
Bile acid–binding resins	Mildly increased LDL	↓ LDL ↑ HDL ↓ TG	10–20% 3–8% 10–15%	Remnant removal disease TG >500 ? TG >200	Cholestyramine	Questran Questran Light	4–24 g (divided)	39.71–238.23 (packets)
					Colestipol (granules)	Colestid	5–30 g (divided)	35.69–209.82 (packets)

?, relative contraindication; TG, triglycerides; LDL, low density lipoprotein-cholesterol; HDL, high density lipoprotein-cholesterol; Lp(a), lipoprotein (a).
*Average wholesale price, 1995 *Drug Topics Red Book.*

coronary artery disease, but the benefit of lowering these levels with medication (also achievable with nicotinic acid) has not been shown.

Elevations of cholesterol in patients aged 70 years and older who do not have symptomatic coronary disease are generally not treated unless the LDL-cholesterol level is extremely high (> 250 mg/dL). In general, therapy should emphasize lifestyle modifications. Medication may be considered in individuals with known coronary disease and may be continued in those currently on lipid-lowering therapy. A decision to use medical therapy should take into account the increased sensitivity to medication side effects seen in this age group, potential drug interactions, limited benefits due to the increased risk of death from noncardiac causes, and the burden that the expense of medication and monitoring imposes on the individual.

Pancreatitis may occur in patients with triglyceride levels greater than 2000 mg/dL. A low-fat diet, such as instant breakfast mix with skim milk, is indicated acutely. Continued therapy includes a low-fat diet, correction of contributing factors (including poor control of diabetes and use of implicated medications or alcohol), and, if needed, a fibric acid derivative. In severe hypertriglyceridemia, some studies suggest that gemfibrozil is more effective than clofibrate.

Monitoring of Treatment. Patients on lipid-lowering medications need periodic monitoring to assess the efficacy and adverse effects of the treatment. The first follow-up LDL-cholesterol determination and assessment for potential drug side effects should be done 6 to 8 weeks after initiating drug therapy with HMG-CoA reductase inhibitors, fibrates, or bile acid–binding resins and 4 to 6 weeks after achieving a stable dose (1.5 g) of nicotinic acid. During monotherapy with HMG-CoA reductase inhibitors, dose-dependent, generally asymptomatic elevations of liver functions to greater than three times the upper limit of normal occur in 0.4% to 1.9% of patients. Myopathy is uncommon (less than 0.1%) on this medication; it is dose dependent and noted with increased frequency when this medication is combined with cyclosporine, nicotinic acid, fibrates, and erythromycin. Side effects of nicotinic acid requiring monitoring include elevations of liver function tests and increases in glucose and uric acid. With fibrate therapy, there is a slightly increased risk of biliary lithogenicity, myositis, and liver function test abnormalities.

Repeat measurement of lipids should be performed in another 6 weeks, then every 3 months initially. Once stabilized, individuals on diet or drug therapy should have biannual evaluation. Patients should be instructed in the symptoms of hepatotoxicity and myopathy and the need for immediate evaluation if either develops.

Cross-References: Periodic Health Assessment (Chapter 8), Alcohol Problems (Chapter 10), Obesity (Chapter 15), Angina (Chapter 78), Cholesterol Screening (Chapter 150), Common Thyroid Disorders (Chapter 153), Diabetes Mellitus (Chapter 154).

REFERENCES

1. Andrade SE, Walker AM, Gottlieb LK, Hollenberg NK, Testa MA, Saperia GM, Platt R. Discontinuation of antihyperlipidemia drugs—Do rates in clinical trials reflect rates in primary care settings? N Engl J Med 1995;332:1125–1131.

An increased rate of discontinuation of antihyperlipidemia drugs in primary care practice was found as compared with those in randomized clinical trials; rates due to adverse effects ranged from 7% with lovastatin to 26% with niacin.

2. Brown G, Albers JJ, Fisher LD, Schaefer SM, Lin JT, Kaplan C, Zhao XQ, Bisson BD, Fitzpatrick VF, Dodge HT. Regression of coronary artery disease as a result of increased lipid lowering therapy in men with high levels of apoprotein B. N Engl J Med 1990;323:1289–1298.

This landmark study showed angiographic evidence of atherosclerotic plaque regression and decrease in cardiac events with aggressive lipid lowering.

3. Havel RJ, Rapaport E. Management of hyperlipidemia. N Engl J Med 1995;332:1491–1498.

The authors provide a comprehensive review of what is and is not known about treating primary hyperlipidemia.

4. Shepherd J, Cobbie SM, Ford I, Isles CG, Lorimar AR, et al. Prevention of coronary heart disease with pravastatin in men with hypercholesterolemia. N Engl J Med 1995;333:1301–1307.

This study showed reduction in cardiac mortality with treatment in men without coronary artery disease. Notably, it showed treatment to be safe in populations at low risk for coronary artery disease. An accompanying editorial questions the arbitrariness of categorizing primary and secondary prevention based on cardiac events and not on degree of underlying atherosclerosis.

5. Walsh JE, Grady D. Treatment of hyperlipidemia in women. JAMA 1995;274:1152–1158.

Evidence is reviewed on treatment of hypercholesterolemia as primary and secondary prevention in women.

153 Common Thyroid Disorders

Problem

LINDA E. PINSKY

Patients with thyroid disease may present with symptoms related to a deficiency or excess of thyroid hormone (i.e., hypothyroidism and hyperthyroidism, respectively), ophthalmologic or dermatologic symptoms associated with a specific type of hyperthyroidism (Graves' disease), or thyroid nodules or enlargement.

THYROID DYSFUNCTION

Epidemiology. Thyroid disease, the second most prevalent endocrine disorder, occurs in 10% to 15% of the population older than age 40. Two percent to 5% of patients admitted to geriatric units have undiagnosed thyroid disease.

The overall prevalence of overt hypothyroidism is 1% to 3%, rising as high as 10% in women. Most cases of hypothyroidism present after the age of 50. In the otherwise healthy elderly person, the prevalence of hypothyroidism is estimated at 1% to 5%, with a reported incidence ranging from 1% to 17%.

The annual incidence of overt hyperthyroidism is 0.05% to 0.1% in adults. One third of thyrotoxicosis cases are in individuals older than 60. Hyperthyroidism occurs in 0.5% to 3% of the elderly population, more frequently in women than men.

Subclinical disease is defined by a mildly abnormal thyroid-stimulating hormone (TSH) level and a normal thyroxine (T_4) level in an asymptomatic person. Subclinical hypothyroidism occurs in an estimated 3% of the general population and in up to 10% of postmenopausal women. The annual rate of evolution from subclinical to overt disease is 5% per year overall and 20% to 24% per year in those older than age 65 with antithyroid antibodies.

In contrast, the approximate prevalence of subclinical hyperthyroidism is 1%; the incidence increases with age and occurs in 0.2% to 5% of the elderly. Progression to overt thyrotoxicosis occurs at a rate of 1% to 5% per year. Individuals with subclinical hyperthyroidism who have an autonomous thyroid adenoma or nodular goiter are at the greatest risk of developing overt disease.

Rationale. Routine screening of the general population for thyroid dysfunction is not cost-effective. In addition, there is no definitive evidence that overall morbidity or mortality is decreased by presymptomatic detection and treatment. However, in the elderly, there is an increased incidence of thyroid disease, and the diagnosis is frequently missed due to subtle or atypical presentations of hypothyroidism or hyperthyroidism in this age group. The consequences of not diagnosing, and thus not treating, symptomatic disease in this age group are serious and include cardiac and cognitive dysfunction.

The clinical significance of subclinical thyroid disease is unclear, and early diagnosis and treatment in the asymptomatic phase have not been shown to improve clinical outcomes.

Strategy. Although routine screening for overt thyroid disease is not recommended, selective annual or biennial screening is indicated in individuals at higher risk for thyroid disease. Individuals at higher risk are the elderly, especially women; those with previous thyroid disease or thyroid surgery; and those with other autoimmune diseases. Screening of asymptomatic patients for subclinical disease is not indicated.

The preferred screening test (T_4 vs. TSH) for thyroid function has been questioned, owing to issues of cost-effectiveness. In general, TSH is favored, because T_4 has a higher rate of false-positive results, misses 5% of cases of hyperthyroidism due to triiodothyronine (T_3) toxicosis, and, by definition, cannot detect subclinical disease. Concomitant use of both tests is clearly not indicated.

Individuals with even limited clinical evidence of thyroid disease, such as fatigue, change in weight, hypercholesterolemia, cognitive dysfunction, or unexplained depression, should undergo appropriate diagnostic testing. If subclinical thyroid disease is detected, clinicians should observe these patients closely, given the relatively high rate of progression to overt disease.

HYPOTHYROIDISM

Etiology. The prevalence of hypothyroidism in the general population is 1% to 3%, with increasing prevalence with age and in women. The prevalence in women older than 50 years is approximately 5%, with an incidence reported as high as 17%. Primary thyroid gland failure due to chronic autoimmune thyroiditis (Hashimoto's thyroiditis) is the most common cause of hypothyroidism. Other frequent causes are previous radioactive iodine therapy for hyperthyroidism and thyroid surgery. Subclinical hypothyroidism, defined as a mildly elevated TSH and a normal T_4 in an otherwise asymptomatic individual, occurs in 3% of the general population and in up to 10% of postmenopausal women. It is most commonly due to autoimmune thyroiditis or to inadequate correction of hypothyroidism.

Signs and Symptoms. The overt and subtle presentations of the associated abnormalities in thyroid, cardiac, gastrointestinal, neuropsychiatric, and reproductive function are presented in Table 153–1. Goiter, periorbital edema, and dry skin are common but nonspecific. Loss of the lateral third of the eyebrow and a delayed relaxation phase of the deep tendon reflexes are highly sugges-

Table 153–1. CLINICAL EVIDENCE OF THYROID DYSFUNCTION

Hypothyroidism	Hyperthyroidism
Risk Factors	
Family or personal history of thyroid disease	Family or personal history of thyroid disease
Goiter or history of goiter	Goiter or history of goiter
Prior or current thyroid hormone use	Prior or current thyroid hormone use
History of other autoimmune disease	History of other autoimmune disease
	Recent iodine exposure
Clinical Findings	
Fatigue	Fatigue
Weight gain	Weight loss without change in appetite
Cold intolerance	Heat intolerance
Depression or memory impairment	Depression or nervousness, irritability, anxiety, or agitation
Menstrual irregularities (menorrhagia), infertility	Menstrual irregularities (oligomenorrhea)
Weakness, muscle cramps, joint pains	Weakness, tremor
Bradycardia	Tachycardia, palpitations
Hypersomnolence	Exertional dyspnea
Xerosis	Insomnia
Constipation	Moist palms (increased perspiration)
Periorbital puffiness	*Thickening of skin, especially pretibial***
Delayed relaxation phase, deep tendon reflex	Hyperdefecation
Dry coarse hair or alopecia	Bulging eyes (lid retraction or *proptosis*), unblinking stare
Hoarseness	*Eye irritation, periorbital edema, diplopia, change in visual acuity*
Nonpitting edema	Hyperreflexia
The elderly may present atypically with isolated symptoms of fatigue, constipation, weight gain, or depression	Anterior neck pain
	The elderly may present atypically, with "apathetic hyperthyroidism" symptoms resembling hypothyroidism in younger patients; with isolated unexplained weight loss; or with cardiac abnormalities (atrial fibrillation or congestive heart failure)

Italic type indicates signs specific to Graves' disease.
*Infiltrative dermopathy of Graves' disease, confusingly referred to as pretibial myxedema.

tive of hypothyroidism. Because the examination is generally not helpful for diagnosis, there should be a low threshold for laboratory testing in patients with nonspecific symptoms such as fatigue, constipation, and menstrual irregularities.

Clinical Approach. The physical examination should include inspection and palpation of the thyroid gland as well as examination for other signs as discussed earlier. The clinical diagnosis is supported by laboratory testing with the ultrasensitive (third-generation) TSH assay. If the TSH level is elevated, repeat testing may identify transient elevations due to nonthyroidal illnesses. After the TSH elevation is confirmed, a free T_4 level is assessed, either measured directly by T_4 radioimmunoassay or estimated by obtaining a total T_4 and a T_3-resin uptake. Cost determines the choice of methods. The interpretation of test results is presented in Table 153–2.

Initial testing with both TSH and T_4 does not improve the diagnostic accuracy for primary hypothyroidism and is not cost-effective for screening for central hypothyroidism due to the rarity of this condition.

Table 153–2. LABORATORY DIAGNOSIS OF HYPOTHYROIDISM: INTERPRETATION OF TEST RESULTS

Initial Thyroid-Stimulating Hormone (TSH) Test Results and Repeat Results	Implication	Action
Nonspecific Symptoms (e.g., Fatigue, Weight Gain, Constipation)		
Normal	Hypothyroidism unlikely	Seek other causes If high clinical suspicion of subclinical disease, consider retest in 6 mo
Elevated; repeat normal	Transient nonthyroidal illness	
Elevated; repeat elevated < 10 mU/L	Hypothyroidism unlikely Possible subclinical disease	Consider repeat testing in 6 mo
Elevated; repeat elevated 10–15 mU/L	Possible subclinical disease	Consider repeat testing in 6 mo Consider treating if thyroxine is decreased or antithyroid antibodies are positive
Elevated; repeat elevated > 20 mU/L	Subclinical or overt disease	Check free thyroxine: If decreased, treat If normal, consider repeat testing in 6 mo or treat if antithyroid antibodies are positive
Clinically Hypothyroid		
TSH low to normal	? Central hypothyroidism ? Apathetic hyperthyroidism in elderly	Check free thyroxine: If decreased, check thyroid-releasing hormone and refer for endocrine studies If increased, evaluate for hyperthyroidism
TSH elevated; repeat elevated	Primary hypothyroidism	Treat

Antithyroid antibodies are diagnostic of chronic autoimmune thyroiditis, and their presence indicates a high rate of progression from subclinical to overt disease. However, assays for antithyroid peroxidase antibodies have a sensitivity of 85% in patients with Hashimoto's thyroiditis and are insensitive to low levels of antibody in early disease. Thus, the use of this test should be confined to cases of subclinical hypothyroidism in which the presence of antibodies would argue for beginning treatment.

Management. Generic levothyroxine is not recommended for replacement therapy; consistent use of a particular brand of replacement therapy results in more consistent clinical results. Younger patients need 75 to 150 μg/d (1.5 to 1.7 μg/kg) and may begin with a full dose, usually 100 μg/d. In patients older than 50 and those with heart disease or chronic illness, precipitation of heart disease is a concern. These patients should be started on 25 to 50 μg/d. The dose should be increased by 25 μg every 1 to 2 months up to a dose of 75 to 100 μg.

Therapy with levothyroxine should be monitored using TSH (Table 153–3). Early testing may lead to overreplacement, owing to premature efforts to normalize the TSH. Many patients feel better on a dose 50 μg higher than needed to normalize TSH secretion, but overreplacement promotes osteoporosis and may precipitate heart disease.

Poor compliance is the most common reason for inadequate replacement. Other causes include malabsorption or the concomitant use of medications that affect the metabolism of T_4 (e.g., phenytoin, carbamazepine, amiodarone) or interfere with its absorption (e.g., ferrous sulfate, cholestyramine, and antacids).

Appropriate thyroid replacement therapy may correct many of the complications of hypothyroidism, including hypercholesterolemia. Changes in heart rate, weight, and facial puffiness occur after a few weeks of treatment. Hoarseness, hair and skin problems, and anemia may require several months of therapy to normalize. Anemia that is severe or persists after adequate thyroid replacement requires evaluation for other causes, including an associated autoimmune pernicious anemia.

Occasionally a treated patient with "a long history of hypothyroidism" questions the initial diagnosis and the need to continue treatment. Current recommendations are to continue therapy and confirm the diagnosis by means of previous medical records or the presence of antithyroid antibodies. This strategy is preferable to stopping therapy and performing a radioactive iodine uptake and thyroid scan 1 month later. Of note, discontinuation of levothyroxine taken for more than 1 year in an initially misdiagnosed euthyroid patient may result in transient, acute hypothyroidism, secondary to a suppressed pituitary-thyroid axis, which requires 6 weeks to 3 months to correct.

If subclinical thyroid disease is detected, clinicians should follow these patients closely, given the relatively high rate of progression to overt disease. Although the need for treatment of subclinical hypothyroidism is debated, 25% to 50% of affected patients report feeling better while taking levothyroxine.

HYPERTHYROIDISM

Etiology. In the general adult population, hyperthyroidism has an annual incidence of 0.05% to 1%, occurring with an increased frequency in women and

Table 153–3. MONITORING L-THYROXINE THERAPY

Clinical Status	Test Results	Implication	Action
*Initiating Therapy**			
Euthyroid	TSH normal	Adequate replacement or early testing	No change in dose; retest in 6 mo or if symptomatic
	TSH decreased but still elevated	TSH normally corrects slowly	No change in dose; retest in 2–6 mo
Hypothyroid	TSH very elevated	Underreplacement	Patient education; retest in 2–6 mo
	TSH and T_4 elevated	Probable noncompliance	Patient education; retest in 2–6 mo
		Underreplacement	
		Probable noncompliance with increased dosage just before visit	
Hyperthyroid or euthyroid	Suppressed TSH	Overreplacement	Decrease dose; retest in 2–6 mo
On Stable Dose†			
Euthyroid	TSH normal	Adequate replacement	No change in dose; retest in 1 year or if symptomatic
	TSH very elevated	Underreplacement	Patient education; retest in 2–6 mo
		Probable noncompliance	
	TSH slightly elevated < 10 mU/L	Individual or laboratory variation or transient nonthyroidal illness	No change in dose; retest in 1 year or if symptomatic
	TSH mildly elevated > 10 mU/L	Probable underreplacement	Increase dose if no evidence of noncompliance; retest in 2–6 mo
	TSH suppressed	Probable overreplacement	Decrease dose; retest in 2–6 mo; consider testing T_3 if persistent
Hypothyroid	TSH elevated	Underreplacement	Increase dose if no evidence of noncompliance; retest in 2–6 mo
		Possible noncompliance	
	TSH normal	Possible underreplacement	Consider increasing dose; retest in 2–6 mo
		Nonconfirming laboratory test not definitive	
Hyperthyroid	TSH suppressed or normal	Probable overreplacement	Decrease dose; retest in 2–6 mo

TSH, thyroid-stimulating hormone; T_4, thyroxine; T_3, triiodothyronine.

*Check laboratory tests after initiating therapy: 1–3 months, only if noncompliance suspected; 3–6 months, routine.

†Check laboratory tests annually or with symptoms of underreplacement or overreplacement.

the elderly. Hyperthyroidism in individuals over the age of 60 accounts for one third of all cases of thyrotoxicosis. The most common cause of hyperthyroidism is Graves' disease (an immunologically mediated toxic goiter). The peak incidence is in the third and fourth decades with an overall female-to-male ratio of 5:1. Individuals with hyperthyroidism caused by Graves' disease are more likely than control subjects to be smokers (odds ratio, 1.9; 95% confidence interval of 1.1 to 3.2), and an increased incidence and severity of ophthalmopathy is seen in patients with Graves' disease who smoke (odds ratio, 7.7; 95% confidence interval of 4.3 to 13).

In the elderly, toxic nodular goiter is more common than Graves' disease. Other causes of hyperthyroidism include toxic adenoma, postpartum thyroiditis, and exogenous thyroid hormone ingestion.

Subacute thyroiditis is a self-limited disease of viral origin that often follows an upper respiratory tract infection. Transient postpartum thyroid dysfunction occurs in approximately 5% of women in the first 3 to 6 months post partum. Women with preexisting chronic autoimmune thyroiditis are at greatest risk. Postpartum thyroiditis, a self-limited disease, increases the risk of developing primary hypothyroidism.

Signs and Symptoms. The signs and symptoms of hyperthyroidism are attributable to increased adrenergic activity and excess circulating thyroid hormone. The presentation varies, depending on the cause of disease and the age of the patient (see Table 153–1). During the physical examination, special attention should be paid to the presence of lid lag, proximal muscle weakness, tremor, and, if present, the pattern of thyroid enlargement (diffuse in Graves' disease, nodular in toxic nodular goiter). Infiltrative ophthalmopathy or dermopathy, specific to Graves' disease and not present in toxic nodular goiter, should be sought. Subacute thyroiditis commonly presents as local or referred pain and occasionally as fever. The thyroid is tender to palpation, and the erythrocyte sedimentation rate is elevated. Postpartum thyroiditis is generally asymptomatic in both its hyperthyroid and hypothyroid phases. If symptomatic, thyrotoxic symptoms are more likely. Common symptoms of the hypothyroid phase are depression and fatigue. Unlike in subacute thyroiditis, the erythrocyte sedimentation rate is not elevated.

Clinical Approach. Generally, the diagnosis of hyperthyroidism is clinical and is confirmed by laboratory testing. The most effective initial laboratory screening test is an ultrasensitive TSH assay. A high free T_4 (estimated or directly measured) supports the diagnosis. Occasionally, elderly individuals with toxic nodular goiter have a low TSH, a normal free T_4, but an elevated free T_3.

Antithyroid antibodies, seldom necessary to diagnose Graves' disease, may aid in differentiating it from toxic nodular goiter, in which the antibodies are not present. If the cause remains in doubt, measurement of radioactive iodine uptake (increased in Graves' disease and toxic nodular goiter; decreased in thyroiditis or exogenous ingestion) may be helpful. Exogenous thyroid hormone use suppresses thyroglobulin production; suspicions of surreptitious ingestion can be confirmed by low serum thyroglobulin levels.

Management. In hyperthyroidism of any etiology, hyperadrenergic symptoms can be controlled with β-blockers (propranolol, 20 mg three times a day).

In subacute thyroiditis, pain control is achieved with nonsteroidal anti-inflammatory drugs or prednisone, 20–40 mg/d. The hypothyroid stage of postpartum thyroiditis, often misdiagnosed, generally responds to 4 to 6 weeks of levothyroxine replacement therapy.

Consultation with an endocrinologist is generally helpful when treating Graves' disease or toxic nodular goiter. Thyroid ablation with radioactive iodine, antithyroid medication, or surgery is effective. In the United States, radioactive iodine is favored. The major complication is subsequent hypothyroidism in 70% to 100% at 10 years after treatment. No increased risk of leukemia or other cancers as a result of radioactive iodine treatment has been seen. Pregnancy and lactation are contraindications.

Antithyroid medications (methimazole, 10 to 40 mg/d, and propylthiouracil, 100 to 600 mg/d), which block hormone production and conversion of T_4 to T_3, can be used as primary therapy in young or middle-aged patients, during pregnancy (propylthiouracil), or in mild hyperthyroidism. They may also be used to lower hormone levels in preparation for definitive treatment by ablation or surgery. The most common side effects are rash and pruritus; the most serious, agranulocytosis, requires monitoring with a white blood cell count obtained at baseline and after 3 to 6 weeks of therapy. In urgent situations, iodine blocks hormone release immediately.

Surgery is generally reserved for patients who have thyroid cancer or who decline radiation therapy. Complications of surgery include hypoparathyroidism and injury to the recurrent laryngeal nerve.

GOITER

Epidemiology and Etiology. Goiter refers to diffuse or nodular thyroid enlargement irrespective of the underlying function of the thyroid. Nontoxic goiter is the most common, with a prevalence of 4% to 8% of the adult American population. It has an annual incidence of 0.1% to 1.5%, with greater prevalence in women (4:1) and with advancing age. Common causes of goiters associated with thyroid dysfunction include Graves' disease and Hashimoto's thyroiditis. Less common causes of goiter are hyperthyroidism of other causes, goitrogens including iodine and lithium, familial goiter, and malignancy. Due to dietary iodine supplementation, iodine deficiency goiter is rare in the United States; it is more common internationally, particularly in rural, inland areas.

Signs and Symptoms. Most goiters, particularly small ones, are asymptomatic; however, symptoms may range from a mild cosmetic annoyance to mechanical compression or displacement of the trachea and esophagus with symptoms of neck discomfort, choking, or cough that may worsen when the arms are raised overhead. Tracheal deviation may be observed on the chest radiograph. Sudden hemorrhage into a nodule may induce pain and worsening mechanical compression. If the goiter is associated with thyroid dysfunction, symptoms of hyperthyroidism or hypothyroidism may be present.

Clinical Approach. The mean weight of the thyroid gland in an iodine-supplemented population is 10 g or less with an upper-normal size of 20 g, or a volume of approximately 2 to 4 teaspoons. Clinical examination should include anterior and lateral inspection and palpation of the thyroid, to categorize the gland as "goiter ruled out" (normal size or small [one to two times normal] with lateral prominence 2 mm or less), "goiter ruled in" (large [> two times normal] or lateral prominence > 2 mm), or "inconclusive." If a goiter is clinically detectable, the positive likelihood ratio of one's being present by ultrasound evaluation is 3.8 (95% confidence interval of 3.3 to 4.5); if one is clinically not present, there is a negative likelihood ratio of 0.37 (95% confidence interval of 0.33 to 0.40). The pattern of thyroid enlargement, diffuse or with a distinct nodule or nodules, should be noted. Thyroid function should be assessed with an ultrasensitive TSH assay.

Management. Correction of underlying thyroid function abnormality including replacement therapy for hypothyroidism may cause the gland size to normalize. Suppressive doses of thyroid hormone may shrink the goiter of autoimmune thyroiditis and possibly prevent disease progression. Data on the efficacy of suppressive therapy in reducing the size or rate of growth of solitary, benign nodules (which spontaneously regress in 30% to 50% of cases) are conflicting. A trial period of therapy for 6 months to 1 year is reasonable except in postmenopausal women, elderly men, and other patients at risk for osteoporosis or heart disease.

Untreated multinodular goiter tends to progress to hyperthyroidism over 15 to 25 years because of the growth in number and size of autonomously functioning nodules. Suppressive therapy with thyroid hormone should not be used in a patient with a nodular goiter and low-to-normal TSH concentrations because the additional thyroid hormone may precipitate hyperthyroidism. If treatment is needed in these patients, radioactive iodine therapy or surgery is indicated.

THYROID CANCER

Epidemiology and Etiology. Thyroid cancer is rare (annual incidence of 0.004%), with low associated morbidity and mortality. In the United States there are 12,000 new cases of thyroid cancer and 1,000 thyroid cancer–related deaths annually. The most common and least aggressive type of thyroid cancer is papillary (75%), followed, in order of decreasing frequency and increasing invasiveness, by follicular (15%), medullary (5%), and anaplastic (3%). Almost all thyroid cancer (95%) presents as a thyroid nodule or a neck mass.

Thyroid nodules are common (prevalence 4%). Half of the thyroid glands examined by ultrasound or direct visualization (surgery or autopsy) have nodules. Physical examination detects approximately 10% of the nodules found by these methods. Nodules increase in frequency with age and are four times more likely in women than men. Less than 5% of all nodules are cancerous.

Rationale for Screening. The incidence of cancer in a solitary nodule in an individual with prior head, neck, or chest irradiation, other than radioactive ablation of the thyroid, is approximately 50%. The incidence of cancer attributable to prior radiation exposure of the thyroid to doses of 6.5 to 1500 rads ranges from 0.11% to 7%, respectively. Lesser risk factors include a family history of thyroid cancer or familial polyposis, male gender, and extremes of age (< 20 or > 60 years old).

Screening Strategy. Annual clinical examination of the thyroid is indicated in adults with a history of radiation to the head or neck.

Clinical Approach. Because most nodules are asymptomatic, the history should assess risk factors. Explicit questioning may elicit a history of therapeutic radiation, used in the past to treat adenoiditis, tonsillitis, otitis media, acne, and tinea capitis. On physical examination, a firm solitary nodule or an enlarged regional lymph node is suspicious. A palpable, hypofunctioning nodule found in a patient with Graves' disease is likely to be malignant. Rapid tumor growth and signs of local invasion (hoarseness, dysphasia, or obstruction) are rare but strongly suggestive of cancer.

A fine-needle aspiration biopsy, done by an experienced practitioner, is the most cost-effective initial evaluation of a solitary nodule. An ultrasensitive TSH assay should be obtained to detect unsuspected hyperthyroidism.

Management. Patients with malignant cytology or significant obstructive or compressive symptoms should be referred for surgery. Suppressive therapy with levothyroxine, resulting in a TSH level of 0.1 or lower, is indicated after thyroid cancer surgery to prevent thyrotropin stimulation of any remaining cancerous cells.

An inadequate sample on fine-needle aspiration requires repeat testing. A patient with indeterminate results should undergo radionuclide scanning to determine the function of the nodule. A cold or warm functioning nodule requires surgery, whereas a hot nodule can be observed.

A nodule with benign cytology may be observed clinically, with consideration of repeat fine-needle aspiration in the future. The use of suppressive therapy with thyroid hormone for these nodules remains controversial.

Cross-References: Hyperlipidemia (Chapter 152), Management of Depression (Chapter 189), Thyroid Disorders in Pregnancy (Chapter 216), Preoperative Endocrine Problems (Chapter 220).

REFERENCES

1. Gharib H, Goellner JR. Fine needle aspiration biopsy of the thyroid: An appraisal. Ann Intern Med 1993;118:282–289.

   Fine-needle aspiration was found safe, accurate, and cost-effective as an initial test for thyroid nodules.

2. Helfand M, Crapo LM. Monitoring therapy in patients taking levothyroxine. Ann Intern Med 1990;113:450–454.

   One study showed average TSH after 4 months of therapy was elevated at 25 mU/L; another showed that changes based on this TSH finding resulted in overtreatment in 40% of patients.

3. Schectman JM, Pawlson LG. The cost-effectiveness of three thyroid function testing strategies for suspicion of hypothyroidism in a primary setting. J Gen Intern Med 1990;5:9–15.

   Analysis of cost-effectiveness recommends first testing for suspected hypothyroidism with TSH due to greater sensitivity (TSH [sensitivity = 99%, specificity = 98%] vs. T_4 [sensitivity = 93%, specificity = 68%]) with only a small increase in cost. This is consistent with findings of the American Thyroid Association, the American Association of Clinical Endocrinologists, and the American College of Endocrinology but differs from those of the American College of Physicians, which finds equal sensitivity of tests and decreased cost with T_4 in most cases.

4. Schneider DL, Barrett Connor EL, Morton DJ. Thyroid hormone use and bone mineral density in elderly women: Effects of estrogen. JAMA 1994; 271:1245–1249.

Osteopenia secondary to thyroxine doses of greater than 200 μg/d was negated by estrogen in postmenopausal women. Whether a thyroxine-induced decrease in bone mineral density translates into an increased fracture rate is still unknown.

5. Siminoski K. Does this patient have a goiter? JAMA 1995;273:813–817.

This article describes a rational clinical exam for goiter and reasons for doing it.

6. Singer PA, Cooper DS, Levy EG, Ladenson PW, Braverman LE, Daniels G, Greenspan FS, McDougall IR, Nikolai TF. Treatment guidelines for patients with hyperthyroidism and hypothyroidism. Standards of Care Committee, American Thyroid Association. JAMA 1995;273:808–812.

A comprehensive review of current expert-based guidelines for clinical practice is presented.

7. US Preventive Task Force. Guide to clinical preventive services, 2nd ed. Baltimore, Williams & Wilkins, 1996.

This provides up-to-date evidence-based recommendations for screening.

■ ■

154 Diabetes Mellitus

Problem

DAWN E. DeWITT

Epidemiology and Etiology. Diabetes mellitus is a common chronic illness, affecting 6% to 8% of the general population older than age 40. Patients with diabetes often develop complications including retinopathy, nephropathy, neuropathy, and cardiovascular disease. Type 1 diabetes, or insulin-dependent diabetes (IDDM), accounts for approximately 10% of all cases. The prevalence of type 2 diabetes, or non–insulin-dependent diabetes (NIDDM), is estimated at over 14 million cases, with over half this number thought to be relatively asymptomatic and therefore often undiagnosed.

Diabetes is generally classified as type 1 diabetes if patients require insulin to prevent ketoacidosis. Type 1 diabetes usually presents before age 30 in lean individuals. The pathophysiology of type 1 diabetes is thought to involve both a genetic predisposition and an environmental trigger event, such as a viral illness, resulting in autoimmune destruction of the pancreatic islet beta cells. Although not recommended routinely, insulin levels can be obtained and should be low in type 1 diabetes.

Type 2 diabetes is associated with obesity, especially central adiposity, and peripheral insulin resistance with abnormal, but not absent, insulin secretion. Onset is typically after age 30. A family history of diabetes in first-degree relatives is common. Other risk factors include previous gestational diabetes (3% of all pregnancies with up to 50% of patients developing overt diabetes at 7 years), race (Native American, Hispanic, black), a history of glucose intolerance, hypertension, and significant dyslipidemia. Many drugs, including corticosteroids, thiazides, niacin, and β-blockers, may produce glucose intolerance.

Criteria for diagnosis in adults include a single plasma glucose level greater than or equal to 200 mg/dL with any symptom such as polydipsia, polyuria, polyphagia, or weight loss; or a fasting plasma glucose greater than or equal to 126 mg/dL on two occasions. Blood glucose meters are accurate only within ± 20 mg/dL; values that suggest diabetes should be verified with plasma glucose measurements. Glycated hemoglobin assays are too insensitive to use for diagnosis. Oral glucose tolerance tests may be used to confirm a diagnosis but are generally not indicated except for screening for gestational diabetes. Care should be taken when evaluating hospitalized or ill patients or those on medications known to cause glucose intolerance. Because the average duration of type 2 diabetes before diagnosis is 10 to 12 years, the American Diabetes Association recommends screening high-risk individuals with one or more risk factors (obesity, age > 45, family history) every 3 years. Screening of the general population is not recommended. Ideally, screening should include risk factor evaluation with fasting plasma glucose testing (if the result is ≥ 115 mg/dL, the patient should be referred for follow-up and surveillance testing). The US Preventive Services Task Force does not recommend screening of nonpregnant, asymptomatic adults but notes that surveillance may be appropriate in persons who are morbidly obese, those with a family history of diabetes, or women with a history of gestational diabetes; it cites poor sensitivity of screening with random or fasting glucose levels and conflicting evidence regarding progression of disease with early hypoglycemic therapy.

Symptoms and Signs. Patients younger than 20 years old with type 1 diabetes usually present with an abrupt illness, often ketoacidosis, precipitated by an acute stressor such as a bacterial infection. They may complain of nausea, vomiting, and abdominal pain with polyuria and polydipsia. Patients may be obtunded with Kussmaul's breathing, acetone breath, hypotension, and tachycardia. Laboratory findings include hyperglycemia, an anion-gap acidosis, elevated serum acetone, and hyperkalemia. Older patients may describe malaise, weight loss, polydipsia, and polyuria over a longer time period.

Patients with type 2 diabetes more commonly present with polyuria, polydipsia, weight loss, or symptoms caused by end-organ complications such as retinopathy, nephropathy, or neuropathy. Many patients are asymptomatic, and hyperglycemia is detected with random blood glucose measurements. Ketoacidosis is rare. Hyperosmolar coma is a life-threatening condition caused by dehydration due to osmotic diureses in conjunction with poor oral intake. The patient, often elderly, is usually confused or comatose and must be admitted for hydration and insulin therapy because mortality is high.

Clinical Approach. Initial evaluation should include a thorough history with special attention to the onset of symptoms, current symptoms, family history, risk factors for cardiovascular disease, other medical diagnoses, previous treatment, medications, diet, history of ketoacidosis or hypoglycemia, weight control, and previous studies, such as glycated hemoglobin results, eye examinations, and assessment of proteinuria. The physical examination should focus on weight (growth for adolescents) and body type, an eye examination for retinopathy, a thyroid examination, a cardiovascular examination including blood pressure, an abdominal examination, a skin and foot examination for deformities or lesions such as ulcers, evidence of acanthosis nigricans (indicates insulin resistance), skin infections, lipohypertrophy from insulin injections, and a neurologic examination with monofilament testing for sensory loss. Laboratory testing should include glucose, creatinine, and electrolyte determinations; urinalysis for 24-hour protein measurements or spot albumin/creatinine ratios; fasting lipid levels; and thyroid function tests. A standardized glycated hemoglobin level, also commonly referred to (incorrectly because they are not technically equal) as glycosylated hemoglobin or HgbA$_{1c}$, should be obtained as a baseline.

Management. In the Diabetes Control and Complications Trial (DCCT), patients with type 1 diabetes who were treated with intensive therapy were 50% to 75% less likely to have progression of retinopathy, nephropathy, and neuropathy than those receiving conventional treatment. These results have led to the recommendation that all patients with type 1 diabetes be treated with the goal of near-normalization of blood glucose level and a glycated hemoglobin value less than or equal to 7% (plasma glucose of approximately 150 mg/dL) when normal is 4% to 6% ($<$ 115 mg/dL). Treatment should be individualized for each patient and should include frequent self-monitoring of blood glucose level, attention to diet with nutrition counseling, regular exercise, multiple insulin injections, and education regarding complications of type 1 diabetes and hypoglycemia. A glycated hemoglobin level should be obtained two to four times per year, and a dilated eye examination for retinopathy and testing for nephropathy should be conducted at least annually after 5 years of diabetes. Although urinalysis will detect macroalbuminuria (1+ equals 300 mg/24 h), a timed urine collection is needed to accurately detect and quantify microalbuminuria (30–300 mg/24 h). Screening may be accomplished with an albumin/creatinine ratio. False-positive results for microalbuminuria may occur in patients with poor glycemic control or after heavy exercise. Foot examinations should be done at least annually, and patients should check their feet daily.

Intensive diabetes therapy for type 1 diabetes uses a team approach with multiple insulin injections, frequent self-monitoring of blood glucose levels, and careful attention to nutrition and exercise. Insulin regimens and algorithms have become more sophisticated, and insulin pumps (continuous subcutaneous insulin infusion) are now available. Pharmacokinetic issues are important to understanding insulin use. In general, human insulin has a quicker onset of action and a shorter duration of action than animal insulin. Insulin absorption varies widely (25%–50%) among persons and from injection to injection in any given patient. Insulin is absorbed most quickly from the abdomen and more slowly (in decreasing order) from the arm, thigh, and buttock. Lipohypertrophy may increase absorption duration. Lag time refers to the amount of time from the injection of insulin to the consumption of food. Varying injection sites and lag times can aid in blood glucose control. For example, because insulin is most effective when blood glucose is already falling, a patient with a high fasting blood glucose level before breakfast might inject insulin in the abdomen and use a relatively long lag time before eating. The use of an insulin pump circumvents many of these pharmacokinetic issues by providing one type of insulin (i.e., usually regular) at a consistent site.

Patients with new-onset type 1 diabetes may need to be referred to a specialist for initiation of therapy. Some patients may need hospitalization.

Newly diagnosed patients generally require less insulin because endogenous insulin secretion may continue for weeks, months, or even years. When beginning a patient on a new insulin regimen, the dosage should be estimated on weight with approximately half to two thirds of the total daily insulin dose designed to cover basal needs, primarily gluconeogenesis, and the rest to cover caloric intake from meals and snacks. Table 154–1 summarizes insulin formulations and the cost of insulin and supplies. Most patients should be started on 0.5 to 1.0 unit/kg, although active patients near ideal body weight often require smaller doses. Many regimens are available, including twice-daily "split-mix" regimens, multiple daytime regular insulin injections with bedtime intermediate insulin, basal ultralente insulin with multiple regular insulin injections at mealtimes, and continuous subcutaneous insulin infusion. Which regimen is best depends on the patient's willingness to perform frequent self-monitoring of blood glucose levels and use multiple injections, the risk of hypoglycemia, and the patient's lifestyle. Continuous subcutaneous insulin infusion may be useful for patients who wish to achieve near-normal glycemia (although studies have not shown a significant improvement with continuous infusion versus multiple injections) or for those with gastroparesis or hypoglycemia unawareness in whom predictable, higher target glucose levels may be needed. In general, insulin doses should be raised no more often than every few days. Close communication between health care provider and patient

Table 154–1. INSULIN FORMULATIONS AND PHARMACOKINETICS AND INSULIN SUPPLIES

Drugs and Supplies	Action	Onset (h)	Peak (h)	Duration (h)	Quantity	Cost ($)*
Insulin, lispro†	Very rapid	5–15 min (0.1–0.25 h)	0.5–1.5	≤ 5	100 U/mL 10 mL	26.25‡
Insulin, regular (Humulin R)	Rapid	0.5–1	1–5	5–8	100 U/mL 10 mL	17.42
Insulin, NPH (Humulin N)	Intermediate	1–4	4–12	24–28	100 U/mL 10 mL	17.42
Insulin, ultralente (Humulin U)	Prolonged	2–6	7–10	24–26	100 U/mL 10 mL	17.42
Insulin 70/30 (Humulin 70/30)	Intermediate/rapid	1–3	6–15	22–28	100 U/mL 10 mL	17.42
Lancets (Monojet)					Box of 200	12.80‡
Basic glucometer§					1	50.00
Strips§					Box of 50	38.85‡
Alcohol wipes					Box of 200	5.60‡
Insulin syringes (LoDose)¶					0.5 mL (50 units) Box of 100	21.47
Insulin syringes (1 mL)¶					1 mL (100 units) Box of 100	21.47

*Average wholesale price, 1995 *Drug Topics Red Book.*
†Available by prescription only.
‡UW price; may be less than average wholesale price owing to direct buying contracts with manufacturers.
§One Touch.
¶B-D MicroFine syringes.

regarding therapy decisions should include attention to exercise, diet, intercurrent illness, and concurrent medications that affect insulin needs. The patient and family should be educated about hypoglycemia and the use of glucose or glucagon to reverse hypoglycemia.

There are only small trials similar to the DCCT to guide therapy for type 2 diabetes. However, the pathophysiology of diabetes complications is similar, and experts now recommend similar treatment goals (glycated hemoglobin ≤ 7.0), allowing for individualization of treatment. Treatment should initially be based on dietary management, weight loss, and exercise. The ideal diet for type 2 diabetes is high in complex carbohydrates and low in refined sugars and fat. The importance of caloric restriction cannot be overstated. Sulfonylureas and insulin may be added when indicated but have been associated with weight gain and therefore increased management problems. In most patients with type 2 diabetes, initial therapy may include diet and an oral agent such as a sulfonylurea, metformin, or acarbose. Table 154–2 summarizes commonly used oral agents. The main goals of treatment should include relief of symptoms and minimizing the risk of complications.

Patients who are asymptomatic, are near ideal body weight, have no complications, and present with a fasting glucose level of 200 mg/dL or less may do well with dietary management alone. Conversely, patients who are symptomatic,

Table 154–2. ORAL AGENTS FOR TREATMENT OF TYPE 2 DIABETES

Agent	Site and Action	Side Effects	Dosage	Cost ($)*
Sulfonylureas†	Pancreas: ↑ insulin secretion	Hypoglycemia, weight gain	Chlorpropamide, 100–500 mg/d	100 mg: 2.39
			Glyburide, 1.25–20 mg/d	2.5 mg: 9.63
			Glipizide, 2.5–40 mg/d	5 mg: 9.17
Metformin (biguanides)†	Liver and muscle: ↓ hepatic glucose output, ↑ muscle glucose uptake	Anorexia, nausea, diarrhea, lactic acidosis (rare)	1000–2550 mg/d divided bid–tid	500 mg: 13.88 850 mg: 23.60
Acarbose (α-glucosidase inhibitor)†	Small intestine: delays carbohydrate digestion, ↓ HgBA$_{1e}$ by 0.5–1%	Flatulence, diarrhea, abdominal discomfort (↓ symptoms over time) ↑ AST, ALT, bilirubin (rare)	12.5–300 mg qd–tid; begin with 12.5–25 mg tid with first bite of meal and increase to 50–100 mg tid	50 mg: 13.68 100 mg: 17.64
Troglitazone (thiazolindinediones)	↓ Hepatic glucose output, ↓ insulin resistance, ↑ peripheral glucose uptake (must be taken with food)	Nausea, vomiting, diarrhea, skin rash (ineffective in 25% of patients)	200–400 mg qd	400 mg: 160.20

AST, aspartate transaminase; ALT, alanine transaminase.
*Cost per month. Average wholesale price, 1997 *Drug Topics Red Book.*
†Contraindicated in pregnancy.

have complications, or present with fasting glucose measurements over 300 mg/dL often respond poorly to oral agents, and insulin, in addition to diet, is appropriate initial therapy. Approximately one third of patients with type 2 diabetes will eventually need insulin therapy; despite initial resistance, many patients feel better on insulin and will achieve better glycemic control.

Nonobese patients who need more than dietary treatment should be started on sulfonylureas, which stimulate pancreatic insulin secretion and decrease insulin resistance. First-generation sulfonylureas, such as chlorpropamide, although inexpensive, are used infrequently, due to their very long half-life and risk of hypoglycemia, especially in the elderly. Low doses should be used, and care should be taken in elderly patients or those with impaired renal or hepatic function. Medication doses should be increased weekly with self-monitoring of blood glucose levels; if after several weeks control is still poor on moderate doses of sulfonylureas, insulin or combination therapy should be considered. Weight gain is a problem with both sulfonylureas and insulin. Institution of bedtime lente or NPH insulin in combination with sulfonylureas or metformin may be helpful and may result in less weight gain than twice-daily insulin alone. Combination oral therapy (e.g., sulfonylureas plus metformin) has been somewhat effective in obese patients, and consultation may be necessary to determine the best combination of doses and medications. The presence of intercurrent illness and medications that exacerbate hyperglycemia may necessitate short-term insulin use. Self-monitoring of blood glucose levels should be performed on a daily basis by all patients on insulin therapy (usually two to four times a day depending on the insulin regimen). Patients on oral agents should monitor their glucose level as needed for dose adjustment and control. Glycated hemoglobin should be measured semiannually for patients who are stable on oral agents and quarterly for those on insulin.

Patients with type 1 or type 2 diabetes need careful counseling and surveillance for complications of microvascular and macrovascular disease. In addition to the recommendations given earlier for type 1 diabetes, all patients with type 2 diabetes should be screened at diagnosis for complications (10% to 15% have neuropathy and 37% have retinopathy at diagnosis) and then yearly thereafter. Because coronary artery disease (present at diagnosis in 50% of patients with type 2 diabetes) may present with atypical symptoms, silent myocardial infarction is common, and over 58% of patients with type 2 diabetes die of cardiovascular disease, careful attention should be paid to cardiovascular or respiratory complaints. Smoking cessation should be stressed.

Angiotensin-converting enzyme (ACE) inhibitors and aggressive control of hypertension (goal, 130/85 mm Hg) have been shown to markedly reduce the progression of nephropathy. β-blockers and thiazide diuretics are poor choices for initial treatment of hypertension in patients with diabetes due to their adverse effects on glycemic control and lipids. Dietary protein restriction is controversial. Hyperlipidemia should be treated aggressively; fibrates and HMG-CoA reductase inhibitors are used most commonly. Gastroparesis is most commonly treated with metoclopramide or cisapride. Erythromycin, a gastric irritant, may be helpful. Painful diabetic polyneuropathy may respond to topical capsaicin cream, tricyclic antidepressants, antiseizure medications, or mexiletine. Skin infections and foot lesions should be treated aggressively to prevent significant morbidity.

Follow-Up. Patients should be seen at least twice a year if stable on oral agents and at least quarterly if stable on insulin. Education plays a key role for the patient and the clinician in the management of diabetes. All patients should be evaluated for complications at follow-up visits and have a glycated hemoglobin measurement to assess glucose control over the preceding 2 to 3 months. The patient's feet should be examined at every visit. Referrals to a nurse educator, nutritionist, podiatrist, or subspecialist should be made as needed. All patients with diabetes who become pregnant, patients with gestational diabetes, patients with advanced nephropathy, and patients with retinopathy should be referred to a specialist.

Cross-References: Obesity (Chapter 15), Unintentional Weight Loss (Chapter 17), Diabetic Retinopathy (Chapter 44), Ophthalmoscopy (Chapter 46), Diarrhea (Chapter 91), Constipation (Chapter 93), Ankle and Foot Pain (Chapter 112), Diabetic Foot Care Education (Chapter 124), Leg Ulcers (Chapter 133), Local Care of Diabetic Foot Lesions (Chapter 134), Peripheral Neuropathy (Chapter 147), Erectile Dysfunction (Chapter 169), Chronic Renal Failure (Chapter 179), Proteinuria (Chapter 181), Diabetes Mellitus in Pregnancy (Chapter 212), Gestational Diabetes Mellitus (Chapter 213), Preoperative Endocrine Problems (Chapter 220).

REFERENCES

1. American Diabetes Association. Clinical practice recommendations. Diabetes Care 1995;18(suppl 1):1–96.

   Update of the ADA's position statement with practical guidelines for care includes insulin administration, blood glucose monitoring, treatment of hospitalized patients, and consensus statements.

2. Diabetes Control and Complications Trial Research Group. The effect of intensive treatment of diabetes on the development and progression of long-term complications in insulin-dependent diabetes mellitus. N Engl J Med 1993;329:977–986.

   A large prospective randomized trial demonstrated that intensive diabetes therapy decreased the rates of microvascular and neuropathic complications of diabetes in patients with type 1 diabetes.

3. Diabetes Mellitus in America, 2nd ed. NIH publication No. 95–1468, Bethesda, MD, National Institutes of Health and National Institute of Diabetes and Digestive and Kidney Diseases, 1995.

   This is a compendium of current information on diabetes mellitus.

4. Hirsch IB. Implementation of intensive diabetes therapy for IDDM. Diabetes Rev 1995;3:288–307.

   A detailed, practical review of intensive therapy includes a detailed discussion of insulin regimens and algorithms. The bibliography is extensive.

5. Report of a Joint Working Party of the British Diabetic Association, The Research Unit of the Royal College of Physicians, and the Royal College of General Practitioners. Guidelines for good practice in the diagnosis and treatment of non–insulin-dependent diabetes mellitus. J R Coll Phys 1993;27:259–266.

   A practical guide is presented for treatment of type 2 diabetes, with blood glucose goals and review of methods and medications.

6. The Expert Committee on the Diagnosis and Classification of Diabetes Mellitus. Report of the Expert Committee on the Diagnosis and Classification of Diabetes Mellitus. Diabetes Care 1997;20(7):1183–1197.

   These new guidelines for diagnosis and classification are considered standard of care by most groups. Guidelines for screening and testing are discussed.

155 Female Infertility

Problem

TERRIE MENDELSON

Epidemiology and Etiology. Infertility has a prevalence of 10% to 15% in industrially developed countries, and half of infertile couples will never bear as many children as they desire. There has been no significant change in the incidence of infertility over the past several decades, but the absolute number of couples seeking evaluation has increased dramatically because the large "baby boom" generation is reaching its late reproductive years and American women are increasingly choosing to delay childbearing. One in five American women is delivered of her first child after age 35, when the prevalence of infertility is 33%; it rises to over 50% after age 40. Episodes of primary or secondary infertility occur in 25% of women, causing significant psychological and economic hardship in many cases.

Infertility refers to the inability of a heterosexual couple to achieve pregnancy after 1 year of frequent, unprotected intercourse. Primary infertility is diagnosed in an infertile couple when there is no prior pregnancy history, whereas secondary infertility denotes that the female partner has previously been pregnant. The term *sterility* connotes an absolute inability to conceive. In describing rates of pregnancy and childbirth, *fecundability* defines the probability of achieving pregnancy within one menstrual cycle, whereas *fecundity* refers to the likelihood of achieving live birth.

Fertility is maximal in both women and men in the early 20s. Age-associated decreases in fecundability and fecundity in women are substantial after age 40. The average pregnancy rate for fertile young couples having frequent, unprotected intercourse is 25% in the first month, 57% by 3 months, 70% at 6 months, and 85% within 1 year. Half of all couples presenting after 1 year of infertility will become pregnant without treatment during the following year. The 25% fecundability rate for women at age 20 falls to 15% at age 30 and 10% by age 35; fecundity falls even more rapidly as the result of a spontaneous abortion rate that reaches 34% by the early 40s.

Among infertile couples, male factors account for 35% of cases, and 10% remain unexplained. Causes of female infertility include tubal obstruction or pelvic pathology (40%), ovulatory dysfunction (40%), and cervical mucus or anatomic causes (10%). Infertility is polyfactorial in many cases.

Symptoms and Signs. Thorough histories from both partners should focus on symptoms and signs that suggest the etiology of the infertility (Table 155–1). The female's ovulatory function should be assessed by menstrual cycle length and regularity and by inquiring about indirect indicators of ovulation such as mittelschmerz, midcycle cervical mucus change, and molimina. A history of hirsutism, obesity, and menstrual irregularity suggests polycystic ovary disease

Table 155-1. DIFFERENTIAL DIAGNOSIS: FEMALE INFERTILITY

Ovulatory Dysfunction	*Uterine Dysfunction*
Age-related oligo-ovulation	Leiomyoma
Inadequate follicle development	Asherman's syndrome
Pituitary tumor	Bicornuate uterus
Premature ovarian failure	
Luteal phase deficiency	*Cervical Dysfunction*
Polycystic ovaries	Abnormal cervical mucus
Hypothyroidism	Inflammation/infection
Hypothalamic dysfunction	Antisperm antibodies
Tubal Dysfunction	
Pelvic inflammatory disease	
Pelvic adhesions	
Endometriosis	

or adrenal hyperplasia. Galactorrhea and infrequent menses may indicate a prolactin-secreting pituitary adenoma. A history of prior abdominopelvic surgery, use of an intrauterine device, complicated ectopic pregnancy, sexually transmitted disease, and pelvic inflammatory disease are risk factors for tubal obstruction. Pelvic pain may indicate endometriosis. Symptoms of hypothyroidism or hyperthyroidism may correlate with ovulatory dysfunction. Social habits, including the use of marijuana, cocaine, tobacco, alcohol, and caffeine, should be assessed. Only very high doses (> 700 mg/d) of caffeine are associated with subfertility. Physical examination should assess for evidence of thyroid dysfunction, hirsutism, and uterine, adnexal, or cervical anatomic abnormalities.

Clinical Approach. Before embarking on an extensive workup, the clinician should provide a realistic estimate of the prognosis for conception based on the couple's medical history, age, and desired level of therapeutic aggressiveness. Because infertility services are not covered by most health plans, many couples may opt for empirical therapy rather than an expensive evaluation that may be inconclusive. At the initial visit, the frequency and timing of coitus should be discussed and the couple should be encouraged to maintain a frequency of intercourse of three to four times per week without undue focus on precise timing. Further evaluation of infertility relies on an adequate understanding and investigation of the requirements for normal fertility (Table 155-2). A minimal evaluation assesses sperm count and motility, ovulatory adequacy, and tubal patency.

If the medical histories are unrevealing, the initial workup should be

Table 155-2. REQUIREMENTS FOR NORMAL FERTILITY

1. Sufficient number of progressively motile sperm to penetrate the cervical mucus and reach the ampulla of the fallopian tube to fertilize the oocyte
2. Normal cervical mucus and uterine/tubal transport
3. Timely release of a mature oocyte
4. Effective uptake and transport of the oocyte by normal fallopian tubes
5. Normal hormonal production by the ovary to support endometrial development and implantation

focused on the male partner, because the differential diagnosis is short and the evaluation relatively easy and inexpensive. Semen analysis should be performed on a freshly collected sample obtained after 2 or 3 days of abstinence and should be evaluated for sperm count, motility, and morphology according to the World Health Organization criteria; abnormalities should be confirmed on a second sample (see Chapter 156, Male Infertility).

Laboratory evaluation for the female should include a screening Papanicolaou smear, determination of thyroid-stimulating hormone level, and tests for infection with *Chlamydia trachomatis* or *Neisseria gonorrhoeae,* as indicated. Serum gonadotropin (follicle-stimulating hormone [FSH] and luteinizing hormone [LH]) and prolactin levels are indicated if menses are infrequent or irregular. Day 3 FSH and estradiol levels are the best predictors of fertility potential; an FSH level greater than 25 mIU/L or estradiol of more than 80 pg/mL correlates with a poor prognosis for spontaneous pregnancy or response to ovulation induction. Androgen panels are useful only if hirsutism is present. Although female antisperm serum antibodies are detectable in a small percentage of women, their evaluation is not recommended because they correlate poorly with pregnancy rates. Pelvic ultrasound is indicated only for evaluation of palpable uterine or adnexal enlargement.

Ovulation is most easily and inexpensively monitored by basal body temperature charting: the woman is instructed to measure and record her sublingual temperature on first awakening each morning before any physical activity. A biphasic pattern with a 0.5- to 1.0-degree temperature rise during the luteal phase allows retrospective identification of probable ovulation, although the technique is inadequately accurate for use as a guide to timed intercourse because correlation with the LH surge varies by as much as 2 or 3 days. Basal body temperature charts are useful, however, in estimating luteal phase length and may confirm ovulation in women with regular menses and biphasic temperature patterns. Ovulation predictor kits using enzyme-linked immunosorbent assays are accurate and widely available but expensive ($25–$50 per month) and inconvenient, requiring urine testing on 4 or 5 sequential days beginning 3 to 4 days before ovulation. A midluteal serum progesterone level greater than 10 ng/mL provides good evidence for an ovulatory cycle. Endometrial biopsy is seldom required to confirm ovulation.

Luteal phase deficiency (LPD), a recurrent postovulatory deficiency in corpus luteum progesterone production (or, rarely, in endometrial sensitivity to progesterone), results in an inadequate hormonal milieu for implantation and maintenance of early pregnancy. LPD is associated with recurrent pregnancy loss and is thought to be a common cause of infertility. Evaluation for LPD should include measurement of both luteal phase length and progesterone production. Luteal phase length is estimated by calculating the time between ovulation (identified by basal body temperature or LH surge) and onset of subsequent menses; normal luteal phase length is 14 days. A shortened luteal phase should not be considered significant unless present for two or more consecutive cycles. A single midluteal phase serum progesterone level of less than 10 ng/mL is 86% sensitive and 83% specific for diagnosing LPD; three assays totaling less than 30 ng/mL during the 5 to 9 days after the LH surge are 100% sensitive and 80% specific.

The postcoital test is designed to evaluate the quality and quantity of cervical mucus, as well as the ability of sperm to penetrate and survive passage through the mucus barrier. The test is performed during the immediate pre-ovulatory period, as predicted by basal body temperature or ovulation predictor kits, and involves examination of cervical mucus within 2 to 8 hours of unpro-tected coitus. An adequate cervical mucus sample should be at least 2 cm in length, demonstrate spinnbarkeit (stretchability) to 8 to 10 cm, and demon-strate prominent ferning when dried on a slide. The finding of more than 20 motile sperm per high-power field denotes a favorable prognosis and correlates well with a sperm concentration of more than 20 million/mL. Although the test is inexpensive and simple to perform, its clinical utility has been called into question, because the therapeutic implications of both normal and abnor-mal tests are identical (intrauterine insemination).

Because up to 50% of women with tubal obstruction have no identifiable risk factors, the hysterosalpingogram is essential to evaluate tubal patency. It also identifies uterine anatomic abnormalities. The procedure is performed by injecting radiopaque dye into the endometrial cavity through a small catheter inserted into the cervical os to fill the uterus and tubes and observe spillage into the peritoneum. If at least unilateral tubal patency is not clearly demonstrated, exploratory laparoscopy is indicated as the final diagnostic procedure for detection of pelvic adhesions or unrecognized endometriosis. The diagnosis and severity of endometriosis discriminates poorly in terms of pregnancy out-come, but therapeutic lysis of adhesions or relief of distal tubal obstruction may result in a 50% or greater pregnancy rate after the procedure.

The pace of evaluation is highly dependent on the age of the woman: in a woman younger than age 30, establishment of the ovulatory pattern by history and basal body temperature monitoring over a 3- to 6-month period is suggested before proceeding with any further evaluation. In a woman older than age 35, fertility may decline rapidly during the course of a prolonged evaluation. After a normal initial evaluation including semen analysis, addi-tional tests may be carried out in any convenient order over a time course dictated by the couple's wishes, financial situation, prognosis, and age (Table 155–3).

Management. If the serum FSH is less than 40 mIU/L and endogenous estrogen is adequate, therapy begins with clomiphene citrate (Clomid), which induces ovulation in 90% of such women. From an initial dosage of 50 mg/d on days 5 through 10 of the menstrual cycle, the dose is increased to 150 mg/d if pregnancy is not achieved, at which point human chorionic gonadotropin (hCG) may be given intramuscularly 1 week after ovulation to facilitate follicle release. Forty percent of oligo-ovulatory women will become pregnant with clomiphene therapy. Complications include nausea, dizziness, headache, and

Table 155–3. INFERTILITY EVALUATION TIMING

Menses	Cycle days 1–5
Hysterosalpingogram	Cycle days 6–10
Postcoital test	Cycle days 12–14
Serum progesterone	Cycle days 21–23
Laparoscopy	Cycle days 2–10

minor abdominal discomfort, as well as a higher than average multiple birth rate (8% to 10%—almost always twins). Women with polycystic ovary disease should be observed carefully because they are at risk for ovarian hyperstimulation, which involves painful ovarian enlargement and, rarely, capillary leak with ascites, pleural effusions, renal hypoperfusion, and hypercoagulability and which may lead to ovarian rupture. Clomiphene costs $5 to $10 per tablet and at higher doses may require ultrasonographic monitoring and serum estradiol measurements. hCG costs $30 to $40 per vial.

In women who have low endogenous estrogen levels or who fail to respond to high clomiphene dosage, gonadotropin-releasing hormone (GnRH) therapy may be administered to stimulate follicle development. hCG must be added to induce subsequent ovum release. Complications include multiple births (20%), gastrointestinal discomfort, and ovarian hyperstimulation, which occurs in mild to moderate degree in approximately 20% of women. GnRH therapy costs more than $500 monthly plus the costs of serial ultrasonography and serum hormone assays.

Treatment of luteal phase deficiency with progesterone by intramuscular injection or vaginal suppositories may facilitate implantation and prevent spontaneous abortion, although this therapy has not been rigorously studied. In cases in which LPD is due to deficient FSH in the follicular phase, clomiphene may be effective.

Although endometriosis may diminish fertility by causing pelvic adhesions or tubal obstruction or impairing tubal transport, the degree to which mild or moderate cases contribute to infertility is the subject of considerable debate. Management of endometriosis and associated infertility with GnRH or surgery requires referral to an appropriately trained specialist.

Intrauterine insemination with the male partner's sperm is most effective when infertility is due to hypospadias, retrograde ejaculation, male sexual dysfunction, or cervical factors. Fecundability rates with both fresh and frozen sperm are approximately 10%. All donor sperm is frozen to allow baseline and follow-up human immunodeficiency virus testing before use. Women who choose to conceive without male partners usually do so through intrauterine insemination of frozen donor sperm. If the woman has normal ovulatory cycles, her fecundability will match that of an age-matched couple practicing frequent unprotected intercourse.

In vitro fertilization with embryo transfer (IVF-ET) and gamete/zygote intrafallopian transfer (GIFT/ZIFT) are highly technologic therapies used in cases of tubal obstruction, severe endometriosis, cervical mucus abnormality, or persistent unexplained infertility. Male factor infertility is especially responsive to IVF with intracytoplasmic sperm injection. Outcome data are typically reported as the live birth rate per oocyte retrieval or embryo transfer, but the cumulative conception rate represents the most clinically useful information. Unfortunately, published data suffer from a lack of uniform acceptance criteria for couples undergoing this therapy. Success rates for fertile ovum transfer with IVF-ET are approximately 20% live births per retrieval cycle, 26% with GIFT, and 23% with ZIFT. The birth rate per oocyte retrieval is only 4% for women older than age 40, as contrasted to a 31% rate with the use of donor oocytes from younger women. The incidence of multiple gestation varies according to the program policy on number of embryos transferred; with the typical transfer of three or four embryos, 20% to 25% of pregnancies will be multiple gestations.

Psychological and Ethical Aspects. Infertility evaluation and treatment is almost invariably associated with significant anxiety and stress for both partners. Appropriate counseling by the primary health care provider may help the couple to avoid common feelings of guilt and blame, to realistically consider diagnostic and therapeutic alternatives, and to know when to quit. Groups such as Resolve have local chapters for peer support and information.

The advent of assisted reproductive technology, while allowing many previously infertile couples to achieve parenthood, has ushered in a host of ethical and legal dilemmas. Because infertility treatment is seldom a covered health benefit, patients of higher socioeconomic status are likely to gain greater access to its use: the estimated cost incurred for each ovum retrieval cycle is over $6500, and the cost per successful delivery is $66,000 to $114,000. Legal ownership and disposition of frozen embryos, as well as the delineation of legal parenthood in cases of IVF-ET and surrogacy, have posed complex legal problems. Finally, the ethical considerations involved in the decision to undergo fetal reduction in greater-than-twin multiple gestations have only begun to be understood and explored.

Cross-References: Male Infertility (Chapter 156), Pelvic Inflammatory Disease (Chapter 166), Erectile Dysfunction (Chapter 169).

REFERENCES

1. Abyholm T, Tanbo T. GIFT, ZIFT and related techniques. Curr Opin Obstet Gynecol 1993;5:615.

    The authors present a concise description of assisted reproductive techniques.

2. Collins JA, Crosignani PG. Unexplained infertility: A review of diagnosis, prognosis, treatment efficacy and management. Int J Gynecol Obstet 1992;39:267.

    This is an excellent review of the approach to diagnosis and management in unexplained infertility.

3. Feichtinger W. Results and complications of IVF therapy. Curr Opin Obstet Gynecol 1994;6:190.

    The author provides an up-to-date review of current assisted reproductive technology.

4. Healy DL, et al. Female infertility: Causes and treatment. Lancet 1994;343:1539.

    This is an outstanding and highly readable review of this complex topic.

5. Neumann PJ, et al. The cost of a successful delivery with in vitro fertilization. N Engl J Med 1994;331:239.

    A fascinating discussion, this article delineates the costs of reproductive technology.

6. Rivlin M, ed. Handbook of Drug Therapy in Reproductive Endocrinology and Infertility. Boston, Little, Brown, & Co, 1990.

    This text is an excellent source of information about commonly prescribed infertility drugs.

156 Male Infertility

Problem

BRADLEY D. ANAWALT

Epidemiology and Etiology. *Infertility* is usually defined as inability to conceive within a 1-year period of unprotected intercourse. Approximately 15% of couples are infertile by this definition, although about half of these "infertile" couples will successfully conceive without medical intervention after a second year of unprotected intercourse. A male factor contributes to or causes infertility in 30% to 50% of these couples. Causes of male infertility can be divided into three categories: (1) potentially treatable infertility (12.5%), (2) subfertility (75%), and (3) untreatable infertility (12.5%). Potentially treatable problems include genital tract obstruction, gonadotropin deficiency, coital disorders, reversible toxin exposures, and varicoceles.

Symptoms and Signs. The testes have two primary functions: production of male sex hormones (androgens) and production of sperm. Most infertile men have no symptoms other than inability to conceive because of isolated defects in sperm production. However, some infertile men also have defects in androgen production and will present with decreased body hair, weakness, gynecomastia, and decreased libido.

Clinical Approach. The primary question in the evaluation of male infertility is whether the testes are potentially capable of producing adequate numbers of normally functioning sperm. If infertility is due to diseases that affect the testes primarily, then usually no effective treatment exists (Table 156–1). On the other hand, diseases that affect the stimulation of sperm production and transport of sperm to the ovum may be treatable (Table 156–2).

The history should focus on previous fertility (including conception with other partners), any possible damage to the testes (undescended testes, torsion, orchitis, trauma, cytotoxic drugs, and radiotherapy), and coital frequency. Many significant systemic illnesses can also impair fertility. The most important aspect of the physical examination is measurement of the testes. The testes are mainly composed of seminiferous tubules, the sperm-producing units. Therefore, the volume of the testes generally corresponds with the ability to produce sperm

---

Table 156–1. CONDITIONS THAT CAN CAUSE UNTREATABLE MALE STERILITY FROM IRREVERSIBLE FAILURE OF SPERM PRODUCTION

Klinefelter's syndrome (XXY karyotype)
Testicular atrophy due to trauma, orchitis, radiation therapy, toxins, or cytotoxic drugs
Undescended testes (cryptorchidism)
Orchidectomy (e.g., therapy for prostate cancer)
Idiopathic

Table 156–2. POTENTIALLY TREATABLE CAUSES OF MALE INFERTILITY

Genital tract obstruction
  Congenital
  Acquired
    Inflammatory: tuberculosis, gonorrhea
    Surgery: vasectomy
Gonadotropin deficiency
  Idiopathic hypogonadotropic hypogonadism
  Pituitary tumor
  Hemochromatosis
Coital disorders
  Inadequate frequency
  Incorrect timing in relation to female ovulation
  Impotence
  Retrograde ejaculation
Reversible toxins
  Systemic illness
  Drugs: corticosteroids, alcohol, marijuana, tobacco
Varicocele

and can be determined by comparison with a Prader orchidometer (a set of ovoids of known volume) or estimated by measuring the length of each testis. The normal size is volume greater than 15 mL or length greater than 4 cm. Very small testes (volume < 4 mL or length < 2 cm) generally confer a poor prognosis for fertility regardless of etiology. The patient's scrotum should also be carefully palpated for a varicocele. Although many men with varicoceles are fertile, men with varicoceles tend to have lower sperm counts and a greater rate of infertility than men without varicoceles.

The laboratory evaluation should include serum testosterone and gonadotropin (follicle-stimulating hormone [FSH] and luteinizing hormone [LH]) levels as well as semen analysis. The most important laboratory datum is the serum FSH level. The FSH level can vary because of the pulsatile secretion of FSH from the pituitary. Therefore, abnormal FSH levels should be corroborated with another measurement at least once. Elevated FSH levels generally indicate an irreversible failure of sperm production. On the other hand, low serum testosterone and gonadotropin levels suggest gonadotropin deficiency that can be successfully treated. The most important feature of semen analysis is the sperm concentration. If no sperm are seen on semen analysis, either sperm transport is blocked (potentially treatable) or sperm production is severely impaired (untreatable unless due to gonadotropin deficiency). Thus, a man with normal testosterone and FSH levels but no sperm on semen analysis is likely to have a potentially reversible obstruction of the genital tract.

Infertile men whose only defect is subnormal sperm concentrations (< 20 million/mL) or defects in sperm motility and morphology are categorized as subfertile. Semen analysis should be done after abstinence from ejaculation for at least 48 hours (recent ejaculation decreases subsequent sperm concentrations) and may have to be repeated several times because of the normal extreme variation in sperm counts.

Management. A key feature of treatment of male infertility is counseling and appropriate psychological support. Infertility can be distressing for the affected couple. Efforts should be made to correct any identified treatable cause of male infertility, and the female partner must also be carefully evaluated for infertility (see Chapter 155, Female Infertility). Although rarely a cause of infertility, coital disorders should be addressed. Vaginal intercourse three times a week appears to optimize the odds of conception. Gonadotropin deficiency can be successfully treated with gonadotropin replacement therapy; appropriate therapy of gonadotropin deficiency generally results in very high rates of fertility (> 80% success). Genital tract obstruction can sometimes be successfully corrected with surgery. Microsurgical reversal of vasectomy, the most common acquired cause of male genital tract obstruction, restores fertility in only 30% to 50% of patients. Cessation of exposure to testicular toxins such as alcohol, tobacco, and marijuana is recommended but rarely results in dramatic improvement in fertility. Varicocele ligation may be helpful in up to 50% of infertile men with a varicocele and no other identifiable cause of infertility.

For most men with infertility, effective medical therapy does not exist; options for these men include adoption. For infertile and subfertile men with some normal sperm production, assisted reproductive technology might be useful. Assisted reproductive technology is very expensive and includes in vitro fertilization with or without intracytoplasmic sperm injection. The intracytoplasmic sperm injection technique consists of aspirating sperm from the epididymis or testis of the infertile man and injecting it into a surgically removed ovum. There have been no controlled trials of assisted reproductive techniques. The largest uncontrolled studies have shown successful delivery rates of less than 15% per attempt in couples using in vitro fertilization for treatment of male infertility factor. The use of intracytoplasmic sperm injection and in vitro fertilization in couples with a male infertility factor might raise the successful delivery rate to 35% per attempt. Because assisted reproductive technology is very expensive and because many couples will conceive after a second year of unprotected intercourse, this technology should be reserved for couples who have not conceived after 2 years of unprotected intercourse.

Cross-References: Female Infertility (Chapter 155), Erectile Dysfunction (Chapter 169), Scrotal Mass (Chapter 183).

REFERENCES

1. Baker HW. Male infertility. Endocrinol Metab Clin North Am 1994;23:783–793.

   The author presents a sensible approach to diagnosis and management of male infertility.

2. Bhasin S, DeKretser DM, Baker HW. Pathophysiology and natural history of male infertility. J Clin Endocrinol Metab 1994;79:1525–1529.

   This is a detailed review of the effect of in vitro fertilization on natural history of male infertility and the molecular pathophysiology of male infertility.

3. Hibbert ML, Wolf DP. In vitro fertilization and the oligozoospermic male. Endocrinologist 1994;4:383–390.

   Readable explanations and assessment of assisted reproductive technology are presented.

4. Howards SS. Treatment of male infertility. N Engl J Med 1995;332:312–317.

   This article is a good review of medical and surgical treatments of male infertility.

5. Keye WR, Chang RJ, Rebar RW, Soules MR. Infertility: Evaluation and Treatment. Philadelphia, WB Saunders, 1995.

   This is an up-to-date text on male and female infertility with excellent diagrams, graphs, and photographs.

SECTION XIV
Women's Health

. . . .

157 Cervical Cancer Screening

Screening

ANNE W. MOULTON and JULIE F. DeLEO

Epidemiology. Cervical cancer is the fourth most common malignant cancer among women in the United States. In 1994, there were 15,000 new cases of invasive cervical cancer and approximately 4600 deaths. An average woman has a lifetime risk of 0.7% for developing invasive cervical cancer and 2% for developing carcinoma in situ. The incidence has increased in younger women, with 27% of cases occurring in women younger than age 50, attributable to the onset of sexual activity at progressively younger ages. Twenty-five percent of cervical cancer occurs in women older than 65, but most of these women have not had regular screening. In third world countries, cervical cancer is the leading cause of cancer deaths in women. Black, Hispanic, and Native American women have approximately twice the risk of white women. The majority of cervical cancer is squamous cell carcinoma. Adenocarcinoma, which accounts for 5% to 10% of cases, has a significantly worse prognosis.

Risk factors for developing cervical dysplasia include multiple sexual partners, early age of first intercourse, tobacco use, lower socioeconomic status, a history of sexually transmitted diseases including human papillomavirus (HPV), immunosuppression such as after organ transplantation or infection with human immunodeficiency virus (HIV), vitamin or betacarotene deficiency, a history of in utero diethylstilbestrol exposure, and a high-risk male partner. A high-risk male partner is defined as one having multiple sexual partners, HPV or HIV infection, or a previous sexual partner with cervical dysplasia or cancer.

HPV is the most prevalent viral sexually transmitted disease in the United States. HPV types 6 and 11 are found in condylomata and in low-grade dysplasia. The risk of malignant transformation with HPV 6 and 11 is low because they do not integrate into host DNA. In contrast, lesions containing HPV 16, 18, 45, and 56 can progress from dysplasia to invasive cancer within 1 year because the HPV DNA does integrate into host DNA.

Rationale. The long preinvasive stage of cervical cancer and the availability of a relatively inexpensive screening test make cervical cancer ideal for screening. The evidence on the efficacy of screening comes from many large screening programs in Scandinavia, Canada, and the United States. In the United States, the incidence of cervical cancer has declined by more than 35% since the advent of screening programs. The most important anatomic area of the cervix to be screened is the squamocolumnar junction, where most clinical neoplasia arises. A sample from the endocervical canal combined with a cervical scraping provides the lowest false-negative rate. The probability that a Papanicolaou (Pap) test will fail to detect a significant lesion because of technical factors (e.g., sampling and laboratory issues such as slide preparation, misdiagnosis, or erroneous reporting) ranges from less than 5% to greater than 50%. Use of a cervical brush produces the lowest false-negative rates for endocervical disease. False-positive smears are infrequent (1% to 9%) and usually result from errors in laboratory reporting.

Strategy. Screening should begin at age 18 or when the patient first becomes sexually active. After three or more satisfactory normal annual examinations, the Pap test should be performed every 3 years, provided that the individual remains in the low-risk category. For individuals with risk factors, annual screening is recommended. HIV-seropositive females should be screened semiannually.

Despite controversy about when screening should be safely discontinued, testing at age 65 is no longer required if the patient has been regularly screened, has had normal Pap tests, and has no new risk factors.

There is also disagreement about patients who have had a hysterectomy. If the surgery was for cervical cancer, there is a 2% to 12% risk for recurrence, and regular testing is indicated. If the surgery was for a benign condition, testing every 3 years is sufficient. Despite best efforts, Pap tests will lack endocervical cells in 2% to 4% of smears and especially in postmenopausal women because the squamocolumnar junction moves up the endocervical canal. When a Pap test fails to contain endocervical cells, a repeat test should be performed as soon as possible.

A comparison of reporting schemes is provided in Table 157–1. The original system (classes I–IV), although still in use in some laboratories, does not reflect the current understanding of cervical neoplasia. The cervical intraepithelial neoplasia (CIN) system was added to improve classification of precancerous lesions. In 1988, the Bethesda classification system for Pap tests was developed to facilitate standardized reporting. Depending on the laboratory, Pap test reports may contain information from one or all of the classification systems.

Action. Any patient with a suspicious cervical lesion should be referred for further evaluation even if a Pap test is negative because of the possibility of a false-negative result. If the Pap smear report notes inflammation but is considered satisfactory, the test should be repeated in 1 year. If the Pap smear is labeled unsatisfactory, antibiotic therapy is instituted and the test is repeated within 3 months.

Patients with atypical Pap smears can be divided into two groups: those with atypical squamous cells of undetermined significance (ASCUS) and those with atypical glandular cells of undetermined significance (AGCUS). All patients in either of these groups and with risk factors for cervical cancer must be referred for colposcopy. Patients with ASCUS and no risk factors should have a repeat Pap smear. If ASCUS is persistent, the patient needs colposcopy.

**Table 157–1. CLASSIFICATION AND COMPARATIVE
NOMENCLATURE OF CERVICAL SMEARS**

	Original Classification	CIN System	Bethesda System
Class I:	Normal smear No abnormal cells		
Class II:	Atypical cells present below the level of cervical neoplasia		Atypical squamous cells of undetermined significance
Class III:	Smear contains abnormal cells consistent with dysplasia	Mild dysplasia = CIN 1 Moderate dysplasia = CIN 2	Low-grade SIL (changes associated with HPV and CIN 1)
			High-grade SIL (CIN 2)
Class IV:	Smear contains abnormal cells consistent with carcinoma in situ	Severe dysplasia and carcinoma in situ = CIN 3	High-grade SIL (CIN 3)
Class V:	Smear contains abnormal cells consistent with carcinoma of squamous cell origin		Squamous cell carcinoma

CIN, cervical intraepithelial neoplasia; SIL, squamous intraepithelial lesion (Bethesda System, 1988); HPV, human papillomavirus.

Patients with dysplasia (CIN 1–3), carcinoma in situ, and both grades of squamous intraepithelial lesion should be referred directly for additional evaluation. If there is a visible lesion on the cervix, it should be sampled; otherwise, the patient should have colposcopy. Additional diagnosis and treatment will be dictated by the findings.

After treatment, follow-up Pap tests should be performed every 3 months for the first year and every 6 months thereafter. Patients who have evidence of invasive carcinoma on cervical smear should be referred immediately for evaluation (biopsy or colposcopy) and definitive treatment. After treatment, they should continue to have regular follow-up, including Pap tests.

Cross-References: Periodic Health Assessment (Chapter 8), Abnormal Uterine Bleeding (Chapter 159), Vaginitis (Chapter 164), Contraception (Chapter 165), Sexually Transmitted Diseases (Chapter 176).

REFERENCES

1. Campion MJ, Reid R. Screening for gynecologic cancer in health maintenance strategies. Obstet Gynecol Clin North Am 1990;17:695–727.

   The authors provide an excellent overview of screening for cervical cancer.

2. Eddy DM. Screening for cervical cancer. Ann Intern Med 1990;113:214–226.

   This article is an excellent review of the literature; it includes mathematic models that address the ideal frequency of screening.

3. Koss LG. The Papanicolaou test for cervical cancer detection: A triumph and a tragedy. JAMA 1989;261:737–743.

   A good discussion of the limitations of the Pap test is provided by a pathologist.

4. Neminen P, Kallio M, Hakama M. The effect of mass screening on the incidence and mortality of squamous and adenocarcinoma of cervix uteri. Obstet Gynecol 1995;85:1017–1021.

   This is a good review of the effects of screening on the incidence and mortality of cervical cancer.

5. US Preventive Services Task Force. Screening for cervical cancer. In: Guide to Clinical Preventive Services, 2nd ed. Alexandria, Virginia, International Medical Publishing, 1996.

   Screening recommendations are presented in this good short review.

. . . .

158 Breast Cancer Screening

Screening

MARY B. LAYA

Epidemiology. Breast cancer is the most common cancer diagnosed in women, accounting for 32% of all new cancers. Although 56% of breast cancer deaths occur in women 65 and older, it is also the leading cause of cancer mortality in women 15 to 54 years of age. The annual incidence of breast cancer increases with age from 127/100,000 for women 40 to 44 years of age to 450/100,000 for women 70 to 74 years of age. As women of the "baby boom generation" age, the absolute numbers of breast cancer cases and deaths are expected to rise substantially. Epidemiologic risk factors for breast cancer include family history of breast cancer, early menarche, late menopause, nulliparity, and late age at first full-term birth. However, only 30% of women who develop breast cancer have known risk factors for the disease. All women are potentially at risk, and this risk increases as a woman ages.

Rationale. Breast cancer is a disease that meets the standard criteria for effective screening (see Chapter 7, Principles of Screening). It is a major cause of morbidity and mortality, and there is often a long preclinical phase during which early detection and treatment may have a positive impact on disease mortality. Three potential methods of early detection exist: screening mammography, the clinical breast examination, and breast self-examination.

The accuracy of mammography has been demonstrated within the context of eight randomized controlled trials. Sensitivities for cancers in women aged 50 to 59 at entry range from 73% to 88%, and specificities range from 82% to 98%. Mammograms appear to be less accurate in women 40 to 49 years of age at entry. Sensitivity for these women ranges from 53% to 81% and is probably lower owing to the greater radiographic density of premenopausal breast tissue. Specificities are similarly lower, which translates into more false-positive results and more diagnostic tests per cancer detected (43.9 per cancer in women aged 40 to 49 versus 21.9 per cancer detected in women aged 50 to 59).

No randomized controlled trials are available regarding the sensitivity and specificity of clinical breast examination used alone. Four of the eight trials of screening for breast cancer included clinical breast examination as part of the screening protocol, and most have not reported separate performance characteristics. Sensitivity of clinical breast examination in the Canadian National Breast Screening Study-2 was 63% for women 50 to 59 years of age and was 10% lower for women 40 to 49 years of age. Three percent to 10% of cancers not detected by screening mammography are detected by clinical breast examination; therefore, it is complementary to mammography.

Breast self-examination is a third potential screening modality. Indirect evidence of its usefulness is based on observational studies that reveal a lower stage at diagnosis for women who practice breast self-examination. Randomized trials in Shanghai and Leningrad, where breast self-examination is being compared with no screening, are ongoing.

Strategy. Recommended breast cancer screening strategies developed by several North American groups are listed in Table 158–1. These recommendations are based on interpretations of the same studies (the eight randomized clinical trials of screening and the observational studies of breast self-examination performance). The groups generally agree on the use of mammography and clinical breast examination to screen women aged 50 and older based on a consistently demonstrated reduction in breast cancer mortality in screened women in the 50- to 65-year age group.

The groups differ in their interpretation of the data and thus in screening recommendations for women 40 to 49 years of age. None of the randomized trials, taken individually or in the aggregate, demonstrate a statistically significant reduction in mortality in women in this age group. Proponents argue that although studies were not statistically significant, they do suggest benefit: 6 of 7 studies that included women aged 40 to 49 at entry showed relative risk of less than 1, and most studies are able to demonstrate earlier stage at diagnosis in screened women. In addition, advocates of screening this group cite potential methodologic and technical flaws in the randomized clinical trials encompassing this age group and the demonstration of benefit of one large nonrandomized trial, the Breast Cancer Detection and Demonstration Project.

Groups that do not support breast cancer screening for women in their 40s point out that even pooling of the randomized clinical trials for this age group does not reveal a statistically significant reduction in mortality. The only large study designed to specifically address the question of screening in women aged 40 to 49 (the Canadian National Breast Screening Study-1) did not show any benefit of screening. Finally, these groups note that screening is not without risk. It results in physical risk resulting from workup of false-positive findings as well as psychological costs to individuals and economic costs to society.

Limited data exist on the effectiveness of screening women 70 and older, although breast cancer rates continue to increase. Performance characteristics of screening mammography (sensitivity and specificity) do not appear to deteriorate with increasing age, so screening is likely to remain beneficial for older women.

The role of breast self-examination in screening for breast cancer is another source of controversy and conflicting recommendations. In the absence

Table 158-1. BREAST CANCER SCREENING RECOMMENDATIONS BY NORTH AMERICAN ORGANIZATIONS*

Group or Organization	Age Group	Mammography	Clinical Breast Examination	Breast Self-Examination
US Preventive Services Task Force (1996)	40–49	Consider if high risk, or per patient preference	Consider if high risk, or per patient preference	No recommendation
	50–69	Every 1–2 years	Every 1–2 years	
	≥ 70	Every 1–2 years if reasonable life expectancy	Every 1–2 years if reasonable life expectancy	
US Consensus Statement (1993)†	40–49	Every 1–2 years	Annually	Monthly starting at age 20
	≥ 50	Annually	Annually	
American College of Physicians (1996)	40–49	Not recommended	Not recommended	No recommendation
	50–74	Every 2 years	Every 2 years	
	> 75	Not recommended	Not recommended	
Canadian Task Force on the Periodic Health Exam (1994)	< 50	Not recommended	Not recommended	
	50–69	Annually	Annually	
American Academy of Family Physicians (1994)	30–39	Not recommended	Every 1–3 years	Recommended
	40–49	Not recommended	Annually	
	> 50	Annually	Annually	

*The National Cancer Institute (NCI) Consensus Panel and the NCI advisory board met in 1997 and disagree about whether mammograms should be obtained for all women 40–49 every 1–2 years.
†American Cancer Society, American College of Radiologists, American College of Obstetricians and Gynecologists, American Medical Association, and others.

of methodologically sound studies on the question of the usefulness of breast self-examination, groups are divided on the basis of their estimation of the risks of this form of screening (e.g., the importance of false-positive findings with its attendant costs, especially among younger women).

Action. For women 50 years and older, mammography and clinical breast examination every 1 to 2 years are indicated based on existing data. Low-risk women 40 to 49 years of age should be informed of the lack of consensus on screening effectiveness in their age group and the rationales of opponents and proponents of screening. A similar discussion with women older than age 70 should also take into account co-morbid conditions. Even groups that do not support screening of women in these age groups recognize the need to take the patient's personal preferences and breast cancer risk factors into account.

Cross-References: Principles of Screening (Chapter 7), Periodic Health Assessment (Chapter 8), Initial Evaluation of a Breast Mass (Chapter 162), Breast Pain in Nonlactating Women (Chapter 163), Mammography and Breast Imaging (Chapter 167).

REFERENCES

1. Fletcher SW, Black W, Harris R, Rimer B, et al. Report of the International Workshop on screening for breast cancer. J Natl Cancer Inst 1993;85:1644–1656.

   This report of the working group's review of clinical trial data (including the Canadian studies) on breast cancer screening discusses the evidence and lack of demonstrated effectiveness of screening women aged 40 to 49.

2. Mettlin C, Smart C. Breast cancer detection guidelines for women aged 40–49: Rationale for the American Cancer Society reaffirmation of recommendations. CA Cancer J Clin 1994;44:248–255.

   The American Cancer Society's stand on screening of women in their 40s is summarized.

3. US Preventive Services Task Force. Screening for Breast Cancer. Guide to Clinical Preventive Services, 2nd ed. Baltimore, Williams & Wilkins, 1996.

   This evidence-based guide to breast cancer screening contains an excellent review of the literature on breast cancer screening and an explanation for the recommended interventions.

159 Abnormal Uterine Bleeding

Symptom

BETH SKRYPZAK

Epidemiology and Etiology. Abnormal uterine bleeding is a common reason women seek out a primary care provider. The causes are numerous, and the differential diagnosis depends on age and the specific pattern of bleeding. The terminology and definitions of bleeding patterns are briefly reviewed in Table 159–1. The possibility of pregnancy must always be considered, even if a woman has been sterilized. Tubal ligations have a 1 in 300 failure rate, and ectopic pregnancy remains a possibility, albeit a rare one.

Beyond pregnancy, most of the causes can be categorized as neoplasia-related (cervix or endometrial), hormonal (also frequently called dysfunctional uterine bleeding), or anatomic (leiomyomas, polyps, or adenomyosis). Leiomyomas occur in about 1 in 4 or 5 white women and 1 in 3 black women. Less than 0.1% are malignant. The possibility of cancer should be eliminated early in the evaluation. Dysfunctional uterine bleeding is a *diagnosis of exclusion* and should not be assumed until other causes have been considered.

On average, menarche begins at 13 years of age, and menopause begins at 51 years of age. The usual cycle interval is 28 (± 7) days with 4 (± 2) days of flow, and an average loss of 35 mL of blood per menses. Bleeding at *regular* intervals for more than 7 days or using more than 6 maxipads per day (> 80 mL blood per menses) is considered *menorrhagia*.

Clinical Approach. In general, *metrorrhagia*, defined as bleeding at irregular intervals, suggests neoplasia, hormonal abnormalities, or polyps. Menorrhagia often suggests uterine abnormalities such as leiomyomas or adenomyosis.

Table 159–1. TERMINOLOGY AND DEFINITIONS OF ABNORMAL UTERINE BLEEDING

Term	Definition
Amenorrhea (secondary)	No menses for 6 months or more if preceded by normal cycles
Dysfunctional uterine bleeding	Abnormal uterine bleeding unrelated to organic causes
Hypomenorrhea	Light regular menstrual bleeding
Menometrorrhagia	Heavy or prolonged irregular and frequent menstrual bleeding
Menorrhagia (hypermenorrhea)	Heavy or prolonged regular menstrual bleeding
Metrorrhagia	Bleeding at irregular intervals or intermenstrual bleeding
Midcycle spotting	Related to physiologic decrease in estradiol; normal, no evaluation needed
Oligomenorrhea	Menstrual interval greater than 35 days; can be normal for some women
Polymenorrhea	Menstrual interval less than 21 days

The provider should ascertain that the bleeding is from the vagina and not the rectum, bladder, or urethra. Any type of pregnancy should be excluded (i.e., spontaneous abortion or gestational trophoblastic pregnancy). Up to 20% of adolescents with menorrhagia have a coagulation disorder (such as von Willebrand's disease), and appropriate laboratory testing including prothrombin time, partial thromboplastin time, platelet count, and bleeding time is needed. Screening for symptoms of iron deficiency anemia is also important. Hyperthyroidism can occasionally cause excessive bleeding. Endometritis should be considered if an intrauterine device is present. Rarely, cervicitis causes spotting. Pelvic pain, dyspareunia, and menorrhagia can be suggestive of an enlarging leiomyoma or adenomyosis. Adenomyosis, defined as the presence of endometrial glands within the myometrium, is often associated with endometriosis. Pelvic ultrasonography should be ordered if the examination is inadequate or if a mass is suspected. Cervical neoplasm should be excluded with a Papanicolaou smear. Table 159–2 summarizes diagnostic testing.

Endometrial biopsy should be performed on any woman older than age 40 with menometrorrhagia or metrorrhagia to exclude endometrial neoplasia. If she has a history of oligomenorrhea or chronic anovulation, this age cutoff should be decreased to age 30. This procedure can be performed by the primary care provider after a small amount of training. Endometrial biopsy is a good screening test for endometrial carcinoma with a sensitivity of 95% to

Table 159–2. DIAGNOSIS AND MANAGEMENT OF ABNORMAL UTERINE BLEEDING

Step 1 (Diagnosis)
  Pelvic examination, Papanicolaou smear
  Hematocrit
  Urine pregnancy test
  Possible prothrombin time, partial thromboplastin time, platelet count, bleeding time
  Possible thyroid-stimulating hormone
  Possible cervical cultures
  Possible endometrial biopsy
  Possible ultrasonography

Step 2 (Initial Management)
  Medroxyprogesterone acetate (Provera) or oral contraceptives
  Nonsteroidal anti-inflammatory drugs
  Rarely intravenous estrogen
  Possible antibiotic therapy
  Possible iron therapy

Step 3 (Ongoing Management)
  Long-term medroxyprogesterone acetate (Provera) or oral contraceptives
  Medroxyprogesterone acetate (Depo-Provera)

Step 4 (Refractory)
  Gynecologic consultation
    Hysteroscopy, dilatation and curettage
    Endometrial ablation
    Hysteroscopic resection of leiomyomas
    Abdominal myomectomy
    Hysterectomy (abdominal/vaginal)
    Gonadotropin-releasing hormone agonist (Lupron)

97%. However, if the biopsy is inadequate or if the bleeding continues, gynecologic referral for hysteroscopy and dilatation and curettage should be considered.

When endometrial biopsy cannot be easily accomplished owing to cervical stenosis or patient discomfort, studies suggest that transvaginal ultrasonography can be helpful in determining endometrial thickness, especially after the menopause. If the lining is thin, 5 mm or less, the clinician can be fairly reassured that neoplasia is not present. If the lining is greater than 5 mm, histologic sampling should be pursued in the operating room.

Management. Interventions should be undertaken when a woman's bleeding pattern is affecting her lifestyle. Table 159–2 reviews some therapies, and drug dosages are outlined in Table 159–3. If pregnancy is not desired and endometrial biopsy is not necessary, initial therapy involves use of medroxyprogesterone acetate (Provera) during the luteal phase or monophasic oral contraceptives and/or nonsteroidal anti-inflammatory drugs. Nonsteroidal agents can reduce blood loss by 30% by their antiprostaglandin effect. Oral contraceptives are more helpful if bleeding has been excessive. Rarely, intravenous estrogen is necessary and should be given with gynecologic consultation.

Endometritis responds to doxycycline. If endometritis is found on biopsy in the menopause, repeat biopsy is necessary after antibiotic therapy to exclude cancer underlying the endometritis.

Long-term hormonal therapy for dysfunctional uterine bleeding includes ongoing oral contraceptives, monthly luteal phase medroxyprogesterone acetate, or possibly depo-medroxyprogesterone acetate. Initially with use of depo-medroxyprogesterone acetate there can be some metrorrhagia, but 50% of patients achieve amenorrhea by 1 year of use.

For persistent bleeding unresponsive to these measures, referral to a gynecologic consultant for possible surgery is warranted. Endometrial ablation with a "roller-ball" technique or hysteroscopic resection of leiomyomas may obviate some hysterectomies. Also, gonadotropin-releasing hormone agonist (Lupron) therapy preoperatively can shrink some leiomyomas and allow a vaginal hysterectomy (with an easier recovery) instead of an abdominal hysterectomy.

Table 159–3. MEDICATIONS FOR TREATMENT OF ABNORMAL UTERINE BLEEDING

Medication	Dose	Cost ($)*
Medroxyprogesterone acetate (Provera)	10 mg PO qd × 10 days in luteal phase every month	9.38 for 3 months
Monophasic oral contraceptives (any type)	1 PO bid or tid for 1 week (acute bleeding), then 1 PO qd	Average 25/month
Ibuprofen	600 mg PO qid × 2–3 days (acutely)	4.48 for 30 tablets (3 months)
Doxycycline (if endometritis)	100 mg PO bid × 1 week	5.43 for 1 week
Medroxyprogesterone acetate (Depo-Provera)	150 mg IM q 3 months	53.67 every 3 months (price includes injection fee)

*Prices for generic where available. Average wholesale price, 1996 *Drug Topics Red Book.*

Follow-Up. Care should include clinical assessment of the effectiveness of hormonal therapies and evaluation for anemia. If initial diagnostic tests do not identify a cause of the bleeding, or if the woman is not responding to medications, gynecologic consultation is recommended. After 3 to 6 months of medications, a trial period off medications will distinguish between transient and ongoing problems. If her problem recurs, medications can be restarted.

Cross-References: Abdominal Pain (Chapter 94), Female Infertility (Chapter 155), Contraception (Chapter 165), Bleeding (Chapter 195), Anemia (Chapter 199), Diagnosis of Pregnancy (Chapter 210).

REFERENCES

1. Herbst AL, Mishell DR, Stenchever MA, Droegemueller W. Comprehensive Gynecology. St. Louis, CV Mosby, 1992.

   This is a basic gynecology textbook that addresses abnormal bleeding patterns.

2. Lemcke DP, Pattison J, Marshall LA, Cowley DS, Skrypzak B. Approach to abnormal vaginal bleeding. In Primary Care of Women. Los Altos, CA, Lange, 1995.

   This is a more in-depth discussion of abnormal bleeding.

3. Lin MC, et al. Endometrial thickness after menopause: Effect of hormone therapy. Radiology 1991;180:427.

   This article addresses the use of ultrasound to exclude neoplasia.

4. Speroff L, Glass RH, Kase NG: Clinical Gynecologic Endocrinology and Infertility, 5th ed. Baltimore, Williams & Wilkins, 1994.

   This endocrinology text addresses hormonal pathophysiology and bleeding.

■ ■

160 Pelvic Pain in Women

Symptom

BETH SKRYPZAK

Epidemiology and Etiology. Pelvic pain is difficult to diagnose and treat, largely because of the many possible causes, including those considered gastrointestinal, urologic, musculoskeletal, gynecologic, and psychological. Acute pelvic pain affects many women in the reproductive age group and is a common reason women seek medical attention. Generally, acute gynecological pain is due to pregnancy, infection, or ovarian cysts. It is estimated that 1 million women in the United States are diagnosed with pelvic inflammatory disease each year and that about 25% require hospitalization. Chronic pelvic pain is associated with endometriosis, adhesions, or a history of sexual or physical abuse. About half of women with chronic pelvic pain and a negative laparoscopy have a history of childhood sexual abuse. Ten percent of outpatient gynecologic visits, 40% of laparoscopies, and 12% of hysterectomies are for chronic pelvic pain. Gynecologic cancers rarely produce pain until the disease is advanced.

Clinical Approach. Obtaining the necessary history in patients with pelvic pain can be time-consuming, but it is important for specific diagnosis and successful treatment. Questions should identify location, duration, and nature of the pain. Fever, associated bowel or urinary symptoms, and the relationship of the pain to the menstrual cycle are important features. Sexual and contraceptive histories and a history of prior gynecologic problems or operative procedures are helpful. Endometriosis is associated with a classic triad of dysmenorrhea, deep dyspareunia, and infertility.

Evaluating the possibility of pregnancy with the use of a sensitive serum or urine pregnancy test is imperative early in the evaluation. Sterilization failure is always a possibility, so testing is needed in sterilized patients also. Owing to the risk of ectopic pregnancy, early gynecologic consultation is needed in sterilized patients with a positive pregnancy test.

Bilateral pain is more common with pelvic inflammatory disease or prostaglandin-associated dysmenorrhea. Unilateral pain is suggestive of appendicitis or adnexal pathology. If a mass is found on physical examination, the differential diagnosis includes ovarian torsion, tubo-ovarian abscess, or neoplasia (usually benign physiologic ovarian cysts). If no mass is appreciated on examination, a common diagnosis is ruptured ovarian cyst. However, this is a *diagnosis of exclusion*, after pregnancy, infection, and masses have been considered. Diagnostic criteria for pelvic inflammatory disease are addressed in Chapter 166.

The hallmarks of chronic pelvic pain include (1) pain duration greater than 6 months, (2) incomplete relief with previous treatments, (3) impaired function at home or work, (4) vegetative signs of depression, (5) pain out of proportion to definable pathology, and (6) altered family roles.

During the pelvic examination, cervical cultures should be obtained before the bimanual examination. A careful distinction between pain elicited by the abdominal versus pain elicited by the vaginal hand can help separate gynecologic and nongynecologic causes. Complete blood cell count can help evaluate infection and intraperitoneal hemorrhage. Ultrasound should be used when the patient's tenderness precludes an adequate examination. Free peritoneal fluid, when a mass is detected on examination or when the diagnosis is uncertain, suggests a recently ruptured ovarian cyst.

For chronic pain, the pelvic examination is often less helpful. Endometriosis and adhesions can be definitively established only with laparoscopy. Laparoscopy should be used judiciously, because 39% of women with chronic pain have normal findings on laparoscopy and 28% of asymptomatic women have "abnormalities," such as adhesions (17%) or endometriosis (5%).

Management. As long as there is no suspicion of significant hemoperitoneum, ruptured or unruptured simple ovarian cysts less than 5 cm can initially be managed on an outpatient basis with nonsteroidal anti-inflammatory medications or, occasionally, with narcotics. Prostaglandin inhibitors decrease peritoneal inflammation from the cyst fluid and are also helpful with dysmenorrhea.

If a mass is present, one should be aware of the possibility of adnexal torsion, which is a surgical emergency. If diagnosed in a timely manner, torsion can be corrected during the laparoscopy, thus saving the adnexa.

Oral contraceptives can be used to suppress ovulation and can be used long term for recurrent pain from ruptured cysts. Traditionally, oral contraceptives have also been used to treat unruptured simple cysts (less than 5 cm) as they are being watched expectantly. However, data show that oral contraceptive use in this situation has little benefit over observation alone.

In a premenopausal woman, if a simple cyst is greater than 5 cm, if there is any solid or complex component to it on ultrasonography, or if it persists after 1 to 2 months of observation, then gynecologic consultation is needed for surgical management. Any postmenopausal woman with an adnexal abnormality on ultrasonography requires an immediate gynecologic referral.

When treating chronic pelvic pain, if the examination is benign, the history is vague, and fertility is not desired, a trial of nonsteroidal anti-inflammatory agents or oral contraceptives along with simultaneous gynecologic and mental health evaluation is appropriate initially. When indicated, laparoscopy with laser therapy can be used to treat endometriosis or adhesions. Often an approach that emphasizes "management" of the pain rather than "cure with definitive surgery" is optimal for the patient in this situation. Narcotic pain medications should be strongly avoided.

Follow-Up. Acute pain from an ovarian cyst or infection should resolve within 2 to 3 days. If it does not, the need for surgery or intravenous antibiotics should be assessed. Chronic pain requires regular visits (e.g., every 2 to 4 weeks) until it is under control.

Cross-References: Chronic Nonspecific Pain Syndrome (Chapter 14), Pelvic Inflammatory Disease (Chapter 166), Urinary Tract Infections in Women (Chapter 175), Screening for Depression (Chapter 185), Diagnosis of Pregnancy (Chapter 210).

REFERENCES

1. Howard FM. The role of laparoscopy in chronic pelvic pain: Promise and pitfalls. Obstet Gynecol Surv 1993;48:357–387.

   The poor correlation between pathology and pain perception is discussed.

2. Lemcke DP, Pattison J, Marshall LA, Cowley DS, Klotz MM. Dysmenorrhea, endometriosis, and pelvic pain. In Primary Care of Women. Los Altos, CA, Lange, 1995.

   This article provides an in-depth discussion of causes of pelvic pain.

3. Steege J. Telinde's Operative Gynecology Updates, vol 1, No. 2. Philadelphia, J.B. Lippincott, 1992:1–9.

   The author discusses the assessment and treatment of chronic pelvic pain.

4. Walker E, et al. Relationship of chronic pelvic pain to psychiatric diagnoses and childhood sexual abuse. Am J Psychiatry 1988;145:75–79.

   This classic article was the first to highlight this important correlation.

161 Menopausal Symptoms

Problem

ELIZA SUTTON

Epidemiology. Menopause, the cessation of menses due to ovarian failure, is a universal event for women in midlife and has both short- and long-term physiological effects. Because the associated symptoms result from decreased ovarian hormone production, they also occur in women who are amenstrual due to hysterectomy. Oophorectomy induces "surgical" menopause, which is sudden and is usually associated with marked symptoms. "Natural" menopause typically occurs between the ages of 48 and 55, although the changes and symptom-complex can begin years earlier and often span 4 to 10 years. At the average age at menopause, 51 years, life expectancy for a white woman in the United States is now about 28 years. There are about 40 million postmenopausal women in the United States, and this number will grow owing to increasing longevity.

Osteoporosis and cardiovascular disease are accelerated by years of low estrogen levels and cause the bulk of serious morbidity and mortality associated with menopause. Osteoporosis contributes to 1.5 million fractures annually, and 90% of those with osteoporosis are postmenopausal women. Evidence of vertebral fractures (often asymptomatic) is found in 25% of white women by age 60 and in 50% to 80% of those older than age 75. Cardiovascular disease is also a leading cause of serious morbidity, and 50% of women eventually die of cardiovascular disease. Long-term use of estrogen replacement therapy after menopause decreases the risk of hip and vertebral fractures by 25% to 50% and of cardiovascular disease (nonfatal and fatal events) by 35% to 50%.

Breast cancer incidence probably rises with long-term use of estrogen replacement therapy, possibly by 20% to 25%. Although the magnitude of this effect is still controversial, it is a significant concern to many women considering estrogen replacement therapy. For women who do not have personal or familial factors placing them at high risk for breast cancer, mortality from breast cancer is about one twelfth that from cardiovascular disease. Use of estrogen for not longer than 5 years does not appear to increase the risk of breast cancer or to provide significant long-term benefits against osteoporosis and cardiovascular disease. Unopposed estrogen increases the risk of endometrial cancer by about eightfold, to about 1% per year of use.

Symptoms and Signs. Symptoms during the climacteric, the time of transition around menopause, stem from the response of various estrogen-sensitive tissues to diminishing estrogen levels.

Before menses cease, cycles become irregular. Shortened follicular phases lead to shorter cycles, and anovulation results in longer cycles and often heavier menstrual flow.

Vasomotor symptoms (hot flushes and sweats) are episodes of cutaneous vasodilation that occur as a result of declining estrogen levels, possibly through a hypothalamic trigger. Women experience a sensation of intense heat, followed by flushing of the face and upper body and then profuse sweating. Hot flushes may last for seconds or minutes and in some women occur very frequently (20 or more times per day). Vasomotor symptoms occur in about 70% of women, begin before the cessation of menses in most, and typically persist for 1 or 2 years. In at least 25% of women, symptoms persist 5 years or more, and occasionally they are lifelong. Vasomotor symptoms may impair sleep and have been correlated with mood changes. Only 30% of women seek medical attention for vasomotor symptoms.

Urogenital symptoms of estrogen deficiency include atrophic vaginitis (vaginal dryness, dyspareunia, and recurrent vaginitis) and urinary changes (increased urinary frequency, stress incontinence, and recurrent urinary tract infections). Pelvic floor tone is influenced by estrogen levels, and laxity of these tissues may result in prolapse of the uterus or bladder, with associated symptoms. About 25% of women present for evaluation of urogenital symptoms.

Clinical Approach. Once 12 months have passed since the last menstrual period in a woman in her mid-40s or older, menopause can be assumed. In a woman of that age who describes irregular menses along with vasomotor or urogenital symptoms, the climacteric is likely. Diagnostic testing may be helpful to confirm the clinical suspicion in this case or to evaluate a younger woman whose menses have ceased. A more challenging situation is the woman in her mid-40s or younger with an isolated symptom that could be an early perimenopausal change. Diagnostic testing is likely to be normal at this stage, and evaluation to rule out other processes causing her symptom may well be appropriate before reassuring her and considering a therapeutic trial of hormones.

Signs of menopause are limited to the vaginal mucosa, which is often thinned and dry. A cystocele or uterine prolapse may be present, skin may be thinned and fragile, or mood changes may be evident; however, none of these signs is diagnostic of, or specific to, menopause.

The diagnosis of menopause is most often made on clinical grounds. The follicle-stimulating hormone level rises, and the estradiol level drops with ovarian failure, but these values remain within the normal range in some perimenopausal women who are still cycling. Hormone levels are more likely to be diagnostic in a woman who has stopped cycling, as is a 10-day medroxyprogesterone acetate challenge (in which absence of withdrawal bleeding suggests a hypoestrogenic state). Cervical or vaginal cytology may reveal a low maturation index from decreased estrogen.

Management. Treatment in menopause has two distinct goals: to alleviate perimenopausal symptoms and to reduce long-term risk of associated diseases. Estrogen replacement therapy is the basis of treatment in menopause for both short- and long-term therapy, with the specific choice of route and regimen based on other factors (Table 161–1).

MANAGEMENT OF SPECIFIC SYMPTOMS. Menorrhagia should be evaluated in the same manner as for nonmenopausal women and can be managed in the short term with low-dose oral contraceptives if the woman has no risk factors

Table 161–1. COMMONLY USED ESTROGENS AND PROGESTINS*

Agent	Side Effects	Doses†	Cost ($ per Month)‡
Oral Estrogens			
Conjugated equine estrogen (Premarin)	All systemic estrogens: breast tenderness, nausea, endometrial stimulation (including carcinoma), thromboembolism, gallbladder disease	0.3 mg	6.80
		0.625 mg	8.90
		0.9 mg	11.00
		1.25 mg	16.20
		2.5 mg	28.00
Esterified estrogens (Estratab)		0.3 mg	6.24
		0.625 mg	8.69
		1.25 mg	11.89
		2.5 mg	20.60
Estradiol (Estrace)		0.5 mg	7.39
		1 mg	9.85
		2 mg	14.40
Estropipate (Ogen)		0.625 mg	15.39
		1.25 mg	21.43
		2.5 mg	37.30
(Ortho-Est)		0.625 mg	9.95
		1.25 mg	13.61
Oral Estrogens + Testosterone			
Conjugated estrogens (CEE) and methyltestosterone (MT) (Premarin with methyltestosterone)	As for oral estrogens, plus: virilization, acne, male pattern baldness, edema, changes in libido, liver changes including cholestatic jaundice and peliosis hepatis	0.625 mg CEE + 5.0 MT	23.82
		1.25 mg CEE + 10.0 mg MT	40.09
Esterified estrogens (EE) and methyltestosterone (Estratest)		0.625 mg EE + 1.25 mg MT	18.63
		1.25 mg EE + 2.5 mg MT	23.19
Transdermal Estrogen			
Estradiol (Estraderm)	As for oral estrogens, plus irritation at patch site	0.05 mg/d (3.5 days)	12.74
		0.1 mg/d (3.5 days)	13.88
(Vivelle)		0.0375 mg/d (3.5 days)	
		0.05 mg/d (3.5 days)	
		0.075 mg/d (3.5 days)	
		0.1 mg/d (3.5 days)	
(Climara)		0.05 mg/d (7 days)	
		0.01 mg/d (7 days)	

Table 161–1. COMMONLY USED ESTROGENS AND PROGESTINS* *(Continued)*

Agent	Side Effects	Doses†	Cost ($ per Month)‡
Oral Progestins			
Medroxyprogesterone acetate			
(Cycrin)	Fluid retention, premenstrual-like syndrome, weight gain, alopecia, spotting/bleeding, acne, rash	2.5 mg 5 mg 10 mg (cyclic: 12–14 days/mo)	8.80 13.30 7.53 (14 days)
(Provera)		2.5 mg 5 mg 10 mg (cyclic: 12–14 days/mo)	10.17 15.34 8.87 (14 days)
Norethindrone (Aygestin)		5 mg	14.62
Oral Estrogens + Progestin (Combined)			
Conjugated estrogens and medroxyprogesterone acetate (MPA)			
(Prempro)	As for oral estrogens and oral progestins	0.625 mg CEE qd + 2.5 mg MPA qd	14.30 (28 days)
(Premphase)		0.625 mg CEE qd + 5 mg MPA qd × 14 days	13.11 (28 days)
Topical (Vaginal) Estrogens			
Conjugated equine estrogens (Premarin Cream)	Some systemic absorption may occur, with side effects as for systemic estrogens	0.625 mg/g (0.5–2 g cream qd)	32.46/42.5-g tube
Estradiol (Estrace Cream)		0.01% (1–2 g cream, one to three times per week)	25.68/42.5-g tube
Estropipate (Ogen Cream)		1.5 mg/g (2–4 g cream qd)	37.61/42.5-g tube

*This table lists noninjection forms including many commonly prescribed brands. It does not include every available brand. In some cases, generic preparations are also available. Injectable forms may be preferred by some physicians and patients.

†All doses are given per day continuously unless otherwise noted.

‡Based on daily dosing unless otherwise noted. Prices based on 1995 *Drug Topics Red Book*, for brand names.

for cardiovascular and thromboembolic complications other than age. Short-term systemic estrogen is quite effective at relieving vasomotor symptoms and should be used in the lowest effective dose for 1 to 2 years, at which time therapy should be reevaluated. Approaches other than estrogen are less effective but include progestins alone, clonidine, or Bellergal-S (belladonna, phenobarbital, ergotamine). For urogenital symptoms, topical (vaginal) estrogen is the most direct approach and has little systemic absorption at usual doses. It may be used alone or can be added to systemic estrogen if symptoms are not adequately controlled.

ESTROGEN REPLACEMENT THERAPY. Most of the studies of estrogen replacement therapy have used oral conjugated equine estrogen at a dose of 0.625 mg, which is the most widely prescribed form. Other oral estrogens are available, including estradiol, esterified estrogens, and plant-derived estropipate. Oral estrogens undergo first-pass metabolism in the liver and have more beneficial effects than the transdermal preparations on low and high density lipoprotein–cholesterols, although they raise triglyceride levels. Transdermal estradiol avoids first-pass metabolism and may be better for women with hypertriglyceridemia, hepatobiliary disease, or history of thromboembolism (if estrogen replacement therapy, relatively contraindicated in these situations, is pursued) and for smokers (in whom circulating estradiol levels are lower, owing to induction of its hepatic metabolism). Some women find transdermal estrogen easier or more acceptable to use. Its main drawbacks are skin irritation, which may be reduced by rotating the site used, and higher cost. Injected estrogen in depot form is used less commonly than previously, in part because of cost and discomfort. Vaginal estrogen is for treatment of local symptoms only. Systemic estrogen should be used each day; there is no physiologic reason for using it only 25 days per month, and some women will experience hot flushes during the off period if estrogen is withheld. Minor side effects from estrogen include breast tenderness and nausea, which are often dose related.

The major risk of unopposed estrogen is endometrial carcinoma. Progestin is used to protect the endometrium against the effects of estrogen. The most commonly used form is oral medroxyprogesterone acetate. Other progestins, such as norethindrone, are also used. A progestin patch is available in other countries, and progestin-releasing implants or intrauterine devices provide other, less typically used, routes of administration.

Women who have undergone hysterectomy should receive estrogen alone, unless endometrial tissue might still be present (endometriosis, or history of endometrial cancer). Women with intact uteri require protection against endometrial cancer, either with progestin or through periodic endometrial sampling. Combination therapy with a progestin is more typically used now, although unopposed estrogen may be used if progestins are not tolerated or if the maximum benefit of estrogen replacement therapy on lipids is desired and risk of cardiovascular disease is more of an issue. If estrogen is used alone, endometrial monitoring by biopsy should be done at baseline and every 1 to 2 years routinely.

When combined with estrogen therapy, a progestin can be given either cyclically for 12 to 14 days each month (cyclical combined therapy) or daily in low doses (continuous combined therapy). Cyclical therapy generally causes withdrawal bleeding or spotting each month, although the amount of flow diminishes with length of time from menopause, and flow may eventually cease. Monthly periods may not be acceptable to many women, and compliance with complicated regimens may be difficult. Again, there is no need to stop estrogen for part of the month, and the progestin course may be most easily remembered if begun on the first day of each month. Spotting or bleeding that occurs outside the cyclical pattern should be evaluated with endometrial biopsy.

Continuous combined therapy is gaining favor. It has been shown to confer protection on the endometrium, improve the lipid profile, and possibly provide better protection against bone loss than cyclical therapy. Irregular spotting occurs frequently in the first few months of use, but after 1 year 60% to 75% of women taking medroxyprogesterone acetate, 2.5 mg daily (and a higher percentage of those taking 5 mg), will have amenorrhea. Once amenorrhea is established, any spotting should be evaluated for endometrial abnormalities. Combination therapy is not as easy to use as unopposed estrogen, owing to side effects and to compliance problems inherent in a multidrug regimen. A tablet containing both conjugated equine estrogen and medroxyprogesterone is now available in the United States and may improve acceptability and compliance. Patches that contain both estrogen and progestin are used in other countries but are not yet available here. For best compliance with any regimen, women need to understand the potential side effects, particularly the likelihood and expected pattern of any bleeding, before beginning treatment.

Long-term issues should be explicitly discussed. Individual risk factors for breast cancer, osteoporosis, and heart disease should be reviewed for each woman. Advice should be given on lifestyle changes to reduce her risks, and potential risks and benefits from long-term estrogen replacement therapy should be discussed. Every woman should be given the opportunity to consider estrogen replacement therapy and to weigh the probable risks, benefits, and side effects as well as her own attitude about using hormone replacement therapy for 10 years or more. In women who have undergone hysterectomy or who have a high risk of cardiovascular disease, the benefits of estrogen replacement therapy probably outweigh the risks. In women who have a high risk of breast cancer, the risks of estrogen replacement therapy may outweigh the benefits. For any woman, deciding whether to embark on long-term estrogen replacement therapy involves multiple factors and should be made by the patient with support from her physician. For some women, further data (such as bone densitometry) may be helpful in making that decision.

General recommendations for women at menopause include smoking cessation, prudent diet, exercise, and supplementation with calcium (1200–1500 mg per day) and vitamin D (400 IU per day).

Follow-Up. Women on estrogen replacement therapy should undergo an annual review of symptoms, side effects, and ongoing risk factors; evaluation including breast and pelvic examinations; mammography; and endometrial biopsy if indicated for use of unopposed estrogen or for abnormal bleeding. (Abnormal bleeding is any postmenopausal spotting when off estrogen; irregular spotting or bleeding on cyclical estrogen replacement therapy; or spotting when on continuous combined estrogen replacement therapy after amenorrhea is established.) Transvaginal ultrasonography to evaluate the thickness of the endometrium, with biopsy if the lining is thickened (over 4 mm) or irregular, may be a reasonable alternative. Annual endometrial biopsy in the absence of symptoms is no longer standard.

Cross-References: Periodic Health Assessment (Chapter 8), Osteoporosis (Chapter 116), Breast Cancer Screening (Chapter 158), Abnormal Uterine Bleeding (Chapter 159), Mammography and Breast Imaging (Chapter 167), Dysuria (Chapter 170), Screening for Depression (Chapter 185).

REFERENCES

1. American College of Physicians. Guidelines for counseling postmenopausal women about preventive hormone therapy. Ann Intern Med 1992;117:1038–1041.

These guidelines are a useful basis for counseling patients. They summarize in table form the estimated magnitude of potential risks and benefits for many outcomes on estrogen replacement therapy, from minor side effects to changes in life expectancy.

2. Belchetz PE. Hormonal treatment of postmenopausal women. N Engl J Med 1994;330:1062–1071.

The author reviews the effects of estrogen replacement therapy on symptoms and disease outcomes, with recommendations on different regimens, duration of therapy, and monitoring.

3. Evans MP, Fleming KC, Evans JM. Hormone replacement therapy: Management of common problems. Mayo Clin Proc 1995;70:800–805.

This is a practical review of common side effects, with management tips.

4. Grady D, et al. Hormone therapy to prevent disease and prolong life in postmenopausal women. Ann Intern Med 1992;117:1016–1037.

This article includes an extensive literature review of estrogen replacement therapy with meta-analysis to estimate relative risks of disease outcomes, changes in lifetime probability of disease, and changes in life expectancy in users of estrogen replacement therapy. It is the basis of the American College of Physicians guidelines in reference 1.

5. Ravnikar V, ed. Primary care of the mature woman. Obstet Gynecol Clin North Am 1994;21.

This volume covers many aspects of menopause in detail, including sections on pathophysiology, alternative therapies, and compliance issues.

162 Initial Evaluation of a Breast Mass

Problem

MARY B. LAYA

Epidemiology. The detection of a *breast lump* (any dominant, palpable mass or thickening), whether by the patient or by her physician, provokes justifiable concerns about breast cancer, one of the most common forms of cancer among women. In the United States, over 175,000 women are diagnosed with this disease each year, many presenting with a palpable lesion. The most important overall predictor of the likelihood that a lump represents a cancer is the age of the patient; the likelihood that a breast mass is malignant increases with age. The presence or absence of risk factors should not influence the workup of a palpable lump because most women who develop breast cancer have no identifiable risk factors.

Clinical Approach and Management. Whether discovered by the patient or by her physician during an office visit, *a breast mass or asymmetric thickening* must be thoroughly evaluated (Fig. 162–1). Benign and malignant breast lumps cannot be reliably distinguished from one another on the basis of physical examination characteristics alone, although clinical features can be used in conjunction with mammography and fine-needle aspiration to improve diagnostic accuracy. The goal of the evaluation process is to maximize the detection of breast cancers (i.e., sensitivity) while minimizing false-positive results, which may lead to unnecessary biopsies. The primary care provider's role is to determine which lesions are unequivocally benign and which require further evaluation by a breast surgeon.

Because breast cancers are rare in younger women, it may be permissible to follow a clinically benign breast mass through one menstrual cycle before proceeding with further evaluation in women under age 35. Nevertheless, breast cancers do occur in young women, and the clinical approach for a persistent breast mass is the same as for older women.

Three modalities are used to evaluate the malignant potential of a breast mass: physical examination, mammography, and fine-needle aspiration with cytologic examination (see Fig. 162–1). Because none of these tests performs well in isolation, the most effective strategy combines them. Physical examination with careful evaluation of the clinical features of the mass is the first step. One or more of the following features are present in 82% of breast cancers presenting as a mass: irregular margins, nipple retraction, dimpling of the overlying skin, bloody nipple discharge, lack of mobility suggesting fixation to the surrounding structures, or axillary lymphadenopathy. Any one of these findings requires prompt surgical referral. A mass characterized as benign on physical examination (i.e., a well-circumscribed, mobile mass without any worrisome features) may still be malignant. In some series, as many as 30% of cancers had "benign" findings on physical examination.

If the physical examination reveals no signs of malignancy, a diagnostic mammogram is the next step in the evaluation process. Overall, the sensitivity of mammography in the setting of a breast mass is 73%; although sensitivity is lower in younger women, mammography still provides valuable information. Definitely benign lesions corresponding to the area in question might include a densely calcified fibroadenoma or intramammary fat consistent with an oil cyst. The diagnosis of "simple cyst" on mammography is still cause for concern because cancers may present in conjunction with a cyst. A normal mammogram does not rule out breast cancer in the setting of a mass. The false-negative rate for mammography alone in this setting ranges from 10% to 27%. If the mammogram indicates that the lump is suggestive of malignancy, immediate referral to a breast surgeon is indicated. If the mammogram is negative, fine-needle aspiration should be performed to further characterize the mass.

Fine-needle aspiration has supplanted the more invasive cutting needle biopsy and can be performed by primary care physicians. The procedure is most helpful when it yields nonbloody, cystic fluid (serous, gray, or green). Such cysts should be totally drained and the area palpated for residual mass. If the mass completely resolves after aspiration, the patient can be evaluated in 1 to 2 months for recurrence. Nonbloody aspirate need not be sent for cytologic study. Bloody or blood-tinged fluid or the presence of a residual mass is cause

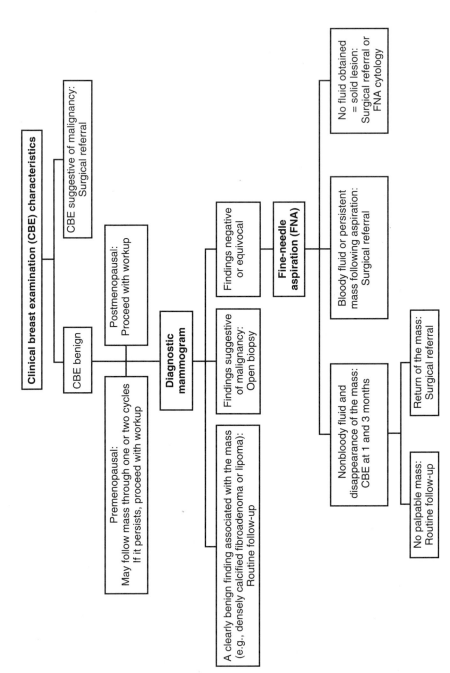

Figure 162–1. Evaluation of a dominant breast mass.

for concern and should prompt referral. Accuracy of fine-needle aspiration for solid lesions depends on the skill of the operator, size of the lesion, cytologic expertise, and type of underlying neoplasm. In one large series, 68% of results were positive by fine-needle aspiration, 14% were falsely negative, and 14% were unsatisfactory for interpretation. Although negative fine-needle aspiration alone is not sufficient to rule out breast cancer in a palpable lesion, it has a false-positive rate of less than 3%. Women with malignant or suspicious cytologic findings should be referred for surgical consultation.

Because of the limitations of physical examination, mammography, and fine-needle aspiration when performed individually, attempts have been made to improve the predictive value by combining the findings into the so-called triple test. In patients with benign findings on examination, a negative mammogram, and a negative fine-needle aspiration based on an adequate sample (a negative triple test), the likelihood that a mass is a cancer is less than 5%. Masses that do not regress in 1 to 2 months should be biopsied. When all three tests suggest cancer, the likelihood that a cancer is present approaches 100%. Other triple test combinations cannot reliably predict which masses are cancer, and the patient should be referred for biopsy.

Cross-References: Breast Cancer Screening (Chapter 158), Breast Pain in Nonlactating Women (Chapter 163), Mammography and Breast Imaging (Chapter 167).

REFERENCES

1. Ciatto S, Cariaggi P, Bulgaresi P. The value of routine cytological examination of breast cyst fluid. Acta Cytol 1987;31:301–304.

   Cytologic examination of 6782 consecutive breast cysts demonstrated that cytologic examination is not necessary for nonbloody cyst fluid.

2. Dahlbeck SW, Donnelly JF, Theriault RL. Differentiating inflammatory breast cancer from acute mastitis. Am Fam Physician 1995;52:929–934.

   The authors present a useful review of this clinical problem.

3. Di Pietr SD, Fariselli G, Bandieramonte, de Yoldi G, et al. Systematic use of the clinical-mammographic-cytological triplet for the early diagnosis of mammary carcinoma. Tumori 1985;71:179–185.

   Performance characteristics of the three diagnostic modalities are described singly and in combination based on 8500 patients presenting with palpable breast lumps.

4. Donegan WL. Evaluation of a palpable breast mass. N Engl J Med 1992;327:937–942.

   This article is a review of breast mass evaluation.

5. Martelli G, Pilotti S, Coopmans de Yoldi G. Viganotti G, et al. Diagnostic efficacy of physical examination, mammography, fine needle aspiration cytology (triple test) in solid breast lumps: An analysis of 1708 consecutive cases. Tumori 1990;76:476–479.

   A large series describes the accuracy of fine-needle aspiration in evaluation of the palpable breast mass. Sample adequacy is dependent on the skill of the operator.

163 Breast Pain in Nonlactating Women

Problem

MARY B. LAYA

Epidemiology. Breast pain is one of the most common breast-related problems encountered in a general practice. Surveys of healthy women demonstrate that 66% experience breast pain (mastalgia) sufficient to interfere with daily activities; as many as 10% of these women may seek care for this complaint. Underlying the decision to seek treatment may be a concern about the possibility of breast cancer. Although only 7% to 10% of cancers present as pain alone, the issue must be addressed in the course of evaluation and treatment of the underlying cause of the pain. Women presenting for evaluation of breast pain are no more likely to suffer from psychiatric illness than patients presenting with other conditions.

Etiology. Breast pain is classified as either acute or chronic. Acute pain (less than 2 months' duration) may be caused by trauma, inflammation, or alterations in the hormonal state (Table 163–1). Trauma to the breast may produce *hematoma, fat necrosis,* or *rupture of a preexisting cyst.* Cyst rupture may also occur during mammographic compression, and the extravasated cyst fluid may cause a localized aseptic chemical inflammation. Symptoms should resolve spontaneously over a week's time. Breast pain and inflammation is also associated with acute *bacterial mastitis.* This condition is rare in nonlactating women and should respond promptly to antibiotics. *Inflammatory carcinoma* should be considered when inflammation involves more than one third of the breast or fails to resolve in 10 days. *Periductal inflammation* represents an infection of ectatic subareolar ducts. It is characterized by a wedgelike area of inflammation emanating from the areola and responds rapidly to antibiotics directed against gram-positive organisms. *Oral contraceptives* or *hormone replacement therapy* may also produce breast pain in some women, although symptoms tend to abate over several months even with continuation of the medication. Diffuse breast pain may also be a presenting sign of an unrecognized early *pregnancy.*

Chronic breast pain (present continuously or intermittently for over 2

Table 163–1. CAUSES OF ACUTE BREAST PAIN*

Traumatic	Homonally Associated	Inflammatory
Hematoma	Oral contraceptives	Mastitis
Fat necrosis	Hormone replacement therapy	Periductal inflammation
Rupture of simple cyst	Pregnancy	Inflammatory cancer

*Breast pain present for 2 months or less.

544

months) is either cyclical or noncyclical. A daily breast pain record used in conjunction with a menstrual calendar helps distinguish these two types. *Cyclical breast pain* occurs in premenopausal women, waxes and wanes with the menstrual cycle, and is worst in the luteal phase (the 7 to 10 days before onset of menses). Palpable nodularity of the breast may increase during this time. The condition begins in the third decade of life and is relieved by menopause, highlighting its relationship to hormonal fluctuations. The pain is often bilateral and may be greatest in the upper outer quadrants. Although symptoms are clearly related to cyclical changes in hormone levels, no consistent sex hormone abnormalities have been observed. Alterations in dynamic prolactin secretion in women suffering cyclical breast pain suggest a role for this hormone in some women. Differences in fatty acid profiles between women with and those without chronic breast pain have led to the use of diet and diet supplement therapy. *Noncyclical chronic breast pain* is less common, occurring with equal frequency in premenopausal and postmenopausal women. The pain may be diffuse or localized. Localized pain may be constant or intermittent and may have an associated trigger point.

Clinical Approach and Management. The physical examination should be used to eliminate chest wall pain as the cause of the complaint and to determine whether a mass is present. If a mass is detected, its evaluation should take precedence. To exclude cancer, mammography should be performed in most women older than age 30 who present with nontraumatic breast pain, especially if the pain is unilateral or well localized. For women younger than age 30 and in women for whom mammography proves too painful, ultrasonography is an alternative imaging procedure. Special effort should be made to exclude cancer in women who present with new onset of localized breast pain.

ACUTE BREAST PAIN. If any of the trauma-associated conditions listed in Table 163–1 fail to resolve within 6 to 8 weeks, evaluation should be as for any breast lump. Similarly, any inflammatory process not responding to treatment 7 to 10 days raises concerns about inflammatory breast cancer, and the patient should be promptly referred to a breast surgeon.

CHRONIC BREAST PAIN. For many women with chronic breast pain, reassurance after the exclusion of breast cancer may be all that is required. Pain that interferes with normal daily activities can be treated with a variety of modalities (Table 163–2). A well-fitting support bra chosen with the aid of a professional fitter significantly improves symptoms in as many as 75% of patients. Diet and dietary supplements may be tried next. Both a reduction in caffeine intake and a decrease in the amount of dietary fat to 15% of calories reduces breast pain in some women. Gamolenic acid (120 mg twice daily), an essential fatty acid sold as evening primrose oil (1.5 g twice daily), has been shown in a small controlled trial to significantly improve cyclical mastalgia. A response to treatment may be delayed for up to 4 months. The supplement is available in health food stores. Short-term side effects are minor, but treatment is expensive ($60–$80 per month); long-term effects of use are not known.

Hormonal treatments are effective but may be associated with troublesome side effects, unknown long-term effects, and significant expense. Hence, hormonal therapy should be limited to women with truly debilitating breast pain unresponsive to nonpharmacologic therapy. Danazol, an inhibitor of pituitary

Table 163–2. TREATMENT OF CHRONIC BREAST PAIN*

Modality	Therapy	Side Effects	Cost ($)†
Mechanical support	Professionally fitted support bra	None	20–30
Dietary measures	Caffeine avoidance	None	0
	Low-fat diet (15–20% of total calories)	None	0
	Evening primrose oil 1.5 g PO bid	Abdominal bloating	60–80/mo
Hormonal therapy‡	Danazol, 200 mg/d × 2 mo then 100 mg/d × 2 mo then 100 mg during the luteal phase only	Weight gain, irregular menses, nausea, vomiting, androgenic effects	50–100/mo
	Bromocriptine, 1.25 mg/d titrated up to 2.5 mg bid over 2 wk	Nausea and vomiting, headache, postural hypotension	25–95/mo
	Tamoxifen, 10 mg/d × 3 mo	Irregular menses/ammenorhea, hot flushes	45/mo

*Symptoms present for 2 months or longer.
†Average wholesale price for prescription medication, 1995 *Drug Topics Red Book.*
‡Hormonal therapy should be reserved for those with debilitating symptoms not responsive to other modalities. Long-term effects are not established.

gonadotropins with antiestrogenic/progestogenic effects, is the most effective hormonal therapy, but 30% of patients treated experience significant side effects. The effectiveness of bromocriptine has also been demonstrated, but side effects severe enough to cause discontinuation occur in 36% of women. Tamoxifen, in a dose of 10 mg/d, may also be tried, but hot flushes, menstrual irregularity, and a potential increase in the risk of endometrial carcinoma make long-term use problematic. Therapies for which there is anecdotal evidence, but for which effectiveness has not been demonstrated in randomized trials, include vitamins E and B_6, diuretics, and medroxyprogesterone acetate.

For diffuse, noncyclical breast pain, the same treatments used for cyclical breast pain may also be helpful, although they are often less effective.

REFERENCES

1. BeLieu RM. Mastodynia. Obstet Gynecol Clin North Am 1994;21:461–477.

   A practical review is provided of the pathophysiology and treatment of chronic breast pain.

2. Fentiman IS, Caleffi M, Hamed H, Chaudary MA. Dosage and duration of tamoxifen treatment for mastalgia: A controlled trial. Br J Surg 1988;75:845–846.

   Tamoxifen at 10 mg/d was found to be as effective as when given at higher doses. Relapse rates were also similar after discontinuation (48% and 39%), suggesting a need for long-term therapy, the safety of which has yet to be established.

3. Gately CA, Miers M, Mansel RE, Hughes LE. Drug treatments for mastalgia: 17 years experience in the Cardiff mastalgia clinic. J R Soc Med 1992;85:12–15.

   A large experience with drug treatment of cyclical and noncyclical mastalgia is described with details regarding therapeutics and side effects.

4. Harrison BJ, Maddos PR, Mansel RE. Maintenance therapy of cyclic mastalgia using low-dose danazol. J R Coll Surg Edinb 1989;34:79–81.

   The authors describe the initial use of conventional doses of danazol (100 mg/d) to induce remission followed by conversion to a luteal phase regimen for women who require long-term treatment.

164 Vaginitis

Problem

JANE SCHWEBKE

Epidemiology and Etiology. Vaginal infections account for 50% of all patient visits to private gynecologists and 28% of visits by women to sexually transmitted disease clinics.

The three main causes of vaginitis in order of frequency of occurrence are bacterial vaginosis, candidiasis, and trichomoniasis. Of these, only infection with *Trichomonas* is proven to be sexually transmitted. Candidiasis most likely represents an overgrowth syndrome triggered by factors such as broad-spectrum antibiotic use, estrogens, and diabetes. Chronic or frequently recurring vaginal candidiasis should raise suspicion of human immunodeficiency virus infection. The etiology of bacterial vaginosis is unknown, but it is found almost exclusively in sexually active women. Data have implicated bacterial vaginosis in infectious complications, including preterm birth.

Symptoms and Signs. The classic symptoms and signs of each type of vaginitis appear in Table 164–1. Women with trichomoniasis and bacterial vaginosis may be asymptomatic, and mixed infections may occur.

Clinical Approach. A speculum examination is necessary to determine whether discharge in the vaginal vault is the result of vaginitis or cervicitis. A diagnosis based on a clinical impression of the characteristics of the vaginal discharge is frequently in error; microscopic diagnosis is required.

The diagnostic approach includes determining the pH of the vaginal fluid, performing a "whiff test" (the addition of 10% potassium hydroxide [KOH] to the vaginal fluid produces a fishy odor if amines are present), and microscopic examination of a saline preparation (wet prep) for fungal elements, clue cells, motile trichomonads, and polymorphonuclear leukocytes. Examination of a KOH preparation and Gram-stained specimen may also be helpful. In general,

Table 164-1. CLINICAL AND LABORATORY FEATURES OF VAGINITIS

	Candida	Trichomonas	Bacterial Vaginosis
Symptoms	Vulvar pruritus; discharge	Pruritus; discharge	Fishy odor, especially after intercourse; discharge
Signs			
Discharge	White, "cottage cheese"	Yellow, thick, occasionally frothy	White-gray, homogeneous
Vulvar dermatitis	Common (erythema, fissures)	Occasional	Rare
Laboratory Findings			
pH of discharge*	<4.5	>4.5	>4.5
Amine odor with 10% KOH	Negative	Often positive	Positive
Wet prep, saline, or 10% KOH†	Leukocytes; budding yeast and pseudohyphae	Leukocytes; motile trichomonads	Clue cells‡§
Gram stain	Leukocytes; yeast and pseudohyphae	Leukocytes; may see fixed trichomonads	Clue cells‡, decreased numbers of lactobacilli; increased gram-variable rods, gram-positive cocci, and gram-variable curved rods (*Mobiluncus*)

*Not reliable during menses or after recent intercourse or douching.
†KOH is useful in this setting only for detection of yeast.
‡Clue cells are squamous epithelial cells with large numbers of adherent bacteria.
§Leukocytes are not present in bacterial vaginosis itself, but they may be present if a concurrent cervical infection such as infection with *Neisseria gonorrhaeae* or *Chlamydia* is present.

cultures for yeast should not be performed, because many women normally harbor small numbers of yeast in the vagina. Culturing for *Trichomonas* may increase the sensitivity of laboratory diagnosis by up to 25%. Because bacterial vaginosis is a mixed infection composed of increased numbers of anaerobic bacteria, *Gardnerella,* and *Mycoplasma,* culture of the vagina is not recommended. Table 164–1 provides further details on laboratory diagnosis.

Management. Appropriate therapy for each infection is outlined in Table 164–2. Women with trichomoniasis or bacterial vaginosis should also be screened for infection with *Chlamydia* and *Neisseria gonorrhoeae,* because they may be at risk for multiple sexually transmitted infections. Treatment of partners is generally limited to those patients with trichomoniasis. The partner should be examined for other sexually transmitted diseases before treatment. Occasionally, partners of women with bacterial vaginosis are treated if the couple is monogamous and bacterial vaginosis is recurring frequently. There are no data to support the theory of a reservoir for bacterial vaginosis in the male.

Follow-Up. Follow-up of vaginal infections is generally not required unless symptoms do not resolve.

Table 164–2. TREATMENT OF VAGINITIS

	Primary	Alternatives	Cost ($)*	Cure Rate
Candida	Clotrimazole 1% vaginal cream/ suppositories qhs × 3–7 d		12.00	80–90%
	Miconazole 2% vaginal cream/ suppositories qhs × 3–7 d		12.85	
	Butaconazole 2% cream, 3-day prefilled		20.16	
	Teraconazole 0.4% cream qhs × 7 d, 0.8% cream qhs × 3 d		23.34	
		Fluconazole, 150 mg PO × one dose	10.63	80–90%
Trichomonas	Metronidazole, 2 g PO in a single dose†		1.20	95%
		Metronidazole, 500 mg PO bid × 7 d†	4.18	95%
Bacterial vaginosis	Metronidazole, 500 mg PO bid × 7 days‡		4.18	85–95%‡
		Metronidazole gel, 0.75%, intravaginally bid × 5 d	24.00	80–90%‡
		Clindamycin, 300 mg PO bid × 7 d	26.15	85–95%‡
		Clindamycin, 2% cream intravaginally qhs × 7 d	23.36	80–95%‡

*Generic price given, when available. Average wholesale price, 1995 *Drug Topics Red Book.*
†Contraindicated in first trimester of pregnancy.
‡Recurrence of disease is common.

Cross-Reference: Dysuria (Chapter 170).

REFERENCES

1. Centers for Disease Control. 1993 Sexually transmitted disease treatment guidelines. MMWR 1993;42(RR-14):67–75.
   Current treatment options are outlined.

2. Krohn MA, Hillier SL, Eschenbach DA. Comparison of methods for diagnosing bacterial vaginosis among pregnant women. J Clin Microbiol 1989;27:1266–1271.
   The authors provide an up-to-date review of bacterial vaginosis.

3. Martius J, Eschenbach DA. The role of bacterial vaginosis as a cause of amniotic fluid infection, chorioamnionitis and prematurity: A review. Arch Gynecol Obstet 1990;247:1–13.
   A review of bacterial vaginosis and prematurity is presented.

4. Rein MF, Holmes KK. "Nonspecific vaginitis," vulvovaginal candidiasis, and trichomoniasis: Clinical features, diagnosis, and management. Curr Clin Topics Infect Dis 1983;4:281–315.
   This article is a general review.

5. Sweet RL. Importance of differential diagnosis in acute vaginitis. Am J Obstet Gynecol 1985;152:921–923.
   The importance of an accurate diagnosis is emphasized.

165 Contraception

Problem

KIRK K. SHY

Epidemiology. The National Survey of Family Growth (1988), the most recent national contraceptive survey, indicated that 78% of women of reproductive age (15–44 years) had had intercourse in the preceding 3 months (43% of women aged 15–19 years). At first intercourse, 35% of women do not use contraception. This percentage is high regardless of race (white, non-Hispanic = 31%). In this survey, 28% of all births were mistimed, and an additional 12% were unwanted. Less than 4% of women of reproductive age actively seek pregnancy. Among all sexually active women (15–44 years), the choice of contraceptive is as follows: sterilization, 33% (male = 19%, female = 14%); oral contraceptives, 32%; condoms, 17%; withdrawal, 6%; and periodic abstinence, 4%. The remainder use other barrier methods.

Clinical Approach. Clinicians should discuss the ranges of contraceptive effectiveness, side effects, and user satisfaction for all contraceptive methods, particularly for the newer methods (e.g., cervical cap, Norplant) that may be unknown to the patient. Table 165–1 reports failure rates in married women, 25 years or older, who were observed for several years (other sources of contraceptive failure data typically overestimate failure with barrier methods). The patient interview should focus on prior contraceptive use, frequency of intercourse, and the patient's viewpoint regarding management of an unplanned pregnancy.

Management. Because latex condoms are associated with significant reductions in transmission of sexually transmitted diseases, they should be used for all sexual relationships that are new or not assuredly mutually monogamous. Polyurethane condoms are available for individuals with latex allergy, but breakage is much more common. Natural membrane (skin) condoms do not prevent transmission of hepatitis B virus and human immunodeficiency virus. "Dry" silicon-based lubricants are most popular. Others use water-based surgical jelly. Oil-based lubricants should be avoided because they weaken condoms and increase breakage. Although contraceptive foam (a vehicle for spermicides: nonoxynol-9 or octoxynol) increases the effectiveness of condoms, the principal contraceptive effect is from the condom itself. Couples should not decide against condoms because the addition of foam is too much effort. Alone, foam, contraceptive suppositories, and the contraceptive sponge are considerably less effective than condoms. Some condoms are coated with nonoxynol-9. Whether it improves contraceptive effectiveness is uncertain. However, nonoxynol-9 may cause vaginal and penile irritation and increase the risk of urinary tract infection in women. Many women choose to use both condoms (to diminish the risk of sexually transmitted diseases) and oral contraceptives (to diminish the risk of pregnancy). Data concerning the effectiveness and acceptability of the

Table 165–1. CONTRACEPTIVE EFFECTIVENESS*

Method	Failure Rate (per 100 Woman-Years)
Chance	85.0
Condom (male)	3.6
Condom (female)	15.0
Diaphragm	1.9
IUD (Paragard [TCu-380A] [Copper])	< 0.8
Norplant (subdermal levonorgestrel implant)	< 0.6
Oral contraceptive	
Combination (< 50 µg estrogen)	0.27
Progestin only	1.2
Rhythm	15.5
Spermicides	11.9
Sterilization	
Female	0.13
Male	0.02
Withdrawal	6.7

*These data are from married women, 25 years or older, who were followed for an average of 9½ years at British family planning clinics.

Data are from Vessey M, Lawless M, Yates D. Efficacy of different contraceptive methods. Lancet 1982;1:841–842, except for data concerning the female condom (from Bounds W, Guillebaud J, Newman GB. The female condom [Femidom]. A clinical study of its use effectiveness and patient acceptability. Br J Fam Plann 1992;18:36), the Copper-TCu-380A (from Trussel J, Hatcher RA, Cates W, et al. Contraceptive failure in the United States: An update. Studies Fam Plann 1990;21:51–54), and Norplant (from Shoupe D, Mishell DR. Norplant: Subdermal implant system long-term contraception. Am J Obstet Gynecol 1989;160:1286–1292).

female condom are limited. Cost of the female condom is relatively high (about $9.00 for a box of three).

Training is necessary to properly fit the cervical cap or diaphragm. The largest diaphragm ring that is comfortable and not distorted by the vagina is best. Almost all women can be fitted for a diaphragm and taught to insert it correctly, but a significant minority of women cannot be fitted for a cervical cap. Contraceptive jelly must be included between the cervix and diaphragm or cervical cap. The diaphragm should remain in place for at least 6 to 8 hours after intercourse, and it should be removed within 24 hours. The cervical cap can remain in place and is effective for 48 hours.

Oral contraceptives are contraindicated if the patient has the following conditions (or a history of them): thromboembolic disease, cerebrovascular accident, coronary artery disease, impaired liver function, hepatic cancer/adenoma, breast cancer, and estrogen-dependent neoplasia. They are also contraindicated during pregnancy and in patients with cholestasis during a previous pregnancy. Strong relative contraindications include vascular headaches, hypertension, forced immobility, and heavy smoking at age 35 years or older. Relative contraindications to oral contraceptives must be considered in the context of the feasibility of alternative contraception and the patient's ability to respond to unplanned pregnancy.

The clinician should initially choose a pill with a daily dosage of 35 µg of estrogen (Table 165–2). Lower dosages are associated with higher rates of troublesome endometrial bleeding, which may affect continuation rates. Higher

Table 165–2. ORAL CONTRACEPTIVES

Clinical Setting	Oral Contraceptive Agent	Estrogen Dosage	ProgestinDosage	Cost ($ per Month)*
Initial choice	Norinyl 1/35	EE, 35 μg	NE, 1.0 mg	22.24
Initial choice	Ortho-Novum 1/35	EE, 35 μg	NE, 1.0 mg	23.14
Initial choice	Brevicon	EE, 35 μg	NE, 0.5 mg	22.94
Initial choice	Modicon	EE, 35 μg	NE, 0.5 mg	23.28
Initial choice	Ortho-Novum 7/7/7†	EE, 35 μg	NE, 0.5/0.75/1.0 mg	23.29
Initial choice	Tri-Levlen†	EE, 35 μg	NG, 0.05/0.75/0.125 mg	19.73
Initial choice	Tri-Norinyl†	EE, 35 μg	NE, 0.5/0.75/1.0 mg	21.15
Initial choice	Triphasil†	EE, 30/40 μg	NG, 0.05/0.75/0.125 mg	25.02
History of acne or hirsutism	Desogen	EE, 30 μg	DG, 0.15 mg	19.55
History of acne or hirsutism	Ortho-Cept	EE, 30 μg	DG, 0.15 mg	22.20
History of acne or hirsutism	Ortho-Cyclen	EE, 35 μg	NGM, 0.25 mg	22.20
History of estrogen side effect‡	Loestrin 21 1/20	EE, 20 μg	NA, 1.0 mg	25.24
History of estrogen side effect‡	Micronor§	None	NE, 0.35 mg	29.22
History of estrogen side effect‡	Nor-Q-D§	None	NE, 0.35 mg	18.05
History of estrogen side effect‡	Ovrette§	None	NG, 0.075 mg	17.52
History of OC failure	Norinyl 1/50	EE, 50 μg	NE, 1.0 mg	22.24
History of OC failure	Ortho-Novum 1/50	EE, 50 μg	NE, 1.0 mg	23.14
Postcoital contraception‖	Ovral	EE, 50 μg	NE, 0.5 mg	32.90

OC, oral contraceptive; EE, ethinyl estradiol; NE, norethindrone; NG, norgestrel; DG, desogestrel; NGM, norgestimate; NA, norethindrone acetate.

*Average wholesale price, 1995 *Drug Topics Red Book.*

†Triphasic oral contraceptive with weekly variation in progestin dosage.

‡Estrogen-related side effects include breast tenderness, nausea, and cyclical weight gain.

§Progestin-only oral contraceptives are taken daily without a medication-free week. Pregnancy rates are somewhat greater with progestin-only oral contraceptives compared with monophasic products.

‖Administration is two Ovral tablets within 72 hours of intercourse, followed by two additional tablets 12 hours later.

dosages should be reserved for women with contraceptive failure at 35 μg. Progestin dosage should be 1 mg or less of norethindrone, or 0.15 mg or less of norgestrel. Triphasic oral contraceptives (Ortho-Novum 7/7/7, Tri-Norinyl, Triphasil) offer the theoretic advantage of lower complication rates because of lower estrogen dosage. However, compared with standard monophasic oral contraceptives (Ortho-Novum 1/35, Norinyl 1/35, Modicon), the dosage reduction is small. Norgestimate and desogestrel are two progestins available in the newest oral contraceptive formulations. These progestins have less androgenic activity and may be preferable in women with acne or hirsutism. Progestin-only oral contraceptives may be useful for women who are breast feeding (estrogen inhibits lactation) or for women with estrogen-related side effects (e.g., breast tenderness, nausea, cyclical weight gain) or estrogen-related risk factors (e.g., history of thrombophlebitis). Progestin-only oral contraceptives have some drawbacks: less predictable menstruation, and pregnancy rates about five times greater than with estrogen-progestin combination oral contraceptives.

There are several options for timing the beginning of oral contraceptives. They may be started (1) immediately (may cause unwanted vaginal bleeding), (2) 5 days after the start of the next period, (3) on the first day of the next period, or (4) on the first Sunday after the onset of the next menstrual period, which generally results in menstruation-free weekends. Except for the first option, effective contraception begins immediately.

Side effects of oral contraceptives include the following:

1. Intermenstrual bleeding, which generally resolves spontaneously in 3 months
2. Nausea, which declines during the first 3 months of use. If persistent, nausea may improve with an oral contraceptive with 20 μg of estrogen (Loestrin 21 1/20) or a progestin-only pill.
3. Light periods (or amenorrhea), which affect most patients but do not adversely affect health.
4. Weight gain (unusual).
5. Chloasma (increased facial pigmentation), which is a cosmetic indication for stopping oral contraceptives.

Medroxyprogesterone acetate in oil (Depo-Provera) and levonorgestrel (Norplant) are effective long-acting progestin-based contraceptives. The contraceptive effect of both of these agents begins immediately, and failure rates approach those of sterilization. The absolute contraindications (acute liver disease, history of liver tumor, acute thrombophlebitis, history of breast cancer, unexplained vaginal bleeding) for both are fewer than for oral contraceptives. Depo-Provera, 150 mg, is administered intramuscularly every 3 months. Menstrual disturbance (initially metrorrhagia and later amenorrhea) occurs for most women. Weight gain averages 1 to 5 kg during the first year of use. Cost for Depo-Provera is approximately $55 for 150 mg, including injection fee.

Norplant consists of six hollow Silastic rods filled with the progestin levonorgestrel and designed for subdermal implantation in the medial aspect of the upper arm. Insertion is simple and largely painless, but some instruction in technique is necessary. Removal is technically difficult but is necessary after 5 years, when the implants lose effectiveness. The major side effect is irregular uterine bleeding, which for some women is continuous throughout use of the implant. Cost of the device (approximately $350), insertion (approximately $250), and removal (approximately $200) varies.

The principal intrauterine device (IUD) is the Paragard (TCu-380A), a T-shaped, copper-covered, polyethylene IUD with 10 years of effectiveness. Pregnancy rates are similar to those with oral contraceptives. Pelvic inflammatory disease is substantially less common with this IUD than with its predecessors; nonetheless, because of this problem, IUDs should be used only by women in mutually monogamous relationships. Contraindications include a history of menorrhagia or dysmenorrhea, immunosuppression, valvular heart disease, or previous pelvic inflammatory disease. Insertion should be by trained practitioners. Cost of the IUD (approximately $150) and insertion (approximately $125) varies.

Postcoital contraception with IUD insertion within 5 days after intercourse or with oral contraceptives within 72 hours after intercourse is effective (Ovral, two tablets initially, followed in 12 hours by two additional tablets). Before treating, however, the clinician should consider the possibility of a preexisting early pregnancy from another recent episode of unprotected intercourse.

Follow-Up. To increase compliance, most patients with prescription contraception should have a return appointment in 4 weeks. The clinician should monitor oral contraceptive users for increased blood pressure. One should also consider following serum lipid levels in women with hyperlipidemia who use hormonal contraception. IUD users should be examined for evidence of pelvic inflammatory disease and for string lengthening or shortening, which indicates potentially improper IUD placement.

Cross-References: Abnormal Uterine Bleeding (Chapter 159), Pelvic Inflammatory Disease (Chapter 166), Urinary Tract Infections in Women (Chapter 175), HIV Infection: Disease Prevention and Antiretroviral Therapy (Chapter 203), Diagnosis of Pregnancy (Chapter 210).

REFERENCES

1. Darney PD. The androgenicity of progestins. Am J Med 1995;98(1A):1045–1105.
   This article provides a discussion of this topic.

2. How reliable are condoms? Consumer Reports 1995 May:1–6.
   A thorough review of varieties, breakage rates, and cost is presented.

3. Mishell DR. Contraception. N Engl J Med 1989;320:777–787.
   A general review is provided.

4. Sivin I. International experience with Norplant and Norplant-2 contraceptives. Studies Fam Plann 1988;19:81–94.
   The author gives a balanced review of the subdermal implant for contraception.

· ·

166 Pelvic Inflammatory Disease

Problem

EMILY Y. WONG

Epidemiology. Pelvic inflammatory disease (PID), also known as salpingitis, affects approximately 1 million American women every year. Up to 25% of these women will develop long-term sequelae associated with the infection, such as infertility, chronic pelvic pain, and ectopic pregnancy. Direct and indirect costs were estimated at close to $4 billion in 1990.

Established risk factors include adolescence, multiple sexual partners, use of an intrauterine device, and previous history of PID. Vaginal douching, low socioeconomic status, substance abuse, and cigarette smoking have also been associated with an increased incidence of PID. Those women who use condoms and spermicide, the diaphragm, or oral contraceptive pills tend to have a relatively lower incidence of disease.

Symptoms and Signs. Patients most typically present during or immediately after menses with bilateral lower abdominal pain and fever. Vaginal discharge, dysuria, metromenorrhagia, nausea and vomiting, and dyspareunia may also be present. The high incidence of "silent" PID is inferred from the observation that both infertility and ectopic pregnancy are frequently associated with positive serologic evidence for *Chlamydia* infection, despite a negative history for clinical disease.

Pain on palpation of the lower abdomen, cervical motion tenderness, and adnexal tenderness are present in 90% of patients. When present, concurrent findings of an exudative and friable cervix are helpful in supporting the diagnosis. Upper abdominal tenderness and peritoneal signs may also be present in PID; the Fitz-Hugh–Curtis syndrome refers to focal inflammation with involvement of the liver capsule.

Clinical Approach. Recommended laboratory tests include leukocyte count, serum human chorionic gonadotropin (β-hCG level) for pregnancy, and endocervical testing for gonorrhea and chlamydial infection. When lower genital tract disease is clinically detectable, an inflammatory exudate is found on wet-mount examination. Erythrocyte sedimentation rate and C-reactive protein have not proven to be helpful in confirming this difficult diagnosis. The gold standard for diagnosis of PID is direct visualization of inflamed pelvic structures by laparoscopy. However, less invasive techniques such as endovaginal ultrasonography, culdocentesis, and endometrial biopsy are being evaluated as diagnostic tools.

Because available criteria for the diagnosis of PID are limited in sensitivity and specificity, the decision for treatment is often made on a clinical basis. The presence of pelvic organ tenderness and mucopurulent cervicitis is highly suggestive, and antibiotic therapy should be initiated presumptively. Adnexal fullness on bimanual examination should be followed up with a pelvic ultrasound examination to rule out tubo-ovarian abscess. Absence of lower genital tract involvement broadens the range of diagnostic possibilities to include ruptured ovarian cyst, ectopic pregnancy, appendicitis, diverticulitis, and endometriosis. Genital testing for infection with *Neisseria gonorrhoeae* and *Chlamydia trachomatis* should still be undertaken, with treatment directed at upper tract disease if findings are positive. Testing for other concurrent sexually transmitted diseases with an asymptomatic phase, such as human immunodeficiency virus (HIV) infection, should also be considered at this time.

Management. Although the majority of cases of PID involve *N. gonorrhoeae* or *C. trachomatis,* polymicrobial infection is also frequently present. A large variety of microorganisms, often endogenous to the vaginal or bowel flora, have been implicated. Broad-spectrum antibiotic therapy targets the aforementioned sexually transmitted organisms, as well as *Mycobacterium hominis, Ureaplasma urealyticum, Escherichia coli, Streptococcus pyogenes, Streptococcus pneumoniae, Bacteroides* species, and anaerobic cocci. Pelvic rest has been advocated as adjunctive therapy. Sexual partners should be evaluated for sexually transmitted diseases and treated presumptively for asymptomatic infection. Table 166–1 lists the antibiotic regimens recommended in the Centers for Disease Control and Prevention (CDC) guidelines for ambulatory treatment of PID.

PID is most commonly treated in the outpatient primary care setting;

Table 166–1. OUTPATIENT ANTIBIOTIC TREATMENT OF PID

Drug	Dosage	Cost ($)*
Ceftriaxone†	250 mg IM one dose	11.44
and		
doxycycline	100 mg PO bid × 14d	4.79
	or	
Cefoxitin,	2 g IM one dose, *plus*	18.39
concurrent probenicid	1 g PO one dose	0.32
and		
doxycycline	100 mg PO bid × 14 d	4.79
	or	
Ofloxacin	400 mg PO bid × 14 d	102.42
and		
clindamycin	450 mg PO qid × 14 d	147.83
or metronidazole	500 mg PO bid × 14 d	8.39

*Average wholesale price, 1995 *Drug Topics Red Book*.
†Or equivalent third-generation cephalosporin.

however, urgent gynecologic consultation or hospitalization for parenteral therapy and close observation may be required in some instances. Guidelines developed by the CDC for inpatient management are as follows:

1. When the diagnosis is uncertain
2. If the possibility of surgical emergencies such as appendicitis or ectopic pregnancy cannot be excluded
3. If a pelvic or tubo-ovarian abscess is suspected
4. When the patient is pregnant
5. When the patient is an adolescent
6. When severe illness precludes outpatient management
7. When the patient either cannot follow or cannot tolerate an outpatient regimen
8. When the patient is not responding to outpatient therapy
9. When follow-up cannot be arranged within 72 hours

In addition, patients with a complex underlying illness such as HIV infection or diabetes or patients on immunosuppressive agents may benefit from inpatient therapy.

Follow-Up. Follow-up should be arranged in 24 to 48 hours to assess response to therapy. Failure to respond may be an indication for admission or for further diagnostic testing with ultrasonography or laparoscopy.

An estimated 25% of women will develop long-term sequelae from PID, including infertility, ectopic pregnancy, and chronic pelvic pain. Tubal factor infertility develops in 8% of women after the first episode of PID, in 19.5% after the second episode, and in 40% after the third episode. Chronic pelvic pain has been found to be present in 18% of women after resolution of acute PID. The incidence of ectopic pregnancy was six times higher than in women without evidence of prior upper genital tract infection. Although prompt and effective antibiotic therapy is thought to prevent tubal damage, further study is required to support this theory.

Cross-References: Abdominal Pain (Chapter 94), Female Infertility (Chapter 155), Abnormal Uterine Bleeding (Chapter 159), Pelvic Pain in Women (Chapter 160), Contraception (Chapter 165), Dysuria (Chapter 170), Sexually Transmitted Diseases (Chapter 176), HIV Infection: Disease Prevention and Antiretroviral Therapy (Chapter 203), HIV Infection: Office Evaluation (Chapter 204), HIV Infection: Evaluation of Common Symptoms (Chapter 205), Diagnosis of Pregnancy (Chapter 210).

REFERENCES

1. Centers for Disease Control. 1993 Sexually transmitted diseases treatment guidelines. MMWR 1993;42(RR-14):75–81.

   Updated recommendations from the CDC are presented.

2. McCormack WM. Pelvic inflammatory disease. N Engl J Med 1994;330:115–119.

   This is a succinct and clinically relevant review.

3. Peterson HB, Walker CK, Kahn JG, Washington AE, Eschenbach DA, Faro S. Pelvic inflammatory disease: Key treatment issues and options. JAMA 1991;266:2605–2611.

   Available data on antimicrobial therapy are reviewed.

4. Soper DE. Pelvic inflammatory disease. Infect Dis Clin North Am 1994;8:821–841.

   More detailed discussion of postulated pathogenic mechanisms and diagnostic criteria is presented.

5. Westrom L, Joesoef R, Reynolds G, Hagdu A, Thompson SE. Pelvic inflammatory disease and fertility. Sex Transm Dis 1992;19:185–192.

   A large cohort study examined the incidence of tubal factor infertility and ectopic pregnancy in women with and without laparoscopic evidence of PID.

167 Mammography and Breast Imaging

Procedure

MARIANN J. DRUCKER

Indications and Contraindications. Mammography is the primary means of screening for occult breast neoplasms as well as for evaluating signs or symptoms that suggest breast disease. Despite the development of many newer forms of imaging, mammography continues to be the most important diagnostic modality. Alternative imaging examinations, which include ultrasonography, magnetic resonance imaging, and stereotactic or ultrasound-guided needle biopsies, are employed primarily to resolve questions elicited by mammography or clinical examination.

Screening mammography reduces breast cancer mortality for women between 50 and 69 years of age. Considerable controversy exists regarding the use of screening mammography in women younger than the age of 50. A screening mammogram usually consists of two standard views of each breast. If an abnormality is detected, additional evaluation may be required to further characterize the finding. This assessment may include additional mammographic views (e.g., spot compression or magnification) or ultrasonography. The rate of "abnormal mammograms" varies among radiologists and different patient populations but generally is in the range of 5% to 15%. Only 1% to 2% of screening mammograms actually require biopsy, and only 1 in 200 screening mammograms actually result in a diagnosis of malignancy. The degree to which mammography can provide definitive information depends on the pretest probability of disease (i.e., on a quantitative assessment by the physician concerning the likelihood of malignancy and on the sensitivity and specificity of the mammogram) (see Chapter 7, Principles of Screening).

A diagnostic mammogram, as the name suggests, is designed to evaluate and diagnose the cause of signs or symptoms that suggest breast disease, such as a lump or thickening that is detected by a woman during breast self-examination or by her clinician during a physical examination. The goals of diagnostic mammography are therefore different from those of screening mammography. Diagnostic mammography attempts to resolve a specific diagnostic dilemma or, if not, to provide a specific recommendation toward closure or diagnosis. Other symptoms for which mammography is employed include breast pain, skin or nipple changes, nipple discharge, and axillary adenopathy. In any woman older than age 30, a diagnostic mammogram should be obtained for either characterization of a palpable lump or documentation of normal breast tissue if clinical suspicion for significant pathology is low. A negative mammogram, however, should never deter a clinician from further evaluation of a clinically suspicious lump or discharge. Such situations require judicious use of other diagnostic tests, ranging from ultrasonography or magnetic resonance imaging to fine-needle or large-core biopsy, before deciding to simply "follow" the patient or to perform an excisional biopsy.

Rationale. A mammographically detected malignancy typically presents as an irregularly marginated mass, as a mass that is either new or has increased in size, or as a cluster of calcifications. Microcalcifications and dense masses usually attenuate or absorb more of the x-ray beam than the surrounding normal fibroglandular tissue. However, adjacent dense tissue can occasionally obscure a mass. This partially explains why the sensitivity of screening mammography is 85% rather than 100%.

Ultrasonography, when used as an adjunct to mammography, improves on the specificity of both physical examination and mammography. In one report it was demonstrated that ultrasonography can reduce the number of excisional biopsies by a third, thereby decreasing morbidity and cost.

Methods. Nearly all breast imaging facilities perform low-dose film-screen mammography, which uses lower energies than most other radiologic examinations. By using lower-energy x-rays, it is possible to provide images with high contrast. The total average glandular dose per breast in a screening mammogram may not exceed 600 mrad but is usually about 250 mrad per breast. Patients can more easily understand the radiation dose by the following comparisons:

1. Natural radiation in New York is 135 mrad per year.
2. Natural radiation in Denver is 200 mrad per year.
3. Dental radiographic series is 400 mrad.
4. Chest radiograph is 100 mrad.

Mammography requires that the patient be able to sit or stand, with some acceptable limitations by body habitus or arm disability such as in stroke or frozen shoulder. Breast compression is imperative. Although uncomfortable, compression rarely causes excruciating pain or skin breaks. Women who have experienced unacceptable pain can be permitted to control the degree of compression, often with the same results as those produced by a trained technologist.

Breast ultrasonography has become widely accepted as a secondary diagnostic test that gives no ionizing radiation. The patient may be scanned in any position but is usually supine. Compression is not required. Ultrasonography is widely used for needle-directed biopsy and cyst aspiration. The disadvantages of breast ultrasonography are that it is operator dependent, cannot detect malignant microcalcifications or small masses in fatty breast tissue, and is not easily reproducible from examination to examination, therefore rendering it inappropriate as a screening modality.

Stereotactic biopsy has gained wide acceptance as a means for histologic diagnosis of nonpalpable lesions. It is a radiography-guided method using either a standard upright mammography unit or a prone table mammography apparatus for localizing and sampling breast lesions discovered on mammography. Core biopsy using a 14-gauge needle has a sensitivity of approximately 95% for breast cancer detection. Modern stereotactic breast biopsy is comparable in sensitivity to surgical biopsy and is quicker, less expensive, and easier than the standard practice of preoperative mammographically guided localization followed by surgical biopsy. Stereotactic core biopsy is valuable because it can render a benign diagnosis for 75% of indeterminate lesions, frequently eliminating the need for excisional biopsy. It also provides tissue for histologic diagnosis, allowing for consideration of management options before definitive surgical treatment.

Cost and Quality Control. Quality control and quality assurance have played significant roles in mammography since the enactment of the Mammography Quality Standards Act of 1992. Mammography facilities and personnel must provide thorough documentation of equipment performance, technologist and physicist quality control tests, medical audits, outcome analysis, and personnel qualification records. They must also pass a rigorous on-site inspection by the Food and Drug Administration before receiving accreditation.

The cost of a screening mammogram varies widely, ranging from $55 to $200. Current Medicare reimbursement is approximately $80. Diagnostic mammogram fees are higher because of the need for additional views and the active involvement of the radiologist and technologist. The cost of breast ultrasonography varies widely, between $100 and $250, again depending on the complexity of the examination and the time required. Stereotactic biopsies cost between $400 and $800, with cost expected to drop somewhat as expensive biopsy units are paid off. Magnetic resonance imaging is costly, ranging from $400 to $1500. Because magnetic resonance imaging cannot provide a definitive diagnosis, this test is most commonly applied to evaluation of breast implants or as a secondary diagnostic test in patients with known breast cancer.

Cross-References: Principles of Screening (Chapter 7), Breast Cancer Screening (Chapter 158), Initial Evaluation of a Breast Mass (Chapter 162), Breast Pain in Nonlactating Women (Chapter 163).

REFERENCES

1. Evans W-P: Breast masses: Appropriate evaluation. Radiol Clin North Am 1995;33(6).
   An in-depth discussion of the radiologic approach to breast imaging, including algorithms, is presented.

2. Houn F, Brown ML: Current practice of screening mammography in the United States: Data from the National Survey of Mammography Facilities. Radiology 1994;190:209–215.
   Quality assurance issues are addressed.

3. Logan-Young WW, Yanes-Hoffman N. Breast Cancer: A Practical Guide to Diagnosis, vol 1. Rochester, New York, Mount Hope Publishing Company, 1994.
   A practical, clinical approach to diagnosis from a radiologic perspective is presented.

4. Parker SH, Jobe WE, eds. Percutaneous Breast Biopsy. New York, Raven Press, 1993.
   This is a good review of this topic.

5. Sickles EA, Kopans DB. Mammographic screening for women aged 40 to 49 years of age: The primary care practitioner's dilemma. Ann Intern Med 1995;122:534–538.
   The authors present an opinionated review of a controversial topic.

Genitourinary and Renal Disorders

168 Cancer of the Genitourinary Tract

Screening

RICHARD E. GREEN, MICHAEL K. BRAWER, and RICHARD M. HOFFMAN

Nearly half (44%) of all male cancers occur in the genitourinary tract, and 22% to 33% are metastatic at the time of diagnosis. There are suggestions that screening for genitourinary neoplasms has improved survival since 1960, but this may simply represent finding tumors at an earlier stage without substantially altering their long-term course (i.e., lead-time bias). Only screening for prostate cancer has been widely embraced, and its value remains controversial.

PROSTATE CANCER

Epidemiology. Prostate cancer is the most frequently diagnosed visceral cancer and the second leading cause of cancer death in men. In 1996, prostate cancer was detected in over 300,000 men and caused about 40,000 deaths. The incidence of prostate cancer has risen by 40% in recent years, whereas the age-adjusted mortality has risen by 24%. Increased screening has inflated the incidence rate by detecting latent cancers; nonetheless, more than 30% of prostate cancers are metastatic when diagnosed.

Rationale. Prostate-specific antigen (PSA) is better able to detect organ-confined prostate cancer than digital rectal examination (DRE). The prognosis for prostate cancer is better when the cancer is confined to the organ rather than being extraprostatic (as is often found in the absence of screening), and patients with organ-confined disease can be offered curative surgery or radiation therapy. Consequently, the American Urological Association (AUA) and the American Cancer Society (ACS) recommend annual PSA testing and DRE for high-risk men (i.e., blacks, those with a family history of prostate cancer) older than age 40 and for all men older than age 50. The US Preventive Services Task Force and the National Cancer Institute, however, do not recommend prostate cancer screening because PSA has a high false-positive rate, there is no clinical trial evidence guiding treatment selection, and the benefit of treating screening-detected cancers is unknown. Randomized trials of screening and treatment (including watchful waiting) are in progress, but results will be unavailable for many years.

Various approaches have been proposed to improve the specificity of PSA testing, including measuring velocity (change in PSA level over time), density (PSA level in relation to prostatic volume), and isoforms (the ratio of free to total PSA). Because PSA increases with age, age-specific levels have been derived to reduce false-positive results in older patients and reduce false-negative results in younger patients. The utility of these approaches has not been prospectively tested in screening trials, and the optimal use of PSA results remains to be determined.

Strategy. A practitioner who elects to screen for prostate cancer should adhere to AUA and ACS guidelines. Patients with elevated PSA levels and DRE abnormalities should be referred to a urologist for transrectal ultrasound-guided biopsies. The most appropriate PSA threshold is 4.0 ng/mL. Although the predictive value of PSA levels between 4 and 10 ng/mL is about 30%, two thirds of detected cancers are confined within the gland. The predictive value is higher when PSA is above 10 ng/mL, but most cancers identified are extraprostatic and carry a much worse prognosis.

Action. Although screening for prostate cancer is controversial, PSA testing is widely used. Before ordering a PSA test, practitioners should discuss with patients the limitations of screening tests, the need for biopsy to diagnose cancer, and the potential risks and benefits of treatment options. In general, screening and aggressive management should be restricted to men with at least a 10-year life expectancy because prostate cancers, especially in the elderly, are often indolent.

CARCINOMA OF THE TESTIS

Epidemiology. Testicular cancer is the leading cause of cancer death among males aged 15 to 35. There are approximately 7100 new cases annually with 400 deaths. Cryptorchidism is a well-established risk factor. Although occupational radar use, vasectomy, spina bifida, and a family history of other cancers have been suggested as risk factors, their role is less clear.

Rationale. Testicular self-examination remains the best method for detecting testicular carcinoma. Although many common, nonmalignant abnormalities such as spermatoceles, varicoceles, hematoceles, and hydroceles may be mistaken for cancer, men should promptly report any new abnormality to a physician, because delays as short as 16 weeks after discovery are associated with shortened survival.

Strategy. The ACS recommends monthly testicular self-examination, whereas other groups, including the US Preventive Services Task Force, do not recommend screening because of uncertain benefits. Clinicians may choose to show their patients, particularly younger men, how to perform self-examination. In younger men, testicular examination should be part of the regular physical examination.

Action. Any man with a palpable scrotal mass should be referred immediately to a urologist, who may perform ultrasonography. This technique has a sensitivity of 82% in detecting testicular carcinoma. Whereas extratesticular masses are rarely malignant, all intratesticular or equivocal lesions require surgical exploration. Treatments include chemotherapy or orchiectomy.

BLADDER CANCER

Epidemiology. Carcinoma of the bladder is the second most common genitourinary neoplasm, with an estimated annual incidence of 50,500 new cases and 11,200 fatalities. Men are affected at approximately three times the rate of women. Exposures to industrial carcinogens and smoking are risk factors for transitional cell carcinoma, whereas chronic infection predisposes to squamous cell cancer.

Rationale. Approximately 20% of men with hematuria have carcinoma detected when evaluated. Cytology is effective in detecting more advanced cancers. A new test, the bladder tumor antigen, appears to provide results that are comparable or superior to cytology at a greatly reduced cost.

Strategy. Some physicians recommend that patients with an identified risk factor have routine urinalyses to screen for hematuria. The US Preventive Services Task Force and other authoritative sources do not presently recommend routine screening for hematuria based on the lack of prospective trials demonstrating improved outcomes among screened populations.

Action. There are many reasons that hematuria may be detected. Individuals with clinically significant gross or persistent microscopic hematuria in the absence of urinary tract infection should be evaluated with urine cytology, intravenous urography, and cystoscopy.

Cross-References: Principles of Screening (Chapter 7), Periodic Health Assessment (Chapter 8), Dysuria (Chapter 170), Scrotal Pain (Chapter 171), Prostate Cancer (Chapter 173), Hematuria (Chapter 180), Proteinuria (Chapter 181), Benign Prostatic Hyperplasia (Chapter 184).

REFERENCES

1. Catalona WJ, Smith DS, Wolfert RL, et al. Evaluation of percentage of free serum prostate-specific antigen to improve specificity of prostate cancer screening. JAMA 1995;274:1214–1220.

   The authors report that using a free PSA cutoff of 23.4% or lower would reduce negative biopsies by 31.3%.

2. Clore ER. A guide for the testicular self-examination. J Pediatr Health Care 1993;7:264–268.

   This article reviews the anatomy of the male reproductive system, discusses testicular cancer, and provides the process of the testicular self-examination, emphasizing the role of nurse practitioners in teaching.

3. Gohagan JK, Prorok PC, Kramer BS, Cornett JE. Prostate cancer screening in the prostate, lung, colorectal and ovarian cancer screening trial of the National Cancer Institute. J Urol 1994;152:1905–1909.

   This article describes the design of an ongoing 15-year multicenter trial to determine whether screening with DRE and PSA reduces prostate cancer mortality.

4. Kramer BS, Elrown ML, Prorok PC, Potosky AL, Gohagan JK. Prostate cancer screening: What we know and what we need to know. Ann Intern Med 1993;119:914–923.

   The authors provide an evidence-based evaluation of prostate cancer and conclude that the net benefit of widespread screening at this time is unclear.

5. Messing EM, Young TB, Hunt VB, Gilchrist KW, Newton MA, Bram LL, Hisgen WJ, Greenberg EB, Kuglitsch ME, Wegenke JD. Comparison of bladder cancer outcome in men undergoing hematuria home screening versus those with standard clinical presentations. Urology 1995;45:387–396.

   In a nonrandomized trial, home screening for hematuria appeared to detect high-grade cancers before they became invasive and thus to reduce mortality.

6. Moul JW, Paulson DF, Dodge RK, Walther PJ. Delay in diagnosis and survival in testicular cancer: Impact of effective therapy and changes during 18 years. J Urol 1995;43:520–523.

   Based on a review of the records of 148 patients, the average interval between onset of symptoms and diagnosis was 21 weeks and did not appear to vary during the 18-year period of review. An increasing interval was associated with worse outcomes in tumors other than seminomas but not in seminomas.

7. Oesterling JE, Jacobsen SJ, Chute CG, et al. Serum prostate-specific antigen in a community-based population of healthy men. JAMA 1993;270:860–864.

   The investigators present the derivation of age-specific reference ranges for PSA.

8. Polak V, Hornak M. The value of scrotal ultrasound in patients with suspected testicular tumor. Int J Urol Nephrol 1990;22:467–473.

   In this prospective review of 56 patients using surgical pathology as the reference standard, the sensitivity of ultrasonography was 95% and the specificity was only 58%, indicating that ultrasonography alone is inadequate to rule out the presence of an intratesticular neoplasm.

9. Sarosody MF, DeVere White RW, Soloway MS, Sheinfeld J, Hudson MA, Schellhammer PF, Jarowenko MV, Adams G, Blumenstein BA. Results of a multicenter trial using the BTA test to monitor for and diagnose recurrent bladder cancer. J Urol 1995;154:379–384.

   Studying 499 patients with previously resected bladder cancers, the investigators found that the assay for bladder tumor antigen identified 61 cases of recurrent cancer compared with only 25 detected by voided cytology.

10. Woolf SH. Screening for prostate cancer with prostate-specific antigen. N Engl J Med 1995;333:1401–1405.

    Controversies over screening are summarized and counseling patients about risks and benefits of PSA testing is recommended.

169 Erectile Dysfunction

Symptom

BRADLEY D. ANAWALT

Epidemiology. Erectile dysfunction, the inability of the male to attain and maintain an erection sufficient to allow sexual intercourse, affects 10 to 20 million men in the United States. Erectile dysfunction increases with age, occurring in less than 1% of men before age 30, less than 3% of men before age 45, about 7% of men between ages 45 and 55, 25% to 40% of men older than age 60, and more than 60% of men older than age 80. Important risk factors for erectile dysfunction include conditions that affect penile neurovascular function such as hyperlipidemia; medications; central and peripheral neurologic disorders; trauma to the nervous system, pelvis, or penis; chronic illnesses; and systemic illnesses such as diabetes mellitus. Elevated high density lipoprotein (HDL)-cholesterol levels may protect against erectile dysfunction.

Etiology. Penile erection results from relaxation of penile smooth muscle and dilatation of penile arteries with engorgement of the venous sinuses of the penile corpora. As these sinuses fill with blood, intrapenile pressure increases, venous outflow through the long subtunical venules is blocked, and blood is trapped in the venous sinuses. The resultant venous engorgement coupled with contraction of the ischiocavernosus muscle of the penis results in a complete erection. Neurologic regulation of this process includes a centrally mediated pathway from the brain and a local reflex arc involving the lower spinal cord. Thus, erectile dysfunction can occur from lack of sexual desire (hypogonadism or psychiatric factors), dysfunction of neural pathways from the brain and the spinal cord to the penis (neurologic disorders and trauma), decreased arterial blood flow (atherosclerosis), and inability to occlude penile venous outflow (penile venous leak) (Table 169–1).

Clinical Approach. Although there are many sophisticated diagnostic tools for erectile dysfunction, a simple, goal-oriented approach to the diagnosis and management of erectile dysfunction is usually successful. The patient interview should review the patient's sexual history, the relationship between the patient and his partner, the degree of motivation of the patient and his partner for treatment, systemic diseases, history of pelvic surgery or trauma, and medication history. Smoking habits, alcohol intake, and use of recreational drugs such as marijuana should be investigated. The absence of morning and nocturnal erections generally suggests organic disease. The physical examination should focus on detection of signs of endocrine, vascular, neurologic, or genital abnormalities. Normal androgen function is assessed by the presence of secondary sexual characteristics and careful palpation of the testes for size and consistency. The penis should be carefully examined and palpated for the presence of fibrosis (Peyronie's disease). Vascular integrity is assessed by palpation of the

Table 169–1. COMMON CAUSES OF ERECTILE DYSFUNCTION

Systemic Diseases
  Atherosclerosis
  Diabetes mellitus
  Hypertension
  Renal failure
  Cirrhosis

Neurogenic
  Cerebrovascular disease
  Multiple sclerosis
  Spinal cord trauma
  Pelvic surgery and radiation

Endocrine
  Hypogonadism
  Hyperprolactinemia

Penile
  Peyronie's disease
  Epispadias
  Trauma

Psychiatric
  Depression
  Relationship discord

Hematologic
  Leukemias
  Sickle cell anemia

Infections
  Acquired immunodeficiency syndrome
  Tuberculosis

Drugs
  Phenothiazines
  Antihypertensives*
  Spironolactone
  Gemfibrozil
  Anticonvulsants
  Marijuana
  Opiates

*Calcium channel blockers and angiotensin-converting enzyme inhibitors have been less commonly reported to cause erectile dysfunction.

peripheral pulses. Measurement of the blood pressure of the penile artery is a poor screening test. Assessment of neurologic function should focus on assessment of sensation in the sacral dermatomes and penis and genital reflexes (anal wink, cremasteric reflex, and bulbocavernosal reflex).

Laboratory evaluation should include a complete blood cell count and serum creatinine and glucose values. A serum total testosterone level should be measured in all patients with erectile dysfunction because clinical assessment of hypogonadism is insensitive, coincident hypogonadism is common in the population of patients with erectile dysfunction, and some hypogonadal patients report improved erectile function with androgen replacement therapy. Serum gonadotropin and prolactin levels should be measured in patients with low serum testosterone levels. Additional testing with a nocturnal penile tumescence test (Rigiscan [Dacomed Corporation, Minneapolis, MN]) is generally unwarranted. The time-honored "stamp test" (application of a roll of perforated stamps around the penis of the patient at bedtime and checking for a break in the perforation in the morning) is not a good method for assessing the presence of nocturnal erections because a break in the perforation might be due to movement of the patient and because some erections that would be adequate for intercourse may not have sufficient force to break the perforations. The best method of assessing penile arterial blood flow is a duplex Doppler scan of the deep penile arterial blood flow; but this test is generally unnecessary because most patients with arterial disease causing erectile dysfunction are treated with medical measures. Assessment of penile venous function is done only in the rare patient who is young and has no other obvious cause of erectile dysfunction.

The best simple test of vascular function and response to medical therapy is the combined intracavernosal injection and stimulation test. The patient is injected with 10 μg of the potent vasodilator prostaglandin E_1 intracavernosally, and he is assessed for tumescence in 15 minutes. A prompt, sustained erection virtually excludes significant arterial or venous insufficiency and predicts an excellent response to self-injection therapy with prostaglandin E_1. Asking the patient to self-stimulate with masturbation helps increase the likelihood for a normal erection. The absence of a normal erection after intracavernosal injection and self-stimulation may be due to the anxiety of doing such an intimate activity in a relatively public setting.

Management. Treatment of erectile dysfunction includes sex therapy for the patient and his partner when the cause of erectile dysfunction is of psychogenic origin. Oral medications such as yohimbine and trazodone are generally not very useful, although a small subset of patients with primarily psychogenic erectile dysfunction may benefit. The only blinded study of yohimbine failed to show any effect. The dose of yohimbine is 5 to 10 mg three times a day, and the dose of trazodone is 50 to 100 mg at bedtime.

A vacuum constriction device that consists of a pump that is placed over the penis causes tumescence by drawing blood into the penis by negative pressure. An elastic ring around the base of the penis maintains the veno-occlusion and tumescence. This device can be useful in many men. Androgen replacement therapy should be initiated in men with proven hypogonadism.

Alprostadil, a formulation of prostaglandin E_1, has been approved by the Food and Drug Administration (FDA) for intracavernosal injection in men with erectile dysfunction. Patients can be taught to self-administer prostaglandin E_1. The primary side effect is mild to moderate pain, which occurs in about 10% of injections. Priapism occurs in less than 0.5% of patients, and penile fibrosis is generally mild and reversible. The usual dose of alprostadil is 2.5 to 20 μg per erection; the dose is titrated to consistently produce erections that last 30 to 60 minutes. Patients with erectile dysfunction from high spinal cord trauma often require low doses, whereas patients with diabetes mellitus often require higher doses for complete erections. About 70% of patients are able to obtain erections consistently with intracavernosal therapy. The cost is $15 to $30 per erection. It should not be used more than two or three times per week. Studies have shown that patient satisfaction is high with intracavernosal therapy, but 20% to 50% of patients stop using it after 1 year. Papaverine and phentolamine have been used with alprostadil in intracavernosal therapy, but neither is FDA-approved for this use, and papaverine is associated with high rates of penile fibrosis and significant rates of priapism requiring urgent urologic intervention.

Surgical options for erectile dysfunction include venous and arterial reconstruction, but these operations are reserved for selected patients. The success rate of the vascular reconstruction surgery for erectile dysfunction is about 50%. Various penile implants are available for treatment of erectile dysfunction, but implants are reserved for patients who fail less invasive options. Furthermore, penile implants may fail to operate properly over time and are potential niduses for infection.

Cross-References: Alcohol Problems (Chapter 10), Smoking Cessation (Chapter 12), Essential Hypertension (Chapter 85), Peripheral Arterial Disease (Chapter

132), Peripheral Neuropathy (Chapter 147), Diabetes Mellitus (Chapter 154), Screening for Depression (Chapter 185), Generalized Anxiety (Chapter 186).

REFERENCES

1. Akpunonu EB, Mutgi AB, Federman DJ, York J, Woldenberg LS. Routine prolactin measurement is not necessary in the initial evaluation of male impotence. J Gen Intern Med 1994;9:336–338.

   Evaluation was done of 299 consecutive patients with impotence in a general medicine clinic. Fifty-one patients had low serum testosterone levels. Only 3 patients had hyperprolactinemia, and 2 of these 3 had low serum testosterone levels; none had pituitary tumors. Prolactin level determination is indicated only if serum testosterone levels are low.

2. Anawalt BD, Matsumoto AM. Medical treatment of erectile dysfunction. Curr Opin Endocrinol Diabetes 1996;3:472–477.

   This is a recent review of current and investigational medical therapies for erectile dysfunction.

3. Impotence—NIH Consensus Conference. JAMA 1993;270:83–89.

   This consensus statement gives a nice overview of the epidemiology, diagnosis, and management of erectile dysfunction.

4. Korenman SG. Advances in the understanding and management of erectile dysfunction. J Clin Endocrinol Metab 1995;80:1985–1988.

   This review includes a practical approach to the treatment of erectile dysfunction.

5. Linet OI, Ogrinc FG. Efficacy and safety of intracavernosal alprostadil in men with erectile dysfunction. N Engl J Med 1996;334:873–877.

   A study was done of 577 men with erectile dysfunction who were evaluated after home intracavernosal injection therapy. Eighty-seven percent of the 471 who completed the 6-month study reported that injection therapy resulted in satisfactory sexual activity. Side effects included penile pain (50%) and priapism (1%). The minimum effective dose was 2 μg.

·······································

170 Dysuria

Symptom

STEPHAN D. FIHN

Epidemiology and Etiology. Dysuria is one of the 15 most frequent reasons for visits to primary care physicians by women in the United States. Eight percent to 14% of women have symptoms of dysuria or urinary frequency in any given year, although most episodes are not reported to physicians.

In 70% to 90% of women with dysuria, the cause is urinary tract infection (UTI). Approximately one half of these infections are characterized by growth of between 10^2 and 10^5 bacteria/mL in a midstream culture. The onset of symptoms owing to UTI is typically sudden and accompanied by urgency, frequency, and occasionally suprapubic pain and gross hematuria. UTI should be suspected in women with dysuria who use a diaphragm. In 10% to 20% of women, the cause of dysuria is vaginitis, most often bacterial vaginosis due to anaerobes (nonspecific vaginitis). These patients frequently also complain of vaginal discharge, "external" dysuria, and vulvar pruritus. In sexually active young women, chlamydial cervicitis or urethritis is the cause of dysuria in 2% to 5% of cases; gonococcal infection occurs much less often. These entities should be suspected when the onset of symptoms is gradual, when the patient has had a recent change in sexual partners, and when the urinalysis demonstrates pyuria but is negative for bacteria. Uncommon causes of acute dysuria include herpetic infection and allergic reactions. In up to 10% of cases, no pyuria is present, and the cause of symptoms is obscure.

Women who have chronic dysuria without evidence of infection may have a poorly characterized syndrome of interstitial cystitis. There are no standard criteria for this diagnosis and no proved beneficial therapy.

Dysuria is less common among males. In younger, sexually active men, the most common cause is urethritis. Gonococcal urethritis is frequent among homosexual men and those with a history of prior gonorrhea. Nongonococcal urethritis is due to *Chlamydia trachomatis* in 30% to 50% of cases and *Ureaplasma urealyticum* in 15% to 20% of cases; in the remaining cases, a definite pathogen is not isolated. Nongonococcal urethritis is several times more common than gonococcal infection among most general heterosexual populations, although 25% of men with *Chlamydia* are co-infected with *Neisseria gonorrhoeae*.

In older men, dysuria often signifies UTI. However, in as many as half of men with dysuria or other irritative symptoms such as frequency and urgency, the cause may be conditions other than infection, including benign prostatic hypertrophy.

Clinical Approach. In many instances, the history alone may be sufficient to make a diagnosis of UTI with a high degree of confidence. Younger women who have had prior UTIs are more than 90% accurate in identifying recurrences and can often be treated for a presumptive recurrence without confirmation by examination of the urine. Lacking an unequivocal history, proper diagnosis depends on laboratory studies. Ideally, a quantitative urinary leukocyte count should be performed using a hemocytometer counting chamber along with a microscopic examination of uncentrifuged urine (Table 170–1). If pyuria (≥ 10 leukocytes/mm^3 or more than 10 per high-power field) and bacteria are present, the likelihood of a UTI is approximately 90%, particularly if the patient uses a diaphragm. If facilities for microscopic examination of urine are unavailable, dipstick tests for leukocyte esterase, bacterially generated nitrate, or a combination of the two are a reasonable substitute. The performance of these tests is slightly poorer than direct microscopy. Like microscopy, these tests are most accurate in detecting UTIs characterized by colony counts exceeding 10^4 bacteria/mL and are less useful for detecting infections with lesser degrees of bacteriuria.

If pyuria is present without bacteriuria, a pelvic examination should be performed, if appropriate, to detect mucopurulent cervicitis and obtain cultures for *C. trachomatis* and *N. gonorrhoeae*, as well as rapid diagnostic tests for *Chlamydia* when available. A pelvic examination is warranted if symptoms suggest vaginitis.

Table 170–1. PERFORMANCE CHARACTERISTICS OF TESTS FOR URINARY TRACT INFECTION IN WOMEN WITH DYSURIA

Laboratory Finding	Sensitivity	Specificity	Predictive Value Positive	Predictive Value Negative
Midstream Culture				
Any coliforms	1.00	0.71	0.79	1.00
$\geq 10^2$ coliforms/mL	0.95	0.85	0.88	0.94
$\geq 10^5$ coliforms/mL	0.51	0.59	0.98	0.65
Microscopy				
2 + visible bacteria	0.70	0.85	0.86	0.69
3 + visible bacteria	0.37	0.97	0.94	0.55
Positive Gram stain	0.81	0.88	0.90	0.79
Visible leukocytes	0.95	0.71	0.80	0.92
≥ 8 leukocytes/mm^3	0.91	0.50	0.67	0.83
≥ 20 white blood cells/mm^3 and visible bacteria	0.50	0.95	0.94	0.54
Rapid Tests				
Leukocyte esterase strips	0.75–0.90	0.95	0.50	0.92
Nitrite dipsticks	0.35–0.85	0.95	0.96	0.27–0.70
Leukocyte esterase/nitrite strips	0.75–0.90	0.70	0.75–0.93	0.41–0.95

Young men with dysuria should be closely questioned about sexual exposures. The clinician should determine whether a urethral discharge is present. In gonococcal urethritis, the discharge is often copious and purulent, whereas that from chlamydial infection is more often scant and mucoid. Symptoms may be more pronounced in the morning, especially with chlamydial infection. A specimen of urethral discharge should be obtained from all patients with suspected urethritis by milking the urethra or by swab, as described in Chapter 176, Sexually Transmitted Diseases.

Older men with dysuria should be questioned about signs or symptoms of prostatism. In most cases a urine culture should be performed. Presence of 10^3 bacteria/mL or more indicates infection.

Management. Management of patients with UTI, vaginitis, and urethritis is accomplished as described in the specific chapters on these disorders (see Cross-References).

Cross-References: Abdominal Pain (Chapter 94), Pelvic Pain in Women (Chapter 160), Vaginitis (Chapter 164), Pelvic Inflammatory Disease (Chapter 166), Urinary Tract Infections in Women (Chapter 175), Sexually Transmitted Diseases (Chapter 176), Urinary Tract Infections in Men (Chapter 177), Bacteriuria in the Elderly (Chapter 178), Hematuria (Chapter 180), Benign Prostatic Hyperplasia (Chapter 184), Bacteriuria in Pregnancy (Chapter 211).

REFERENCES

1. Berg AO, Heidrich FE, Fihn SD, et al. Establishing the cause of genitourinary symptoms in women in a family practice: Comparison of clinical examination and comprehensive microbiology. JAMA 1984;251:620–625.

In a prospective study of women coming to a family medicine clinic with a variety of genitourinary symptoms, a diagnosis was made in 34% using simple tests and in 66% using sophisticated tests. The positive predictive value of dysuria for UTI was 67%.

2. Hurlbut TA, Littenberg B, and the Diagnostic Technology Assessment Consortium. The diagnostic accuracy of rapid dipstick tests to predict urinary tract infection. Am J Clin Pathol 1991;96:582–588.

   After reviewing 1017 citations, the authors concluded that while the leukocyte esterase test was a better indicator of bacteriuria, the best diagnostic accuracy was achieved when a positive result on either strip was considered to indicate bacteriuria.

3. Lipsky BA, Ireton RC, Fihn SD, et al. Diagnosis of bacteriuria in men: Specimen collection and culture interpretation. J Infect Dis 1987;155:847–854.

   This study demonstrated that voided specimens from adult men are highly accurate and the best diagnostic criterion for bacteriuria is $10^3/mL$ or more. Irritative symptoms often indicated bladder infections but occurred in several men who did not have infection.

4. Stamm WE, Wagner KF, Amsel R, et al. Causes of the acute urethral syndrome in women. N Engl J Med 1980;303:409–412.

   This is the earliest study to demonstrate the importance of sexually transmitted diseases, especially Chlamydia, as causes of dysuria, and of pyuria as an important indicator of bladder or urethral infection.

5. Wathne B, Hovelius B, Mardh PA. Causes of frequency and dysuria in women. Scand J Infect Dis 1987;19:223–229.

   In a community-based prospective study, over 80% of women presenting with dysuria and urinary frequency were found to have UTI. Chlamydial infection was diagnosed in 10% of women without bacteriuria, 93% of whom had pyuria.

• •

171 Scrotal Pain

Symptom

STEVEN R. McGEE

Epidemiology. Both testicular torsion and testicular cancer affect men between the ages of 15 and 35. The incidence of testicular torsion peaks during puberty. Epididymitis affects men of all ages.

Etiology. The important causes of scrotal pain are listed in Table 171–1. In men older than 20 presenting with an acutely inflamed scrotum, epididymitis is the most common diagnosis, outranking torsion 10 to 1.

   Testicular torsion occurs when the testis, lacking the normal fixation to the posterior scrotal wall, freely twists on the spermatic cord. If this is not treated, necrosis of the testis occurs in 10% to 20% of patients after 6 hours of

Table 171–1. CAUSES OF SCROTAL PAIN

Disease within scrotum	Disease distant from scrotum
Torsion	Abdominal aortic aneurysm
Of spermatic cord	Renal pain
Of testicular appendage	Radicular pain
Epididymitis	Prostatic pain
Orchitis	Prostatitis
Testicular tumor	Prostatodynia
Polyarteritis nodosa	
Drugs	
Desipramine	
Mazindol	
Amiodarone	

symptoms and in more than 90% after 24 hours. *Epididymitis* results from bacterial infection of the epididymis. Heterosexual men younger than 35 usually have associated urethritis from *Chlamydia trachomatis* or *Neisseria gonorrhoeae.* In heterosexual men older than 35 and in all homosexual men, epididymitis is associated with bacteriuria, usually from Enterobacteriaceae. Most men older than 35 also have associated urinary tract abnormalities, typically benign prostatic hypertrophy. *Orchitis* is usually due to viral infections, especially mumps.

In addition, scrotal pain may result from diseases distant to the scrotum, either along the course of the genitofemoral nerve in the retroperitoneum (abdominal aortic aneurysm, ureterolithiasis, retrocecal appendicitis) or along the posterior scrotal nerves (prostatic pain, radicular pain).

Clinical Approach. Although testicular tenderness may occur in patients with either local or distant disorders, the finding of scrotal redness, swelling, or mass always indicates an intrascrotal condition (see Table 171–1). Routine laboratory tests include a urinalysis, urine culture, and, in the sexually active patient, urethral Gram stain and culture.

In patients with acute scrotal pain, redness, and swelling ("acute scrotum"), radionuclide scanning of the testis accurately distinguishes torsion from epididymitis. Although some studies tout the accuracy of Doppler ultrasonography, the results are very operator dependent. Real-time ultrasonography is inappropriate because it does not reliably discriminate between epididymitis and torsion.

In patients younger than 40 who have an acute scrotum, the evaluation must be prompt to distinguish testicular torsion, a surgical condition in which delay increases the chances of necrosis, from epididymitis, a nonsurgical condition. Patients with three of the following six findings should receive treatment for presumptive epididymitis: (1) gradual onset (days) of pain; (2) dysuria, urethral discharge, recent cystoscopy, or urethral catheter; (3) fever greater than 38.3°C (101°F); (4) previous urinary tract infections; (5) induration localized to the epididymis; and (6) pyuria (> 10 white blood cells/high-power field). In those with fewer than three of these findings, the approach depends on the duration of the patient's pain. In those with less than 24 hours of pain, testicular salvage is possible, and nothing—including radionuclide scanning—should delay urologic consultation. If the pain has persisted beyond 24 hours, testicular radionuclide scanning is reasonable; even if torsion is diagnosed, surgery is less urgent because its only purpose is to remove the necrotic testis and fix the contralateral one.

Renal colic begins gradually, is continuous (not colicky), and rarely lasts longer than 24 hours. In all men older than 50 who have unexplained testicular pain or who have suspected renal colic, the clinician should consider the diagnosis of abdominal aortic aneurysm.

Management. In patients with epididymitis, the choice of antibiotic is based on the likely organism, as described earlier, and the results of Gram stains of the urethra or urine (see Chapter 176, Sexually Transmitted Diseases, and Chapter 177, Urinary Tract Infections in Men). Bed rest with scrotal elevation, scrotal support when ambulatory, and analgesics help relieve the pain. Referral to a urologist is mandatory for all patients with epididymitis that fails to respond to treatment; surgical exploration may reveal unsuspected tumors, abscesses, vasculitis, or tuberculosis. Up to 50% of documented testicular tumors are initially misdiagnosed as epididymitis.

Cross-References: Abdominal Pain (Chapter 94), Peripheral Arterial Disease (Chapter 132), Cancer of the Genitourinary Tract (Chapter 168), Dysuria (Chapter 170), Nephrolithiasis (Chapter 174), Sexually Transmitted Diseases (Chapter 176), Urinary Tract Infections in Men (Chapter 177).

REFERENCES

1. Berger RE, Alexander ER, Harnisch JP, et al. Etiology, manifestation and therapy of acute epididymitis: Prospective study of 50 cases. J Urol 1979;121:750–754.

   The bacterial causes of epididymitis are defined based on the age of the patient.

2. Edelsberg JS, Surh YS. The acute scrotum. Emerg Med Clin North Am 1988;6:521–546.

   The authors present an excellent review of testicular torsion, epididymitis, and other less common causes of the acutely inflamed scrotum.

3. Knight PJ, Vassy LE. The diagnosis and treatment of the acute scrotum in children and adolescents. Ann Surg 1984;200:664–673.

   This is the best study of clinical features that distinguish epididymitis from torsion (395 patients), although it includes only patients 17 years of age or younger.

4. McGee SR. Referred scrotal pain: Case reports and review. J Gen Intern Med 1993;8:694–701.

   Referred scrotal pain may result from an abdominal aortic aneurysm, ureterolithiasis, nerve root or bone disorders, appendicitis, retroperitoneal tumors, or pelvic floor disorders.

172 Urinary Incontinence

Symptom

CRAIG V. COMITER, MARYROSE P. SULLIVAN,
and SUBBARAO V. YALLA

Epidemiology. Urinary incontinence that is bothersome enough for patients to seek medical attention affects 0.1% of men and 0.2% of women aged 15 to 64 and 1.3% of men and 2.5% of women older than 65. Less bothersome and relatively unrecognized incontinence affects 2% of men and 8% of women between the ages of 15 and 64 and 6% of men and 13% of women older than 65. Approximately 5% of these persons will experience wetness sufficiently to require an extra change of clothing on a daily basis. Half of the institutionalized elderly are incontinent.

Etiology. *Transient incontinence* is common in the elderly, causing a third of cases of community-dwelling incontinence and half of cases of hospitalized incontinence. Causes include urinary tract infection, atrophic vaginitis or urethritis, medications directly or indirectly affecting the lower urinary tract, fecal impaction, excessive urine output, restricted mobility, and altered sensorium.

The causes of more permanent forms of incontinence can conveniently be divided into those related to the bladder (overactivity vs. underactivity) and those related to the outlet (incompetence vs. obstruction).

Urge incontinence results from a phasic involuntary rise in detrusor pressure during bladder filling that cannot be inhibited. When this detrusor overactivity is due to neurologic causes such as stroke, Parkinson's disease, multiple sclerosis, Alzheimer's disease, and suprasacral spinal cord lesions, it is termed *detrusor hyperreflexia*. Overactivity due to non-neurologic causes, such as cystitis, tumors, stones, and outlet obstruction, is referred to as *detrusor instability*.

Overflow incontinence, which accounts for 5% to 10% of all incontinence, is associated with a failure to empty the bladder and is caused by continuous or episodic increases in intravesical pressure that exceed urethral closure pressure. Incomplete bladder emptying can develop with detrusor underactivity or bladder outlet obstruction or both. *Detrusor underactivity*, characterized by a hypocontractile or even areflexic bladder, can be caused by mechanical injury to the nerves (herniated disc, tumor, surgery), autonomic neuropathy (diabetes, tabes dorsalis, alcohol abuse), detrusor muscle fibrosis, or various medications. Bladder *outlet obstruction*, most commonly caused by prostatic enlargement, may result in detrusor decompensation and overflow incontinence, in addition to post-void dribbling and detrusor instability.

Stress urinary incontinence refers to the involuntary loss of fluid during physical exertion (coughing, sneezing) in the absence of a detrusor contraction. Stress urinary incontinence typically occurs in women when a laxity of the pelvic musculature allows the bladder neck and proximal urethra to descend below the urogenital diaphragm, whereby increases in intra-abdominal pressures are no longer protectively acting to occlude the proximal urethra. Another cause of stress urinary incontinence is intrinsic weakness of the smooth muscle sphincter, secondary to diabetic neuropathy, operative trauma, hypoestrogenic atrophy (loss of the vascular cushion), or sympathetic neural injury. A different form of *outlet incompetence* is urethral instability—a reflex-mediated relaxation of the urethra occurring alone or in concert with detrusor overactivity. In men with stress urinary incontinence, outlet incompetence may occasionally be due to traumatic neural injury but most commonly follows surgical injury to the sphincter mechanism. Transurethral or suprapubic prostatectomy can occasionally produce total outlet incompetence with subsequent stress urinary incontinence, owing to the loss of proximal (bladder neck) and distal intrinsic sphincter mechanisms. Although these patients have passive incontinence due to the loss of intrinsic smooth muscle sphincter mechanisms, they are able to voluntarily interrupt their urinary stream due to the presence of an intact periurethral striated muscle (external sphincter). Stress urinary incontinence can also be a distressing sequela of radical prostatectomy, which results in the loss of the entire proximal smooth muscle sphincter mechanism (bladder neck and prostatic urethra) and potential compromise to the distal sphincter (both smooth and striated muscle components) or their nerve supply.

Clinical Approach. The initial evaluation should exclude any of the transient causes of incontinence, such as cystitis, atrophic vaginitis, acute retention, restricted mobility, fecal impaction, acute delirium, or adverse drug effects (most commonly α-adrenergic agents, anticholinergics, sedatives, narcotics, and diuretics).

History should assess the frequency and severity of the incontinence and the clinical situation surrounding urine loss. For example, patients with *urge incontinence* are unable to suppress involuntary bladder contractions. Urge incontinence is usually indicative of bladder outlet obstruction, neurologic disease, or intrinsic vesical pathology. Patients with *stress urinary incontinence* lose urine when increases in intra-abdominal pressure are insufficiently transmitted to the bladder neck and proximal urethra, such as during coughing, straining, or sneezing. In severe cases, simply standing up can cause urinary leakage. A lack of sensation before voiding may indicate a *sensory neurogenic bladder.* Total incontinence (i.e.. constant leakage without urgency) suggests outlet incompetence or a fistula (vesicovaginal or ureterovaginal) if the patient has undergone surgery or irradiation. In either case, normal voiding is usually possible despite continual wetness.

Frequency, urgency, and nocturia, also known as irritative symptoms, may indicate an unstable bladder with or without obstruction. Hesitancy, decreased force of urinary stream, and a feeling of incomplete emptying (often referred to as obstructive symptoms) may indicate a hypocontractile, areflexic, or obstructed bladder. These complaints may be more appropriately termed *lower urinary tract symptoms.* These symptoms cannot be used to reliably distinguish between an obstructive or nonobstructive cause. Other causes of lower urinary tract symptoms should be sought, such as infection (usually with dysuria), interstitial cystitis (usually with pelvic pain relieved by voiding), carcinoma of the bladder (usually with hematuria), or carcinoma in situ.

A focused neurologic history should include inquiries about pelvic trauma, back injury, fecal incontinence or constipation, impotence, ejaculatory dysfunction, prior surgery, alcohol abuse, and diabetes mellitus.

Physical examination of women should include a vaginal examination, with particular attention paid to the urethral meatus (caruncle, stenosis) and vaginal mucosa (atrophic vaginitis). The anterior vaginal vault should be examined for the presence of a cystocele, enterocele, urethral diverticulum, uterine prolapse, or urinary fistula. A rectocele may protrude through the posterior wall. Asking the patient to increase intra-abdominal pressure while the examiner's finger is in the vagina may demonstrate posterior movement of the proximal urethra or bladder base with overt leakage of urine. A cotton-tipped applicator stick placed in the urethral meatus may demonstrate hypermobility during abdominal straining. If gentle elevation of the vaginal fornices on both sides of the urethra prevents urine loss (Marshall test), stress urinary incontinence is likely. Leakage in the absence of such urethral hypermobility suggests an incompetent sphincter, a fistula, or an uninhibited detrusor contraction.

In men, the penis is examined for phimosis, meatal stenosis, or other obvious abnormality. Rectal examination should assess anal tone, rule out fecal impaction, and identify the size and consistency of the prostate. An enlarged prostate does not necessarily imply bladder outlet obstruction, even in the setting of significant lower urinary tract symptoms.

Neurologic evaluation may reveal decreased anal sphincter tone, which usually implies neurologic disease but may be due to previous surgery or chronic overstretching. Sacral reflexes may be assessed by testing the bulbocavernosus reflex, in which the perineal muscles normally contract with stimulation of the clitoris or glans. An absent bulbocavernosus reflex does not differentiate between afferent and efferent neurologic lesions. Voluntary contraction of the anal sphincter can be elicited to indirectly evaluate urethral striated sphincter function because both responses are mediated by the same spinal cord segment.

Laboratory data should include urinalysis and urine culture to rule out infection. Microhematuria may suggest carcinoma in situ among other disorders and should be further investigated. Urine cytology should be obtained in all patients with urgency or microhematuria who have obvious other causes, such as infection. Elevated serum glucose levels may indicate diabetes mellitus, often associated with polyuria and neurologic sequelae. Blood urea nitrogen and creatinine levels may be elevated in patients with obstructive uropathy.

Uroflowmetry provides information about the integrated function of the detrusor and bladder outlet. Peak flow should normally exceed 15 mL/s. A low flow rate may be due to obstruction or detrusor hypocontractility. The normal voiding time varies from 10 to 20 seconds for a volume of 100 mL to 25 to 35 seconds for a 400-mL volume. Visual inspection of the flow curve is vital for assessing whether a patient voids with the aid of abdominal straining, experiences detrusor instability, or has striated sphincter dyssynergia. Post-void residual should be determined by ultrasonography or by straight catheterization. A large residual volume (i.e., more than one third of bladder capacity on three occasions) with a low uroflow may indicate obstruction or hypocontractility. More detailed multichannel *urodynamic studies* are indicated when empirical treatment has failed, in patients with neurologic disease, and to diagnose bladder outlet obstruction.

Management. Transient incontinence usually resolves when the aggravating factor is treated, such as antibiotic treatment of any infection, estrogen replacement for atrophic vaginitis, disimpaction of the rectum, reversal of delirium, and withdrawal of offending medications. Incontinence due to impaired mobility or impaired cognition should be treated with timed and assisted voiding, possibly in combination with bladder relaxants. Any urinary fistula requires surgical repair.

A patient with an overactive detrusor, often presenting with urge incontinence, can frequently be managed with pharmacologic therapy. There are many different types of bladder suppressants (Table 172–1). Anticholinergics such as propantheline increase the volume to the first involuntary contraction, decrease the magnitude of detrusor contractions, and increase bladder capacity. Direct smooth muscle relaxants (e.g., flavoxate and dicyclomine) often have mild anticholinergic effects. Oxybutynin is an anticholinergic agent that also acts as a smooth muscle relaxant and local anesthetic and has been shown to reduce detrusor overactivity. Tricyclic antidepressants (e.g., imipramine) not only work as direct detrusor relaxants but also have anticholinergic and α-adrenergic enhancing (contracting) effects. Finally, β-adrenergic agonists have been anecdotally associated with improvement in urge incontinence.

More drastic measures to treat hyperreflexia include afferent pudendal reflex arc simulation, sacral rhizotomy, peripheral bladder denervation, and sacral root stimulation. Bladder capacity can be improved by augmentation cystoplasty. A program of scheduled voiding may be combined with any of the above treatments. In intractable cases of bladder overactivity, an external collecting device or even an indwelling catheter may be necessary.

Table 172–1. PHARMACOLOGIC TREATMENT OF INCONTINENCE

Drug	Initial Dose	Indication	Adverse Effects	Contraindications
Anticholinergic Agent				
Propantheline	7.5 mg bid	Urge incontinence	Dry mouth, blurred vision, tachycardia, constipation	Narrow-angle glaucoma, obstructive uropathies
Oxybutynin	2.5 mg tid			
α-Adrenergic Agonist				
Phenylpropanolamine	25 mg bid	Stress incontinence	Hypertension, anxiety, insomnia, headache, tremors, arrhythmias	Documented benign prostatic hypertrophic obstructions, cardiovascular diseases
Direct Smooth Muscle Relaxants				
Flavoxate	100 mg tid	Urge incontinence	Dry mouth, blurred vision, tachycardia, constipation	Obstructive uropathies, obstructive disease of the gastrointestinal tract
Dicyclomine	20 mg tid			
Tricyclic Antidepressant				
Imipramine	25 mg qd	Urge incontinence	Dry mouth, blurred vision, tachycardia, constipation	If on monoamine oxidase inhibitors

In patients with overflow incontinence, outlet obstruction should be considered and treated appropriately with medical management (α-adrenergic blockers) or surgery. Patients with overflow incontinence resulting from a hypocontractile detrusor may also benefit from surgery to reduce outlet resistance. Abdominal straining can facilitate voiding efficiency in these patients after incision or resection of the bladder neck or prostate, thereby reducing residual volume. When hypocontractility and high post-void residuals persist despite outlet surgery, clean intermittent catheterization is recommended. If this is impossible, an indwelling catheter may be indicated.

Mild forms of stress incontinence due to muscle laxity usually respond to pelvic floor (Kegel) exercises. Obesity, chronic cough, or atrophic vaginitis/urethritis should also be treated. α-Adrenergic receptor agonists can often be used to increase outlet resistance. Other options include vaginal cones and electrical stimulation of the pelvic floor musculature. Collagen injection into the suburethral tissues in women with an incompetent bladder neck is often effective. The results of collagen injection in men with postprostatectomy incontinence are less satisfactory. When conservative measures have failed, surgery is often indicated. Bladder neck suspension and sling operations (in women) and artificial sphincter implantation and use of an external urethral clamp (in men) are usually successful, especially when detrusor instability is absent or mild.

Follow-Up. Patients should be referred to a urologist if they (1) have intractable incontinence not easily managed by empirical therapy such as anticholinergic medications, (2) have outlet obstruction or refractory stress incontinence, or (3) have hematuria or positive urine cytology.

REFERENCES

1. McGuire EJ. Evaluation of urinary incontinence. In Yalla SV, McGuire EJ, Elbadawi A, Blaivas JG, eds. Neurourology and Urodynamics: Principles and Practice. New York, Macmillan, 1988.

   This chapter reviews pathophysiology and principles of management of urinary incontinence.

2. Resnick NM. Urinary incontinence in older adults. Hosp Pract 1992;139:602–616.

   This excellent review on urinary incontinence includes guidelines on the use of medications in the elderly and important side effects.

3. Resnick NM, Yalla SV. Management of urinary incontinence in the elderly. N Engl J Med 1985;313:800.

   Epidemiologic and management aspects of urinary incontinence in the elderly are presented.

4. Resnick NM, Yalla SV. Evaluation and medical management of urinary incontinence. In Walsh PC, Retik AB, Stamey TA, Vaughn ED Jr, eds. Campbell's Urology, 6th ed. Philadelphia, WB Saunders, 1992.

   This is a thorough review of etiology and classification of urinary incontinence.

5. Wein AJ. Clinical neuropharmacology of the lower urinary tract. In Yalla SV, McGuire EJ, Elbadawi A, Blaivas JG, eds. Neurourology and Urodynamics: Principles and Practice. New York, Macmillan 1988.

   The pharmacologic treatment of urinary incontinence is reviewed.

6. Yalla SV, Kirsh L, Kearney G, et al. Post-prostatectomy incontinence: Urodynamic assessment. Neurourol Urodyn 1982;1:77–87.

   Urodynamic evaluation of incontinence is discussed.

173 Prostate Cancer

Problem

RICHARD E. GREEN, MICHAEL K. BRAWER,
and RICHARD M. HOFFMAN

Epidemiology. Prostate cancer is the second leading cause of cancer death in men, accounting for 13% of cancer-related deaths. Although autopsies detect histologic cancers in at least 30% of men older than age 50, most of them are clinically unimportant. For a 50-year-old man with a 25-year life expectancy, the lifetime risks of clinical and fatal prostatic cancer are estimated at 9.5% and 2.9%, respectively. Black men and men with a first-degree relative with prostate cancer have the highest risk for being diagnosed with prostate cancer. Less clearly established risk factors include high saturated fat intake, radon and cadmium exposure, vasectomy, and smoking.

Symptoms and Signs. Most early-stage malignancies are asymptomatic, and there may be only subtle alterations in the consistency of the prostate. Hard nodules, however, can often be palpated in patients with higher-stage disease. Locally advanced prostate cancer can cause irritative and obstructive symptoms, dysuria, and hematuria. Metastatic disease often presents as bone pain, especially in the lumbosacral spine; spinal cord compression; anemia; and weight loss.

Clinical Approach. An abnormal digital rectal examination or an elevated prostate-specific antigen test are indications for ultrasound-guided needle biopsy of the prostate.

Management. Decisions regarding treatment of prostate cancer depend on the disease stage as well as the patient's life expectancy and quality of life. Localized prostate cancer may be managed with watchful waiting with or without hormonal therapy, radical prostatectomy, radiation therapy (by external-beam irradiation or surgically implanted radioactive seeds [brachytherapy]), or cryoablation of the prostate. Because each approach has advantages and disadvantages, treatment should be individualized. Many urologic oncologists contend that the morbidity of radical prostatectomy and external-beam irradiation may outweigh the benefits in older men expected to live less than 10 years. The efficacy of the standard curative therapies for prostate cancer (i.e., radical prostatectomy and external-beam irradiation) remains uncertain, but large, randomized, controlled trials are underway. Although surgical techniques have improved, significant postoperative complications still occur, including erectile dysfunction, incontinence, vesicourethral anastomotic strictures, blood loss, and rectal injury. Advances in radiation therapy have also reduced complications, but patients remain at risk for impotence, incontinence, proctitis, cystitis, and urethral stricture. Although cryoablation has reportedly less morbidity than surgical prostatectomy, its long-term efficacy is unknown, and complications include rectourethral fistula and sloughing of the prostatic urethral tissue.

Hormonal therapy is the primary option for treating metastatic cancer. Orchiectomy lowers the testosterone level and eliminates problems with medication compliance but is unacceptable to many men. Gonadotropin-releasing hormone (GnRH) agonists lower testosterone levels as effectively as orchiectomy, although these medications are very expensive. Medical antiandrogen therapy delays disease progression when combined with medical or surgical castration but does not significantly lengthen survival. Cytotoxic therapy has not been effective in this disease.

Follow-Up. After any curative therapy, patients should be followed for recurrent cancer with regular prostate-specific antigen evaluation and digital rectal examination. Patients with advanced disease should be observed for urinary symptoms, bone pain, or neurologic problems suggesting cord compression.

Cross-References: Cancer of the Genitourinary Tract (Chapter 168), Benign Prostatic Hyperplasia (Chapter 184).

REFERENCES

1. Catalona WJ. Management of cancer of the prostate. N Engl J Med 1994;331:996–1004.

   The author provides a succinct overview of current treatments.

2. CancerNet from the National Cancer Institute. PDQ Information for Health Care Professionals. Access by phone: 1-800-422-6237. World Wide Web http://www.nih.gov.

   The NIH frequently updates this information about current treatment recommendations and active clinical trials.

3. Fleming C, Wasson JH, Albertsen PC, Barry MJ, Wennberg JE. A decision analysis of alternative treatment strategies for clinically localized prostate cancer. JAMA 1993;269:2650–2658.

   This careful analysis advances the conclusion that radical prostatectomy and radiation therapy may benefit younger men with high-grade tumors but watchful waiting is appropriate for many older men.

4. Wilt TJ, Brawer MK. The prostate cancer intervention versus observation trial: A randomized trial comparing radical prostatectomy versus expectant management for the treatment of clinically localized prostate cancer. J Urol 1994;152:1910–1914.

   The authors describe the design of an ongoing 15-year multicenter US trial to determine whether curative surgical treatment reduces all-cause and prostate cancer mortality.

5. Prostate Cancer Trialists' Collaborative Group. Maximum androgen blockade in advanced prostate cancer: an overview of 22 randomised trials with 3283 deaths in 5710 patients. Lancet 1995;346:265–269.

   This meta-analysis concludes that maximum androgen blockade does not result in longer survival than conventional castration.

174 Nephrolithiasis

Problem

DONALD J. SHERRARD and STEPHAN D. FIHN

Epidemiology and Etiology. Kidney stones occur three to five times more often in men (approximately 124/100,000 men per year) than in women (36/100,000 women per year). Over 50% of all stones are composed of a calcium salt, most commonly calcium oxalate or calcium phosphate or both. Forty percent of all stones and 50% of calcium stones occur in persons with hypercalciuria. Hyperuricuria potentiates the precipitation of urinary calcium, and 80% of stones in persons with excessive uric acid excretion are composed of calcium oxalate. Hyperuricuria accounts for 20% of all calcium stones and occurs mainly in the elderly, who often cannot alkalinize their urine. Hyperuricuria and hypercalciuria coexist in 10% of stone formers. Hypocitruria leads to renal stones because of the enhanced precipitation of calcium salts with low urinary citrate levels. Like hyperuricuria, this disorder may occur by itself or in conjunction with hypercalciuria. It appears to be about as frequent as hyperuricuria and also occurs in patients with distal renal tubule injury states, such as renal tubular acidosis. Less common causes of stones include hyperoxaluria (due to hyperabsorption after ileojejunostomy or Crohn's disease of the terminal ileum, excessive intake in the form of vitamin C or leafy vegetables, or a congenital disorder); chronic urinary tract infections by urea-splitting organisms such as *Proteus mirabilis,* causing magnesium ammonium phosphate (struvite) stones; or cystinuria, a rare autosomal dominant disorder of amino acid transport.

Forty percent of men who have one calcium stone will not have another. For the remainder, recurrence is maximal at 2 to 3 years and usually occurs within 5 to 10 years.

Symptoms and Signs. Stones usually present as renal colic, which is severe intermittent pain that has an abrupt onset, increasing in intensity over 1 hour or 2 hours and lasting 6 hours or longer. The pain may be centered in the flank, back, or lower abdominal quadrant. Shifting pain suggests passage of the stone across the pelvic brim or into the ureterovesical junction. In males, pain may radiate into the ipsilateral testis. Gross hematuria is common.

Clinical Approach. A renal stone should be suspected in the presence of characteristic pain and hematuria, gross or microscopic. For patients with a history of previous stones, the pain will be familiar. Patients should be questioned about excessive intake of ascorbic acid or leafy vegetables (tea and chocolate are other sources of oxalate) and about a family history of stones. The diagnosis is confirmed by excretory urography, if readily available, or ultrasonography. Both procedures also detect hydronephrosis, if present. All patients should have serum calcium, phosphate, creatinine, and uric acid measurements plus a urinalysis to check for the presence of crystals. Analysis of the stone composition, initially, is not often useful, because almost all the stones are calcium oxalate. However, if the workup for the usual causes is negative, assessing the chemical content of the stone may be useful.

After a second episode of stone formation, investigation should be undertaken to determine the cause. Repeat determinations of serum calcium, uric acid, phosphate, and creatinine should be obtained, along with a spot urine sample for uric acid and a 24-hour urine collection for calcium, oxalate, citrate, and creatinine.

Hypercalciuria is defined as excretion of over 200 mg urinary calcium (or 150 mg of calcium/g of creatinine) per 24 hours. The cause may be classified as renal (idiopathic, due to a renal tubular leak), absorptive (due to excessive gastrointestinal absorption), or excessive filtered load (hyperparathyroidism) (Table 174–1). The first two causes do not need to be distinguished because they are treated the same. The last disorder, hyperparathyroidism, will usually be recognized because of the accompanying hypercalcemia and will usually be treated surgically with parathyroidectomy.

Hyperuricosuria is defined as excretion of over 800 mg of uric acid per 24 hours or by a spot determination demonstrating excretion of more than 0.6 mg of uric acid per deciliter of glomerular filtration rate, computed by dividing the product of the urine urate concentration and the serum creatinine value by the urine creatinine concentration.

Because excretion of calcium and uric acid may be variable, these determinations should be repeated several times if the tests are initially negative. If the tests are persistently negative, 24-hour urine specimens should be collected for citrate and oxalate.

Management. Renal colic is usually controlled with parenteral or oral narcotics, as required. Patients with obstruction, complicated urinary tract infection, or intractable pain should be referred to a urologist for consideration of stone removal with cystoscopy or lithotripsy. Most stones less than 5 mm in diameter will pass without surgical intervention.

For long-term prevention of stones due to hypercalciuria, thiazides are the treatment of choice unless hyperparathyroidism is the cause (Table 174–2). Calcium intake should be reduced to normal if excessive, and adequate fluids should be consumed. In younger persons, stones due to hyperuricosuria should be treated with allopurinol or dietary protein restriction or both; in the elderly, alkali plus an adequate fluid intake is recommended. A low-sodium diet may also be helpful in some patients.

Table 174–1. EVALUATION OF HYPERCALCIURIA (>200 mg/24 h)

Characteristic	Renal	Absorptive	Hyperparathroidism
Serum Ca^{2+}	Normal	Normal	>10.3
Serum PO_4	Normal	Low	<3.1
Parathyroid hormone	Increased	Normal or decreased	Increased
Mechanism	Renal tubular leak of Ca^{2+}	Increased gut absorption of Ca^{2+}	Increased filterd load of Ca^{2+}

Table 174–2. PREVENTION OF RENAL STONES

Etiology	Treatment
Hypercalciuria (absorptive or renal)	Thiazide, chlorthalidone (low doses)
Hyperparathyroidism	Parathyroid surgery
Hyperuricosuria	Allopurinol, alkali, protein restriction
Hypocitruria	Potassium citrate
Hyperoxaluria	Diet, calcium

For hypocitruria, potassium citrate in divided doses with meals (5 to 20 mEq twice daily) will normalize urinary citrate and reduce stone formation. Hyperoxaluria may require a decrease in dietary oxalate, increased calcium intake (calcium oxalate is poorly absorbed), and measures to reduce steatorrhea if fat malabsorption is present.

For patients interested in a nonpharmacologic approach to therapy, a combination of low protein (< 40 g/d), low sodium (< 3 g/d), and high water (> 2 L/d) will reduce calcium and uric acid excretion, enhance citrate excretion, and dilute the urinary oxalate. Thus, all of the common stone causes will be benefitted and stone frequency may be reduced by two thirds overall. Certainly this hygienic approach, on top of the medical measures, will be effective in all but the most difficult (noncompliant) patients.

Follow-Up. In the average patient, no special follow-up is required. Patients will often continue to pass stones for several months after effective therapy is started, but those who continue to form stones after 9 to 12 months despite therapy should be referred to a specialist.

Cross-References: Gout/Hyperuricemia (Chapter 119), Scrotal Pain (Chapter 171), Hematuria (Chapter 180), Electrolyte Abnormalities (Chapter 182).

REFERENCES

1. Coe F, Parks J. Recurrent renal calculi: Causes and prevention. Hosp Pract 1986;21:49–57.

   A detailed strategy is outlined for outpatient evaluation of patients with recurrent stones.

2. Consensus Conference. Prevention and treatment of kidney stones. JAMA 1988;260:977–981.

   This succinct review advocates the conservative approach to evaluation outlined in this chapter and emphasizes the importance of medical therapy to prevent recurrence.

3. Drach GW, Dretler S, Fair W, et al. Report of the United States cooperative study of extracorporeal shock wave lithotripsy. J Urol 1986;135:1127–1133.

   This is a relatively early but large report on the results of lithotripsy in over 2000 patients. In patients with small (< 1 cm) stones, complications were infrequent. Patients with larger or multiple stones more frequently experienced obstruction, increased pain, or need for urologic intervention.

4. Pak CYC, ed. Renal Stone Disease: Pathogenesis, Prevention and Treatment. Boston, Martinus Nijhoff, 1987.

   An exhaustive review is presented in this textbook.

175 Urinary Tract Infections in Women

Problem

STEPHAN D. FIHN

Epidemiology. Approximately 20% of all women will have a urinary tract infection (UTI) during their lifetime. The vast majority of these infections are uncomplicated. The incidence rises sharply with onset of sexual activity and increases slowly thereafter. Three fourths of those having an initial UTI have sporadic recurrences, and 3% to 5% have two to three reinfections each year. Use of a diaphragm and spermicides raises the risk of UTI by twofold to threefold. Some evidence suggests an inherited predisposition to recurrent UTI that is related to presence of mucosal receptors for *Escherichia coli*. Seventy percent to 80% of UTIs in young women are caused by *E. coli,* and 15% to 20% are due to *Staphylococcus saprophyticus*. Infections with *S. saprophyticus* occur most commonly in spring and summer, and upper tract infection results more often than typical infection with gram-negative uropathogens.

Twenty percent to 30% of women older than age 65 have bacteriuria, which may come and go, often without specific treatment. In elderly women, the incidence of bacteriuria is higher in those who are institutionalized or debilitated.

Symptoms and Signs. Dysuria is a cardinal symptom, but urgency and frequency may be more common. Gross hematuria and suprapubic pain or tenderness are highly specific for UTI but occur in only 10% to 20% of cases. Infections due to *S. saprophyticus* are manifested by hematuria and pyuria more often than infections with other pathogens. Nausea, vomiting, fever, chills, and flank pain suggest pyelonephritis. Fever and flank tenderness are usually absent unless pyelonephritis is present. Elderly patients with UTI may lack some of these features and may present with more protean manifestations, such as mental status changes or nonspecific gastrointestinal or respiratory symptoms.

Clinical Approach. In a woman who has no complicating risk factors (see later), who presents with dysuria, and who describes her symptoms as identical to those occurring with prior documented UTIs, a diagnostic test is often unnecessary, and empirical treatment may be prescribed. Under some circumstances, this may be safely done by telephone. If this history is lacking, microscopic evaluation of the urine is the most useful next step. Visible bacteria on Gram stain or direct microscopy is highly specific (> 90%) for UTI but not sensitive (< 50%). Pyuria (defined by the presence of eight or more white blood cells/mm^3 or a quantitative leukocyte count of five cells per high-power field or more) is sensitive (about 90%) but has relatively low specificity

(50%–75%). Microscopically visible bacteria and pyuria are almost always present in acute pyelonephritis unless obstruction is present. Rapid tests for bacteria or pyuria are sensitive for UTIs associated with high levels of bacteriuria but insensitive for infections associated with lower colony counts.

In women with acute dysuria, a clean-catch midstream culture will yield 10^5 bacteria/mL or more in only 50% of those with proved infection. Using 10^2 or more as the criterion for infection is 95% sensitive and provides a positive predictive value of close to 90%. This lower definition of infection is more clinically relevant to the ambulatory setting. A culture is generally required only when urine microscopy is negative or there are complicating factors, including recent urinary tract instrumentation, childhood UTI, anatomic abnormality of the urinary tract, recent use of antibiotics, pregnancy, symptoms present for more than 1 week, diabetes, or immunosuppression.

Management. Antibiotic treatment for 3 days appears optimal for most uncomplicated UTIs, although many low-risk women can be safely treated with only a single dose. In the presence of complicating factors, longer therapy is warranted (Table 175–1). For the past two decades, trimethoprim-sulfamethoxazole has been the drug of choice based on its high cure rates and low incidence of adverse effects. In some settings, however, the prevalence of bacterial resistance to this agent has been rising, making other agents, such as the fluoroquinolones or amoxicillin-clavulanate, preferable. Although very effective, the fluoroquinolones are appreciably more expensive than trimethoprim-sulfamethoxazole or trimethoprim alone, and their widespread use for simple infections is likely to promote increasing resistance to these valuable agents. The decision to use more expensive drugs should be based on local antimicrobial susceptibility patterns.

Women who experience recurrent UTIs should be counseled to void promptly after intercourse, and diaphragm users should be counseled about the possibility of using other contraceptive methods. Prophylactic antimicrobial agents given to women who have had two or more recurrences within a year is cost effective and reduces morbidity from cystitis and pyelonephritis. This should be initiated only after the urine has been sterilized. Prophylaxis may be given on a continuous basis or only after intercourse in women whose infections are clearly related to sexual activity. Continuous prophylaxis is safe and effective for periods as long as 5 years, reducing the rate of cystitis from an average of 1.7 infections per year to 0.03 to 0.5, without increasing emergence of resistant organisms. Responsible women with frequent recurrences may be given the option of taking single-dose treatment on their own, early after the onset of symptoms.

Women with acute pyelonephritis who show signs of toxicity (e.g., high fever, nausea, and vomiting) should be admitted for parenteral therapy. Women with milder symptoms may be appropriately managed as outpatients under close supervision. Two-week therapy for pyelonephritis is as effective as that lasting 6 weeks. However, patients who relapse after a 2-week course should be given an additional 6 weeks of therapy.

Elderly women with symptomatic UTIs can usually be treated in the same fashion as younger women, although the threshold for admission to the hospital for pyelonephritis is lower. In general, asymptomatic bacteriuria in elderly

Table 175–1. TREATMENT OF URINARY TRACT INFECTION (UTI) IN WOMEN*

Clinical Setting	Antimicrobial Agent	Administration	Daily Cost† ($)
Acute UTI, uncomplicated	TMP-SMX (DS—160/800 mg)	1 tablet bid for 3 d (single dose 2 tablets)	0.52
	Trimethoprim	100 mg bid for 3 d (single dose 400 mg)	0.52
	Nitrofurantoin macrocrystals	100 mg qid for 3 d	3.86
	Nitrofurantoin monohydrate	100 mg bid for 3 d	2.46
	Sulfisoxazole	500 mg qid for 3 d	0.40
	Ampicillin	500 mg qid for 3 d	0.54
	Amoxicillin	500 mg bid for 3 d	0.47
	Norfloxacin	400 mg bid for 3 d (single dose 800 mg)	4.68
	Ciprofloxacin	250 mg bid for 3 d (single dose 500 mg)	3.24
	Ofloxacin	200 mg tid for 3 d (single dose 400 mg)	5.88
	Lomefloxacin	400 mg qd for 3 d (single dose 800 mg)	6.41
	Amoxicillin-clavulanate 500	1 tablet q8h for 3 d	7.99
Acute UTI, complicated	TMP-SMX (DS—160/800 mg)	1 tablet bid for 7–14 d	0.52
	Trimethoprim	100 mg bid for 7–14 d	0.34
	Norfloxacin	400 mg bid for 7–14 d	4.68
	Ciprofloxacin	250 or 500 mg bid for 7–14 d	5.60, 6.48
	Ofloxacin	200 mg bid for 7–14 d	5.88
	Lomefloxacin	400 mg qd for 7–14 d	6.41
	Amoxicillin-clavulanate 500	1 tablet q8h for 7–14 d	7.99

Recurrent UTI (regimen to be initiated after therapy of acute infection)	TMP-SMX (SS—80/400 mg)	½ tablet qhs or thrice weekly for 6 mo	0.09, 0.06
	Trimethoprim	100 mg qhs for 6 mo	0.17
	Nitrofurantoin	50 or 100 mg qhs for 6 mo	0.57, 0.97
	First generation cephalosporin (cephalexin)	125 or 250 mg qhs for 6 mo	0.07, 0.12
	Norfloxacin	200 mg qhs	1.27
	TMP-SMX (SS—80/400 mg)	½ or 1 tablet post coitus	0.09
	Nitrofurantoin macrocrystals	50 or 100 mg post coitus	0.57/0.97/dose
	Cephalexin	250 mg post coitus	0.14
	TMP-SMX (DS—160/800 mg)	1 tablet at onset of symptoms	0.27
Acute pyelonephritis, mild symptoms	TMP-SMX (DS—160/800 mg)	1 tablet bid for 14 d	0.52
	Trimethoprim	100 mg bid for 14 d	0.34
	Norfloxacin	400 mg bid for 14 d	4.68
	Ciprofloxacin	250 or 500 mg bid for 14 d	5.60, 6.48
	Ofloxacin	200 or 400 mg bid for 14 d	5.88, 7.32
	Lomafloxacin	400 qd for 14 d	6.41
	Amoxicillin-clavulanate 500	1 tablet q8h for 14 d	7.99

TMP-SMX, Trimethoprim-sulfamethoxazole; DS, double-strength; SS, single strength.

*Therapeutic options given in descending order of general preference. The choice and dose of therapy in any individual patient must be guided by specific clinical factors and by antimicrobial sensitivities when available. Fluoroquinolones may be preferred in settings where resistance to less expensive drugs routinely exceeds 10% to 15%.

†Average wholesale price, 1996 *Drug Topics Red Book.* Prices for generic equivalents are given as available.

women does not require treatment unless the patient is at higher than average risk of upper tract infection or sepsis (see Chapter 178).

Follow-Up. Follow-up of uncomplicated infections is generally not required unless symptoms persist or recur. Women with complicated infections should have a urine culture 2 to 3 weeks after therapy. Recurrent infections after that time are usually reinfections and may be treated with short-course therapy if appropriate.

Women with recurrent UTI do not routinely require excretory urography or cystoscopy unless history, symptoms, or pattern of recurrences suggests structural abnormalities of the urinary tract.

Cross-References: Abdominal Pain (Chapter 94), Pelvic Pain in Women (Chapter 160), Dysuria (Chapter 170), Bacteriuria in the Elderly (Chapter 178), Hematuria (Chapter 180), Bacteriuria in Pregnancy (Chapter 211).

REFERENCES

1. Grüneberg RN. Changes in the antibiotic sensitivities of urinary pathogens, 1971–89. J Antimicrob Chemother 1990;26(suppl F):3–11.

   An 18-year study from one hospital in London documents a fall in susceptibility of common outpatient uropathogens to commonly used antibiotics. During this period, sensitivity to ampicillin fell from 88% to 62% and that to trimethoprim-sulfamethoxazole from 97% to approximately 85%. Similar, though more pronounced, trends were noted for hospital pathogens (ampicillin, 66% to 50%, and trimethoprim-sulfamethoxazole, 84% to 72%).

2. Hooten TM, Stamm WE. Management of acute uncomplicated urinary tract infections in adults. Med Clin North Am 1991;75:339–357.

   This good overview advocates empirical 3-day treatment for most women with presumptive uncomplicated UTI without obtaining an initial culture. The authors also recommend that routine post-treatment cultures be omitted unless complicating factors or upper tract involvement is present.

3. Iravani A, Tice AD, McCarty J, Sikes DH, Nolen T, Gallis HA, Whalen EP, Tosiello RL, Heyd A, Kowalsky SF, et al. Short-course ciprofloxacin treatment of acute uncomplicated urinary tract infection in women. The minimum effective dose. The Urinary Tract Infection Study Group. Arch Intern Med 1995;155:485–494. Published erratum appears in Arch Intern Med 1995;155:871.

   In a careful series of trials that involved nearly 1000 women and compared different dosages and durations of ciprofloxacin, 100 mg twice daily for 3 days, was the minimum effective dose for the treatment of uncomplicated UTI.

4. Stamm WE, Counts GW, Running K, et al. Diagnosis of coliform infection in acutely dysuric women. N Engl J Med 1982;307:463–468.

   The authors provide the basis for using 10^2 bacteria/mL or more as the criterion to diagnose UTI.

5. Stamm WE, McKevitt M, Roberts PL, White NJ. Natural history of recurrent urinary tract infections in women. Rev Infect Dis 1991;13:77–84.

   The extensive clinical experience of a leading research group is summarized; the group, like others, observed marked clustering of infections with a diminishing risk of recurrence as time since the last infection lengthened. Women who had unacceptably frequent infections off prophylaxis were safely maintained on continuous, low-dose antibiotics for as long as 5 years without adverse effects or emergence of resistance. As well as preventing cystitis, prophylaxis appeared to reduce the risk of pyelonephritis.

176 Sexually Transmitted Diseases

Problem

THOMAS M. HOOTON

URETHRITIS

Epidemiology. Urethritis is the most common sexually transmitted disease and affects several million men annually in the United States. Gonococcal urethritis, caused by *Neisseria gonorrhoeae*, is often accompanied by infection with *Chlamydia trachomatis*. *C. trachomatis* had previously been found to cause 20% to 50% of cases of nongonococcal urethritis (NGU), but more recent studies have demonstrated *Chlamydia* in only 15% to 25% of cases. Likewise, *Ureaplasma urealyticum* was generally thought to cause 10% to 40% of cases of NGU, but it probably causes no more than 10% to 20% of cases. Miscellaneous bacteria, *Trichomonas vaginalis*, and herpes simplex virus cause a small proportion of cases. However, in perhaps as many as 50% of patients with NGU, no etiology can be determined. There is a high prevalence of infection with *N. gonorrhoeae* or *C. trachomatis* among female partners of men infected with these pathogens.

Symptoms and Signs. Dysuria with or without urethral discharge is the main symptom of urethritis, and most men have objective evidence of urethral discharge. However, both *N. gonorrhoeae* and *C. trachomatis* may be present in men with no symptoms or signs of urethritis. Patients with gonococcal urethritis tend to have more abrupt symptoms, a shorter incubation period, and a more purulent discharge than NGU, but a clear distinction cannot be made in the individual patient without an examination. Symptoms and signs are most prominent in the morning before urinating, especially with NGU.

Clinical Approach. A Gram stain of discharge (if present) or urethral swab specimen should be examined for evidence of urethral inflammation and gram-negative diplococci. The hallmark of urethritis is the presence of 5 or more leukocytes per oil immersion (1000×) field in a urethral Gram-stained specimen or 15 or more leukocytes per 400× field in the spun sediment of a first-voided urine specimen. The leukocyte esterase test is often used to screen for evidence of urethritis in asymptomatic males, but a positive test should be confirmed with microscopy of a urethral swab or urine. In a symptomatic male, the urethral Gram stain is highly sensitive (95%) and specific (95%) in distinguishing gonococcal from nongonococcal urethritis. Although specificity remains high in the asymptomatic patient, sensitivity is approximately 70%. A urethral culture or antigen test is necessary to determine whether *C. trachomatis* is present. Polymerase chain reaction and ligase chain reaction tests using first-voided urine specimens are highly sensitive and specific for *N. gonorrhoeae* and *C. trachomatis*, but their role in the evaluation of patients with sexually transmitted diseases remains to be determined. Because *U. urealyticum* is commonly found in normal sexually active men and women, routine cultures for this organism are not recommended.

Management. Patients with uncomplicated genital or anal gonorrhea should be treated with a single oral dose of cefixime, 400 mg; ciprofloxacin, 500 mg; or ofloxacin, 400 mg; or with a single intramuscular injection of ceftriaxone, 125 or 250 mg. However, if pharyngeal infection is a concern, either ceftriaxone or ciprofloxacin should be used. Cefixime or ceftriaxone should be considered the drugs of choice in areas where resistance of *N. gonorrhoeae* to fluoroquinolones has been reported. In the patient who can tolerate neither cephalosporins nor quinolones, spectinomycin, 2 g, in a single intramuscular injection should be given. Selected alternative gonococcal treatment regimens are listed in Table 176–1; many other antimicrobial agents are effective against *N. gonorrhoeae*. All patients with gonorrhea should also receive treatment for *C. trachomatis* because of the high rate of co-infection. Additionally, patients with sexually transmitted diseases should be offered testing for syphilis and human immunodeficiency virus (HIV) infection.

Patients infected with *Chlamydia* or with a clinical diagnosis of NGU should receive doxycycline, 100 mg orally twice daily for 7 days, or azithromycin, 1 g orally as a single dose. Erythromycin base, 500 mg orally four times daily for 7 days, is also effective against *Chlamydia*. Ofloxacin is effective against *C. trachomatis* but only when used in a regimen of 300 mg orally twice daily for 7 days.

Table 176–1. TREATMENT REGIMENS FOR URETHRITIS

Drug	Dose	Duration	Cost ($)*
Gonococcal Urethritis†			
Ceftriaxone	125 mg IM	Once	5.72
Ceftriaxone	250 mg IM	Once	11.44
Cefixime	400 mg PO	Once	6.32
Ciprofloxacin‡	500 mg PO	Once	3.13
Ofloxacin‡	400 mg PO	Once	3.66
Norfloxacin‡	800 mg PO	Once	5.08
Ceftizoxime	500 mg IM	Once	6.48
Spectinomycin	2 g IM	Once	16.13
Chlamydial or Nongonococcal Urethritis			
Doxycycline	100 mg PO	Twice daily for 7 days	13.16
Azithromycin	1 g PO	Once	18.75
Erythromycin base	500 mg PO	Four times daily for 7 days	7.00

*Average wholesale price for regimens listed, 1995 *Drug Topics Red Book*.

†All regimens should be followed by one of the antichlamydial regimens listed in table to treat possible concomitant *Chlamydia* infection.

‡Ciprofloxacin, ofloxacin, and norfloxacin are contraindicated in pregnant or nursing women and in persons 17 years of age and younger.

Norfloxacin, ciprofloxacin, cephalosporins, and spectinomycin have inadequate activity against infection with *C. trachomatis*.

Recent sexual partners of men with urethritis should be examined, a culture should be obtained, and the gonorrhea or chlamydial infection treated appropriately.

Follow-Up. All men with persistent or recurrent symptoms should be reevaluated for evidence of urethritis. It is very unusual to have persistent infection with *N. gonorrhoeae* or *C. trachomatis* if an appropriate regimen as listed in Table 176–1 was used and if the patient was compliant in taking these antibiotics. Therefore, men with uncomplicated gonorrhea or chlamydial infection who were treated with an appropriate regimen listed earlier and are asymptomatic need not return for follow-up. Likewise, men with NGU require no follow-up if their symptoms resolve. Men with recurrent NGU in whom reinfection is likely should be re-treated with doxycycline, azithromycin, or erythromycin. If reinfection is unlikely (i.e., the patient has not resumed unprotected intercourse), the patient should be treated with a different antibiotic from that used initially: erythromycin or doxycycline for 7 days, depending on what was used for initial therapy. Patients with continued persistence or recurrence of NGU should be considered for re-treatment with several weeks of therapy with erythromycin. Routine evaluation of the prostate gland or cystourethroscopy is not indicated in the patient with persistent or recurrent NGU.

GENITAL ULCERS

Epidemiology and Etiology. In the United States, genital herpes is by far the most common cause of genital ulcer syndrome, followed by syphilis and chancroid. Not infrequently, multiple diseases coexist in patients with genital ulcers. Chancroid is the most common etiology in many underdeveloped countries and is now endemic in several large US cities. Lymphogranuloma venereum and donovanosis are uncommon in the United States. Traumatic ulcers are often confused with those of an infectious etiology. The incidence of genital ulcers in the United States is difficult to estimate because syphilis is the only reportable cause. Genital ulcers place patients at greater risk for HIV infection.

Symptoms and Signs. Genital ulcers may be painful or asymptomatic. The ulcers caused by herpes simplex virus are typically small, multiple, shallow, tender, and relatively free of exudate but may coalesce or become large, tender, and indurated owing to secondary infection. Such lesions may be easily mistaken for those caused by chancroid or syphilis. The lymphadenopathy that frequently accompanies genital herpes is usually bilateral, tender, and only rarely fluctuant.

The classic syphilitic chancre is a solitary, painless, indurated ulcer that is not purulent or undermined and develops and disappears slowly. Multiple ulcers or ulcers with an atypical appearance, however, are as common as the classic chancre in primary syphilis. Chancres are often accompanied by bilateral, nontender, and firm lymphadenopathy.

Chancroid causes one or more painful ulcers, which are usually deep, tender, and friable with ragged, undermined edges. The ulcer base is usually purulent. Painful, tender, inguinal lymphadenopathy is often present; if the adenopathy is suppurative, it is almost pathognomonic for chancroid.

Clinical Approach. The diagnosis of genital ulceration is complicated by the frequent atypical presentations of the different syndromes. Lesions of herpes simplex virus, syphilis, and chancroid can appear identical. Darkfield microscopy is a sensitive and specific method for diagnosing primary syphilis when performed by trained personnel. Because the nontreponemal antibody tests (Venereal Disease Research Laboratories [VDRL] and rapid plasma reagin [RPR] tests) are positive in only 70% of patients with primary syphilis, repeat serologic testing 4 to 6 weeks later may be warranted to document seroconversion. Treponemal antibody tests, such as the fluorescent treponemal antibody absorbed (FTA-ABS), are more specific and, if positive, exclude biologic false-positive nontreponemal antibody tests. A cerebrospinal fluid evaluation should be performed in all patients with latent syphilis who have neurologic or ophthalmic signs or symptoms, evidence of tertiary syphilis, treatment failure, HIV infection, or a VDRL test result of 1:32 or greater, or if nonpenicillin therapy is planned.

Culture is the most sensitive diagnostic method for herpes simplex virus but has a sensitivity of less than 60% during the ulcerated stage of the disease. In the setting of a darkfield microscopy–negative ulcer and absence of characteristic vesicles, a culture or antigen detection test for herpes simplex virus is warranted.

Haemophilus ducreyi is a fastidious gram-negative organism that requires a selective medium for isolation. Gram stain evaluation of ulcers is neither sensitive nor specific in diagnosis.

HIV testing should be performed in patients with genital ulcers, especially those patients with syphilis or chancroid.

Management. Selected effective treatment regimens for these genital syndromes are listed in Table 176–2. Some patients with genital ulcers, especially those with lesions suggestive of syphilis or chancroid, may warrant empirical therapy before a definitive diagnosis can be made. Patients with herpes simplex virus and HIV infections may benefit from higher doses of acyclovir, such as 400 mg three to five times daily, until lesions disappear. Treatment of recurrent herpes simplex virus infection is generally ineffective unless started early in the course of the recurrence (within 2 days of onset of lesions). Topical acyclovir is less effective than oral acyclovir. Patients should keep involved areas dry and avoid occlusive underwear.

The proper treatment of primary, secondary, and early latent (less than 1 year) syphilis is benzathine penicillin, 2.4 million units given intramuscularly once. Patients with syphilis of longer duration or unknown duration without evidence of neurologic involvement should receive benzathine penicillin, 2.4 million units intramuscularly every week for 3 weeks. Neurosyphilis documented by cerebrospinal fluid findings warrants extended high-dose intravenous penicillin therapy. Patients treated for syphilis at any stage should be warned about the possibility of an acute febrile reaction (Jarisch-Herxheimer reaction). Expert advice should be sought for treatment of penicillin-allergic patients.

Patients with chancroid and HIV infection heal more slowly and should be treated with the erythromycin 7-day regimen shown in Table 176–2.

Table 176–2. TREATMENT REGIMENS FOR GENITAL ULCER SYNDROMES

Syndrome	Drug	Dose	Duration	Cost ($)*
Primary herpes simplex virus infection	Acyclovir	200 mg PO 5× daily	7–10 d	35.70 (7 d)
		400 mg PO tid	7–10 d	41.79 (7 d)
Recurrent herpes simplex virus infection	Acyclovir	200 mg PO × daily	5 d	25.50
		400 mg PO tid	5 d	29.85
		800 mg PO bid	5 d	38.70
Syphilis < 1 y	Benzathine penicillin G	2.4 million units IM	Once	26.85
Syphilis < 1 y in penicillin-allergic patients	Doxycycline	100 mg PO bid	14 d	26.32
	Tetracycline	500 mg PO qid	14 d	6.16
Syphilis > 1 y or unknown duration	Benzathine penicillin G	2.4 million units IM	Once weekly for 3 weeks	80.55 (3 wk)
Neurosyphilis	Aqueous crystalline penicillin G	2–4 million units IV q4h	10–14 d†	18.30 (10 d, 3 million units)
	Procaine penicillin G *plus*	2.4 million units IM once daily	10–14 d†	109.00 (10 d)
	Probenecid	500 mg qid		
Chancroid	Azithromycin	1 g PO	Once	18.75
	Ceftriaxone	250 mg IM	Once	11.44
	Erythromycin base	500 mg PO qid	7 d‡	7.00

*Average wholesale price for regimens listed, *Drug Topics Red Book* 1995.
†Follow with benzathine penicillin G weekly for 3 weeks.
‡Some experts recommend this regimen for treating persons infected with human immunodeficiency virus.

Follow-Up. Patients with genital herpes do not require routine follow-up. Patients treated for early syphilis should be reexamined at 3 and 6 months and for longer periods if they have more advanced stages of syphilis. More frequent follow-up is indicated in patients who are HIV positive. The VDRL titer should decrease at least fourfold within 3 months of treatment for primary and secondary syphilis. The VDRL response seen with syphilis of longer duration is more variable. Unless reinfection is likely, failure of the VDRL titer to fall or persistence of signs or symptoms indicates treatment failure; the patient should undergo examination of the cerebrospinal fluid and be re-treated appropriately.

Chancroid ulcers generally improve within 7 days after institution of therapy, whereas the lymphadenopathy may resolve more slowly. Patients should be observed until the ulcer is completely healed. Fluctuant lymphadenopathy may require needle aspiration through adjacent intact skin. Poor response to therapy in the compliant patient suggests misdiagnosis, antimicrobial-resistant *H. ducreyi*, or co-infection with another sexually transmitted disease (including infection with HIV).

CERVICITIS

Epidemiology. Cervicitis can be caused by *N. gonorrhoeae, C. trachomatis,* or herpes simplex virus, although in most cases no pathogen can be identified. The incidence of cervicitis in the United States is unknown because nongonococcal causes of cervicitis are not reportable. Pelvic inflammatory disease (PID) and its serious sequelae, discussed in Chapter 166, may result from spread of pathogens from the cervix to the upper genital tract.

Symptoms and Signs. Compared with urethritis in men, cervicitis is more often asymptomatic and the diagnostic criteria are less well defined. The patient may complain of vaginal discharge, dyspareunia, or vaginal odor. Cervicitis is manifested by a purulent endocervical discharge, friability of the endocervix, and edematous cervical ectopy or some combination thereof. Vesicles or ulcerations on the ectocervix suggest the diagnosis of herpes simplex virus infection. Fever, lower abdominal pain or tenderness, or a pelvic mass suggests PID.

Clinical Approach. Mucopurulent cervicitis is characterized by a yellow endocervical exudate visible in the endocervical canal or on an endocervical swab specimen. An endocervical Gram stain should be performed to look for evidence of inflammation (> 30 leukocytes per $1000\times$ field on a cervical Gram stain) and for gram-negative diplococci. Although highly specific, a Gram stain is insensitive for detection of infection with *N. gonorrhoeae,* and a cervical culture is necessary. A urethral culture or antigen test should be obtained to determine whether *C. trachomatis* is present. Both *N. gonorrhoeae* and *C. trachomatis* may be present in the cervix of a woman who has no symptoms or signs of cervicitis. Polymerase chain reaction and ligase chain reaction tests using first-voided urine specimens are highly sensitive and specific for *N. gonorrhoeae* and *C. trachomatis,* but their role in the evaluation of patients with sexually transmitted diseases remains to be determined.

Management. The patient with cervicitis is usually treated empirically for both *N. gonorrhoeae* and *C. trachomatis* infections or, if the likelihood of *N. gonorrhoeae* is low, for *Chlamydia* infection alone; or treatment is delayed until test results become available. Cervical gonorrhea or chlamydial infection should be treated with any of the regimens described for treatment of gonococcal or chlamydial urethritis in a male (see Table 176–1). Patients with gonorrhea should also receive therapy for chlamydial infection. Ofloxacin, 300 mg orally twice daily for 7 days, is an effective alternative regimen against *Chlamydia.* The quinolones are contraindicated in pregnant or nursing women and in persons aged 17 years or younger. Nongonococcal cervicitis should be treated with doxycycline, 100 mg orally twice daily for 7 days, or azithromycin, 1 g orally as a single dose, or with alternative regimens as recommended for NGU in a male (see Urethritis earlier in this chapter). Patients with signs of PID should be treated accordingly (see Chapter 166). Cervicitis caused by herpes simplex virus should be treated with acyclovir (see Table 176–2). Male sexual partners should be examined, cultured, and treated for gonorrhea or chlamydial infection as appropriate.

Follow-Up. All women with persistent or recurrent symptoms should be reevaluated for evidence of cervicitis. It is very unusual to have persistent infection with *N. gonorrhoeae* or *C. trachomatis* if an appropriate regimen listed earlier was used, and if the patient was compliant in taking these antibiotics. Therefore, women with uncomplicated gonorrhea or chlamydial infection who were treated with an appropriate regimen listed earlier and are asymptomatic need not return for follow-up. Likewise, women with nongonococcal cervicitis require no follow-up if their symptoms resolve. Some experts recommend rescreening women several months after treatment of chlamydial infection to detect reinfection and reduce morbidity.

Cross-References: General Approach to Arthritic Symptoms (Chapter 106), Pelvic Pain in Women (Chapter 160), Pelvic Inflammatory Disease (Chapter 166), HIV Infection: Disease Prevention and Antiretroviral Therapy (Chapter 203), HIV Infection: Office Evaluation (Chapter 204), HIV Infection: Evaluation of Common Symptoms (Chapter 205).

REFERENCES

1. Bowie WR. Urethritis in males. In Holmes KK, Mardh P-A, Sparling PF, et al., eds. Sexually Transmitted Diseases, 2nd ed. New York, McGraw-Hill Book Company, 1989:627–639.

   This chapter is a general review of urethritis.

2. Centers for Disease Control and Prevention. 1993 Sexually transmitted diseases treatment guidelines. MMWR 1993;42(No. RR-14):1–102.

   Succinct treatment guidelines and rationale are presented.

3. Holmes KK. Lower genital tract infections in women: Cystitis, urethritis, vulvovaginitis, and cervicitis. In Holmes KK, Mardh P-A, Sparling PF, et al., eds. Sexually Transmitted Diseases, 2nd ed. New York, McGraw-Hill Book Company, 1989:533–540.

   This is a general review of infections in women.

4. Hooton TM, Wong ES, Barnes RC, Roberts PL, Stamm WE. Erythromycin for persistent or recurrent nongonococcal urethritis: A randomized, placebo-controlled trial. Ann Intern Med 1990;113:21–26.

   Erythromycin significantly decreased pyuria in men with persistent or recurrent NGU, especially in those with evidence of prostatic inflammation.

5. Piot P, Plummer FA. Genital ulcer adenopathy syndrome. In Holmes KK, Mardh P-A, Sparling PF, et al., eds. Sexually Transmitted Diseases, 2nd ed. New York, McGraw-Hill Book Company, 1989:711–716.

   This is a good general review of genital ulcers.

177 Urinary Tract Infections in Men

Problem

BENJAMIN A. LIPSKY

Epidemiology and Etiology. In community surveys, the frequency of bacteriuria is age related. It is rare in young men (prevalence $\leq$ 0.1%), occurs in about 5% of those aged 65 to 85 years (one third of the rate in women), and is found in about 15% of those older than age 85 years (two thirds of the rate in women). Bacteriuria is found in about 5% of adult male outpatients and in over 25% of elderly hospitalized or institutionalized men. A risk factor for urinary tract infection in infants, and perhaps young men, is lack of circumcision. Sexual activity appears to predispose to urinary tract infections (UTIs) in men, as does infection with the human immunodeficiency virus. The major factor contributing to UTIs in older men is believed to be prostatic hypertrophy, which results in bladder outlet obstruction. This predisposes to infection directly, by creating a residual of urine in the bladder after voiding, and indirectly, by leading to genitourinary instrumentation for its evaluation or treatment.

Gram-negative bacilli cause about 75% of UTIs in men. Unlike in women, however, *Escherichia coli* is responsible for only 25% to 50% of the infections, whereas *Proteus* and *Providencia* species cause most of the rest. UTIs in men are occasionally caused by other gram-negative bacilli, streptococci (especially enterococci), staphylococci (both coagulase-positive and -negative), or, rarely, fastidious organisms such as *Gardnerella vaginalis* or *Haemophilus influenzae*. Men who are institutionalized, who require a urinary catheter, or who have received recent courses of antibiotics are likely to have uropathogens that are resistant to commonly prescribed antibiotics.

Symptoms and Signs. Genitourinary symptoms of a UTI are usually primarily irritative (i.e., dysuria, frequency, urgency, strangury) but may also be obstructive (i.e., hesitancy, nocturia, slow stream, and dribbling). Systemic symptoms (e.g., fever, malaise) are infrequent; when present they suggest involvement of the epididymis, prostate, or kidney. Infection in these sites can often be detected by physical examination. A urethral discharge usually indicates urethritis rather than a UTI.

Clinical Approach. A urine culture should be obtained for all men with symptoms suggesting a UTI, as well as for men in whom bacteriuria must be excluded (e.g., before genitourinary instrumentation). A voided specimen from a man is much less likely to be contaminated than that from a woman. Several

All of the material in Chapter 177 is in the public domain, with the exception of any borrowed figures and tables.

studies have shown that factors such as the man's circumcision status or use of meatal cleansing or midstream sampling have little effect on the accuracy of urine cultures; thus, the clean-catch midstream void technique is usually unnecessary for men. The best laboratory criterion for diagnosing true (i.e., bladder) bacteriuria in men is growth of 10^3 colony-forming units (CFU)/mL or more of a single or predominant species. In one study this criterion had a sensitivity and specificity of 0.97. Defining bacteriuria as greater than or equal to 10^5 CFU/mL will miss true bacteriuria in about a third of bacteriuric men.

When a specimen of bladder urine is needed, suprapubic aspiration is generally easier, more accurate, and less painful than urethral catheterization. Specimens from a man wearing a condom catheter should be obtained by collecting the first 10 to 20 mL of urine produced after applying a clean catheter and collection bag; bacteriuria of 10^5 CFU/mL or more has a positive predictive value of over 90% if the same organism is found in two consecutive specimens.

Localizing the site of infection in bacteriuric men is usually unnecessary. Pyelonephritis is generally diagnosed clinically, and it is only rarely necessary to know which kidney is infected. Acute bacterial prostatitis presents as an acute febrile illness with an exquisitely tender prostate. Determining when chronic prostatic infection is present is more difficult; clinical diagnosis is inaccurate, the recommended four-cup test is a cumbersome and rarely used procedure, and immunologic methods are not routinely available.

Management. All symptomatic men with bacteriuria should receive antibiotic treatment, but the appropriate duration of therapy is debated. Single-dose or short-course therapy probably has no role in bacteriuric men. Available data suggest that 7 to 10 days of treatment with any one of several antibiotics cures uncomplicated cystitis in most men. For those with a UTI complicated by pyelonephritis, prostatism, or another anatomic or functional genitourinary problem, more prolonged treatment (2 to 3 weeks) may be necessary. Men with recurrent bacteriuria, most of whom probably have a prostatic focus of infection, require at least 6 weeks of antibiotic therapy. When prostatic infection is believed to be present, an agent that penetrates the prostate (e.g., trimethoprim, erythromycin, doxycycline, or a fluoroquinolone) is needed. When recurrent UTIs are frequent or severe, they can be effectively suppressed by daily low-dose antibiotic treatment (e.g., cotrimoxazole, 1 regular-strength tablet a day).

Follow-Up. For patients in whom it is important to eradicate bacteriuria, a follow-up urine culture should be obtained 2 to 3 weeks after completing treatment. Earlier recurrences are usually relapses; later ones are usually reinfections. The indications for a urologic diagnostic evaluation in a man with bacteriuria are not well defined. Although genitourinary abnormalities are frequent in bacteriuric men, the clinical and prognostic significance of many of these findings is undetermined. Certainly, men presenting with evidence of urinary tract obstruction or those with recurrent infections, progressive renal dysfunction, or other complicating features should be evaluated. The workup should usually include renal ultrasonography and, if necessary, excretory urography, cystoscopy, or urodynamic studies.

Cross-References: Dysuria (Chapter 170), Scrotal Pain (Chapter 171), Urinary Tract Infections in Women (Chapter 175), Bacteriuria in the Elderly (Chapter 178).

REFERENCES

1. Lipsky BA. Urinary tract infections in men. Epidemiology, pathophysiology, diagnosis, and treatment. Ann Intern Med 1989;110:138–150.

   A thorough review that includes a discussion of diagnosis and treatment algorithms and 107 references.

2. Lipsky BA, Ireton RC, Fihn SD, et al. Diagnosis of bacteriuria in men: Specimen collection and culture interpretation. J Infect Dis 1987;155:847–854.

   Data are presented from 76 comprehensive evaluations of 66 bacteriuric and nonbacteriuric men demonstrating that voided specimens are highly accurate and that the best diagnostic criterion for bacteriuria is greater than or equal to 10^3 CFU/mL.

3. Richmann M, Goetzman B, Langer E, et al. Risk factors for bacteriuria in men. Urology 1994;43:617–620.

   A study of 99 mentally and physically competent nursing home residents found that the presence of bacteriuria did not correlate with any of the presumed risk factors, including post-void residual volume.

4. Schaeffer AJ. Urinary tract infection in men: State of the art. Infection 1994;22(suppl 1):S19–S21.

   This review, from a urologist's point of view, is followed by commentaries from a panel of international authorities.

5. Sugarman ID, Pead LJ, Payne SR, et al. Bacteriological state of the urine in symptom-free adult males. Br J Urol 1990;66:148–151.

   Voided specimens from 120 asymptomatic men yielded no aerobic organisms in pure growth; 26% had fastidious organisms but none in counts of greater than or equal to 10^4 CFU/mL.

178 Bacteriuria in the Elderly

Problem

BENJAMIN A. LIPSKY

Epidemiology and Etiology. In the elderly, urinary tract infections (UTIs) are the most common cause of bacteremia and one of the leading causes of fever and hospitalization. The prevalence of bacteriuria increases with age and debility (Table 178–1). Rates of infection are highest in hospitalized or institutionalized patients. Factors contributing to bacteriuria in the elderly include (1) in men, prostatic hypertrophy and age-related decrements in antimicrobial activity of prostatic secretions; (2) in women, fecal incontinence and age-related changes in vaginal secretions and bladder function; and (3) in both sexes, bladder catheterization and other coexisting diseases (especially those interfering with bladder emptying). Bacteriuria is often intermittent (even without therapy), and the infecting organism may change over time. Among patients with asymptomatic bacteriuria, repeat cultures 1 to 5 years later are negative in

**Table 178–1. APPROXIMATE PREVALENCE OF
BACTERIURIA IN ELDERLY SUBJECTS (%)**

Population	Men	Women
Community based		
Ages 65–85 y	5	15
Age ≥ 85 y	13	25
Patient based		
Inpatients age < 70 y	8	30
Inpatients age > 70 y	25	30
Institutionalized	> 30	> 30

about 80% of men and 50% of women. Among those with sterile cultures, about 10% of men and 20% of women develop bacteriuria.

Although *Escherichia coli* is the most frequent cause of UTIs in the elderly, other gram-negative bacilli, such as *Proteus, Providencia, Klebsiella, Enterobacter, Pseudomonas,* and *Serratia* species, are isolated more often than in younger patients. Polymicrobial infections are also more common in the elderly and account for 25% to 33% of cultures in noncatheterized residents of long-term care facilities. Uropathogens from institutionalized, instrumented, or recurrently infected patients are often resistant to antibiotics.

Symptoms and Signs. Most elderly bacteriuric subjects have no urinary or systemic symptoms. With an acute UTI, most elderly patients have typical irritative genitourinary symptoms of dysuria, frequency, urgency, or incontinence. Diagnosing a UTI in the elderly is made more difficult by the fact that some patients present with only urinary incontinence or generalized symptoms (e.g., a change in mental status, anorexia, malaise), and many nonbacteriuric elderly patients have irritative urinary symptoms. If symptoms are of recent onset or are accompanied by dysuria, a UTI should be considered.

Low-level pyuria is frequently unrelated to bacteriuria in elderly ambulatory women, although its absence strongly suggests the absence of bacteriuria. Among elderly institutionalized women, however, the finding of a quantitative urine leukocyte count of $20/mm^3$ or more has a positive and negative predictive value of about 80% for upper tract infection.

Clinical Approach. In asymptomatic patients, bacteriuria is defined as growth of greater than or equal to 10^5 CFU/mL from a voided specimen on two separate cultures. In elderly, especially institutionalized, patients, pyuria does not differentiate infection from colonization, nor is it a reliable diagnostic test for bacteriuria. Genitourinary symptoms should not be automatically attributed to bacteriuria; other causes, such as prostatic hypertrophy or vaginitis, should be considered. A urine culture is indicated only if there is an intent to treat bacteriuria if it is detected.

Bacteriuria, whether symptomatic or not, may reflect more than uncomplicated cystitis. Half or more of elderly bacteriuric women have upper UTIs, and about half of bacteriuric elderly men have prostatic infections. Twenty percent of cases of acute pyelonephritis are initially misdiagnosed in elderly patients because attention is focused on nonurinary symptoms. Bacteremia and shock are more frequent with pyelonephritis in elderly patients than in younger patients. Up to half of patients 65 or older hospitalized with a complicated UTI will be bacteremic, and over half of the etiologic agents will likely be resistant to ampicillin.

Management. All symptomatic patients with bacteriuria should receive antibiotic treatment. Because single-dose or short-course therapy has an unacceptably high failure rate (up to two thirds) in elderly patients, 1 to 2 weeks of therapy are recommended (see the recommendations in Chapters 175 and 177). Patients with indwelling bladder catheters inevitably develop bacteriuria but do not require treatment unless they develop urinary symptoms or fever. Elderly patients with acute pyelonephritis should be hospitalized to exclude bacteremia, to identify the etiologic organism, and to monitor the initial response to therapy.

A major issue in elderly patients is whether to treat asymptomatic bacteriuria. Despite earlier studies to the contrary, asymptomatic bacteriuria per se is probably not associated with premature mortality or other long-term adverse outcomes but is simply a marker for other serious medical problems, particularly dementia. In the absence of obstruction, treatment of asymptomatic bacteriuria appears to provide no improvement in survival or reduction in the rate of symptomatic UTIs. In view of the expense of detection and treatment of bacteriuria, the potential for adverse reactions to antimicrobial agents (which occur in up to a fourth of elderly patients), and the frequent spontaneous disappearance of asymptomatic bacteriuria, routine treatment is not warranted. Treatment should be considered for patients who are immunologically compromised or who will be undergoing genitourinary instrumentation or placement of a prosthetic device. In these patients, 3 days of therapy may be sufficient. Studies in hospitalized patients have shown that recurrence rates of asymptomatic bacteriuria after antimicrobial treatment are high.

Follow-Up. The indications for diagnostic evaluation of the urinary tract are discussed in Chapters 175 (for women) and 177 (for men).

Cross-References: Fever (Chapter 16), Urinary Tract Infections in Women (Chapter 175), Urinary Tract Infections in Men (Chapter 177).

REFERENCES

1. Armitage KB, Salata RA, Landefeld CS. Urosepsis in the elderly in clinical and microbiologic characteristics. Infect Dis Clin Pract 1993;2:260–266.

   Among 105 patients aged 65 years or older admitted to a university-affiliated hospital with urosepsis, bacteremia was present in 50% and was predicted by the presence of hypotension. The etiologic agents were gram-negative rods in 95%, but 56% were ampicillin resistant.

2. Boscia JA, Abrutyn E, Levison ME, et al. Pyuria and asymptomatic bacteriuria in elderly ambulatory women. Ann Intern Med 1989;110:404–405.

   Cultures and urinary leukocyte counts of voided urine specimens from 317 asymptomatic women revealed a positive predictive value for bacteriuria of pyuria of 39% and a negative predictive value for no pyuria of 96%.

3. Gleckman RA. Urinary tract infection. Clin Geriatr Med 1992;8:793–803.

   An excellent up-to-date overview is presented of the available information in this area, with 39 references.

4. Nicolle LE. Urinary tract infections in long-term care facilities. Infect Control Hosp Epidemiol 1993;14:220–225.

   This is a thoughtful review of a common problem by a recognized authority.

5. Nicolle LE, Muir P, Harding GKM, et al. Localization of urinary tract infection in elderly, institutionalized women with asymptomatic bacteriuria. J Infect Dis 1988;157:65–70.

   In 51 women with asymptomatic bacteriuria, bladder washout localized the infection to the kidney in two thirds of patients. The positive and negative predictive values of the antibody-coated bacteria test were 82% and 43%, respectively, and the quantitative leukocyte count of 20/mm³ or more was 80% and 88%, respectively.

- -

179 Chronic Renal Failure

Problem

MINDY A. COOPER

Epidemiology and Etiology. Chronic renal failure (CRF) refers to a variety of pathologic processes that are characterized by the gradual loss of renal function. A subset of patients with CRF will progress from asymptomatic decreases in renal reserve to end-stage renal disease (ESRD), which requires some form of renal replacement therapy. Approximately 200,000 patients are on dialysis in the United States, with costs averaging $57,000 per patient-year of therapy. The incidence of ESRD is three times higher in blacks than whites and is 30% to 40% higher in men than women. The leading causes of ESRD in the United States are hypertension, diabetes, glomerulonephritis, and polycystic kidney disease.

Symptoms and Signs. Patients who have lost 25% to 50% of their renal function are usually asymptomatic. *Renal insufficiency* refers to the loss of 50% to 75% of renal function. Blood urea nitrogen (BUN) and serum creatinine concentrations are increased (1–4 mg/dL), whereas calcium, phosphorus, and potassium homeostasis remain intact. Patients usually have no symptoms of renal disease. Patients with *renal failure* typically have less than 25% of renal function associated with an elevated BUN and creatinine value (> 4 mg/dL). Symptoms, if present, are mild. There may be hypocalcemia and hyperphosphatemia and a normochromic, normocytic anemia. When residual renal function is no longer able to sustain normal body function and composition, *uremia or ESRD* ensues. Uremic symptoms include nausea, vomiting, malaise, sleep disturbances, and pruritus. Bleeding due to platelet dysfunction, severe hypocalcemia, and hyperparathyroid bone disease inducing pathologic fractures may occur. These patients require chronic dialysis or renal transplantation to survive.

Clinical Approach. The clinician should (1) quantify the degree of renal failure, (2) attempt to diagnose the etiology of renal failure, and (3) identify any potential reversible disorders. Several methods are available for assessing renal function. The steady-state concentration of serum creatinine provides a reasonable estimate (Table 179–1). In general, each time the steady-state creatinine doubles, renal function decreases by 50%. Another simple and fast way to assess renal function is to calculate the creatinine clearance with the Cockcroft and Gault formula:

$$\text{creatinine clearance} = \frac{(140 - \text{age}) \times \text{body weight (kg)}}{72 \times \text{serum creatinine}}$$

This formula can be multiplied by 0.85 for women to correct for lean body mass. The formula is especially useful for estimating renal function in elderly patients in whom small increments in serum creatinine level reflect large impairments in renal function. Creatinine clearance can also be determined using 24-hour urine collection.

Diagnosis of the cause of renal failure starts with a thorough history and physical examination as well as a careful analysis of the urine sediment. Carotid, femoral, or renal artery bruits suggest a renovascular cause. Careful retinal examination may reveal diabetic or hypertensive changes that correlate with renal involvement. Bilateral abdominal masses can be palpated in advanced polycystic kidney disease. Renal ultrasonography should be obtained on initial evaluation of the patient with CRF. Bilateral small kidneys (less than 9 cm) indicate irreversible loss of kidney function. Asymmetric kidney size may suggest renal artery stenosis as the cause of renal failure. Congenital kidney disease and obstruction can also be diagnosed by renal ultrasonography.

Conditions that worsen preexisting renal impairment include volume depletion, congestive heart failure, urinary obstruction (especially if associated with infection), nephrotoxic agents (nonsteroidal anti-inflammatory agents, aminoglycosides, radiocontrast dyes), and hypercalcemia.

Management. Management of the patient with CRF usually focuses on the following areas.

FLUID AND ELECTROLYTE BALANCE. There is loss of fine tuning of both sodium and water balance in patients with renal failure. Conditions that would otherwise be well tolerated in patients with normal renal function can cause devastating abnormalities in patients with CRF. Sodium excretion cannot be readily altered by the kidney; thus, patients can exhibit evidence of intravascular volume depletion because of overzealous diuretic use, vomiting, fever, or diarrhea. In addition, there is a limited ability to excrete a sodium load, such that

Table 179–1. ESTIMATING GLOMERULAR FILTRATION RATE FROM THE STEADY-STATE SERUM CREATININE CONCENTRATION

Creatinine (mg/dL)	Glomerular Filtration Rate (mL/min)
1	100
2	50
4	25
8	12.5
16	6.25

acutely increasing sodium intake can rapidly expand extracellular fluid volume and result in pulmonary edema. The diseased kidney has a limited ability to concentrate and dilute the urine, thus predisposing to hypernatremia and hyponatremia when there is variable access to water. Patients must be advised to judiciously monitor sodium and water intake.

METABOLIC ACIDOSIS. Prolonged metabolic acidosis can cause calcium wasting as well as bone disease. Treatment with sodium bicarbonate or sodium citrate is indicated if the serum bicarbonate level drops below 16 mEq/L.

HYPERTENSION. Hypertension is present in up to 80% of patients with a glomerular filtration rate of less than 25%. Treatment is essential, because it has been well documented that hypertension accelerates the progression of renal disease. Hypertension in most azotemic patients is sodium dependent; therefore, treatment should begin with dietary sodium restriction (2 g/d). Addition of a diuretic is often required. Subsequent addition of a β-blocker, calcium antagonist, or angiotensin-converting enzyme (ACE) inhibitor may be warranted. At this time ACE inhibitors are the treatment of choice for diabetic nephropathy. Close monitoring of diabetic patients for hyperkalemia is indicated because many have a coexistent type IV renal tubular acidosis and cannot tolerate the further diminution of potassium excretion associated with ACE inhibitor–induced hypoaldosteronism.

HYPERPARATHYROIDISM. Dietary phosphate should be restricted to less than 1000 mg/d to maintain the serum phosphate level below 6 mg/dL. Phosphate-binding antacids (calcium carbonate or calcium acetate) should be given with meals if dietary measures are unsuccessful. Initial doses of 500 mg with meals can be titrated to achieve serum calcium levels in the high-normal range. If these steps are ineffective, 0.25 μg/d calcitriol (1,25-dihydroxyvitamin D) should be added.

ANEMIA. The hematocrit begins to decrease when the glomerular filtration rate reaches 30 mL/min owing to the loss of the kidney's ability to produce erythropoietin. Treatment of the anemia with erythropoietin has been shown to increase exercise tolerance and quality of life in patients. Iron studies should be watched closely because patients with renal insufficiency are frequently iron deficient secondary to ongoing gastrointestinal blood loss.

DRUG DOSING. It is imperative to carefully monitor drug dosing and administration. Standard tables of drug dosing guidelines for patients with renal failure are available. Patients should be advised to avoid over-the-counter medications, such as nonsteroidal anti-inflammatory agents, that can worsen renal function.

UREMIA. The definitive treatment of uremia is with dialysis or transplantation. Indications for initiating renal replacement therapy include uremic symptoms, resistant hypertension, pericarditis, neuropathy, and encephalopathy. In addition, when hyperkalemia, metabolic acidosis, and congestive heart failure are refractory to medical therapy, dialysis may be required.

Follow-Up. Patients with CRF should be vaccinated against influenza and pneumococcus. The frequency of follow-up depends on the stage of renal failure and the severity of the patient's symptoms. When the creatinine clearance drops to 30 mL/min, the patient should be referred to a nephrologist for discussion of treatment options.

Cross-References: Anorexia (Chapter 18), Fatigue (Chapter 21), Pruritus (Chapter 23), Essential Hypertension (Chapter 85), Diabetes Mellitus (Chapter 154), Proteinuria (Chapter 181), Electrolyte Abnormalities (Chapter 182), Benign Prostatic Hyperplasia (Chapter 184).

REFERENCES

1. Bennett W, et al. Drug Prescribing in Renal Failure—Dosing Guidelines for Adults. Philadelphia, American College of Physicians, 1994.

   This book is the most commonly used resource for drug dosing in patients with renal insufficiency and renal failure.

2. Cockcroft DW, Gault MH: Prediction of creatinine clearance from serum creatinine. Nephron 1976;16:31.

   The authors describe the estimation of creatinine clearance using age, weight, and serum creatinine.

3. Eschbach JW, Adamson JW. Guidelines for recombinant human erythropoietin therapy. Am J Kidney Dis 1989;14(suppl 1):2–8.

   This article is a practical review of indications, dosages, and complications of recombinant human erythropoietin therapy.

4. Kimmel PL. Management of the patient with chronic renal disease. In Primer on Kidney Diseases. San Diego, National Kidney Foundation, 1994:281–287.

   Prevention of progression is discussed with other management issues in patients with chronic renal failure.

180 Hematuria

Problem

SHIN-PING TU

Epidemiology. The prevalence of hematuria ranges from 13% to 22% depending on the definition of hematuria and age of the study population.

Etiology. Hematuria may result from strenuous exercise and various genitourinary disorders: urinary tract infection, trauma, renal calculi, tuberculosis, polycystic kidney disease, and sickle cell disease. Other causes include interstitial nephritis, vasculitis, and the glomerulonephropathies. In younger persons, IgA nephropathy is the most common cause of microscopic hematuria. In older persons, the incidence of urologic malignancies (i.e., bladder, renal, and prostate cancers) increases and the disease may present as gross or microscopic hematuria. Ureteral cancer may also present as hematuria, but this malignancy is uncommon.

Clinical Approach. The history and physical examination should focus on indicators of urinary infection (dysuria, urgency, frequency, fever, suprapubic tenderness), stones (flank pain), trauma, glomerulonephritis (rash, recent respiratory tract infection, hypertension, hepatitis, or human immunodeficiency virus infection), and interstitial nephritis (medications). A family history of polycystic kidney disease or sickle cell disease is helpful for diagnosis. In patients older than age 60, risk factors for urologic malignancies include tobacco use, occupational exposure to dyes or rubber compounds, pelvic irradiation, analgesic abuse, and cyclophosphamide treatment.

Initial laboratory testing should include a dipstick urinalysis and sediment examination. Determinations of blood urea nitrogen, serum creatinine, urine culture, and urinary protein and a complete cell blood count should also be considered (Fig. 180–1).

When evaluating hematuria, the following should be considered:

1. *Isolated versus intermittent or persistent hematuria?* There are numerous causes of transient microscopic hematuria: physical exercise, viral illnesses, men-

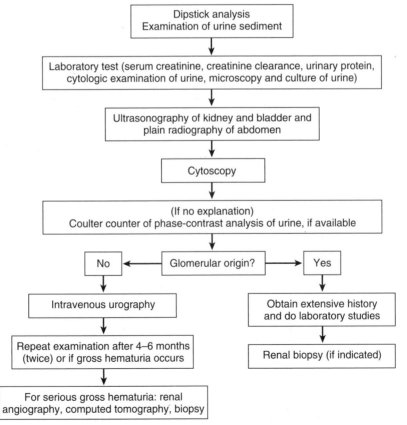

Figure 180–1 Algorithm of diagnostic tests recommended for microscopic hematuria. (Redrawn from Shroder F. Microscopic hematuria. BMJ 1994;309:70–72.)

struation, and mild trauma. One approach is to initiate an evaluation if the urinalysis shows more than 100 red blood cells per high-power field on one occasion or more than 3 red blood cells per high-power field on two of three occasions. In the presence of urologic risk factors, all episodes of hematuria should be evaluated even if there are fewer than 3 red blood cells per high-power field.

2. *Ultrasonography versus intravenous urography?* Ultrasonography and intravenous urography have similar sensitivity and specificity for lesions greater than 3 cm. For lesions less than 3 cm, ultrasonography combined with a single plain abdominal film may be more cost-effective and safer with minimal decrease in accuracy. Intravenous urography must be performed in patients with urine cytology suggestive of urothelial malignancy or a history of bladder neoplasia. Some radiologists recommend performing computed tomography in conjunction with intravenous urography to improve sensitivity to stones or other lesions.

3. *Glomerular versus nonglomerular origin?* The morphology of urinary sediment assessed by phase-contrast microscopy may assist with localization of the bleeding site. Dysmorphic red blood cells that appear deformed by passage through the renal tubules suggest a renal origin, whereas normal-appearing red blood cells suggest a nonglomerular site. Because this test is highly dependent on the training and diligence of the laboratory technician, reliability of this technique has been challenged. The red cell volume distribution curve has been suggested as an alternative method for distinguishing bleeding that is from a glomerular origin. This technique uses automated blood cell analyzers to measure the mean corpuscular volume of urinary red blood cells. A distribution curve of red blood cells with low mean corpuscular volume suggests a glomerular etiology and is reported to be 97% sensitive and 80% specific.

4. *Role of renal biopsy.* A biopsy is often recommended when a glomerular origin of the bleeding is suspected. Some authorities argue that biopsies should be performed more often in younger patients because renal abnormalities are more prevalent (e.g., IgA nephropathy, global or segmental mesangial proliferative glomerulonephritis, interstitial nephritis, membranous nephropathy, thin membrane nephropathy, vascular changes secondary to hypertension). On the other hand, no therapy exists for most of these disorders. Thus, this decision must be individualized.

5. *Anticoagulation.* Anticoagulation usually provokes hematuria from preexisting lesions rather than causing it de novo. Therefore, the same rules for evaluation of other patients apply to patients taking anticoagulants.

Management. Antibiotic treatment should be prescribed for UTI. Patients with renal calculi need analgesics, should strain their urine, and should drink plenty of fluids. Stones less than 5 mm usually require no treatment. For larger stones, urologic evaluation is recommended. Possible inciting factors for conditions such as interstitial nephritis should be eliminated. Vasculitis may respond to anti-inflammatory or immunosuppressive therapy. Referral to a specialist is indicated when a patient has been diagnosed with vasculitis, glomerulonephritis, severe trauma, urologic malignancies, acute deterioration of renal function, or significant proteinuria.

Follow-Up. If evaluation of the hematuria is negative, the patient should be retested for hematuria at 6 months and then again at 1 year. Occult cancers will usually become clinically apparent within 1 year.

Cross-References: Cancer of the Genitourinary Tract (Chapter 168), Dysuria (Chapter 170), Scrotal Pain (Chapter 171), Prostate Cancer (Chapter 173), Nephrolithiasis (Chapter 174), Urinary Tract Infections in Women (Chapter 175), Urinary Tract Infections in Men (Chapter 177), Bacteriuria in the Elderly (Chapter 178), Proteinuria (Chapter 181), Benign Prostatic Hyperplasia (Chapter 184), Bleeding (Chapter 195), Thrombocytopenia (Chapter 197), Chronic Anticoagulation (Chapter 201).

REFERENCES

1. Corwin H, Silverstein M. The diagnosis of neoplasia in patients with asymptomatic microscopic hematuria: A decision analysis. J Urol 1988;139:1002–1006.

   This study determined that intravenous urography did not add significantly to the diagnostic accuracy, but was more costly and resulted in greater morbidity.

2. Greenberg A. Primer on Kidney Diseases. San Diego, Academic Press, 1994.

   There is a concise chapter on hematuria in this textbook.

3. Mariani A, et al. The significance of adult hematuria; 1000 hematuria evaluations including risk benefit and cost effectiveness analysis. J Urol 1989;141:350–355.

   The authors recommend evaluating patients with more than 3 red blood cells per high-power field on two of three properly collected urinalyses, more than 100 red blood cells per high-power field on one urinalysis, or one episode of gross hematuria.

4. Schroder F. Microscopic hematuria. BMJ 1994;309:70–72.

   An algorithm is presented for the evaluation of microscopic hematuria.

5. Sutton J. Evaluation of hematuria in adults. JAMA 1990;263:2475–2480.

   In this review the author recommends the incorporation of risk factors for evaluation of hematuria.

181 Proteinuria

Problem

MINDY A. COOPER

Epidemiology and Etiology. Proteinuria is arbitrarily defined as urine excretion of more than 150 mg of protein in 24 hours. The etiology of proteinuria is diverse and may reflect renal manifestations of systemic disease (e.g., diabetes, lupus erythematosus, or human immunodeficiency virus infection) or primary renal diseases (e.g., glomerulonephritis, minimal change disease, or IgA nephropathy). Proteinuria can also occur in the absence of recognized disease processes, for example, as a transient response to physical stress such as exercise.

Table 181–1. CAUSES OF FUNCTIONAL PROTEINURIA

Fever	Exposure to cold
Emotional stress	Orthostatic proteinuria
Acute medical illness	Congestive heart failure
Exercise	Hypertension

Symptoms and Signs. Proteinuria is usually first detected on routine urinalysis and is often an unsuspected finding. Patients may be completely asymptomatic or may present with a spectrum of signs and symptoms depending on the magnitude of proteinuria as well as on the level of renal function. Classic presentation of the nephrotic syndrome includes edema, hypertension, hypoalbuminemia, and hypercholesterolemia. Patients with glomerulonephritis may be asymptomatic or present with hematuria, new-onset edema, hypertension, renal insufficiency, or pulmonary involvement.

Clinical Approach. Proteinuria may be classified based on whether the proteinuria is transient (functional) or persistent (fixed). *Functional proteinuria* is the term used for transient increases in protein excretion that occur in the absence of renal disease (Table 181–1). The patient is usually asymptomatic, and the urine sediment is otherwise unremarkable. Functional proteinuria is common in adolescents and young adults and may be caused by exercise, superimposed medical illness, or a benign condition called orthostatic proteinuria. The prognosis is good, and patients rarely develop renal insufficiency.

Fixed proteinuria is a term that encompasses several different causes of proteinuria (Table 181–2). Coexistent abnormalities in the urinalysis (red blood cells, white blood cells, casts) are common. Renal manifestations of systemic diseases, as well as primary renal disorders, make up this category of proteinuria. Prognosis is based on the underlying disease process.

Table 181–2. CAUSES OF FIXED PROTEINURIA

Primary renal disease
  Focal glomerular sclerosis
  Minimal change disease
  Membranous glomerulonephritis
  IgA nephropathy
  Hereditary nephritis
Secondary renal disease
  Glomerular
    Diabetes mellitus
    Amyloidosis
    Systemic lupus erythematosus
    Human immunodeficiency virus–associated nephropathy
    Heroin nephropathy
    Postinfectious glomerulonephritis
  Tubulointerstitial disease
    Chronic pyelonephritis
    Chronic intestitial nephritis (chronic obstruction, sickle cell disease)
    Allergic interstitial nephritis (nonsteroidal anti-inflammatory drugs, penicillin)
Miscellaneous
  Bence Jones proteinuria
  Monoclonal gammopathies

It is important to measure how much protein is being excreted. Proteinuria is most commonly detected by urine dipstick, which measures protein concentration (30–500 mg/dL) on a semiquantitative scale of 0 to 4. Because the urine protein concentration is affected by urine volume, measurement by dipstick does not predict daily protein excretion. Moreover, the dipstick measures only negatively charged proteins such as albumin, missing positively charged proteins such as light chain immunoglobulins, which are excreted in multiple myeloma.

The most accurate means of quantitating the degree of proteinuria is a 24-hour urine collection; however, this is a cumbersome procedure even for the most motivated patient. The simplest way to make sure a patient has provided a complete 24-hour collection is to check the creatinine excretion. Daily creatinine production (and excretion) is constant, based on muscle mass. Men and women should excrete approximately 20 mg/kg and 15 mg/kg creatinine per day, respectively. These values decrease to approximately 10 mg/kg in the elderly.

A convenient alternative to the 24-hour urine collection is to compare the concentrations (in milligrams per deciliter) of protein and creatinine on a random spot urine specimen. Because urinary excretion of creatinine is relatively constant, the urine protein/creatinine ratio can help detect and quantify proteinuria. A protein/creatinine ratio of less than 0.2 reflects daily protein excretion of less than 200 mg, whereas a ratio of 1 reflects approximately 1 g of protein excretion per day, and a ratio of greater than 3.5 suggests excretion of greater than 3.5 g of protein per day.

Nephrotic range proteinuria is defined as excretion of protein greater than 3.5 g/d. Patients with functional proteinuria usually excrete less than 1 g/d of protein.

Determining what kind of protein is being excreted is also often helpful. The normal glomerulus filters 500 to 1500 mg of low molecular weight proteins each day, which are subsequently reabsorbed and metabolized by the renal tubular cells. Total daily excretion of protein should not exceed 150 mg. When excess protein is detected in the urine, serum and urine protein electrophoreses can identify the type of protein and help to determine the underlying disease process (Table 181–3). Glomerular disorders, the most common cause of abnormal proteinuria, result in increased excretion of albumin. In tubulointerstitial diseases (e.g., chronic pyelonephritis), there is a diverse array of low molecular weight proteins in the urine. In monoclonal gammopathies and multiple myeloma, excess quantities (sometimes up to 10 g/d) of low molecular weight plasma proteins can be excreted in the urine.

The history should focus on identifying an underlying systemic disease

Table 181–3. TYPE OF PROTEIN EXCRETION BASED ON URINE PROTEIN ELECTROPHORESIS

Disease Process	Predominant Protein Excreted
Glomerular	Albumin
Tubulointerstitial	Multiple low molecular weight proteins
"Overflow" proteinuria	Monoclonal globulin

that can be associated with renal involvement and should include information on medications and family, sexual, and drug histories. A history of recent infection, weight change, fever, hemoptysis, skin changes, or hematuria should also be elicited. Physical findings such as hypertension, rash, edema, or arthritis also may suggest a specific cause of proteinuria.

A urinalysis including the microscopic examination of the sediment should be repeated before an extensive workup for proteinuria. Patients should be advised to abstain from intense physical exertion for 24 hours before the examination to rule out exercise-induced proteinuria. If the patient is young and otherwise asymptomatic, a simple workup for orthostatic proteinuria can be undertaken. A spot urine protein/creatinine ratio obtained from a first-voided specimen should be compared with that obtained from a midday specimen. The former should have a ratio of less than 0.2 and the latter a ratio of less than 1. Orthostatic proteinuria is a benign condition and usually disappears after 10 years. No further workup is required.

All patients with fixed proteinuria should have a serum creatinine determination to assess renal function. Patients at greatest risk for serious renal disease are those with renal insufficiency, nephrotic range proteinuria, or red blood cell casts. These patients should generally be referred to a nephrologist for further evaluation. If the patient has no evidence of renal insufficiency or secondary causes of renal disease (see Table 181–2), renal ultrasonography may be helpful in excluding other causes of proteinuria, such as chronic obstruction. Often the cause of non-nephrotic range proteinuria remains elusive.

Management. Management of the patient with proteinuria depends on the underlying cause and coexistent conditions. Although diabetic patients with proteinuria benefit from angiotensin-converting enzyme inhibitors, this has not yet been demonstrated in other types of renal disease. There is much controversy about dietary protein restriction in patients with nephrotic syndrome, and this is not universally recommended at this time. Patients should be monitored and treated for hypertension. Renal function should be assessed yearly.

Cross-References: Osteoporosis (Chapter 116), Hyperlipidemia (Chapter 152), Diabetes Mellitus (Chapter 154), Chronic Renal Failure (Chapter 179), Pregnancy and Hypertension (Chapter 214).

REFERENCES

1. Abuelo JG. Proteinuria: Diagnostic principles and procedures. Ann Intern Med 1983;98:186–191.
   A discussion of a general evaluation of proteinuria is presented.

2. Bernhard D, Salant D. Clinical approach to the patient with proteinuria and the nephrotic syndrome. In Jacobson H, Striker G, Klahr S, eds. The Principles and Practice of Nephrology, Philadelphia, BC Decker, 1991:250–261.
   This chapter is a general review describing proteinuria and the nephrotic syndrome.

3. Schwab SJ, Christensen RL, Dougherty K, Klahr S. Quantitation of proteinuria by the use of protein-to-creatinine ratios in single urine samples. Arch Intern Med 1987;147:943–944.
   The protein/creatinine ratio is described as a means of quantitating 24-hour urine protein levels.

182 Electrolyte Abnormalities

Problem

BESSIE A. YOUNG

DISORDERS OF POTASSIUM

Physiology

Potassium is the major intracellular electrolyte (intracellular concentration of 120–140 mEq/L), with 2% of potassium found extracellularly. Normal extracellular concentrations are between 3.5 and 5.0 mEq/L. Ninety percent of dietary potassium is excreted by the distal tubule of the kidney (principal cell), with the rest excreted in stool, which can increase up to 35% if renal insufficiency is present.

Hypokalemia

Epidemiology. Defined as a serum potassium level less than 3.5 mEq/L, hypokalemia is the most common ambulatory electrolyte abnormality. Usually asymptomatic, hypokalemia is not clinically apparent until the potassium level is less than 2.5 mEq/L.

Etiology. The diagnosis can be divided into three main categories: (1) transcellular shifts from plasma into cells; (2) low potassium diet; and (3) potassium loss from the gastrointestinal tract, skin, or kidneys (Table 182–1).

Transcellular potassium shifts represent minimal alterations in total body potassium concentration. Metabolic alkalosis and, less commonly, respiratory alkalosis cause hypokalemia through a transcellular exchange of hydrogen for potassium (0.1–0.4 mEq/L of potassium for every 0.1-unit change in serum pH). Insulin, large dextrose loads, and β-adrenergic stimulation (e.g., β-adrenergic drugs, physiologic stress, acute myocardial infarction, or delirium tremens) can induce intracellular transfer of potassium.

Decreased potassium intake rarely causes hypokalemia except when prolonged (e.g., "tea and toast" diet, alcoholism, and anorexia with vomiting), because most foods contain some potassium. Clay ingestion (geophagia) induces hypokalemia by chelating potassium and preventing intestinal absorption.

Potassium loss can occur through the skin, gastrointestinal tract, or kidney. Extrarenal loss through the gastrointestinal tract occurs with vomiting and diarrhea. Gastric losses must be enormous to cause significant potassium losses (gastric fluid contains 5–10 mEq/L of potassium), with hypokalemia more common through lower intestinal secretion (up to 75 mEq/L). Extrarenal losses may also occur through the skin from excessive sweating and extensive burns. Renal loss occurs with diuretic use and vomiting but can also be

Table 182–1. ETIOLOGY OF HYPOKALEMIA

Transcellular potassium alterations
  Metabolic alkalosis
  Respiratory alkalosis
  Insulin
  β-Adrenergic stimulation: drugs, acute myocardial infarction,
    delirium tremens
  Barium salts
  Hypokalemic periodic paralysis
  Treatment for vitamin B_{12} deficiency
Decreased potassium intake
  Alcoholism
  Anorexia with vomiting
  "Tea and toast" diet
  Geophagia
Potassium loss
  Gastrointestinal tract: vomiting, diarrhea
  Renal: diuretic use, renal tubular acidosis, hypomagnesemia, primary
    hyperaldosteronism, Bartter's syndrome
  Skin: excessive sweating, extensive burns

associated with renal tubular acidosis, primary hyperaldosteronism (in patients with hypokalemia and hypertension), hypomagnesemia (cisplatin therapy, hyperaldosteronism), aminoglycoside therapy, Bartter's syndrome, or nonreabsorbable anions such as carbenicillin and bicarbonate.

Symptoms and Signs. Most patients are usually asymptomatic, but clinical abnormalities (e.g., muscle weakness, cramps, and paresthesias) occur when the potassium concentration drops rapidly or is less than 2.5 mEq/L. Low potassium concentrations hyperpolarize cell membranes, leading to an increased susceptibility to reentrant arrhythmias (particularly with digoxin therapy) and even to sudden death. Rhabdomyolysis occurs with tissue hypoperfusion. Hypokalemia can lead to polyuria and polydipsia, producing a type of nephrogenic diabetes insipidus. Electrocardiographic findings initially include ST segment depression, decreased amplitude of T waves, increased amplitude of the U wave (which sometimes is mistaken for the T wave in more severe hypokalemia), and prolongation of the TU interval.

Clinical Approach. An accurate history should address the patient's symptoms and medication list. A standard laboratory evaluation should include determination of levels of blood urea nitrogen, creatinine, electrolytes, and magnesium; arterial blood gas analysis (to determine serum pH for acid–base status); and determination of urine levels of electrolytes (sodium, chloride, potassium). If the urine potassium excretion is greater than 30 mEq/24 h, a urinary cause of potassium excretion is more likely. Lower levels indicate either other causes of potassium loss or diuretic therapy that has been discontinued. Metabolic alkalosis may be secondary to diuretic therapy, vomiting, or diarrhea associated with volume depletion. Hypokalemia may exacerbate hypertension in some patients, but primary hyperaldosteronism (check renin-to-aldosterone ratio) or other forms of hyperadrenalism (cortisol level) must be ruled out.

Management. Mild hypokalemia (3.0–3.5 mEq/L) may be managed by increasing potassium in the diet or by ingesting small amounts of oral potassium chloride (10–20 mEq/d). If a patient is symptomatic, therapy should be aimed at rapid correction of potassium loss to avoid cardiac arrhythmias (especially, if the patient is taking digoxin) and to correct neuromuscular effects. Each 1-mEq/L decrease in serum potassium concentration corresponds to a 200- to 400-mEq decrease in potassium stores until the serum potassium level is less than 2.0 mEq/L, which is equal to a potassium deficit greater than 1000 mEq/L. Repletion of potassium may be done orally or parenterally, depending on the patient's clinical status. Oral repletion in asymptomatic patients can be done using 40 to 60 mEq/d of potassium chloride in divided doses, with frequent monitoring of levels (every 2 to 3 days until the patient's condition is stable). However, if a diuretic is the cause, substitution or addition of a potassium-sparing diuretic may be adequate to reverse the hypokalemia.

If rapid correction of the potassium concentration is needed, parenteral potassium chloride at a concentration not greater than 40 mEq/L may be used peripherally at 10 mEq/h, or through a central line (subclavian or femoral) 20 to 40 mEq/h. In patients requiring correction of potassium loss through a central line, electrocardiographic monitoring in an intensive care unit should be considered. Glucose-containing solutions can cause further hypokalemia and should be avoided. In refractory cases, the patient should be referred to a nephrologist for renal abnormalities or to an endocrinologist if an endocrinopathy is suspected.

Hyperkalemia

Epidemiology. Hyperkalemia is defined as a potassium level greater than 5.5 mEq/L, but most patients remain asymptomatic until the potassium concentration is greater than 6.5 mEq/L. Hyperkalemia is less common in the ambulatory setting but occurs in renal insufficiency or with alterations of the renin-angiotensin-aldosterone axis.

Etiology (Table 182–2). Pseudohyperkalemia is caused by the release of potassium from clotted blood and occurs with increased frequency in traumatic blood drawing, blood clotting in the presence of thrombocytosis or leukocytosis, and red cell hemolysis. This represents no threat to the patient and can be eliminated as the cause by redrawing the blood sample in a heparinized tube to prevent clotting.

Redistribution of potassium occurs with acid–base abnormalities, as described earlier. Acidemia forces an intracellular exchange of potassium for hydrogen. Hyperkalemia occurs with insulin deficiency and hyperosmolality secondary to hyperglycemia. Cell breakdown secondary to rhabdomyolysis, trauma, or chemotherapy (tumor lysis syndrome) can increase serum potassium levels significantly. Nonspecific β-blockers such as propranolol or drugs such as succinylcholine or arginine can cause hyperkalemia by interference with the Na^+/K^+ pump. Massive ingestion of digoxin can cause fatal hyperkalemia, also by inhibiting Na^+/K^+ ATPase. Hyperkalemic periodic paralysis is a rare cause of hyperkalemia.

Increased potassium intake either orally or parenterally may cause hyperkalemia, but only in the setting of decreased or altered renal function. Hidden sources of potassium include penicillin potassium salts, salt substitutes that contain potassium chloride, stored blood, or potassium supplements in a per-

Table 182-2. ETIOLOGY OF HYPERKALEMIA

Pseudohyperkalemia
  Thrombocytosis
  Leukocytosis
  Clotted blood
Transcellular potassium alterations
  Metabolic acidosis
  Insulin deficiency
  Hyperosmolarity: hyperglycemia, mannitol, urea
  Cellular breakdown: rhabdomyolysis, trauma, chemotherapy
  Na^+/K^+ ATPase interference: digitalis, propranolol, arginine, succinylcholine
  Increased potassium intake
Impairment of the renin-angiotensin-aldosterone system
  Diabetes mellitus
  Type IV renal tubular acidosis
  Type I renal tubular acidosis: sickle cell disease, obstructive uropathy
  Drugs: nonsteroidal anti-inflammatory drugs, angiotensin-converting enzyme
    inhibitors, cyclosporine
  Adrenal insufficiency

son with renal insufficiency or on potassium-sparing medication (angiotensin-converting enzyme inhibitor, potassium-sparing diuretic, nonsteroidal anti-inflammatory agents).

Impairment in the renin-angiotensin-aldosterone system occurs commonly with nonsteroidal anti-inflammatory drugs, angiotensin-converting enzyme inhibitors, cyclosporine, and pentamidine. Asymptomatic hyperkalemia with mild renal insufficiency commonly occurs in hyporeninemic hypoaldosteronism, which occurs with type IV renal tubular acidosis (found in diabetes mellitus), renal interstitial disease, aging, the acquired immunodeficiency syndrome, and occasionally distal type I renal tubular acidosis (sickle cell disease or obstructive uropathy). Less commonly, primary adrenal insufficiency (Addison's disease) may cause hyperkalemia.

Symptoms and Signs. Most patients are asymptomatic, but clinical manifestations are similar to those seen with severe hypokalemia and include muscle weakness, paresthesias, areflexia, and ascending paralysis. Electrocardiographic findings depend on the concentration of potassium and usually begin with peaked T waves and shortened QT interval (5.5–6.0 mEq/L), prolonged PR interval, and QRS widening (6.0–7.5 mEq/L), progressing to flattening of the P waves and further widening of the QRS complex until a biphasic sine wave appears (8.0 mEq/L), which can quickly deteriorate to ventricular fibrillation or asystole.

Clinical Approach. The history should include medications and diet. Orthostatic blood pressures help diagnose volume depletion. Pseudohyperkalemia is excluded by a repeat blood test with a heparinized sample. Renal insufficiency is identified with serum blood urea nitrogen and creatinine assessment. Other laboratory tests should include evaluation of electrolyte levels, a complete blood cell count, liver function tests, and determination of glucose level, arterial blood gases, urine pH, urinary sodium concentration, and, when clinical circumstances dictate, a serum aldosterone level. If the aldosterone level is low, a cortisol level should be drawn to rule out adrenal insufficiency.

Management. Asymptomatic hyperkalemia (5.5–6.0 mEq/L) may respond to removal of exogenous potassium from the diet (oral potassium chloride replacement, certain fruits and vegetables) or discontinuation of potassium-sparing diuretics, angiotensin-converting enzyme inhibitors, or nonsteroidal anti-inflammatory drugs. Outpatients may initially respond to a thiazide or loop diuretic, but volume status must be monitored. Acute therapy should be instituted for clinical manifestations of hyperkalemia (electrocardiographic changes) or if the potassium level is greater than 6.5 mEq/L.

Cation exchange resins may be given orally or per rectum for complete potassium removal. Effects start in 30 to 60 minutes and last for several hours, with diarrhea the most common side effect. Sodium polystyrene sulfonate (Kayexalate), 15 to 30 g in 50 to 100 mL of 20% sorbitol orally (or 50 g of sodium polystyrene powder in 200 mL of 20% dextrose solution given as an enema), should be repeated every 4 hours up to three to four doses per day in the ambulatory setting, with daily monitoring of serum potassium levels until the patient's condition is stable.

Other emergent therapy for hyperkalemia (potassium > 6.5 mEq/L) consists of parenteral calcium (which temporarily antagonizes the cardiac and neuromuscular manifestations of hyperkalemia); glucose with insulin, if needed; or bicarbonate, which should be reserved for the inpatient setting with cardiac monitoring. Referral to a nephrologist for hemodialysis is indicated for severe hyperkalemia associated with renal failure when these measures are not adequate.

DISORDERS OF CALCIUM

Physiology

Calcium homeostasis depends on the interactions of three systems—gastrointestinal, renal, and skeletal—and is regulated by parathyroid hormone (PTH) and vitamin D_3. After hydroxylation of vitamin D_3 in the liver, 25-hydroxyvitamin D_3 is then hydroxylated to 1,25-dihydroxyvitamin D_3 (calcitriol or $1,25(OH)_2D_3$) in the kidney under the regulation of PTH. Calcitriol increases absorption of calcium from the intestines for deposition in bone. PTH increases calcium reabsorption in the proximal tubule and increases reabsorption of calcium from bone. Hypocalcemia and hyperphosphatemia increase PTH secretion, whereas vitamin D_3 responds directly to phosphate levels and PTH.

In hypoalbuminemia, the total serum calcium level must be corrected; for every 1 g/dL the serum albumin level is below normal (4 g/dL), 0.8 mg/dL must be added to the total serum calcium. Normal ranges of serum calcium are 8.5 to 10.5 mg/dL, or for ionized calcium, 2.3 to 2.8 mEq/L (4.5–5.6 mg/dL or 1.1–1.4 mmol/L).

Hypocalcemia

Epidemiology. Hypocalcemia is rarely encountered in the ambulatory setting, with the most common cause being hypoalbuminemia. It is defined as a serum calcium value less than 8.0 mg/dL or an ionized calcium level less than 4.0 mg/dL.

Etiology (Table 182–3). Disorders of parathyroid hormone production cause true hypocalcemia either primarily or secondarily. Primary idiopathic hypoparathyroidism is rare and is usually associated with other autoimmune endocrinopathies such as Hashimoto's thyroiditis, adrenal insufficiency, or pernicious anemia. Post-thyroidectomy hypoparathyroidism occurs when the parathyroid glands are mistakenly removed during surgery. Symptoms, however, may not be apparent until months afterward.

Secondary hypoparathyroidism may also occur with infiltrating systemic diseases, such as amyloidosis, hemochromatosis, and malignancy.

Hypomagnesemia can cause bone and end-organ resistance to PTH, whereas hypermagnesemia (magnesium > 5.5 mg/dL) can suppress PTH secretion, directly leading to hypocalcemia. Drugs that cause renal magnesium wasting (e.g., gentamicin, cisplatin) may also precipitate hypocalcemia.

Vitamin D deficiency can be caused by decreased intake secondary to nutritional deficiency, gastrointestinal malabsorption (partial gastrectomy, short bowel syndrome, or other malabsorptive syndromes), decreased 25-hydroxylation secondary to liver disease (primary biliary cirrhosis, alcoholism), or increased vitamin D metabolism secondary to drugs (phenobarbital, phenytoin). Decreased levels of vitamin D may also occur with renal failure, hyperphosphatemia, or hereditary vitamin D–dependent rickets.

Miscellaneous causes include acute pancreatitis, malignancy (medullary carcinoma of the thyroid), and hyperphosphatemia.

Symptoms and Signs. Symptoms depend on the degree of hypocalcemia present but consist of neuromuscular hyperexcitability including muscle spasm, tetany, and nerve paresthesias (fingers, toes, circumoral). A positive Chvostek's sign may be elicited by tapping the facial nerve anterior to the ear and observing muscle spasms around the mouth. Trousseau's sign consists of development of hand spasms after the inflation of a blood pressure cuff at a pressure above the systolic pressure for 3 minutes. Psychological symptoms may also occur, such as mood swings, depression, delirium, or psychosis. Confusion and lethargy can be seen with severe hypocalcemia, as can carpopedal spasm (leading to tetany), laryngospasm, seizures, and, rarely, papilledema. Cardiac manifestations include hypotension, bradycardia, arrhythmias, and reversible congestive heart failure. Electrocardiographic findings include a prolonged QT interval. Chronic features of hypocalcemia include dry skin, brittle fingernails, patchy hair loss, and cataracts. Basal ganglia calcification and candidiasis may be seen with hypoparathyroidism.

Clinical Approach. The history should be focused on recent head or neck surgery, a history of neck irradiation as a child, or a history of other endocri-

Table 182–3. ETIOLOGY OF HYPOCALCEMIA

Hypoparathyroidism	Electrolyte abnormalities
Idiopathic	Hypomagnesemia
Secondary: amyloidosis, hemochromatosis,	Hypermagnesemia
malignancy	Hyperphosphatemia
Postparathyroidectomy	Vitamin D deficiency
Pseudohypoparathyroidism	Acute pancreatitis

nopathies (Hashimoto's thyroiditis, adrenal failure). Laboratory evaluation is necessary to determine the diagnosis and should include an ionized calcium determination (if unavailable a total serum calcium and albumin level), a complete blood cell count, and determination of electrolyte, creatinine, magnesium, phosphate, PTH, and vitamin D levels.

Management. Asymptomatic hypocalcemia may be treated with increasing dietary sources of calcium, including milk that is fortified with vitamin D and other dairy products (skim milk contains 1 g/L of calcium). Other oral therapy includes calcium carbonate (Tums), 0.5 to 1.0 g twice daily. The underlying cause should be diagnosed and treated. If hypomagnesemia is present, it must be treated initially to correct hypocalcemia. Hypoparathyroidism should be treated with calcium supplementation (calcium carbonate 0.5–1.0 g twice daily) and oral calcitriol at 0.25 to 0.50 μg/d orally. After parathyroidectomy, up to 1.5 μg/d of calcitriol may be necessary to correct hypocalcemia. Calcium and alkaline phosphatase need to be carefully monitored; once bone requirements are met and alkaline phosphatase level decreases, the amount of calcium and calcitriol may be tapered. Serum calcium level, urinary calcium excretion, and renal function must be monitored chronically. Symptomatic patients should be hospitalized and treated emergently with a 10% calcium gluconate solution (90 mg elemental calcium in 10 mL) or 10 to 20 mL intravenously over 10 minutes, followed by a calcium drip.

Hypercalcemia

Epidemiology. Hypercalcemia, defined as a total serum calcium greater than 11 mg/dL, is asymptomatic in most patients until the total serum calcium level is greater than 12.5 to 13 mg/dL. The most common cause of hypercalcemia in ambulatory patients is thiazide diuretic use. Hyperparathyroidism has an incidence of 1 to 2 per 1000 patients found to have hypercalcemia on screening.

Etiology. Hypercalcemia is caused by endocrinopathies, malignancies, granulomatous disease, and renal failure (Table 182–4).

Primary hyperparathyroidism usually occurs in premenopausal women older than 40 years of age and in the elderly (both male and female). It is usually associated with nephrolithiasis, joint disease, and peptic ulcer disease. A primary parathyroid adenoma is the most common cause. Other, less common endocrinopathies that cause hypercalcemia include hyperthyroidism and hypoadrenalism (Addison's disease).

Malignancy produces hypercalcemia by humoral or osteolytic mechanisms.

Table 182–4. ETIOLOGY OF HYPERCALCEMIA

Endocrinopathies	Granulomatous diseases	Acute renal failure
Primary hyperparathryoidism	Tuberculosis	Miscellaneous
Hyperthryoidism	Sarcoidosis	Milk-alkali syndrome
Hypoadrenalism (Addison's disease)	Histoplasmosis	Lithium therapy
Malignancy	Coccidioidomycosis	Vitamin A or D toxicity
Solid tumors	Berylliosis	
Multiple myeloma		
Paget's disease		

Carcinoma of the lung and breast (60% of patients with tumor-associated hypercalcemia), squamous cell carcinomas of the head and neck (10%), or renal cell carcinoma (10% to 15%) usually causes hypercalcemia by producing parathyroid hormone–related peptide, which has amino acid similarities to PTH. Osteolytic hypercalcemia is seen in patients with multiple myeloma almost 100% of the time.

Granulomatous diseases associated with hypercalcemia include tuberculosis, sarcoidosis, histoplasmosis, coccidioidomycosis, and berylliosis. The mechanism is thought to involve hypersensitivity to vitamin D and, at least in sarcoidosis, is glucocorticoid responsive.

Acute renal failure may cause hypercalcemia through decreased excretion of calcium, especially in patients with underlying malignancies such as multiple myeloma. Chronic renal failure is initially associated with hypocalcemia owing to the decreased production of vitamin D, which increases PTH production. Excess PTH production eventually normalizes serum calcium levels or causes hypercalcemia. Secondary hyperparathyroidism develops in patients with chronic dialysis when the parathyroid gland no longer responds to hypercalcemia.

Miscellaneous causes include milk-alkali syndrome, lithium therapy, Paget's disease, and vitamin A or D toxicity.

Symptoms and Signs. Symptoms of hypercalcemia, usually apparent once the serum calcium level is greater than 12 mg/dL, include general malaise, weakness, anorexia, weight loss, and fatigue. Constipation, nausea, vomiting, and pruritus occur occasionally. Elderly patients with milder hypercalcemia may present with confusion. Renal insufficiency, volume depletion, or azotemia may develop. Cardiovascular manifestations include bradycardia, shortened QT interval, arrhythmias, and digitalis toxicity. Chronic symptoms include nephrolithiasis, polyuria, soft tissue calcification, bone cysts, peptic ulcer disease, pancreatitis, and muscle atrophy.

Clinical Approach. The history and physical examination may elicit nonspecific symptoms such as anorexia, fatigue, or weight loss (malignancy, tuberculosis), or more specific symptoms, such as nephrolithiasis, joint disorders, or peptic ulcer disease, which suggest hyperparathyroidism. Laboratory tests should include determination of levels of ionized calcium, albumin, total serum calcium, magnesium, phosphate, electrolytes, blood urea nitrogen, and creatinine; a complete blood cell count; a PTH level with a concurrent calcium level (intact PTH if there is renal failure); and a PTH-related peptide level if there are symptoms suggesting malignancy.

Management. Hypercalcemia related to diuretic use is reversible by stopping the offending drug. Decreasing calcium consumption is useful if the hypercalcemia is associated with oral calcium excess (milk-alkali syndrome) or chronic renal failure but is not useful in malignancies, because most malignancies are associated with low levels of vitamin D.

Intravenous fluid with a saline diuresis may be necessary if the patient is severely symptomatic and has volume depletion. Addition of a loop diuretic (furosemide, bumetanide) increases renal calcium excretion. Calcitonin rapidly lowers calcium by 2 to 3 mg/dL but by 2 to 3 days is associated with a non–glucocorticoid-responsive tachyphylaxis. Plicamycin and diphosphonates directly inhibit bone reabsorption. Etidronate, 7.5 mg/kg/d NS intravenously for 3 days, or pamidronate, 60–90 mg/L NS or D5W intravenously over 4 to 6 hours every 4 weeks, which may have fewer side effects, should be used for bone metastasis or Paget's disease.

Corticosteroids (prednisone, 20 to 50 mg orally twice daily) are effective in hypercalcemia secondary to multiple myeloma, sarcoidosis, vitamin D toxicity, lymphoma, and other malignancies.

Less commonly, intravenous phosphate or gallium nitrate can be used. Parathyroidectomy is the treatment of choice for hyperparathyroidism. Oral phosphates should be used with mild hypercalcemia but avoided in renal failure.

DISORDERS OF PHOSPHATE

Physiology

Phosphorus is essential for most cellular functions, with normal levels between 2.6 and 4.5 mg/dL. Homeostasis is balanced between phosphate intake, gastrointestinal excretion, tissue requirements, and renal excretion and absorption. Total phosphorus stores are 1% of body weight, with 85% found in the skeleton and only 1% found extracellularly. Phosphorus is present in most food, especially meats, dairy products, and vegetables. Regulation of phosphorus occurs primarily in the kidney, where 80% of phosphate reabsorption occurs in the proximal tubule.

Hypophosphatemia

Epidemiology. Less common in the ambulatory care setting, hypophosphatemia occurs primarily in hospitalized patients (30% of surgical patients) and is related to the infusion of glucose-containing solutions.

Etiology. Causes can be divided into redistribution, gastrointestinal losses, and renal losses (Table 182–5).

Table 182–5. ETIOLOGY OF HYPOPHOSPHATEMIA

Redistribution	Renal losses
Glucose solution infusion	Primary or secondary hyperparathyroidism
Respiratory alkalosis	Recovery from acute tubular necrosis
Metabolic alkalosis	Renal transplantation
Salicylate overdose	Fanconi's syndrome
Gram-negative sepsis	X-linked hypophosphatemia
Post parathyroidectomy	Malignancy
Intravenous quinine therapy in	Oncogenic osteomalacia
malaria	Tumors of bone
Gastrointestinal losses	Nutritional
Malabsorption	Total parenteral nutrition
Vomiting	Refeeding after malnutrition
Diarrhea	Vitamin D deficiency
Aluminum-, magnesium-, or	
calcium-containing antacids	

Redistribution occurs with intravenous glucose solution infusion, respiratory or metabolic alkalosis, or recovery from diabetic ketoacidosis (secondary to insulin therapy and glucose infusion). It is usually associated with less than 100 mg/d excretion of phosphorus in the urine. Transcellular shifting may also occur with salicylate overdose, gram-negative rod sepsis, severe burns, and the "hungry bone syndrome" after parathyroidectomy and in patients treated with intravenously administered quinine for malaria.

Gastrointestinal losses occur with malabsorption, vomiting, diarrhea, or aluminum-, magnesium-, or calcium-containing antacids. Urine excretion is less than 100 mg/d.

Renal losses are associated with greater than 100 mg/d urinary phosphate excretion, with the most common cause being primary or secondary hyperparathyroidism. Thiazide diuretics may also cause renal phosphate wasting, as can recovery from acute tubular necrosis, renal transplantation, Fanconi's syndrome (associated with glycosuria and aminoaciduria), and X-linked hypophosphatemia.

Miscellaneous causes of hypophosphatemia include alcoholism and withdrawal, dietary vitamin D deficiency, oncogenic osteomalacia, other tumors of bone, administration of total parenteral nutrition, and refeeding after malnutrition.

Symptoms and Signs. Clinical findings include muscle weakness, lethargy, coma, ataxia, peripheral nerve paresthesias, and interference with bone mineralization. Hypophosphatemia can produce rickets in growing children or osteomalacia in adults. Severe hypophosphatemia (< 1.0 mg/dL) is associated with acute respiratory muscle paralysis, congestive cardiomyopathy, and even rhabdomyolysis. Hemolysis and platelet abnormalities rarely occur.

Clinical Approach. The history and physical examination may lead one to consider many electrolyte abnormalities; thus, diagnosis requires laboratory studies and should include phosphate, calcium, magnesium, potassium, and bicarbonate. Other tests include a complete blood cell count and determination of PTH or vitamin D levels if clinically indicated. Urinary phosphate levels less than 100 mg/d (or a fractional excretion of phosphate [FEPO] $< 10\%$) suggest nonrenal losses of phosphate, whereas levels greater than 100 mg/d (or FEPO $> 20\%$) suggest renal losses.

Management. Moderate hypophosphatemia (1.0–2.5 mg/dL) is usually asymptomatic and can be treated by increasing dietary sources and avoiding phosphate binders (skim milk contains 1 g/L of both phosphorus and calcium). Elemental phosphate may also be used at a dose of 0.5 to 1.0 g orally, two or three times a day. Neutra-Phos (250 mg phosphate/tablet) or Neutra-Phos K (250 mg phosphorus, 14 mEq potassium) or Fleet Phospho-Soda are standard preparations that may be used. Intravenous phosphate should be used in cases of severe hypophosphatemia but should be avoided in treatment of diabetic ketoacidosis or in patients with renal failure unless absolutely necessary. Complications include metastatic calcification, hypotension, and renal failure.

Hyperphosphatemia

Epidemiology. Defined as a phosphate level greater than 5.0 mg/dL, hyperphosphatemia is a rare ambulatory problem, found almost exclusively in patients with mild to moderate renal insufficiency or renal failure.

Etiology (Table 182–6). Hyperphosphatemia develops with renal underexcretion of phosphate, such as that found in acute renal failure (myoglobinuric acute tubular necrosis, after surgery, trauma) or chronic renal insufficiency, but it can also occur in patients with normal renal function who are exposed to a high phosphate load.

Endogenous phosphate loading or transcellular shifting may occur with myoglobinuric acute renal failure or rhabdomyolysis, metabolic or respiratory acidosis, strenuous exercise, tumor lysis syndrome, acute hemolysis, or malignant hyperthermia. Hyperphosphatemia also occurs with diphosphonate therapy (etidronate, pamidronate) and is dose dependent.

Exogenous loading can occur with vitamin D toxicity (milk), phosphate-containing enemas, or infusion of phosphate-containing solutions.

Hypoparathyroidism can cause hyperphosphatemia, as can other *endocrinopathies*, such as hyperthyroidism, acromegaly, glucocorticoid withdrawal, or low-level estrogen replacement in postmenopausal women. Higher levels of estrogen replacement for osteoporosis can cause hypophosphatemia.

Pseudohyperphosphatemia is seen with hyperglobulinemic or hyperlipidemic states.

Symptoms and Signs. Mild hyperphosphatemia is associated with minimal signs and symptoms, but rapid increases can be associated with symptoms that may be induced by hypocalcemia or the rapid deposition of calcium phosphate salts seen in patients with metastatic calcification. Metastatic calcification usually occurs when the calcium phosphate product (total serum calcium level multiplied by the serum phosphate level) is greater than 70 and may lead to renal failure. Anorexia, nausea, and vomiting may occur, as well as cardiac arrhythmias, conduction disturbances, pulmonary congestion, and shock. Secondary hyperparathyroidism occurs in patients on long-term dialysis.

Clinical Approach. A history with medication list is important, but diagnosis depends on laboratory analysis and should include the following: determination of phosphate, magnesium, calcium, PTH, and electrolyte levels; a complete blood cell count; and arterial blood gas analysis.

Management. A low-phosphate diet (1000 mg/d) should be initiated in patients with chronic renal insufficiency and elevated phosphate levels. Oral phosphate binders such as calcium carbonate (0.5 to 1.0 g orally three times a day) or

Table 182–6. ETIOLOGY OF HYPERPHOSPHATEMIA

Transcellular shifting of phosphate (endogenous loading)	Endocrinopathies
Metabolic and respiratory acidosis	Hypoparathyroidism
Myoglobinuric acute renal failure	Hyperthyroidism
Rhabdomyolysis	Acromegaly
Strenuous exercise	Glucocorticoid withdrawal
Tumor lysis syndrome	Pseudohyperphosphatemia
Malignant hyperthermia	Hyperglobulinemia
Exogenous loading	Hyperlipidemia
Vitamin D toxicity	
Phosphate-containing enemas	
Infusion of phosphate-containing solutions	

calcium acetate (667 mg/tablet, 1 to 2 tablets orally three times a day) should be given with meals to bind phosphate at the time of ingestion to prevent gastrointestinal absorption. Aluminum hydroxide avidly binds phosphate but should be avoided in patients with renal disease because of aluminum bone toxicity. Saline diuresis may be used in patients with normal renal function.

Dialysis may be required in severe renal failure but may not be very effective because phosphate is poorly dialyzed. Referral to a nephrologist should be made early for a patient with renal insufficiency to prevent secondary complications (secondary hyperparathyroidism).

DISORDERS OF MAGNESIUM

Physiology

Magnesium is found mostly in bone (50%–60%) and skeletal muscle, with 1% of it being extracellular. Magnesium is not known to be regulated exclusively by any one hormone. Normal levels are between 1.5 and 1.9 mEq/L (1.7–2.2 mg/dL). Magnesium is readily absorbed in the gastrointestinal tract, with the amount absorbed inversely proportional to the amount ingested. It is also freely filtered in the kidney, with reabsorption occurring passively in the proximal tubule (20%–30%) and actively in the thick ascending limb of Henle (65%). Most regulation occurs within the kidney and is based on the amount of magnesium ingested.

Hypomagnesemia

Epidemiology. Defined as a magnesium level less than 1.5 mEq/L, hypomagnesemia is more frequent than hypermagnesemia, but both are chronically under-diagnosed and may be more prevalent in the ambulatory setting than is commonly recognized. In patients admitted to a large city hospital, at least 10% were found to be hypomagnesemic, including 65% in a medical intensive care unit. Hypomagnesemia is common in persons with poor nutrition, such as alcoholics, or in patients with malabsorption syndromes or with extensive bowel resection and may be seen along with hypokalemia in patients on diuretics. Hypomagnesemia may be noted in 25% to 39% of diabetics in the ambulatory setting and increases in patients with diabetic ketoacidosis.

Etiology. Hypomagnesemia is caused by gastrointestinal loss, renal loss, or endocrine and other systemic metabolic disorders (Table 182–7).

Gastrointestinal loss of magnesium occurs in patients with malabsorption syndromes (gluten enteropathy), extensive bowel resection, acute and chronic diarrhea, acute hemorrhagic pancreatitis, or intestinal biliary fistulas. Alcoholism or other states of severe protein-calorie malnutrition may lead to hypomagnesemia. Prolonged nasogastric suctioning is a common cause in hospitalized patients.

Renal loss occurs with drugs such as diuretics, chemotherapeutic agents (e.g., cisplatin), aminoglycosides, and possibly the cardiac glycosides, amphotericin B, and cyclosporine. Hyperosmolar states such as diabetes, high levels of urea, or mannitol infusion can induce an osmotic diuresis with renal magne-

Table 182–7. ETIOLOGY OF HYPOMAGNESEMIA

Gastrointestinal loss
  Malabsorptive syndromes: gluten enteropathy (celiac sprue), extensive bowel resection
  Acute and chronic diarrhea
  Hemorrhagic pancreatitis
  Alcoholism
  Severe protein-calorie malnutrition
Renal loss
  Drugs: diuretics, aminoglycosides, amphotericin B, cyclosporine, cisplatin
  Hyperosmolar states: diabetes mellitus, mannitol, urea
  Chronic pyelonephritis
  Glomerulonephritis
  Postobstructive diuresis
  Acute tubular necrosis in the diuretic phase
  Renal transplantation
Endocrinopathies
  Diabetic ketoacidosis
  Increased extracellular fluid volume: syndrome of inappropriate antidiuretic hormone
    secretion, hyperaldosteronism
  Parathyroidectomy
  Hyperthyroidism
Metabolic and electrolyte disorders
  Metabolic acidosis
  Hypophosphatemia
  Bartter's syndrome

sium wasting. Maganesium deficiency through renal mechanisms may be caused by primary renal diseases such as chronic untreated pyelonephritis, glomerulonephritis or interstitial nephritis, acute tubular necrosis during the diuretic phase, postobstructive diuresis, or renal transplantation.

Endocrine and metabolic disorders cause hypomagnesemia directly or indirectly through renal mechanisms. Metabolic acidosis, the syndrome of inappropriate antidiuretic hormone secretion, and primary aldosteronism cause renal magnesium wasting. Diabetic ketoacidosis and the osmotic diuresis that ensues can also cause magnesium depletion. Resection of the parathyroid gland for hyperparathyroidism or in hyperthyroidism can cause the "hungry bone syndrome," in which rapid bone remodeling after gland resection causes deposition of calcium as well as magnesium. Hypophosphatemia can cause magnesium deficiency, and hypomagnesemia is frequently encountered as part of Bartter's syndrome.

Symptoms and Signs. Magnesium deficiency is usually asymptomatic but can present as a complex clinical picture, because it is associated with and may cause hypokalemia and hypocalcemia. Magnesium depletion can cause neuromuscular hyperexcitability, leading to spontaneous carpopedal spasm, positive Chvostek's and Trousseau's signs, seizures, athetoid and choreiform movements, and other neurologic manifestations, such as lethargy, confusion, ataxia, tremors, and nystagmus. Cardiac manifestations include prolonged PR and QT intervals; U waves (also seen with hypokalemia); atrial tachycardia; premature atrial contractions and fibrillation; junctional arrhythmias; and ventricular arrhythmias, such as tachycardia, fibrillation, premature ventricular contractions, and torsades de pointes. It has also been associated with myocardial infarction.

Clinical Approach. In addition to magnesium levels, levels of calcium, potassium, and other electrolytes (sodium, chloride, bicarbonate) should be obtained to detect concurrent hypocalcemia, hypokalemia, and metabolic acidosis. A history of diarrhea also helps to distinguish gastrointestinal from renal losses of magnesium.

Management. Mild or chronic hypomagnesemia can usually be treated with oral therapy. Elemental magnesium (300–600 mg/d in divided doses) or magnesium oxide 400 mg (240 mg of elemental magnesium/400 mg tablet) once or twice daily may be used but can cause diarrhea. Symptomatic or severe hypomagnesemia can be treated with parenteral or intramuscular magnesium sulfate, given as a 50% solution (4 mEq/mL), 2 to 4 mL intravenously over 15 minutes initially, then continued as an intravenous drip for a total of 48 mEq over 24 hours. In severe hypomagnesemia, treatment should be continued for 3 to 7 days. Magnesium levels must be checked frequently to avoid hypermagnesemia, especially with renal insufficiency, when doses should be halved. Magnesium sulfate may also be given intramuscularly at a dose of 2 g/d, but this method may be painful.

Hypermagnesemia

Epidemiology. Hypermagnesemia in the ambulatory setting is rare but can occur in patients with renal insufficiency or renal failure who may inadvertently be using magnesium-containing laxatives or antacids. It is also probably underdiagnosed and in one study was found in 13% of patients admitted to a large city hospital.

Etiology (Table 182–8). The ability of the normal kidney to excrete magnesium is so effective that hypermagnesemia rarely develops except in those patients with decreased renal function. In those patients, hyperparathyroidism, volume contraction, low-sodium diet, and hypothyroidism can decrease magnesium excretion. In patients with renal insufficiency, ingestion of magnesium from antacids, sucralfate, or laxatives (milk of magnesia, magnesium citrate, Epsom salts) can lead to hypermagnesemia. Hypermagnesemia is found in patients with adrenocortical insufficiency or in dialysis patients if the water is not sufficiently treated.

Table 182–8. ETIOLOGY OF HYPERMAGNESEMIA

Normal renal function
    Iatrogenesis: therapy for preeclampsia or ventricular arrhythmias
    Adrenal cortical insufficiency (Addison's disease)
Renal insufficiency
    Ingestion of magnesium-containing antacids or laxatives
    Hyperparathyroidism
    Volume contraction
    Low-sodium diet
    Hypothyroidism
Renal failure
    High magnesium levels in dialysate water
    Magnesium ingestion

Clinical Findings. Symptoms usually do not become apparent until the serum magnesium level is greater than 4 mEq/L. Magnesium acts as a central and peripheral nervous system depressant and may depress deep tendon reflexes. At levels greater than 8 to 10 mEq/L, flaccid paralysis, cardiac arrhythmias, and respiratory muscle paralysis occur.

Clinical Approach. The history and physical examination, emphasizing a thorough medication history (including over-the-counter laxatives, antacids, or home remedies), and neurologic examination may lead one to think about the diagnosis of hypermagnesemia. The actual diagnosis depends on laboratory tests, including determination of levels of magnesium, electrolytes, blood urea nitrogen, creatinine, calcium, and phosphate.

Management. Magnesium-containing products should be discontinued. Patients with renal insufficiency and renal failure should be advised to avoid magnesium-containing products completely. Patients with normal renal function may be treated with calcium gluconate if symptomatic (to antagonize magnesium) or be given normal saline with calcium gluconate intravenously, to promote excretion through the kidneys. Dialysis may acutely decrease toxic levels in patients with renal failure.

Cross-References: Fatigue (Chapter 21), Chronic Ventricular Arrhythmias (Chapter 83), Essential Hypertension (Chapter 85), Diarrhea (Chapter 91), Constipation (Chapter 93), Abdominal Pain (Chapter 94), Paget's Disease (Chapter 115), Osteoporosis (Chapter 116), Muscular Weakness (Chapter 137), Seizures (Chapter 139), Common Thyroid Disorders (Chapter 153), Diabetes Mellitus (Chapter 154), Prostate Cancer (Chapter 173), Chronic Renal Failure (Chapter 179), Psychosis (Chapter 190), Altered Mentation in the Patient with Cancer (Chapter 206), Preoperative Evaluation (Chapter 217).

REFERENCES

1. Hodgson SF, Hurley DL: Acquired hypophosphatemia. Endocrinol Metab Clin North Am 1993;22:397–409.

   The authors review phosphorus metabolism and the treatment of hypophosphatemia.

2. Narins RG, ed. Maxwell and Kleeman's Clinical Disorders of Fluid and Electrolyte Metabolism, 5th ed. New York, McGraw-Hill Book Company, 1994.

   This text is an excellent in-depth reference for electrolyte and acid–base physiology and clinical abnormalities.

3. Nussbaum SR. Pathophysiology and management of severe hypercalcemia. Endocrinol Metab Clin North Am 1993;22:343–361.

   The pathophysiology, etiology, and therapy of hypercalcemia are reviewed.

4. Rose BD. Clinical Physiology of Acid-Base and Electrolyte Disorders, 4th ed. New York, McGraw-Hill Book Company, 1994.

   This book is another excellent reference of electrolyte physiology and abnormalities.

5. Rude RK. Magnesium metabolism and deficiency. Endocrinol Metab Clin North Am 1993;22:377–395.

   Magnesium metabolism and the causes of magnesium deficiency are reviewed; a discussion of the clinical usefulness of the magnesium tolerance test is included.

183 Scrotal Mass

Problem

STEVEN R. McGEE

Epidemiology. Varicoceles and testicular cancer occur most often between the ages 15 and 35 years, whereas hydroceles and spermatoceles usually affect men older than 30. Varicoceles are found in 9.5% of young healthy men, although most are small and asymptomatic.

Etiology. Hydroceles result from accumulation of fluid between the two layers of the tunica vaginalis, the remnant of peritoneum that descends into the scrotum with the testes during fetal development. Most hydroceles are idiopathic, although some are due to trauma, inguinal surgery, epididymitis, or a testicular tumor. Bilateral hydroceles are common in patients with anasarca (e.g., uncontrolled congestive heart failure, nephrotic syndrome). *Spermatoceles* are sperm-containing cysts on top of the testis that presumably occur because of blockage in the efferent ductules of the rete testis. *Varicoceles*, associated in many studies with abnormal sperm counts, are dilated veins in the pampiniform plexus of the spermatic cord. Seventy-eight percent to 93% of varicoceles appear in the left hemiscrotum; the remainder are bilateral. Right varicoceles are associated with total situs inversus. Most *testicular tumors* are malignant and originate from germ cells.

In surveys of men referred for ultrasonography because of nontender scrotal swellings (inguinal hernias excluded), hydroceles are found in 33% to 56% of cases, spermatoceles in 9% to 29%, cancer in 5% to 18%, varicoceles in 4% to 16%, and miscellaneous diagnoses (e.g., cysts, nontesticular tumors, chronic epididymitis) in 14% to 18%.

Clinical Approach. The approach to the acutely painful and inflamed scrotum is discussed in Chapter 171. In those patients with nontender scrotal swellings, the examination should include bimanual scrotal palpation with the patient standing and supine and transillumination (Table 183–1). The length of the normal adult testis is 3.5 to 5.0 cm.

Any intratesticular mass found on examination should be regarded as testicular cancer until proven otherwise. These patients should be promptly referred to a urologist; ultrasonography may provide additional information but should not delay consultation. All other patients with nontender scrotal swellings—unless inguinal hernia is suspected—require an ultrasound examination to confirm the diagnosis, because (1) ultrasonography is more accurate than clinical examination (up to 28% of cancers identified in some ultrasound surveys were found in patients referred with benign diagnoses) and (2) some

Table 183–1. NONTENDER SCROTAL MASSES: CLINICAL EXAMINATION

Condition	Findings	Transillu-minates?	Supine vs. Standing
Inguinal hernia	Mass extends into inguinal region Unable to get fingers above mass Mass increases with Valsalva maneuver Bowel sounds in mass Sometimes reducible	No	Often smaller supine
Hydrocele	Large pear-shaped anterior mass Skin stretched, shiny, red Penis appears shortened Obscures testis in 90%	Yes*	No change
Spermatocele	Discrete cystic mass on superior testis Usually < 2 cm diameter May be multiple	Yes	No change
Varicocele	Bluish discoloration "Bag of worms" Involves cord May increase with Valsalva maneuver	No	Collapses or disappears in supine position
Tumor	Firm intratesticular mass	No	No change
Sebaceous cyst	Round (size of marble), firm, yellow Confined within scrotal skin	No	No change

*In chronic hydroceles, a thickened wall may prevent transillumination.

patients have more than one diagnosis (e.g., 10% of testicular tumors present as hydroceles that prevent adequate palpation of the testis).

The acute appearance of symptomatic varicoceles in elderly men suggests obstruction of the spermatic veins by retroperitoneal disorders, frequently renal tumors.

Management. Patients with inguinal hernias should be referred to a surgeon. Most hydroceles and spermatoceles require no treatment, but if they become large, uncomfortable, or embarrassing, referral to a urologist for excision is appropriate. Aspiration of hydroceles is a reasonable alternative for the symptomatic patient with contraindications to surgery, but fluid usually appears again within weeks to months. Whether varicocele repair improves abnormal sperm counts is controversial.

Cross-References: Male Infertility (Chapter 156), Cancer of the Genitourinary Tract (Chapter 168), Scrotal Pain (Chapter 171).

REFERENCES

1. Fowler RC, Chennells PM, Ewing R. Scrotal ultrasonography: A clinical evaluation. Br J Radiol 1987;60:649–654.
   Ultrasonography is diagnostically superior to physical examination when evaluating the scrotum.

2. Kromann-Andersen B, Hansen LB, Larsen PN, Lawetz K, Lynge P, Lysen D, Pors Nielsen S, Stokholm KH, Foged P. Clinical versus ultrasonographic evaluation of scrotal disorders. Br J Urol 1988;61:350–353.

In 104 consecutive patients with scrotal abnormalities, the sensitivity/specificity of physical diagnosis, compared with the surgical diagnosis as the "gold" standard, was 0.9/0.81 for cancer, 0.89/0.96 for hydrocele, 0.74/0.94 for spermatocele, and 0.93/1.0 for varicocele.

3. Spittell JA, DeWeerd JH, Shick RM. Acute varicocele: A vascular clue to renal tumor. Mayo Clin Proc 1959;34:134–137.

The initial presentation of left hypernephroma in three men, aged 46 to 58, was an acute symptomatic left varicocele.

4. Zornow DH, Landes RR. Scrotal palpation. Am Fam Physician 1981;23:150–154.

The authors present a nice review of examination techniques and scrotal findings.

184 Benign Prostatic Hyperplasia

Problem

BARAK GASTER and JOHN B. STIMSON

Epidemiology. Eighty-five percent of men older than age 80 have histologic evidence of benign prostatic hyperplasia (BPH). Prostatectomy to treat clinically significant BPH is the second most common surgery performed in men older than age 65. The cause is not known, but the process is clearly androgen dependent.

Symptoms and Signs. Obstructive symptoms of BPH include decreased force of urine stream, hesitancy, intermittent stream, and post-void dribbling. Nocturia, urgency, and frequency are also symptoms seen in BPH but are termed *irritative* because they are believed to reflect detrusor muscle instability rather than a direct effect of obstruction. Irritative symptoms are less likely to abate with surgical treatment. Although acute urinary retention can complicate BPH, it is not necessarily related to the severity of preexisting symptoms and is often precipitated by medications or spontaneous infarction of hyperplastic prostatic tissue. Rarely, patients may present with uremic symptoms from severe bladder outlet obstruction. The American Urologic Association Symptom Index can reproducibly quantify a patient's symptoms and reliably allows their objective assessment over time.

Few useful physical signs exist. Prostate size on rectal examination correlates poorly with symptom severity, although rectal examination is also performed to detect prostate cancer or prostatitis. The bladder may be percussible or palpable in the lower abdomen if it decompensates and becomes distended.

Clinical Approach. Symptoms suggesting BPH can be caused by a number of other conditions. Urinary tract infection, glucosuria, and diuretic therapy cause frequency and nocturia and exacerbate symptoms in those with mild prostatism. Sympathomimetic and anticholinergic medications often worsen the obstructive symptoms of BPH. Neurologic diseases affecting bladder function (e.g., stroke, autonomic neuropathy, multiple sclerosis, Parkinson's disease) may be difficult to differentiate from BPH. A careful medication and neurologic history, neurologic examination, and urinalysis will identify these conditions. Serum blood urea and creatinine values should be obtained. If they are found to be elevated, ultrasonography should be done to exclude hydronephrosis. Cystourethroscopy visually confirms the presence of obstructing prostate tissue and rules out a urethral stricture, but it is routinely used only when there are risk factors for stricture (e.g., a history of frequent instrumentation or urethritis).

Management. Patients without significant retention and tolerable symptoms can be reassured and observed yearly. Symptoms can be minimized by avoidance of diuretics, caffeine, alcohol, sympathomimetics, and anticholinergics. For those whose symptoms significantly impair their quality of life, treatment is appropriate. Although medical therapy is somewhat less effective than surgery, it has a lower complication rate. Medications are now considered first-line therapy for those with moderate symptoms, as well as for those with severe symptoms who either decline surgery or are considered to be too high-risk for surgery due to co-morbidities.

Two classes of agents, α_1-blockers and 5α-reductase inhibitors, have been approved for use in BPH. The α_1-blockers, prazosin (up to 5 mg/d) and terazosin and doxazosin (both up to 10 mg/d), reduce symptoms by 50% and are also effective at lowering blood pressure in patients with coexisting hypertension. Care must be taken to titrate doses slowly to minimize orthostatic hypotension, which occurs in 10% of patients.

The 5α-reductase inhibitor finasteride blocks the conversion of testosterone to its active form, dihydrotestosterone, thereby shrinking the prostate gland. Although early studies performed in men with very large glands found that finasteride decreased symptoms by 25%, a large trial in patients with more moderate prostatic enlargement found finasteride to be no better than placebo. Based upon these results, finasteride's use should probably be limited to men with very large glands who are unable to tolerate an α_1-blocker. Finasteride's only major side effect is impotence, which affects 5% to 10% of patients (vs. 2% to 5% with placebo).

Transurethral resection of the prostate (TURP), the most common surgical approach used, is the most effective treatment available for BPH, reducing symptoms by 70% to 80%. In addition to the risks of the surgery itself, complications include persistent incontinence (0.7% to 1.4%) and impotence (14%), although in one randomized trial no difference was detected in sexual performance in patients after TURP compared with patients who did not undergo surgery.

Transurethral incision of the prostate (TUIP) is a less invasive procedure that can be performed in the outpatient setting under local anesthesia. It avoids the high risk of bladder neck contracture associated with transurethral resection in patients with small prostate glands. It may also have a role in patients with larger glands who wish to preserve antegrade ejaculation, which is often lost after TURP. Several newer, less invasive procedures that are coming into widespread use include the placement of prostatic stents, microwave thermotherapy, and laser prostatectomy. Their efficacy and safety are still under study.

Cross-References: Cancer of the Genitourinary Tract (Chapter 168), Dysuria (Chapter 170), Prostate Cancer (Chapter 173), Urinary Tract Infections in Men (Chapter 177), Bacteriuria in the Elderly (Chapter 178), Chronic Renal Failure (Chapter 179).

REFERENCES

1. Lepor H, Willford WO, Barry MJ, et al. The efficacy of terazosin, finasteride, or both in benign prostatic hypertrophy. N Engl J Med 1996;335:533–539.

   This article describes a large, randomized, placebo-controlled Veterans Affairs trial in 1229 men with moderate to severe BPH symptoms. Finasteride was no better than placebo, whereas terazosin decreased symptom scores by about 40%. The two drugs were equally well tolerated, with only 5% of patients in each group stopping the study drug due to adverse effects (vs. 2% with placebo). Combination therapy offered no advantage over monotherapy.

2. McConnell JD, Barry MJ, Bruskewitz RC, et al. Benign Prostatic Hyperplasia: Diagnosis and Treatment. Quick Reference Guide for Clinicians. No. 8. AH-CPR publication No. 94-0583. Rockville, MD, Department of Health and Human Services, 1994.

   This is a multidisciplinary overview with a meta-analysis of trial results and practical recommendations for treatment of benign prostatic hyperplasia.

3. Oesterling JE, Benign prostatic hyperplasia: Medical and minimally invasive treatment options. N Engl J Med 1995;332:99–109.

   The authors present a thorough review of the topic and include some of the more experimental surgical modalities under investigation.

4. Wasson JH, Reda DJ, Bruskewitz RC, et al. A comparison of transurethral surgery with watchful waiting for moderate symptoms of benign prostate hyperplasia. N Engl J Med 1995;332:75–79.

   In this first rigorously controlled trial of this extremely common procedure, performed by the Veterans Administration, 500 patients were followed for 3 years; there was sustained efficacy and less impairment of sexual function than is usually reported.

SECTION XVI

Psychiatric and Psychosomatic Disorders

185 Screening for Depression

Screening

GREGORY E. SIMON

Epidemiology. Major depression has a prevalence of 2% to 3% among the US population and a prevalence among medical outpatients of 8% to 20%. Depression is an episodic illness, with first onset in adolescence or early adulthood, peak prevalence in middle age, and declining prevalence in later years. Prevalence rates for females are approximately twice those for males in clinical and community samples. Approximately half of US residents treated for depression are managed exclusively in primary care settings. Fewer than one third of community residents with major depression use specialty mental health services.

Rationale. Major depression carries a burden of morbidity and disability equivalent to serious chronic medical illness. Depression also increases mortality through both an increase in suicide rates and a generalized increase in all-cause mortality. Patients with depression accompanying other medical conditions report more severe symptoms and poorer functional outcomes. Depression is also associated with increased use of outpatient medical services. Treatment of depression is effective in approximately 65% of cases, and early treatment appears to reduce the risk of chronicity.

In typical primary care practices, however, in only 50% of patients with major depression, the disorder is recognized with a smaller portion receiving effective treatment. Patients with unrecognized depression and untreated patients tend to be less severely ill and less disabled. Routine screening increases recognition and treatment rates but has not been shown to improve outcomes.

Strategy. Routine screening of all primary care patients is not supported by the available evidence. It may be justified among patients having clinical problems strongly associated with depression in primary care (chronic pain, insomnia, multiple unexplained physical symptoms, and high use of medical services) or those having medical conditions frequently complicated by depression (stroke, Parkinson's disease, and systemic lupus erythematosus).

Several paper-and-pencil screening questionnaires (e.g., Beck Depression

Inventory, Center for Epidemiologic Studies Depression Scale) have shown sensitivities of over 80% with specificities of over 70% when compared with a structured psychiatric interview. Of the widely used questionnaires, none is clearly superior.

Positive responses to screening questions should be followed up with specific questions covering diagnostic criteria for major depression described in Chapter 189, Management of Depression. This examination typically takes less than 10 minutes. Patients with positive screening examinations who do not meet diagnostic criteria for current major depression should be reexamined at the next visit.

Action. See Chapter 189, Management of Depression.

Cross-References: Periodic Health Assessment (Chapter 8), Somatization (Chapter 188), Management of Depression (Chapter 189).

REFERENCES

1. Depression Guideline Panel. Depression in Primary Care: Volume 1. Detection and Diagnosis. Clinical Practice Guideline, No. 5. Rockville, MD, US Department of Health and Human Services, Public Health Service, Agency for Health Care Policy and Research. AHCPR publication No. 93–0550. April 1993.

   This thorough review of relevant literature is accompanied by recommendations for primary care practice. Findings are summarized in the companion Quick Reference Guide for Clinicians. Both publications are available from AHCPR at 800-358-9295.

2. Mulrow CD, Williams JW, Gerety MB, Ramirez G, Montel OM, Kerber K. Case-finding instruments for depression in primary care settings. Ann Intern Med 1995;122:913–921.

   The authors present an up-to-date review of data on various screening instruments.

- -

186 Generalized Anxiety

Symptom

GREGORY E. SIMON

Epidemiology. Clinically significant anxiety affects 2% to 5% of the US general population and approximately 20% of patients in a medical clinic population. Anxiety disorders typically begin in early adulthood and affect women approximately twice as often as men.

Etiology. Anxiety may be a nonspecific response to various biologic, psychological, and social factors. Although anxiety in primary care medical patients may result from undiagnosed medical illness, clinicians should avoid exhaustive efforts to rule out all potential medical causes no matter how rare. Metabolic states associated with anxiety include withdrawal syndromes, medication side effects/intoxication, hyperthyroidism, hypoglycemia, and hypoxia. Specific psychiatric disorders accompanied by anxiety include depression, alcohol or drug abuse/dependence, panic disorder, and phobias. Nonspecific generalized anxiety is the heterogeneous group remaining once these more specific syndromes have been excluded. Generalized anxiety overlaps considerably with depression in presentation, biology, and treatment.

Clinical Approach. After a reasonable medical evaluation (including consideration of prescription and nonprescription medication), evaluation should focus on symptoms of depression, panic attacks, and alcohol or drug use (see Chapter 9, Diagnosis and Management of Drug Abuse; Chapter 189, Management of Depression; and Chapter 191, Panic Disorder). Phobic anxiety occurs in specific feared situations (e.g., bridges, heights, crowds, open spaces), whereas generalized anxiety is more pervasive, although often affected by social stresses.

Management. Treatment should first focus on any specific medical or psychiatric disorder that may contribute to anxiety. Alcohol and drug abuse/dependence take precedence over other diagnoses, and no separate diagnosis of anxiety disorder should be considered until after weeks of abstinence. All patients with generalized anxiety (even those with no pattern of substance abuse) should be advised to avoid all caffeine and alcohol. The short-term anxiolytic effects of alcohol are often followed by withdrawal anxiety. Generalized anxiety associated with depression or panic disorder typically responds well to treatment of those specific problems. For patients with nonspecific anxiety, cognitive and behavioral approaches should be the primary treatments. Good self-help manuals to guide patients through these treatments are available (see References).

Cognitive approaches to anxiety focus on the half-conscious, often unreasonable thoughts associated with anxiety. Patients are asked to focus on the specific thoughts occurring during times of greatest distress. By learning to examine the irrational fears associated with anxiety, patients will gain a sense of calm and self-control. For example, a patient reporting disabling symptoms of fear, ruminative worry, nausea, and tension headaches after starting a new job would be asked to examine out loud the thoughts associated with these anxiety symptoms. After describing fears of failing at work leading to being fired, losing a home, and being left penniless, the patient is asked to sort out reasonable concerns (increased work pressures) from exaggerated ones (bankruptcy and homelessness). Performing this exercise, initially with the help of a calm and concerned physician, will help a patient to gain mastery of anxious thoughts later on his or her own. Practice at home and reinforcement during later visits are critical to building confidence. Anxiety after specific life stresses often responds well to such an approach.

Behavioral approaches to anxiety use relaxation exercises to relieve associated physical symptoms. Typical exercises begin with rhythmic deep breathing followed by visualization of relaxing images and progressive muscle relaxation. Systematically tensing and relaxing specific muscle groups helps patients to focus on relaxation while avoiding distracting fearful thoughts. After initial instruction during an office visit, patients should practice two or three times a day at home to build skill and self-confidence. Exercises focusing on muscle relaxation are especially useful to patients suffering from tension-related physical complaints (headache, muscle stiffness, dyspnea).

Phobic anxiety also calls for strategies to overcome situational fears. Avoidance of feared situations reinforces anxiety and leads to a cycle of increasing anxiety and withdrawal. Physicians should assist patients in developing a plan for gradually increasing exposure to feared situations. For example, a patient with intense fear of shopping in crowded stores is first told to go to the supermarket at an uncrowded time in the company of a friend. Although this may produce some anxiety, the patient should remain until the initial wave of fear passes. This exercise should be repeated daily until it no longer provokes any anxiety. Then the patient should gradually increase the level of exposure (e.g., going into the store alone while a friend remains in view outside). Using this incremental technique, the patient should increase the level of exposure once the lower exposure level can be tolerated without difficulty. With this approach, most phobic patients can confront previously intolerable situations with a manageable level of anxiety.

Benzodiazepine anxiolytics, although useful for management of short-term situational anxiety, should be avoided for management of chronic anxiety states. As-needed use of anxiolytics for generalized anxiety should be confined to periods of 1 month or less and should be avoided completely for patients with histories of alcohol or sedative abuse. Accumulation of benzodiazepines in the elderly carries risks of oversedation, cognitive impairment, and injury due to falls. Shorter-half-life medications carry less risk of tolerance, dependence, and accumulation. Less lipophilic drugs have more gradual onset and thus less reinforcement for frequent use. Lorazepam and oxazepam satisfy both of these criteria (Table 186–1).

If continued pharmacotherapy is necessary, antidepressant drugs should be considered. The limited evidence available suggests they may be as effective as benzodiazepines in relieving generalized anxiety symptoms without risks

Table 186–1. SELECTED ANXIOLYTIC DRUGS

Drug	Starting Dose	Speed of Onset*	Half-Life (h)†	Cost ($ per Day)‡
Diazepam (Valium)	5 mg bid prn	+ + + +	20–100	0.26
Chlordiazepoxide (Librium)	10 mg bid prn	+ +	10–30	0.13
Lorazepam (Ativan)	0.5 mg tid prn	+ +	5–20	0.40
Oxazepam (Serax)	15 mg tid prn	+	5–15	0.75
Alprazolam (Xanax)	0.25 mg tid prn	+ + + +	8–12	1.55
Buspirone (BuSpar)	5 mg bid or tid	0	20–100	1.36

*0 = very delayed onset to + + + + + = very rapid onset.
†May be greatly prolonged in the elderly.
‡Generic prices used, where available; average wholesale price of starting dose listed, 1996 *Drug Topics Red Book.*

of dependence. See Chapter 189 for specific advice regarding prescribing antidepressants.

Buspirone, a nonbenzodiazepine anxiolytic, appears to have little potential for abuse and does not provoke tolerance or dependence. Although quite effective in some patients with generalized anxiety, it appears less universally efficacious than benzodiazepines and provokes agitation in a significant minority. It must be administered regularly for 1 to 2 weeks to achieve therapeutic effect and is thus not suitable for as-needed use. Patients with histories of alcohol or benzodiazepine abuse (the population for whom a nonbenzodiazepine anxiolytic might be most useful) may respond less often to buspirone.

Follow-Up. Cognitive and behavioral techniques require both continued practice by patients and reinforcement by physicians to remain effective. Group programs offering instruction in cognitive and behavioral techniques may be helpful. Psychiatric consultation may be necessary in cases of significant generalized anxiety persisting over 1 month and unresponsive to nonpharmacologic interventions. Both patients and physicians must realize that complete relief of chronic generalized anxiety is an unrealistic goal. Management should focus on relief of symptoms and reduction of functional disability.

REFERENCES

1. Burns DD. The Feeling Good Handbook. New York, Plume Press, 1979.

   This is a good, practical guide to cognitive treatment of anxiety.

2. Crashe M. Mastery of Your Anxiety and Worry. Albany, Greywind Publications, 1992.

   This is the best source of self-treatment of anxiety but is hard to find.

3. Stoudemire A. Epidemiology and psychopharmacology of anxiety in medical patients. J Clin Psychiatry 1996; 57(suppl 7):64–75.

. . . .

187 Insomnia

Symptom

DONALD W. BELCHER

Epidemiology and Etiology. Patients often complain that their sleep is inadequate, is unrestoring, or hinders daytime function. Insomnia is described as either short term (days to weeks) or chronic (more than 1 month). Short-term insomnia, often related to work shift changes, jet lag, bereavement, or other stressors, can be treated with behavioral advice and judicious prescription of hypnotic agents for 1 to 2 weeks.

Chronic insomnia occurs in up to 15% of surveyed adults, with higher rates in patients with medical or psychiatric problems and about one third of elderly adults (as evidenced by decreased deep sleep time, earlier bedtime, more naps). Because insomnia is multifaceted, a structured approach is recommended to understand how specific factors affect sleep onset or sleep maintenance. Treatment includes optimal management of symptoms, adjusting relevant medications, and efforts to improve sleep hygiene.

Clinical Approach. A brief interview with the patient and partner helps to clarify the pattern of chronic insomnia and contributing circumstances. In contrast, the physical examination (mouth, nose, throat, lungs—see Chapter 64, Sleep Apnea Syndromes) is usually unrewarding. The patient should be asked if the problem is falling asleep, frequent or prolonged awakening, or undesirable daytime effects. Individuals who are experiencing anxiety, feeling stressed, or worrying at bedtime often need help to identify and confront these barriers. Stimulants such as caffeine in the evening, nicotine within a half hour of retiring, or use of illicit drugs (e.g., cocaine) may be at fault. A disrupting bedroom environment can interfere with sleeping. Often insomniacs can recite a litany of helps—the value of regular sleep-wake times, restricting nap times, a restful bedroom atmosphere, avoiding stimulants—but they may practice such tactics poorly.

Patients who report either increased awakening or a period of midsleep insomnia should be asked specific questions regarding symptoms associated with awakening (e.g., pain, dyspnea, palpitations, nocturia, nausea). The clinician should ask about the presence of common medical problems (arthritis, esophageal reflux, angina, neuropathy, chronic pain, congestive heart failure, chronic obstructive pulmonary disease, bladder dysfunction) and any related symptoms. Many elderly patients experience frequent awakening unassociated with either causal symptoms or decreased daytime performance. A discussion of age-related sleep changes (less deep stages, more awakenings) may help them modify unrealistic expectations.

Underlying causes should be treated. Furthermore, insomnia due to poorly timed medication schedules or inadequate dosages can be considered. If treatment is optimized (e.g., analgesics, antacids, antianginal agents, diuretics), sleep disruption can be improved. When side effects from current drugs are suspected (e.g., corticosteroids, theophylline), a trial of withholding or changing the medication should be considered.

When the complaint is persistent early awakening, the patient should be asked about a depressed mood and related symptoms (see Chapter 185, Screening for Depression, and Chapter 189, Management of Depression) and current use of alcohol (alcohol shortens latency but disrupts sleep stages). Other causes of sleep interruptions, such as the restless legs syndrome (nocturnal paresthesias relieved by movement) or sleep apnea, may need corroboration by a partner.

Management. Medications have limited use in chronic insomnia. Hypnotics (e.g., benzodiazepines) can be used selectively for 2 weeks or so but may cause oversedation and dependence (Table 187–1). They must be used cautiously in the elderly or patients with renal/liver disease or heavy snorers and are contraindicated in alcoholism, sleep apnea, and pregnancy. Nonhypnotics (e.g., antihistamines, low-dose antidepressants, anxiolytics) have significant anticholinergic side effects that may interfere with ambulation or urination.

Table 187-1. SELECTED DRUGS FOR SLEEP

Indication/Drug	Dose (mg)	Side Effects, Comments	Cost ($ per Week)*
Mild, intermittent			
Diphenhydramine (Benadryl, others; OTC)	25, 50	Anticholinergic side effects can be a problem for elderly	1.52–2.05
Moderate, short term			
Triazolam (Halcion)	0.125, 0.25	Less rebound insomnia at lower dose	4.52–4.94
Temazepam (Restoril, others)	7.5, 15, 30	Can give 1–2 hours before retiring to offset slow onset; lasts 6–8 hours	4.55–5.09
Zolpidem (Ambien)	5, 10	Nonbenzodiazepine; short acting; no rebound, withdrawal, or tolerance; less daytime confusion in elderly	8.72–10.72
Severe, prolonged; associated with depression			
Trazodone (Desyrel, others)	150, 300	Best hypnotic effect; give 1 hour before retiring; dry mouth; rare priapism	12.98–23.11
Doxepin (Sinequan, others)	25, 50	Anticholinergic side effects; orthostatic hypotension	3.06–4.30
Amitriptyline (Elavil, others)	10, 25, 50	Same; these side effects limit use of tricyclic antidepressants in elderly	1.30–2.61–4.64

*Average wholesale price; often lower for generic, if available. From 1995 *Drug Topics Red Book.*

Nonpharmaceutical approaches (behavioral-cognitive) should be encouraged and have been found to improve sleep complaints in at least half of insomniacs. All chronic insomniacs benefit from discussing habits conducive to sleep, including a favorable bedroom environment. The clinician should emphasize that adequate sleep is helped by a regular sleep/awake rhythm, a positive bedroom-sleep association, an ability to relax, and minimizing of external disturbances. Examples of poor sleep hygiene and relevant interventions include (1) irregular sleep schedule due to changes on weekends or after retirement (revise schedule); (2) excessive time in bed (plan to get up at a consistent time; avoid excessive napping); (3) disruptive bedroom environment (too light or noisy; television or reading; uncomfortable temperature—suggest stimulus control, cooler temperature); (4) worrying that prevents sleep (try to confront problems in daytime); (5) anxiety about insomnia (offer relaxation training); or (6) high body temperature (do physical exercise, use hot tub well before bedtime).

Experts recommend use of a daily sleep diary as background information—the time in and out of bed, minutes to fall asleep, number and duration of awakenings, associated symptoms, or potentially offending medications/stimulants—to clarify the pattern and contributing causes. Then each intervention can be tried for a week or so. If neither symptoms nor medications seem at fault but excessive stimuli (e.g., television, worrying) or long daytime naps are issues, one can move the television out of the bedroom, limit naps to less than 1 hour, and try a 10-minute evening "worry time" to identify and confront troubling issues. Underlying depression must be considered as well.

In summary, one should identify and treat underlying causes of insomnia and recommend general hygiene measures that promote sleep. Patients with significant psychiatric components (e.g., major depression, manic disorders, panic attacks, psychoses) often have chronic insomnia, and consultation with a mental health specialist is essential. Patients who prove refractory to management or have potentially serious problems (e.g, sleep apnea) may be referred to a sleep laboratory for additional assessment.

Cross-References: Sleep Apnea Syndromes (Chapter 64), Restless Legs Syndrome (Chapter 113), Screening for Depression (Chapter 185), Management of Depression (Chapter 189).

REFERENCES

1. Guilleminault C, Clerk A, Black J, Labowski M, Pelayo R, Claman D. Nondrug treatment trials in psychophysiologic insomnia. Arch Intern Med 1995;155:838–844.

   All 30 patients showed some improvement with structured sleep hygiene. Although afternoon exercise added little, the use of dawn light therapy improved results, presumably by favorably manipulating the biologic clock.

2. Hartmann PM. Drug treatment of insomnia: Indications and newer agents. Am Fam Physician 1995;51(a):191–194.

   A concise summary of newer hypnotics and their attributes, such as rebound, daytime sedation, and tolerance, is provided.

3. Morin CM, Culbert JP, Schwartz SM. Nonpharmacological interventions for insomnia: A meta-analysis of treatment efficacy. Am J Psychiatry 1994;151:1172–1180.

   In 59 outcome trials involving about 2000 patients, stimulus control and sleep limitation were the most effective and clinical efficacy persisted at 6 months.

4. Murtagh DRR, Greenwood KM. Identifying effective psychological treatments for insomnia: A meta-analysis. J Consult Clin Psychol 1995;63:79–89.

   Psychological treatments, notably stimulus control, were effective in improving sleep latency and patterns, particularly in patients who were not regular users of sedative/hypnotics.

■ ■

188 Somatization

Problem

GEOFFREY H. GORDON

Epidemiology. *Somatization* is broadly defined as emotional distress that is experienced and expressed as physical symptoms. Patients who somatize chronically often make frequent or intense requests for medical care with many unscheduled visits to multiple providers and undergo repetitive but unrevealing work-ups ("much doctoring, little curing"). Somatization can occur in the presence of co-morbid physical illness, with symptoms unrelated or out of proportion to objective findings. Thus, somatization and related psychiatric disorders neither are diagnoses of exclusion nor are confined to the "worried well." The severity of somatization varies from transient amplification of minor physical concerns during times of stress to adoption of illness as a pervasive and disabling lifestyle.

Somatization is an important clinical problem. Half of all patients given psychiatric diagnoses are seen solely by nonpsychiatrists, and three fourths of them present with physical symptoms related to emotional distress. Physical symptoms due to psychosocial distress account for an estimated 25% to 75% of visits to primary care providers.

Clinical Approach. An obscure or persistent physical symptom can represent an unspoken fear of disease or a hidden request for reassurance, information, specific care, or advocacy. It is useful to ask patients what they believe is wrong (or what concerns them the most) and what they think should be done (or how they hope their physician can help). Translators for non–English-speaking patients should explore cultural beliefs about the meaning of the illness in addition to providing literal translations.

Certain psychiatric disorders are particularly prevalent among somatizing patients, but classification of individual patients using the current psychiatric *Diagnostic and Statistical Manual of Mental Disorders (DSM-IV)* can be difficult. In one study, nearly 50% of 100 consecutive somatizing outpatients had major depression. In addition to cognitive and affective symptoms, depressed patients may report somatic symptoms such as headache, dizziness, or abdominal pain. Panic disorder, a type of anxiety disorder, occurs in approximately 6% of primary care patients and presents as cardiac, gastrointestinal, neurologic, or other symptoms that cluster in discrete episodes and are often alarming and misdiagnosed. Depression and anxiety often coexist and are usually overlooked as patients (and their providers) focus on the physical symptoms and dismiss the mood disturbance as a secondary or nonpathologic condition. Alcoholism and substance abuse can cause a variety of physical symptoms or conceal underlying psychiatric disorders.

Four "somatoform disorders" present as physical symptoms that cannot be explained by the presence or severity of a physical disorder. The most valid and reliable of these entities, *somatization disorder*, is characterized by multiple unexplained symptoms in multiple organ systems starting before the age of 30. The *DSM-IV* diagnostic criteria require the presence of four pain symptoms, two gastrointestinal symptoms, one sexual symptom, and one pseudoneurologic symptom from an extended list of possible symptoms. The symptoms must have been present for several years and resulted in treatment-seeking behavior or significant social or occupational impairment. Patients with fewer symptoms ("abridged" criteria) may follow a similar course. The prevalence of somatization disorder is 2% in the general population, 6% in general medical clinics, and 9% among tertiary hospital inpatients. Patients with somatization disorder have an excessive amount of health care utilization and surgical procedures, despite normal mortality rates. Most patients with somatization disorder are women, and the illness usually begins in adolescence. Common co-morbid psychiatric disorders include depression, anxiety, alcohol/substance abuse, and personality disorders. *Conversion* symptoms are medically unexplainable losses or changes in voluntary motor or sensory function (e.g., paralysis or blindness). The symptoms may follow a pattern suggested by the patient's experiences, fears, or expectations about illness. Most conversion symptoms occur in the setting of another psychiatric disorder, usually somatization disorder. Conversion symptoms in the absence of a medical, neurologic, or psychiatric disorder generally have a good psychiatric prognosis, but 12% to 25% of these patients subsequently develop a physical disorder that better explains their symptoms. *Hypochondriasis* is characterized by excessive fear of disease, preoccupation with body function, and conviction that a serious disease is present. Hypochondriasis is more common in middle or old age and affects both sexes equally. Hypochondriac patients misinterpret normal physiologic sensations as evidence of disease, worry about having specific diseases, and are demanding and critical of their physicians. Hypochondriasis accompanies up to 5% of all medical and psychiatric illnesses. Patients with *somatoform pain disorder* are preoccupied with pain that has lasted for at least 6 months with little relation to objective findings. The relationship of this disorder to chronic pain syndrome is poorly defined. The clinical features of the four somatoform disorders overlap with each other and with those of depression, anxiety, alcohol/substance abuse, and the personality disorders.

Management. Chronically somatizing patients are not reassured by a "negative workup" and may experience the news that "nothing is wrong" as an accusation of lying ("I'm not making it up."), being crazy ("You think it's all in my head!"), or threat of abandonment ("Where are you going to send me this time?"). Thus, an important early step in treatment is to legitimize the presence of the symptoms ("I can see this pain is really a problem for you.") and the frustration with multiple attempts to "find it and fix it" ("It must be really frustrating for you to have all these doctors and tests and still not get help for your symptoms.") and to express continued interest and hope ("I'd like to work with you on these problems.").

Convincing yourself and the patient that no physical disease is present is rarely possible or useful. However, it is important to establish that there is no immediate danger or need for further testing. Reaching this level of certainty may be difficult in some circumstances (e.g., functional chest pain in a patient with known coronary disease). Familiarity with the patient over time through a continuing primary care relationship is very useful. Periodic evaluation of chronic symptoms and investigation of new ones should be conservative and logical. Descriptive diagnostic terms are preferable to misleading labels that are hard to prove or disprove and may lead to unnecessary testing and treatment. (For example, "chronic abdominal pain" is preferable to "possible adhesions".) Somatizing patients are generally at greater risk for iatrogenic disease than from missed nonpsychiatric diagnoses.

The treatment plan should focus more on restoring and maintaining function than on removing, reducing, or explaining symptoms ("care, not cure"). Medication and other treatment trials should be time limited and linked to positive functional outcomes. (For example, "This medication will not relieve all of your symptoms, but it may help you do more of the activities you want to do, such as volunteer work. Let's try it for 8 weeks. We'll know whether the medicine is working by counting the days you were able to volunteer successfully.") Disability- and compensation-seeking should be discouraged as contrary to the goal of maximizing function.

Other reasonable treatment goals include fewer unscheduled, catastrophic, or disruptive calls and visits and less doctor shopping. Scheduling brief but regular office visits or telephone contacts reassures patients that they will not be abandoned and demonstrates that they do not have to have worsened symptoms to be seen. Successful functional improvement requires that both physicians and patients not expect a "quick fix." Improvement may be impressive, but often it is slow and may not be appreciated by students and residents who have not seen patients in long-term follow-up.

There are several useful techniques for addressing the psychosocial aspects of the illness. One is to listen carefully to the uninterrupted story of illness, taking note of the patient's spontaneous associations of symptoms with events, circumstances, or other people. Asking patients for details or clarification of their own stories is more effective than taking a stereotyped psychosocial history. Another technique is to "normalize" stress and ask about its effects in the individual ("Everyone has stress in their lives, and we know that stress aggravates most medical conditions. How does stress affect you?"). Still another strategy is to ask about the effect of the symptoms on psychosocial function ("What things have these symptoms kept you from doing?"). This can be presented in a way that broaches treatment options. For example, a physician who wants to elicit symptoms of depression and lay the foundation for biologic treatment might ask a patient, "Sometimes illness causes chemical changes in the nervous system that affect sleep, appetite, energy, or even the ability to enjoy things. Has that happened to you?"

Often the best strategy for dealing with chronic unexplained symptoms is to acknowledge the complexity of the condition and the importance of taking time to consider carefully all potential pieces of information, including biologic and psychosocial factors. Patients can help by keeping a symptom diary, rating the intensity of one or more symptoms on a scale from 1 to 10, and describing related circumstances (e.g., food, activity, other persons) and perhaps their stress level, again on a numeric scale. These ratings can be done twice or three times a day for 1 to 2 weeks and brought in for discussion at the next office visit. Patients should share their diaries verbally, because further history (such as antecedents or consequences of symptoms) may be uncovered. Family members can be interviewed for their perceptions of the patient's illness.

A mental health consultant can help by confirming the diagnosis, providing crisis intervention and support, and recommending effective treatment. However, many somatizing patients refuse mental health consultation. Patients who agree to referral should be told that the purpose is to help understand the illness and to gather new information. They should be told whom they will see and what to expect. ("Dr. Baker is a psychologist who works with medically ill patients. He may be able to help us develop a treatment plan. He will talk with you about your condition and then call me.") They should be reassured of continuity of care ("I'll schedule a visit with you soon afterward so we can discuss his ideas."). In addition to medications for depression and anxiety when indicated, somatizing patients may benefit from cognitive therapy (e.g., identifying and correcting catastrophic thinking), behavior therapy (e.g., monitoring and changing the antecedents and consequences of pain behavior), relaxation training, biofeedback, and group or family therapy.

Follow-Up. In one study, treatment applying the principles outlined markedly reduced the health care utilization of a group of patients with somatization disorder. Physicians should be aware of their own personal reactions, strengths, and weaknesses in working with somatizing patients. Discussing a difficult patient with a colleague is one way to maintain perspective.

Cross-References: Effective Communication in the Ambulatory Care Setting (Chapter 2), Diagnosis and Management of Drug Abuse (Chapter 9), Alcohol Problems (Chapter 10), Chronic Nonspecific Pain Syndrome (Chapter 14), Fatigue (Chapter 21), Acute Chest Pain (Chapter 73), Recurrent Chest Pain (Chapter 74), Abdominal Pain (Chapter 94), Low Back Pain (Chapter 107), Fibromyalgia (Chapter 121), Headache (Chapter 138), Pelvic Pain in Women (Chapter 160), Screening for Depression (Chapter 185), Generalized Anxiety (Chapter 186), Management of Depression (Chapter 189), The Difficult Patient (Chapter 192).

REFERENCES

1. Blackwell B. Sick role susceptibility. Psychother Psychosom 1992;58:79–90.

   The author discusses somatization as chronic illness behavior and describes practical steps to identify symptom amplifiers, decrease rewards of illness, and promote healthy behaviors.

2. Hanner L, Witek JJ, Clift RB. When you're sick and don't know why: Coping with your undiagnosed illness. Minneapolis, DCI Publishing, 1991.

   A useful book for somatizing patients on what medical care can and can't do to help.

3. Kaplan C, Lipkin M Jr, Gordon GH. Somatization in primary care: Patients with unexplained and vexing medical complaints. J Gen Intern Med 1988;3:177–190.

   This is a comprehensive review article.

4. Katon W, Ries RK, Kleinman A. A prospective DSM-III study of 100 consecutive somatization patients. Compr Psychiatry 1984;25:305–314.

   Somatizing patients referred to a psychiatric consultation service had significantly more depression, panic, personality disorders, and psychophysiologic illness than a control group of nonsomatizing referral patients.

5. Quill TE. Somatization: One of medicine's blind spots. JAMA 1985;254:3075–3079.

   The author captures the flavor of the clinical presentation and diagnosis of somatization disorder, reviews barriers to effective care, and outlines a treatment approach.

■ ■

189 Management of Depression

Problem

GREGORY E. SIMON

Epidemiology. Depression is a common, disabling condition in primary care practice. (See Chapter 185, Screening for Depression.)

Symptoms and Signs. The hallmarks of depression are pervasively sad mood and markedly diminished interest or pleasure in almost all activities. These are typically accompanied by physical symptoms of depression (change in weight or appetite, increased or decreased sleep, motor agitation or retardation, and fatigue) as well as cognitive symptoms (feelings of guilt or worthlessness, impaired concentration, and thoughts of death or suicide). Current diagnostic criteria for major depression require a 2-week period of depressed mood or loss of interest accompanied by at least four other symptoms. More severe depression may also be accompanied by psychotic symptoms including hallucinations and delusions.

Depression is typically an episodic illness with onset in the teens or 20s. Episodes often recur, and each recurrence carries a greater risk of chronicity. In bipolar disorder, episodes of depression are associated with one or more episodes of hypomania (elevated mood or irritability, increased energy, impulsivity) or mania (all of the above plus psychosis). Although episodes of depression may appear to be more or less related to stressful life events, classifying depression based on relation to life stresses ("reactive" vs. "endogenous") does not reliably predict clinical course or treatment response.

Clinical Approach. Reports of depressed mood, crying spells, insomnia, fatigue, or loss of interest should prompt the provider to inquire specifically about depressive symptoms. Observations by family members, friends, or physicians might also prompt further examination. Straightforward inquiry about each symptom listed earlier is usually well received (e.g., "Have you noticed any change in your sleeping, either trouble sleeping or sleeping too much?" "Have you noticed trouble concentrating or feeling like your thinking is slowed down?"). Questions about suicide should begin by determining the presence of any suicidal ideas ("Have you been thinking a lot about death or dying?" "Have you been feeling like you might rather be dead?") followed by specific questions to determine the level of risk ("Have you had thoughts about killing yourself?" "Have you made any plans for how to do it?" "Have you taken any steps toward doing it?" "Do you feel now like you would want to kill yourself?" "Are you planning to?"). This diagnostic evaluation typically takes less than 10 minutes.

Four specific areas should always be addressed in evaluating patients with significant depression. First, substance abuse often causes or complicates depression. Alcohol is a potent depressant, and abstinence from cocaine can produce severe symptoms of depression. Substance abuse must be addressed initially, and consideration of independent depression should be postponed until after a few weeks of abstinence. Second, depression may be accompanied by psychosis, which may require specific treatment. Straightforward inquiry about psychotic symptoms is the best approach ("Have you had any trouble with hearing voices or hearing things that might not be there?" "Have you been seeing visions or seeing things that might not be there?" "Have you had any unusual ideas that someone has been interfering with your mind?"). Psychotic depression often involves delusions of guilt or disease. Psychotic symptoms should prompt psychiatric consultation regarding need for antipsychotic medication or hospitalization. Third, patients with current mixed (manic and depressive) symptoms or histories of mania may become manic when treated with conventional antidepressants. Ask specifically about a history of mania ("Have you ever had a period of a week or more when you felt unusually high or energetic, didn't sleep, or acted on impulse, or when a doctor said you were manic?") and about current manic symptoms (mood lability, irritability, impulsivity). Suspicion of mania should prompt psychiatric consultation regarding need for lithium or other pharmacotherapy. Fourth, significant risk of suicide should prompt hospitalization. Patients who report any current intent or plan to attempt suicide should be offered voluntary hospitalization and considered for involuntary treatment. Those reporting suicidal ideas with no current intent or plan do not require hospitalization if they can agree to contact the physician's office, hospital emergency department, or other community resources if suicidal urges appear.

Crisp separation of normal grief from depression is not possible. Grieving may involve all symptoms of major depression, and the distinction must be made according to duration and severity. Bereaved patients with disabling depressive symptoms that persist longer than 2 months or result in threats to health should be considered for the treatments outlined below for depression.

Patients with chronic pain or other "functional" physical symptoms may deny depressed mood and loss of interest while reporting other associated symptoms. Because these patients may benefit from antidepressant medication, such syndromes have been labeled "masked depression." This relabeling, however, tends to irritate patients and focus attention away from the primary complaint. Instead, one should explain that the pharmacologic and nonpharmacologic techniques used in treatment of depression may also relieve a variety of chronic physical symptoms.

Management. Benefits of specific treatment (pharmacotherapy or psychotherapy) are well established for patients meeting diagnostic criteria for major depression and for those with less severe symptoms of prolonged duration (> 12 months). In less severe or chronic cases, spontaneous remission rates are high and active treatments are not clearly superior to "placebo" treatments. If the need for specific treatment is not clear, the patient is offered support and advice (see later) and reassessed after 2 to 4 weeks.

For patients with moderate depression, antidepressant medication and specific psychotherapies (see later) are equally effective in relieving symptoms. Initial choice of treatment should depend on availability and patient preference. Providing both treatments simultaneously is not clearly superior to either treatment alone. For the severely depressed patient, antidepressant medication is recommended.

Drugs used in treatment of depression include tricyclic antidepressants, serotonin-reuptake inhibitors, and other nontricyclic drugs. Primary care physicians should understand the use of at least one drug from each of these groups. Less commonly used treatments (monoamine oxidase inhibitors, augmentation or combination regimens) should be prescribed only by specialists or the especially interested generalist.

Tricyclic antidepressants and newer nontricyclic agents are equal in effectiveness when used in comparable doses. Each is effective in 60% to 70% of patients with major depression, whereas over 80% of major depression will respond to at least one of them. Therapeutic effect is first evident in 1 to 2 weeks, with full effect in 3 to 6 weeks.

Antidepressants differ primarily in their side effects (which unfortunately appear after the first dose). The tricyclic antidepressants have a similar range of side effects that vary in severity (Table 189–1). These include sedation, anticholinergic effects (dry mouth, constipation, urinary retention, tachycardia), and postural hypotension. These effects are usually greater with earlier, tertiary amine tricyclics (amitriptyline, imipramine, doxepin) than with their secondary amine descendents (desipramine, nortriptyline). Newer nontricyclic drugs are generally better tolerated but are considerably more expensive. Serotonin-reuptake inhibitors can cause nausea, headache, increased muscle tension, feelings of agitation, and sexual dysfunction. Trazodone has minimal anticholinergic effect but is highly sedating and may rarely cause priapism (about which all males taking trazodone should be warned). Amoxapine has some neuroleptic activity and has caused extrapyramidal side effects (dystonia, parkinsonism, and tardive dyskinesia).

The cardiac effects of antidepressants have generated the most concern among medical providers. Tricyclic antidepressants have quinidine-like effects on cardiac rhythm. They typically suppress ambient ventricular ectopy but may cause idiosyncratic increases in atrial and ventricular arrhythmias as well as

Table 189–1. CHARACTERISTICS OF SELECTED ANTIDEPRESSANT DRUGS

Drug	Initial Daily Dose	"Target" Dose	Maximal Dose	Sedative Effect	Anticholinergic Effect	Postural Hypotension	Gastrointestinal Upset	Sexual Dysfunction	Cost ($ per Month)*
Amitriptyline (Elavil)	10–25 mg qhs	75–150 mg qhs	300 mg	+ + + +	+ + + +	+ + +	+	+	7.50
Imipramine (Tofranil)	10–25 mg qhs	75–150 mg qhs	300 mg	+ + +	+ + +	+ +	+	+	8.00
Doxepin (Sinequan)	10–25 mg qhs	75–150 mg qhs	300 mg	+ + + +	+ + +	+ + +	+	+	8.00
Desipramine (Norpramin)	10–25 mg qd	75–150 mg qd	300 mg	+	+	+ +	+	+	35.94
Nortriptyline (Pamelor)	10–20 mg qhs	25–75 mg qhs	200 mg	+ +	+	+	+	+	66.59
Trazodone (Desyrel)	25 mg qhs	75–200 mg qhs	400 mg	+ + +	0	+ +	+	+	28.57
Fluoxetine (Prozac)	10 mg qod–qd	10–30 mg qd	60 mg	0	0	0	+ +	+ +	71.42
Sertraline (Zoloft)	25 mg qd	50–100 mg qd	200 mg	0	0	0	+ +	+ +	64.60
Paroxetine (Paxil)	10–20 mg qd	20–40 mg qd	100 mg	+	0	0	+ +	+ +	64.44
Bupropion (Wellbutrin)	75–100 mg qd	75–100 mg tid	450 mg	0	0	0	+ +	0	74.65
Venlafaxine (Effexor)	37.5 mg qd–bid	75–100 mg tid	375 mg	+	+	0	+	+ +	99.88
Nefazodone (Serzone)	75–100 mg bid	100–200 mg bid	600 mg	+ +	0	+	+	0	52.37

*Average wholesale price for 30-day supply of upper "target" dose. Generic prices used, where available; 1996 *Drug Topics Red Book*.
0 = no effect to + + + + = frequent effect.

cause refractory arrhythmias in overdose. Preexisting arrhythmias do not contraindicate use of tricyclics, but one must exercise the same caution one would use in starting treatment with quinidine. Tricyclic antidepressants also can impair atrioventricular conduction, resulting in prolongation of the PR interval or increase in grade of preexisting conduction disturbance. In patients with first-degree atrioventricular block or bundle branch block, dosage should be increased slowly with repeat electrocardiography at each dosage increase. Although tricyclic antidepressants may have a negative inotropic effect in overdose, they do not appear to impair ventricular function in routine clinical use. Postural hypotension is usually the most important adverse cardiovascular effect of tricyclic agents in patients with heart disease. Newer antidepressants (e.g., serotonin-reuptake inhibitors, bupropion, venlafaxine, and nefazodone) usually have minimal effect on cardiac rhythm and conduction.

The selection of an antidepressant should be guided initially by the patient's history of previous treatment. An antidepressant that previously yielded relief of depression without intolerable side effects should be used again. A drug that previously was ineffective (when given in therapeutic dose) or caused intolerable side effects should be avoided. Previous difficulty with either oversedation or overstimulation argues for an antidepressant with the opposite effect. Without prior history of antidepressant treatment, the choice of an initial agent depends on side effects and patient preference. Anticholinergic side effects (constipation, urinary retention, confusion) and postural hypotension are especially problematic among the elderly.

Initiating treatment at low doses and building to therapeutic dose over 7 to 10 days will minimize initial side effects. The doses listed in Table 189–1 represent averages for healthy young or middle-aged patients. Doses in the elderly or chronically ill should initially be reduced by one half, although some elderly patients may require the full doses. The maintenance doses lie in the lower range of therapeutic effect. In general, maintenance doses should be increased after 3 to 4 weeks if side effects are tolerable but depression has not significantly improved. Consultation should be sought before exceeding the "maximum" doses listed. Side effects should be first managed by reducing the dose or slowing the rate of increase before changing medication. Tolerance to side effects often develops with time. A relationship between serum level and drug efficacy is well established for nortriptyline and somewhat established for desipramine. Serum levels for these drugs may be helpful in ill or elderly patients, patients with side effects at low doses, and patients unresponsive to usual doses. For other agents, serum levels are commercially available but of unproven value.

Specific psychotherapies (cognitive therapy, behavior therapy, interpersonal therapy) are effective treatments for moderately severe depression. These treatments are typically delivered in 10 to 15 sessions over 4 months, but less frequent maintenance treatment may sometimes be necessary. Other psychotherapies (e.g., psychoanalytic or psychodynamic psychotherapy) may be effective but are not proven to be so.

Brief primary care counseling can incorporate several of the therapeutic elements of effective psychotherapies. Although this counseling is not a definitive treatment for moderate or severe depression, it may be useful in milder depression or as an adjunct to pharmacotherapy delivered in primary care. Suggested elements of primary care counseling include the following:

- Encourage patients to schedule relaxing or enjoyable activities every day.
- Identify and challenge patients' exaggerated negative or self-critical thoughts.
- Break patients' current life problems into smaller components and identify specific steps for addressing them.

Self-help manuals (see References) provide clear guidance in these techniques.

Follow-Up. Psychiatric consultation is indicated for depression that is unimproved after 6 to 8 weeks of appropriate treatment. Development of significant suicide risk, psychosis, or mania during treatment should also prompt referral. When effective, tricyclic antidepressants should be continued for at least 6 months. Many patients can then taper medication over 4 to 6 weeks with low probability of relapse. Recurrence of depression should prompt resumption of an antidepressant for another 3 to 6 months before another attempted taper of dosage. When tapering antidepressants, the patient should be advised of warning signs of relapse. For patients at high risk of relapse (three or more significant episodes of depression in 5 years), longer-term treatment is recommended. Although cognitive-behavioral techniques are especially helpful in preventing relapse of depression, continued practice is essential.

REFERENCES

1. Burns DD. The Feeling Good Handbook. New York, Plume Press, 1989.

   This is an excellent guidebook for self-treatment of depression using cognitive techniques.

2. Depression Guideline Panel. Depression in Primary Care: Volume 2. Treatment of Major Depression. Clinical Practice Guideline, No. 5. Rockville, MD, US Department of Health and Human Services, Public Health Service, Agency for Health Care Policy and Research. AHCPR publication No. 93-0551. April 1993.

   A thorough review of relevant literature is accompanied by recommendations for primary care practice. Findings are summarized in the companion Quick Reference Guide for Clinicians. Both publications are available from AHCPR at 800-358-9295.

3. Lazarus A. I Can If I Want To. New York, William Morrow & Co, 1992.

   This is a good, brief self-help handbook based on behavioral and cognitive techniques.

190 Psychosis

Problem

GREGORY E. SIMON

Epidemiology. Schizophrenia and the affective psychoses (bipolar disorder and related disorders) have a combined prevalence in the community of 1% to 2%. The average prevalence among medical clinic patients is probably four to five times as high, but rates vary widely according to the type of medical practice. It is much higher in emergency departments or clinics serving socioeconomically disadvantaged populations and lower among more privileged groups. Schizophrenia and related disorders are characterized by psychotic symptoms, impairment of overall function, chronicity, and absence of prominent fluctuations in mood. Affective psychoses typically present with episodes of depression and mania occurring in varying patterns accompanied by varying levels of psychotic symptoms. In practice, the boundaries between schizophrenia and bipolar disorder (in presentation, course, and treatment response) are blurred.

Symptoms and Signs

HALLUCINATIONS. False perceptions are most often auditory but may affect any sensory mode. Visual or auditory hallucinations should raise suspicion regarding an "organic" cause (e.g., intoxication, delirium, atypical seizure disorder).

DELUSIONS. Fixed false beliefs are inconsistent with the patient's cultural and social network. These are typically impervious to evidence and argument. Delusions often concern paranoid suspicions or bizarre communications (e.g., mind reading).

DISTURBED AFFECT. Expressed emotion may be exaggerated, may be constricted, or may appear inappropriate to the situation (e.g., apparently lighthearted discussions of murder or suicide).

THOUGHT DISORDER. Thought and speech may be accelerated or slowed. Connections between thoughts may be loosened, bizarre, or nonexistent.

Clinical Approach. Psychotic disorders are typically chronic, episodic illnesses; history (from patient, records, or other contacts) is critical. "Functional" psychotic disorders (schizophrenia and affective psychoses) cannot be reliably distinguished from organic psychoses (e.g., intoxication, encephalitis) on the basis of acute clinical presentation. Prior history of psychosis makes undiagnosed medical cause of psychotic symptoms less likely, but exacerbations of chronic psychosis may be precipitated by intercurrent medical illness or drug intoxication or withdrawal. In addition, patients with chronic psychotic disorders have high rates of undiagnosed medical illness because of their poor self-care, disorganized lifestyle, impaired communication, and concomitant substance abuse. Consequently, any psychotic presentation requires a reasonable

649

evaluation for drug intoxication or withdrawal or for precipitating medical illness.

Characteristics of the acute presentation also do not discriminate between schizophrenia and bipolar disorder because presenting symptoms may be identical. This distinction, however, is more important to long-term than to acute management.

Initial evaluation should focus on the patients' level of threat to themselves or to others and on the ability to provide for their daily needs. Evaluation of dangerousness includes questioning patients directly about current urges to harm themselves or others, current plan or intent to do so, and previous history of violence. Evaluation of self-care includes observation of a patient's current state (e.g., hygiene, nutrition) and investigation of available family and community supports. Patients who are unable to care for themselves or who pose a significant threat of violence should be hospitalized. Laws regarding criteria for involuntary psychiatric treatment vary by state, but most apply a standard consistent with this approach.

Management. Management of acute psychotic episodes should focus on safety and stabilization. Antipsychotic agents (Table 190–1) are usually effective in reducing agitation, hallucinations, and delusions. They are usually less effective in reducing withdrawal, disorganization of thought, and disturbance of emotional expression. The lowest effective dose should be prescribed. Benzodiazepines (e.g., lorazepam, 1–2 mg orally or intramuscularly) may be useful adjuncts to antipsychotic treatment in acute management. Delusions and hallucinations are by nature impervious to argument. Often it is best to "agree to disagree"—tell the patient that although you appreciate how firmly he believes what he thinks (sees, hears, etc.), you do not agree. Explain that you will continue to care for him as best as you can despite this disagreement. Family members and friends will need support and advice.

Traditional antipsychotics (i.e., neuroleptics) appear equal in effectiveness when given in equivalent doses (see Table 190–1). More potent drugs usually

Table 190–1. SELECTED ANTIPSYCHOTIC DRUGS

Drug	Initial Dose	Maximal Dose*	Sedation†	Extrapyramidal Symptoms†	Cost ($ per Month)‡
Haloperidol (Haldol)	2 mg bid	5 mg qid	+	+ + + +	21.60
Thiothixene (Navane)	5 mg bid	10 mg qid	+	+ + +	22.80
Perphenazine (Trilafon)	8 mg bid	24 mg qid	+ +	+ +	39.60
Chlorpromazine (Thorazine)	100 mg bid	200 mg tid	+ + + +	+	6.60
Thioridazine (Mellaril)	100 mg bid	200 mg tid	+ + + +	+	12.60
Risperidone (Risperdal)	1 mg bid	3 mg bid	+	+	114.00

*Seek consultation if no response.
†Severity ranges from mild and infrequent (+) to profound and common.
‡Generic prices used, where available; average wholesale price for 30-day supply of initial dose.
1996 *Drug Topics Red Book.*

cause less sedation, postural hypotension, and anticholinergic effect at the expense of greater tendency to cause extrapyramidal side effects. Acute treatment should begin with the doses listed, with an increase after 24 to 48 hours if no improvement is evident. Doses of less potent drugs may be limited by sedation and hypotension. Psychiatric consultation should be sought if response is not rapid. Common extrapyramidal effects include acute spasms or dystonia (often involving the tongue, neck, or face), drug-induced parkinsonism, and akathisia (irresistible motor restlessness). Young males appear at highest risk for these complications. Use of prophylactic antiparkinsonian agents is controversial but is often unnecessary with less potent antipsychotics or with lower-risk patients (older or female). Typical antiparkinsonian regimens used prophylactically or therapeutically (after emergence of side effects) include benztropine (Cogentin), 0.5 to 1.0 mg twice daily; trihexyphenidyl (Artane), 1 to 2 mg twice daily; or amantadine (Symmetrel), 100 mg up to twice daily.

Newer antipsychotic agents will probably be prescribed more frequently during the late 1990s. Clozapine, the first "atypical" antipsychotic drug, appears to carry little risk of tardive dyskinesia and may be more effective against symptoms of disorganization and withdrawal ("negative" symptoms). Because it carries significant expense and risk of agranulocytosis (and requires weekly monitoring for hematologic toxicity), it is not a first-line treatment. Risperidone has fewer motor side effects than traditional antipsychotic drugs and may produce greater relief of negative symptoms.

Follow-Up. Long-term management should focus on treatment adherence and rehabilitation. Continued use of antipsychotics raises questions about alternative maintenance treatments (e.g., lithium, antidepressants) as well as risks (especially tardive dyskinesia). Psychiatric consultation should be obtained soon after beginning acute treatment. The guiding principle for continued antipsychotic use is to seek the lowest effective dose. Medication should be continued for at least 4 months after resolution of a first episode of psychosis and longer after any subsequent episode. Patients and families should be advised about the high risk of relapse after premature discontinuation. Patients should be encouraged to function at the highest level that is realistic. Family support organizations (e.g., state chapters of the Alliance for the Mentally Ill) are an important resource.

Cross-References: Diagnosis and Management of Drug Abuse (Chapter 9), Alcohol Problems (Chapter 10), Dementia (Chapter 140), Alcohol Withdrawal (Chapter 142), Management of Depression (Chapter 189), The Difficult Patient (Chapter 192).

REFERENCES

1. Gelenberg AJ. Psychoses. In Bassuk EL, Schoonover SC, Gelenberg AJ, eds. Practitioner's Guide to Psychoactive Drugs. Plenum, New York, 1984.

   This is a good guide to medication selection and side effects.

2. Hyman SE. Acute psychosis. In Hyman SE, ed. Manual of Psychiatric Emergencies. Little, Brown, Boston, 1984.

   This is a concise discussion of emergency evaluation and management.

191 Panic Disorder

Problem

GREGORY E. SIMON

Epidemiology. Panic disorder has a point prevalence of 0.5% among community residents, with a prevalence at least 10 times higher in most medical clinics. Panic disorder is two to three times more prevalent in females, with greatest onset in early adulthood. Because of associated physical symptoms, patients with panic disorder often present in emergency departments as well as in cardiology, neurology, and otolaryngology clinics. Panic disorder often follows an episodic course with symptomatic recurrences precipitated by periods of life stress.

Symptoms and Signs. Panic disorder presents as discrete, unprovoked attacks of fear or discomfort accompanied by various physical symptoms (dyspnea, palpitations, dizziness, tremors, sweating, choking, nausea, paresthesias, chest pain). Either fear or physical symptoms may be most prominent, but questioning usually reveals both. Some physical symptoms of panic (dyspnea, dizziness, palpitations) appear to be mediated by acute hyperventilation. The panic syndrome varies in severity from rare, isolated panic attacks to severe daily attacks with completely disabling phobic fear. Panic attacks are often accompanied by depression and phobic anxiety (especially phobias of crowds, open spaces, waiting in lines, and leaving home alone).

Clinical Approach. Recognition may be difficult because physical symptoms of panic disorder often focus attention (both patients' and doctors') on serious, urgent medical problems. Because panic attacks can be an overwhelmingly powerful stimulus to focus on physical symptoms and disease fears, patients often insistently demand diagnostic testing. Symptoms of panic may resemble symptoms of almost any paroxysmal neurologic or cardiovascular event including angina, pulmonary embolus, arrhythmia, transient ischemic attack, presyncope, or seizure. This does not imply that clinicians should rule out each of these disorders before considering the diagnosis of panic but means that panic disorder should be considered when any of these medical diagnoses are entertained. Among young healthy patients (especially female), the prior probability of panic disorder far exceeds that of malignant arrhythmia or angina. Alcohol withdrawal may also cause attacks of anxiety with associated physical symptoms. In these cases, the initial step should be treatment of the primary alcohol problem.

Management. The intense focus on physical symptoms and medical illness accompanying panic attacks often poses problems for medical providers. Recurrent panic symptoms can rapidly reverse the most careful reassurance and education. Relief of anxiety symptoms offers the best reassurance that no serious undiagnosed medical condition exists.

Cognitive and behavioral techniques (discussed in Chapter 186, General-ized Anxiety) can be very effective in reducing panic symptoms and limiting phobic avoidance. There are simple techniques for "talking through" panic attacks. Patients can remind themselves: "I've been through this many times. It's terribly unpleasant, but it's not dangerous. Although it may seem like forever, it will be better in 15 to 20 minutes." The most important educational message is that avoidance of feared situations reinforces anxiety. Actively con-fronting feared situations (as difficult as that seems) will significantly reduce anxiety symptoms. Good self-help manuals are available (see References). Some panic patients may feel more anxious with breathing or relaxation exercises, so be alert for this paradoxic response.

Both anxiolytic and antidepressant medications are effective in treatment of panic attacks. Anxiolytics offer more immediate relief but carry risks of tolerance and dependence. Patients with rare and uncomplicated attacks or patients unwilling to take scheduled daily medication may be treated with low-dose anxiolytics alone. Higher-potency benzodiazepines may have greater efficacy against panic. Good choices are lorazepam, 0.5 to 1.0 mg up to four times a day (rapid onset, intermediate duration, lowest cost); alprazolam, 0.25 to 0.5 mg up to three times a day (rapid onset, short duration, greater rebound anxiety); or clonazepam, 0.5 to 1.0 mg twice daily (more steady effect but onset too slow for as-needed use). Patients with panic accompanied by depression often respond poorly to anxiolytics alone. These patients with associated depres-sion and others not responding to the anxiolytic doses just listed may require antidepressant treatment. Imipramine is the traditional choice, but all tricyclic antidepressants appear equally effective. Serotonin reuptake inhibitors (fluoxe-tine, sertraline, paroxetine, fluvoxamine) are probably equal to tricyclic antide-pressants. Monoamine oxidase inhibitors may be more effective than tricyclic antidepressants, but risk and inconvenience make these second-line agents in primary care. See Chapter 189, Management of Depression, for guidance on prescribing antidepressants. Initial dosing should be lower than that for depression, and panic disorder may respond to lower doses. Some patients with panic disorder may experience transient increase in agitation or anxiety on starting antidepressants. When this occurs, the usual dosing schedule should be reduced to allow accommodation, and patients should be reassured that this response usually indicates eventual benefit.

Ingrained phobic avoidance may persist even after panic attacks have resolved. These patients will benefit from the behavioral programs for phobia described in Chapter 186 and described in available self-help manuals (see References).

Follow-Up. Psychiatric consultation should be arranged for patients unrespon-sive to the standard treatments just discussed. Patients who respond can usually taper antidepressant medication after 3 to 4 months, although rarer cases may require longer-term treatment. Even for those who respond, panic disorder is often a chronic remitting and relapsing condition. Cognitive and behavioral strategies provide some prophylactic benefit; the patient must be encouraged to continue to practice these strategies. Continued discussion may help avoid exhaustive medical evaluation if anxiety symptoms recur.

Cross-References: Alcohol Problems (Chapter 10), Dyspnea (Chapter 19), Diz-ziness (Chapter 20), Recurrent Chest Pain (Chapter 74), Syncope (Chapter

75), Palpitations (Chapter 76), Dyspepsia (Chapter 95), Tremor (Chapter 136), Alcohol Withdrawal (Chapter 142), Common Thyroid Disorders (Chapter 153), Generalized Anxiety (Chapter 186), Hyperventilation Syndrome (Chapter 194).

REFERENCES

1. Barlow DH, Craske M. Mastery of Your Anxiety and Panic. Albany, NY, Graywind Publications, 1994.

   The authors present an excellent self-help workbook for managing panic attacks and overcoming phobic avoidance.

2. Weekes C. Peace from Nervous Suffering. New York, Bantam Books, 1972.

   This is an excellent self-help manual for treatment of panic attacks and phobias.

. . . .

192 The Difficult Patient

Problem

GREGORY E. SIMON

Symptoms and Signs. Even the most caring and courteous clinicians will experience troubling and unproductive doctor–patient relationships. Although the resulting conflict and disappointment often lead to accusations from both parties, these difficult situations are almost never the result of malice or bad intentions. Doctors and patients usually come together with a shared purpose, mutual trust, and a desire for understanding. When attempts to form a working partnership fail, the clinician must draw on that original trust and good will.

Certain patients have difficulty with practically every provider they see and may experience similar problems in other important interpersonal relationships. These patients often suffer from chronic emotional distress compounded by coping strategies that lead to interpersonal conflict. The hope and authority attached to health care providers can make provider–patient relationships both more powerful and unsettling. For example, a seriously ill patient caught between fear of life-threatening complications and the desire to lead a normal life might try to relieve his or her internal conflict by creating an external one. By acting irresponsibly, he or she might steer a physician into the role of guardian and disciplinarian. This polarization might culminate in an angry conflict in which the patient complains of being treated like a child. This process through which internal distress emerges as interpersonal conflict is characteristic of many difficult patients. The harried physician must recall that these patients are usually just doing the best they can with a difficult situation.

Other doctor–patient difficulties are more idiosyncratic; a particular doctor and patient may have conflicting styles. Most clinicians learn that certain types of patients may be personally difficult. Some physicians are irritated by patients desiring a high level of authority and control, whereas others may be put off by patients who ask for extra reassurance and support. These preferences are no indication of pathologic or psychological difficulty; they simply represent the vagaries of human personality. Early recognition of this pattern can substitute understanding for personal conflict.

When the clinical relationship turns sour, both providers and patients often feel hurt. Discussion shifts from shared attempts at understanding and managing health problems to increasing conflict over authority and support. Physicians find themselves more concerned with their personal adequacy than with medical diagnosis and management. Patients speak more of their dissatisfaction with care than the health concerns that brought them in. The initial complaint can be easily obscured by these recriminations. Physicians may be troubled by unusually strong personal reactions or find themselves straying into unusual patterns of practice (either overly solicitous or unreasonably withholding). This pattern of increasingly personalized interaction (focus on personal conflict, feelings of inadequacy, "special" types of care) should serve as an early warning of trouble ahead.

Clinical Approach. Breakdowns in doctor–patient relationships often result when patients' usual ways of coping are inadequate to manage personal distress. For some patients, this appears to be a chronic condition. For others, coping mechanisms are temporarily overwhelmed when internal stress rises above a manageable level or when personal resources are weakened. Various life stresses can upset this balance, transforming a stressed patient into a difficult one. Because adequate cognitive function is required to effectively manage emotional and interpersonal affairs, any cognitive impairment may precipitate a decompensation. Alcohol or drug intoxication may be the most striking example of transient impairment of interpersonal function. Dementing illness may first manifest as personality change and irritability. Medical illness may cause decompensation by both increasing level of stress and impairing ability to cope. The physician confronted with a difficult patient should try to determine what acute stressful events or insults to coping might contribute to this decompensation. Shifting the focus from personal conflict to the causes of coping failure may help restore mutual trust and cooperation.

Management. Just as difficult doctor–patient relationships suffer from a high degree of personalization, rebuilding those relationships must shift attention away from personal conflict, blame, and feelings of inadequacy. The clinician must first decide that the patient is neither malicious nor defective and then proceed to examine the causes of the conflict. The following are a few practical suggestions.

An intellectual understanding of breakdowns in the doctor–patient relationship may be helpful to the clinician, but it is usually not helpful to the patient. For example, a provider may come to understand that a patient's angry demands for unnecessary diagnostic tests arise from a fear that his or her chest pain is not being taken seriously. A frightened and angry patient, however, will find little comfort in this neat explanation. This understanding, though, will help the clinician to offer the right kind of reassurance. Instead of focusing on the expense, risk, and low yield of the requested diagnostic tests, the provider would express concern about the pain and discuss strategies to relieve it.

The clinician should try to recall a sense of shared purpose by returning to the patient's original concern. In the midst of a conflict in which the physician is portrayed as cruel and heartless and the patient as unreasonably demanding, the original goal of the visit may be lost. All encounters begin with a common purpose: to understand and relieve suffering. It may be helpful to say, "I am concerned that we haven't made much progress helping you with the pain you came here about. Maybe we should go back and work on that again."

It is essential to clarify mutual expectations. Unreasonable expectations often fade when assurances of reasonable care are given. For example, a patient who angrily demands unlimited access may calm considerably when offered clear reassurance that calls will be returned and urgent problems dealt with appropriately. Conversely, a clinician may be less angry with a noncompliant patient after negotiating an agreement about managing at least part of a complex medical regimen.

Conflict over clinically unimportant issues should be avoided. Misplaced hostility can lead to escalating struggles over surprisingly insignificant questions. Disagreement is worthwhile for substantive questions (e.g., chronic use of anxiolytics in a patient with active alcohol abuse), but providers should avoid large struggles over small differences (e.g., a 3-week prescription for anxiolytics instead of only a 2-week prescription).

Increasing a patient's fear or anxiety is almost never helpful. For example, a patient with chest pain in an emergency department who adamantly refuses a necessary intensive care admission is probably too frightened to acknowledge the real threat he or she faces. Emphasizing the risk of death is not likely to change his or her mind. Instead, one should focus on how hospitalization would more rapidly relieve the patient's discomfort and speed his or her recovery.

Setting limits is often necessary but is rarely effective when done in anger. For example, a patient taking narcotics for chronic pain who repeatedly reports losing the prescription and requests early refills may engender a sense of mistrust and irritation. After granting this request several times, a clinician might angrily refuse to prescribe any more narcotics, provoking a confrontation. This might be avoided by setting explicit limits before mounting irritation prompts a sudden shift in care. After the first lost prescription, the patient should be given a refill and told that future prescriptions will have to last for the expected period without exception.

If multiple providers are involved, explicit communication is essential. Any inconsistencies among providers may lead to triangulation (frequently known as "splitting"). Providers often view these interactions as patients' conscious and malicious attempts to divide and conquer. In fact, frightened patients more often feel unsettled by perceived inconsistency and uncertainty. "Splitting" behavior is one way of testing providers' confidence. Communication and consistency can have a settling effect.

Clinicians should remember that idealization and devaluation are two sides of the same coin. A patient who lavishes unreasonable praise on a new physician while vilifying all previous ones will become dissatisfied soon enough. The clinician can best deal with the criticism by acknowledging the patient's disappointment and restating a commitment to providing good care.

On rare occasions, a doctor–patient relationship may fail. A provider and patient may be unable to negotiate a working agreement for continued care. Such a decision should be openly discussed and mutually agreed upon. Avoidance of open disagreement through referral or rejection only reinforces a pattern of disappointment and hostility.

Follow-Up. To a busy primary care physician, energy spent on interpersonal negotiations can seem wasted, a distraction from the supposedly more important issues of diagnosis and treatment. Effective care of distressed patients, however, requires a working doctor–patient relationship. Progress is slow, but meaningful. Maintaining a long-term relationship with a calm and tolerant physician has great therapeutic power. Primary care physicians are uniquely suited to this task.

Cross-References: Effective Communication in the Ambulatory Care Setting (Chapter 2), Diagnosis and Management of Drug Abuse (Chapter 9), Alcohol Problems (Chapter 10), Chronic Nonspecific Pain Syndrome (Chapter 14), Fatigue (Chapter 21), Dementia (Chapter 140), Generalized Anxiety (Chapter 186), Somatization (Chapter 188), Psychosis (Chapter 190).

REFERENCES

1. Groves JE. Taking care of the hateful patient. N Engl J Med 1978;298:883–887.

   This is a classic paper with much practical wisdom.

2. Quill TE. Partnerships in patient care: A contractual approach. Ann Intern Med 1983;98:228–234.

   The author provides an excellent model for building constructive relationships with trying patients.

3. Stoudemire A, Thompson TL. The borderline personality in the medical setting. Ann Intern Med 1982;96:76–79.

   Problems in the care of this most difficult group of patients are described and useful guidelines are offered for inpatient and outpatient medical care.

193 Psychological Assessment

Procedure

EDMUND CHANEY and DIANE GREENBERG

Indications and Contraindications. Psychological assessment is useful in the following situations:

1. When the physician suspects the presence of a psychological condition such as depression, anxiety, or post-traumatic stress that might interfere with a treatment regimen, interact with a disease process, or affect the physician–patient relationship.
2. To evaluate cognitive, affective, and adaptive functioning in patients who have known or suspected cognitive impairment (e.g., memory impairment or cognitive disturbance after head injury or stroke).
3. To provide psychosocial information to guide the physician in counseling to assist in motivating the patient to change toward a more healthy lifestyle.
4. To assist the physician in working with difficult patients.

Rationale. Patients often present with somatic symptoms that may be related in some way to stress, lifestyle, or relationship issues or to more enduring psychological problems, such as mood disorder, personality disturbances, substance use, domestic violence, sexual or physical assault or abuse history, sexual dysfunction, thought disorder, or cognitive changes. Recognition of these problems may be critical in choosing the best treatment course and in supporting patient adherence. If there are high rates of occurrence of specific psychological problems such as substance abuse or depression in the physician's practice, routine preliminary psychological assessment should be considered. In many cases, once relevant psychosocial issues have been identified, the primary care physician can provide the treatment. For more complex or refractory problems, psychological assessment information is helpful in making the appropriate referral for specialized treatment. Structured, quantitative psychological assessment instruments are accurate and time-efficient techniques for gathering information to improve the diagnostic and therapeutic process. Results can be compared with appropriate normative groups, often matched for age, sex, ethnicity, education level, and illness. Some instruments, designed for repeated administration, can identify subtle changes over time.

Methods. Different methods of psychological assessment should be used for preliminary and in-depth evaluation. For preliminary or screening evaluation, paper and pencil instruments can often be introduced and administered by physician support staff in the waiting room (given sufficient privacy) or sent home with the patient for completion. An example of this type of instrument is the PRIME-MD, a 30-item self-report inventory to assess mood, anxiety,

All of the material in Chapter 193 is in the public domain, with the exception of any borrowed figures and tables.

somatoform, and alcohol disorders in the primary care setting. The instrument is congruent with the *Diagnostic and Statistical Manual of Mental Disorders (DSM-IV)* psychiatric diagnosis. Many other instruments are available. The choice of instrument should be guided by its reliability and validity for the intended use in the target population. If the patient's ability to give accurate information is in doubt, for example, when the physician suspects dementia, instruments designed to be completed by a relative are available.

Results of preliminary evaluation through interview, use of a screening instrument, or mental status examination may reveal the need for in-depth assessment of cognitive function, psychopathology, or both. Neuropsychological testing or psychopathology assessment using tests such as the classic Minnesota Multiphasic Personality Inventory (MMPI) or the Millon Clinical Multiaxial Inventory (MCMI) requires referral to a specialist trained in administration and interpretation. Neuropsychological testing measures receptive, expressive, memory, and problem-solving abilities in both verbal and visuospatial domains. Examples of specific areas that can be assessed are basic sensory-perceptual functioning (vision, hearing, tactile sense); motor and visuomotor abilities; attention; language; intelligence; achievement (reading, spelling, arithmetic); memory (learning and retention); abstract reasoning; and flexibility in thinking. Assessment of affect or personality can be directed and limited in scope, such as measuring symptoms of depression, or more lengthy and complex, such as trying to discriminate among the different personality disorders.

Cost and Complications. The cost of psychological assessment involves materials and labor. Materials not requiring expert administration range in cost from free to $50 per administration for some computer-scored instruments. Labor for specialist administration ranges from $100 to $200 an hour, with some comprehensive neuropsychological evaluations such as the Halstead-Reitan battery requiring up to 8 hours of administration time, plus scoring and interpretation time.

Potential complications primarily affect the physician–patient relationship. If not appropriately prepared for psychological assessment, particularly if by referral, the patient may infer that the clinician thinks his or her problem is "all in the head." Prolonged testing can be fatiguing. Even though physically noninvasive, psychological assessment can be perceived as emotionally intrusive. If not presented sensitively and confidentially, results can be perceived as stigmatizing by the patient.

Cross-References: Diagnosis and Management of Drug Abuse (Chapter 9), Alcohol Problems (Chapter 10), Chronic Nonspecific Pain Syndrome (Chapter 14), Dementia (Chapter 140), Screening for Depression (Chapter 185), Somatization (Chapter 188), The Difficult Patient (Chapter 192).

REFERENCES

1. Cushman LA, Scherer MJ. Psychological Assessment in Medical Rehabilitation. Washington, DC, American Psychological Association, 1995.

   The authors review psychological assessment of adults with chronic illnesses or disabilities.

2. Hahn SR, Thompson KS, Wills TA, Stern V, Budner NS. The difficult doctor–patient relationship: Somatization, personality and psychopathology. J Clin Epidemiol 1994;47:647–657.

The role of psychological assessment in understanding difficult physician–patient relationships is discussed.

3. Jamison RN, Rudy TE, Penzien DB, Mosley TH. Cognitive-behavioral classifications of chronic pain: Replication and extension of empirically derived patient profiles. Pain 1994;57:277–292.

The West Haven-Yale Multidimensional Pain Inventory (WHYMPI), a successor to the Minnesota Multiphasic Personality Inventory (MMPI), is useful in encouraging patients with chronic pain to consider lifestyle changes.

4. Lezak MD. Neuropsychological Assessment. New York, Oxford University Press, 1995.

The author comprehensively describes neuroanatomic correlates of behavior, neuropsychological assessment and interpretation, and most significant neuropsychological tests.

5. Spitzer RL, Williams JB, Kroenke K, Linzer M, deGruy FV III, Hahn SR, Brody D, Johnson JG. Utility of a new procedure for diagnosing mental disorders in primary care: The PRIME-MD 1000 study. JAMA 1994;272:1749–1756.

A self-report screening instrument is presented with a brief structured interview for the physician to use to obtain more detail on the issues raised by the screening instrument.

· ·

194 Hyperventilation Syndrome

Problem

ERIKA GOLDSTEIN

Epidemiology. *Hyperventilation syndrome* describes symptoms produced by ventilation in excess of metabolic requirements and excludes physiologic causes of hyperventilation (e.g., pneumonia, heart failure, metabolic acidosis). The incidence of hyperventilation syndrome in the general population reportedly varies between 6% and 11%, although in studies conducted in general medical clinics, up to 30% to 40% of patients have symptoms attributable to it. Most cases occur between ages 20 and 40 years, but hyperventilation syndrome can occur at any age and may be more common in women. The diagnosis of hyperventilation syndrome overlaps considerably with anxiety disorders, and their precise relationship is controversial.

Symptoms and Signs. Acute hyperventilation syndrome is rare (1% of cases) and is characterized by dramatic hyperpnea, anxiety, tetany, and carpopedal spasm. The chronic form is vastly more common (99% of cases) and is often misdiagnosed because the presenting symptoms may be referable to any organ system (Table 194–1). The breathing pattern often appears normal. Signs and symptoms result from metabolic derangements induced by hyperventilation and from anxiety. Most patients present with cardiovascular symptoms (52%) or neurologic symptoms (23%) rather than respiratory complaints (6%).

Clinical Approach. The diagnosis of hyperventilation syndrome relies on the exclusion of organic disease by history and physical examination and is con-

Table 194–1. HYPERVENTILATION SYNDROME: ASSOCIATED SIGNS AND SYMPTOMS

General	Cardiovascular
Irritability	Palpations
Weakness	Chest pain
Exhaustion	Tachycardia
Fatigue	Neurologic
Respiratory	Headache
Sighing and yawning	Dizziness
Shortness of breath	Lightheadedness
Air hunger	Numbness and tingling
Musculoskeletal	Unsteadiness
Arthralgia	Impaired memory/concentration
Tremors	Giddiness
Myalgia	Visual disturbances
Carpopedal spasm	Gastrointestinal
Tetany	Belching
Psychogenic	Flatulence
Apprehension	Dysphagia
Anxiety/panic	Dry mouth
Nervousness	Bloating
Tension	Abdominal distress
Sweating	Anorexia and/or nausea

From Brashear RE: Hyperventilation syndrome. Lung 1983;161:257–273.

firmed by performing a hyperventilation provocation test. A positive test is defined by reproduction of the patient's symptoms within 5 minutes while breathing deeply and rapidly (30–40 breaths/min). The test should be discontinued after 5 minutes or when the patient complains of dizziness. A blood gas determination to confirm hypocapnia is probably unnecessary. Once symptoms appear, rebreathing into a paper bag will terminate symptoms. Provocative testing is contraindicated in patients with chronic obstructive pulmonary disease, chronic hypercapnia, sickle cell anemia, or history of seizures or strokes. In patients with coronary artery disease or spasm, continuous electrocardiographic monitoring should accompany the test. Recently the use of the hyperventilation provocation test has been called into question by a double-blind, placebo-controlled study (see References).

Management. Seventy percent of patients improve dramatically after the relationship between symptoms and the metabolic derangements induced by hyperventilation is demonstrated by provocative testing and explained by the provider. Although rebreathing terminates symptoms acutely, it is not adequate long-term therapy. More effective are psychotherapy, behavior therapy, physical training to correct "bad breathing habits," and drug therapy. Pharmacologic therapies, in order of preference, include imipramine (25–150 mg/d) or other antidepressants, β-blockers (propranolol, 80 mg/d), monoamine oxidase inhibitors (phenelzine, 45–90 mg/d in three divided doses), and benzodiazepines (to be used only for limited periods of time).

Follow-Up. If symptoms resolve after provocative testing and patient education alone, no further follow-up is needed. Psychiatric consultation may be necessary when there is a coexistent anxiety disorder or when psychotherapy, behavior therapy, or assistance with pharmacologic management is required.

Cross-References: Dyspnea (Chapter 19), Dizziness (Chapter 20), Pleuritic Chest Pain (Chapter 61), Syncope (Chapter 75), Palpitations (Chapter 76), Headache (Chapter 138), Screening for Depression (Chapter 185), Generalized Anxiety (Chapter 186), Panic Disorder (Chapter 191).

REFERENCES

1. Cowley DS, Roy-Byrne PP. Hyperventilation and panic disorder. Am J Med 1987;83:929–937.

   This article discusses the relationship of these disorders.

2. Evans RW. Neurologic aspects of hyperventilation syndrome. Semin Neurol 1995;15:115–125.

   The author focuses on neurologic symptoms and signs and includes a very good patient handout.

3. Gardner WN. The pathophysiology of hyperventilation disorders. Chest 1996;109:516–534.

   This is a review with emphasis on the etiology and pathophysiology in relation to signs and symptoms.

4. Hornsveld HK, Garssen B. Fiedeldij Dop MJC, van Spiegel PI, de Haes JCJM. Double-blind placebo-controlled study of the hyperventilation provocation test and the validity of the hyperventilation syndrome. Lancet 1996;348:154–158.

   This article raises questions about the use of the hyperventilation provocation test in diagnosis with implications for our understanding of pathophysiology.

5. Magarian GJ. Hyperventilation syndromes: Infrequently recognized common expressions of anxiety and stress. Medicine 1982;61:219–236.

   This is an excellent review with a particularly good discussion of management issues.

SECTION XVII
Hematologic Disorders

195 Bleeding

Symptom

GERALD J. ROTH

Epidemiology. Bleeding may result from abnormalities of the hemostatic system (platelets, plasma coagulation) or occur after trauma or surgery in patients with normal hemostasis. Hemostatic disorders affect an estimated 30 to 50 individuals per 100,000 in the general population.

Etiology. Hemostasis (Gr. *hemo*, "blood"; *stasis*, "stopping") involves the blood itself, blood flow, and blood vessels (Virchow's triad), but most bleeding problems involve the blood alone, specifically platelets, plasma coagulation, or both.

PLATELETS. Platelet disorders, either quantitative (thrombocytopenia) or qualitative (functional) defects, result in mucocutaneous bleeding: blood loss through the skin (bruising) or mucous membranes (epistaxis, menorrhagia). Thrombocytopenia (platelet count < 150,000/mm³) commonly results from bone marrow and megakaryocyte suppression due to malignancy (i.e., leukemia) or medications such as chemotherapeutic agents. It also occurs when the life span of circulating platelets (normally 10 days) is shortened by premature destruction by agents such as antiplatelet antibodies (idiopathic thrombocytopenic purpura). Platelet function defects are caused by disorders such as von Willebrand's disease or aspirin ingestion and are marked by an inability of platelets to aggregate or secrete normally.

PLASMA COAGULATION. Both congenital (e.g., hemophilia) and acquired (e.g., ingestion of anticoagulants such as warfarin) disorders can affect the plasma coagulation system. The resultant bleeding is characteristically visceral (muscular) or within joints (hemarthrosis).

DISSEMINATED INTRAVASCULAR COAGULATION. Serious systemic illness, particularly gram-negative sepsis, can activate the hemostatic system and lead to consumption of both platelets and plasma coagulation factors. The resultant bleeding disorder includes features of thrombocytopenia and coagulation factor deficiency.

Clinical Approach. The patient interview should focus on the patient's response to prior hemostatic challenges (surgery, trauma, tooth extraction), drug ingestion (particularly aspirin), family history, and associated diseases that

**Table 195–1. CLINICAL FEATURES OF PLATELET
DISORDERS AND PLASMA COAGULATION DEFECTS**

Clinical Feature	Platelet Disorders	Plasma Coagulation Defects
Type of bleeding	Mucocutaneous	Visceral/joint
Onset of bleeding (after trauma, surgery)	Immediate	Delayed
Sex predominance	Females	Males
Family history	Often negative	Often positive

could impair hemostasis (e.g., uremia or lupus erythematosus). The physical examination determines the extent of bruising, the presence of petechiae, the presence of joint deformity, or evidence of associated diseases such as chronic liver disease. This initial assessment indicates the severity of the defect and suggests whether platelets or plasma coagulation factors are responsible (Table 195–1).

Simple, inexpensive laboratory tests should precede more specific, elaborate testing. For example, if the history and physical examination suggest a platelet disorder, a platelet count should be performed; if the count is normal, a bleeding time should be used to assess platelet function. Subsequent workup may include platelet aggregometry to detect a defect in platelet aggregation or secretion. For plasma coagulation, the activated partial thromboplastin time is used to measure the intrinsic system of coagulation (factors XII, XI, IX, VIII, X, V, II), and the prothrombin time screens the extrinsic factors (factors X, VII, V, II). Additional tests, such as specific factor assays, thrombin time, fibrinogen level, and tests for fibrin or fibrinogen degradation products, may be necessary for a more specific diagnosis.

Management. Management of bleeding disorders requires an accurate diagnosis so that therapy can be directed toward a specific abnormality. Examples are platelet transfusion for thrombocytopenia due to inadequate platelet production and specific factor replacement in hemophilia A (factor VIII deficiency) or Christmas disease (factor IX deficiency).

Cross-References: Epistaxis (Chapter 55), Hemoptysis (Chapter 62), Abnormal Uterine Bleeding (Chapter 159), Thrombocytopenia (Chapter 197), Transfusion Therapy (Chapter 202), Preoperative Hematologic Problems (Chapter 219).

REFERENCES

1. Bachmann F. Diagnostic approach to mild bleeding disorders. Semin Hematol 1980;17:292–305.

   A review of the epidemiology of mild bleeding disorders in a well-defined population as assessed by a single coagulation laboratory.

2. Berchtold P, McMillan R. Therapy of chronic idiopathic thrombocytopenic purpura in adults. Blood 1989;74:2309–2317.

   This article is a review of modern management of a common cause of bleeding in adults.

3. Rapaport SI. Introduction to Hematology, 2nd ed. Philadelphia, JB Lippincott, 1987:432–577.

The author presents a concise and lucid discussion of hemostatic mechanisms, common bleeding disorders, and an approach to the evaluation of the bleeding patient.

4. Rapaport SI. Preoperative hemostatic evaluation: Which tests if any? Blood 1983;61:229–231.

An exceptionally practical and pointed discussion is presented of how to estimate and evaluate a patient for bleeding risk before surgery.

5. Roth GJ, Calverley DC. Aspirin, platelets and thrombosis: Theory and practice. Blood 1994;83:885–898.

The mechanism of aspirin's effect on normal hemostasis is reviewed and a discussion is presented of the use of low-dose oral aspirin (100 mg/d) to prevent thrombosis.

196 Lymphadenopathy

Symptom

DAVID C. DALE

Epidemiology. *Lymphadenopathy* or *adenopathy* is a general term for any infectious, inflammatory, or malignant disease involving lymph nodes. Usually lymphadenopathy causes lymph node enlargement and is reactive, occurring because a person has been exposed to new antigens. Children have lymphadenopathy more often than adults, because of both the lack of previous exposures and the more rapid proliferative responses of lymphoid cells in young individuals. With a careful examination, almost all children younger than age 12 years have palpable cervical, axillary, and inguinal lymph nodes. Cervical adenopathy can be detected in about 50% of persons between ages 20 and 50 years; it tends to decline thereafter. Prominent cervical, axillary, or inguinal adenopathy is uncommon in older adults in the absence of a significant underlying disease. However, mild bilateral inguinal adenopathy (i.e., a few discrete, nontender nodes in both groins) is common throughout life.

Individual lymph nodes normally vary from a few cubic millimeters to 2 cm^2. When lymphadenopathy occurs, it is often both the enlarged node and inflammation in surrounding tissues that is palpable.

Etiology. Lymphadenopathy occurs worldwide; its causes follow somewhat distinctive geographic and age-specific patterns. Upper respiratory tract infections and oral and peridontal inflammation are the most common causes for cervical lymphadenopathy. In young adults, cervical lymphadenopathy with pharyngitis and constitutional symptoms suggests infectious mononucleosis. Prominent inguinal adenopathy prompts consideration of sexually transmitted diseases. Generalized lymphadenopathy in sexually active persons may suggest the acute phase of human immunodeficiency virus infection or secondary syphilis. In areas with endemic parasitic infections (e.g., filariasis and trypanosomiasis), these causes should be considered. In older adults, enlarging lymph nodes suggest a malignant process.

The causes of lymphadenopathy are outlined in Table 196–1, including notations of the most frequent causes for a general medical practice in the United States. Frequently, patients recognize their own lymphadenopathy, especially when it occurs acutely, as with most infections, drug reactions, cutaneous injuries, bites, and stings. In the other disorders, when the onset is insidious and the nodes are nontender, the patient may not notice them.

Clinical Approach. Because there are so many causes of lymphadenopathy, the clinical evaluation should always be conducted in stages, tailoring the evaluation to the clinical and epidemiologic circumstances. The time of onset of lymph node enlargement, associated symptoms, and evidence for contiguous inflammation (e.g., pharyngitis, cutaneous abrasions, ulcers, lymphangitis) should be noted. Lymphadenopathy is usually attributable to a regional viral or bacterial

Table 196–1. CAUSES OF LYMPHADENOPATHY

Infections

Bacterial: Group A and other streptococci,* *Staphylococcus aureus,** syphilis,*† cat-scratch
  disease,* oral/dental infections (anaerobic streptococci and other mouth anaerobes*),
  Mycobacterium tuberculosis and other mycobacteria,† brucellosis,† leptospirosis,† mellioidosis,†
  chancroid, plague, tularemia, rat-bite fever
Viral: Adenovirus,* immunodeficiency virus (HIV),*† infectious mononucleosis,*† herpes simplex,*
  measles,† rubella,† cytomegalovirus,† hepatitis,† Kawasaki disease
Mycotic: Sporotrichosis, histoplasmosis,† coccidioidomycosis†
Rickettsial: Rocky Mountain spotted fever,*† scrub typhus†
Chlamydial: Chlamydia trachomatis, lymphogranuloma venereum
Protozoan: Toxoplasmosis,† trypanosomiasis,† kala-azar†
Helminthic: Filariasis,† onchocerciasis

Immunologic

Stings and bites*
Drug reactions*†: phenytoin, hydralazine
Serum sickness*†
Collagen vascular diseases: Rheumatoid arthritis,† dermatomyositis,† angioimmunoblastic
  lymphadenopathy†

Malignancies

Hematologic: Hodgkin's disease,* acute leukemia,† chronic lymphocytic leukemia,† chronic
  myelogenous leukemia,† lymphoma,† myelofibrosis†
Other: Metastatic carcinoma, sarcomas

Endocrine Diseases

Hyperthyroidism†

Histiocytic Disorders

Lipid storage disease,† malignant histiocytosis,† Langerhans' (eosinophilic) histiocytosis

Miscellaneous

Sarcoidosis, amyloidosis,† chronic granulomatous disease, lymphomatoid granulomatosis,
  necrotizing lymphadenitis

*Most common causes in general practice in the United States.
†Usually causes generalized lymphadenopathy.

infection. When such a cause is not readily apparent, a more detailed history, including drug exposures, sexual activity, travel, work, and hobbies, is important.

With the initial examination, the clinician should carefully record the characteristics of the lymphadenopathy: location; size; tender or nontender; discrete or matted together; and hard, soft, or fluctuant. Many soft, tender, discrete nodes suggest a reactive process. Predominantly regional or asymmetric enlargement suggests a localized inflammatory process, although this pattern is also the most frequent presentation of Hodgkin's disease. Very tender, enlarged, and fluctuant nodes may have central necrosis, a finding in some severe bacterial infections such as tularemia. Discrete rubbery lymph nodes are common in chronic lymphocytic leukemia and the lymphomas. Discrete, asymmetric, hard lymph nodes suggest a metastatic malignancy.

During the rest of the physical examination, particular attention should be paid to the skin (rashes, pustules, ulcers, erythema nodosum), eyes (conjunctivitis, iritis), throat (redness, exudate), ears (otitis externa or media, mastoiditis), chest (rales, dullness), heart (murmurs), abdomen (hepatic or splenic enlargement, stool for occult blood), and extremities (bone tenderness, local swelling or pain). In obscure cases, the diagnosis is found only after repeated examinations.

When acute lymphadenopathy is easily attributed to pharyngitis or a skin infection, multiple laboratory tests and follow-up are generally unnecessary. In less clear-cut circumstances, an extensive laboratory investigation may be required. The three most useful initial tests are the complete blood cell count with blood smear examination, bacterial cultures, and a chest radiograph. The complete blood cell count may show anemia (a sign of chronic inflammation), atypical or abnormal blood leukocytes, leukopenia, leukocytosis, or eosinophilia. Throat cultures for β-hemolytic streptococci, skin cultures for *Staphylococcus aureus* or *Corynebacterium diphtheriae,* and cultures of any discrete lesions can be very helpful. The chest radiograph may show infiltrates or hilar adenopathy. In young adults with cervical or generalized adenopathy, a monospot test is often useful. Jaundice, hepatomegaly, or right upper quadrant tenderness mandates liver function tests and serologic tests for hepatitis. In a small proportion of cases, lymphadenopathy cannot be easily explained based on the history, physical examination, or basic laboratory tests. In these instances, and in a few special circumstances, lymph node aspiration or a surgical biopsy is indicated. Before a cervical node biopsy, thorough laryngeal examination (i.e., indirect or direct laryngoscopy) is warranted, particularly in older adults with a history of smoking. With very enlarged or fluctuant adenopathy and a high suspicion of a bacterial pathogen, aspiration and culture for *Francisella, Yersinia,* and other pathogens under careful laboratory conditions (the material can be very infectious) is justified. Tuberculosis may also be diagnosed from aspirated lymph node tissue in some situations (e.g., in association with the acquired immunodeficiency syndrome), but biopsies are generally preferable.

Ordinarily, lymph node biopsy is reserved until it is clear the lymphadenopathy is a manifestation of a serious illness that cannot be diagnosed by examination of the blood or by biopsy of other more accessible tissues. For instance, in patients with suspected granulomatous inflammation (e.g., sarcoidosis, tuberculosis, histoplasmosis), biopsies of the skin, liver, or bone marrow should be considered as alternatives. If a biopsy is necessary, it is better to sample a central rather than a peripheral node. It is always important to discuss the probable diagnoses with the surgeon and pathologist before the biopsy sample is obtained. It is not unusual to obtain nondiagnostic tissue from patients suspected to have a serious infiltrative or malignant disease. In these instances, it is wise to consider a second biopsy soon if the diagnosis remains obscure and the illness persists.

Management. In most cases of lymphadenopathy, the focus is on making a precise diagnosis. It rarely takes more than a few weeks for the lymphadenopathy to resolve or a diagnosis to be made. Empirical therapy with antibiotics is justified when there is a strong suspicion that lymphadenopathy is due to a pyogenic infection; otherwise, antibiotic trials are often confusing and unhelpful. Corticosteroids ameliorate severe lymphadenopathy in patients with infectious mononucleosis and other viral illnesses, but their use is generally not necessary or indicated. Radiation therapy will shrink enlarged nodes but should not be used without a precise indication.

Follow-Up. Acute lymphadenopathy due to infection or inflammation usually resolves within 1 to 3 weeks. Serial physical examinations as well as laboratory evaluation as outlined under Clinical Approach should be done in all patients with lymphadenopathy persisting beyond 3 weeks.

Cross-References: Detection and Initial Management of Oral Cancer (Chapter 47), Pharyngitis (Chapter 54), HIV Infection: Disease Prevention and Antiretroviral Therapy (Chapter 203), HIV Infection: Office Evaluation (Chapter 204), HIV Infection: Evaluation of Common Symptoms (Chapter 205).

REFERENCES

1. Brook I. The swollen neck: Cervical lymphadenitis, parotitis, thyroiditis, and infected cysts. Infect Dis Clin North Am 1988;2:221–236.

   Diagnosis and treatment of common causes of neck swelling is discussed.

2. Grossman M, Shiramizu B. Evaluation of lymphadenopathy in children. Curr Opin Pediatr 1994;6:68–76.

   A good discussion is provided of the diverse causes of lymphadenopathy in children and young adults.

3. Manolidis S, Frenkiel S, Yoskovitch A, Black M. Mycobacterial infections of the head and neck. Otolaryngol Head Neck Surg 1993;109:427–433.

   The authors discuss diagnosing tuberculosis in patients with cervical adenopathy.

4. Pangalis GA, Vassilakopoulos TP, Boussiotis VA, Fessas P. Clinical approach to lymphadenopathy. Semin Oncol 1993;20:570–582.

   This is a clinical guide to evaluating lymphadenopathy.

5. Williamson HA. Lymphadenopathy in a family practice: A descriptive study of 249 cases. J Fam Pract 1985;20:449–452.

   Serious disease was rare in asymptomatic patients, justifying a period of observation.

197 Thrombocytopenia

Problem

STEPHEN H. PETERSDORF

Epidemiology and Etiology. *Thrombocytopenia* is defined as a platelet count of less than 150,000/mm³. There is an increased risk of serious bleeding during surgery or after trauma when the platelet count is less than 50,000/mm³. Spontaneous bleeding usually occurs only when the platelet count is less than 20,000/mm³. Thrombocytopenia is caused by impaired platelet production or increased platelet destruction. Although many agents such as drugs or viruses may cause thrombocytopenia, most people exposed to these agents do not develop a low platelet count. The differential diagnosis of thrombocytopenia is outlined in Table 197–1.

Symptoms and Signs. The tendency to bleed is the primary manifestation of thrombocytopenia. In mild cases, petechiae appear in dependent areas such as the feet or ankles or in the lining of the buccal mucosa. Increasingly severe thrombocytopenia leads to more diffuse petechiae as well as epistaxis, gingival bleeding, ecchymoses, hematuria, and increased menstrual bleeding. The sever-

---

Table 197–1. DIFFERENTIAL DIAGNOSIS OF THROMBOCYTOPENIA

Thrombocytopenia secondary to decreased marrow production (decreased bone marrow megakaryocytes)
Viral infection (mumps, cytomegalovirus, Epstein-Barr virus, hepatitis B)
Alcohol
Drugs (e.g., thiazide diuretics, chemotherapy)
Disorders associated with marrow invasion (e.g., leukemia, infection, metastatic carcinoma)
Disorders associated with ineffective myelopoiesis (e.g., aplastic anemia, myelodysplasia, paroxysmal nocturnal hemoglobinuria)
Hereditary (Fanconi's anemia, Wiskott-Aldrich)

Thrombocytopenia secondary to increased platelet destruction (normal to increased megakaryocytes in bone marrow)
Immune-mediated destruction
  Immune thrombocytopenic purpura
  Post-transfusion purpura
  Infection (human immunodeficiency virus)
  Drug-induced purpura (quinine, gold, heparin)
  Neonatal immune purpura
Nonimmunologic destruction
  Hypersplenism
  Disseminated intravascular coagulation
  Thrombotic thrombocytopenic purpura/hemolytic-uremic syndrome
  Infection (human immunodeficiency virus, *Rickettsia*)
  Pregnancy (preeclampsia)

---

ity of the bleeding may also depend on other hemostatic defects such as coagulopathy, trauma, and vasculitis.

Clinical Approach. Because thrombocytopenia may be caused by decreased production or increased destruction of platelets, the clinical evaluation should determine the cause of thrombocytopenia. The history (drug history, infection, family history, and duration of bleeding), physical examination (location of bleeding, presence of splenomegaly), and laboratory studies (including a complete blood cell count, review of the peripheral smear, and bone marrow evaluation) are necessary parts of the evaluation.

Thrombocytopenia due to decreased production may be associated with infection, drug exposure, or a primary bone marrow problem such as marrow failure or infiltration. There will be decreased megakaryocytes in the bone marrow and possibly other abnormalities seen on the peripheral smear, such as nucleated red blood cells or unusually small or large platelets. Drugs may also cause increased destruction of platelets (Table 197–2). Thrombocytopenia secondary to increased destruction may be associated with a history of recent transfusion or pregnancy, infection with human immunodeficiency virus, or other autoimmune phenomena. The bleeding time is normal in immune thrombocytopenia because the few platelets present are hyperfunctional. On bone marrow examination, megakaryocytes are increased in all cases of thrombocytopenia caused by increased destruction. Nonimmune causes of increased platelet destruction such as thrombotic thrombocytopenic purpura or disseminated intravascular coagulation are characterized by fragmentation of red cells on the peripheral smear as well as thrombocytopenia. Finally, patients with splenic sequestration have splenomegaly on physical examination and normal to increased megakaryocytes in the bone marrow.

Management. Platelet transfusions, with either random donor–pooled platelets or single-donor pheresed platelets, are appropriate in patients with frank bleeding or a platelet count less than $20,000/mm^3$ if the thrombocytopenia is due to decreased production or increased destruction from a nonautoimmune phenomenon. Subsequent management requires removal of the offending agent or treatment of the underlying cause. For patients with autoimmune disorders such as immune thrombocytopenic purpura, transfused platelets have a very short survival and are not of benefit unless the patient has uncontrolled bleeding. Initial treatment of immune thrombocytopenic purpura includes prednisone at a dose of 2 mg/kg/d. If the thrombocytopenia has not resolved after 2 weeks, splenectomy is indicated. Ten percent to 20% of patients with immune thrombocytopenic purpura do not respond to these measures and require immunosuppressive therapy with cyclophosphamide, azathioprine, or

Table 197–2. DRUGS COMMONLY ASSOCIATED WITH THROMBOCYTOPENIA

α-Methyldopa (Aldomet)	Gold salts
Carbamazepine (Tegretol)	Heparin
Cephalosporins	Histamine-2-receptor blockers
Chlorothiazides	Phenytoin (Dilantin)
Diazepam (Valium)	Quinine/quinidine
Digoxin	Sulfa drugs

vincristine or, alternatively, intravenous immunoglobulin (400 mg/kg/d for 5 days). Patients with thrombotic thrombocytopenic purpura should receive exchange transfusion with plasma.

Follow-Up. Thrombocytopenia secondary to decreased production from drugs should correct within 7 to 14 days of removal of the offending agent. Recovery from exposure to quinine takes 3 to 14 days, and recovery after gold exposure may take slightly longer. The thrombocytopenia of patients with either immune or thrombotic thrombocytopenic purpura may have a relapsing course after appropriate initial therapy.

Cross-References: Epistaxis (Chapter 55), Cirrhosis and Chronic Liver Failure (Chapter 99), General Approach to Arthritic Symptoms (Chapter 106), Abnormal Uterine Bleeding (Chapter 159), Anemia (Chapter 199), Transfusion Therapy (Chapter 202), HIV Infection: Disease Prevention and Antiretroviral Therapy (Chapter 203), HIV Infection: Office Evaluation (Chapter 204), HIV Infection: Evaluation of Common Symptoms (Chapter 205), Preoperative Hematologic Problems (Chapter 219).

REFERENCES

1. Berchtold P, McMillan R. Therapy of chronic idiopathic thrombocytopenic purpura in adults. Blood 1989;74:2309–2317.

   The acute and long-term management of adults with idiopathic (immune) thrombocytopenic purpura is reviewed.

2. Kaufman DW, Johannes CB, Kelly JP, et al. Acute thrombocytopenic purpura in relation to the use of drugs. Blood 1993;82:2714–2718.

   Mechanisms of drug-induced platelet destruction are presented.

3. Salama A, Mueller-Eckhardt C. Immune-mediated blood dyscrasias related to drugs. Semin Hematol 1992;29:54–63.

   The authors give a detailed review of the drug-induced immune-mediated causes of thrombocytopenia.

· ·

198 Polycythemia

Problem

STEPHEN H. PETERSDORF

Epidemiology and Etiology. Polycythemia refers to an increased red blood cell concentration. There are three situations associated with an increased red cell concentration:

1. Polycythemia vera, a clonal stem cell disorder characterized by increased production of red cells, granulocytes, and platelets

2. Secondary polycythemia, which represents increased red blood cell mass due to increased erythropoietin production, high-affinity hemoglobin, or a chronic hypoxemic state
3. Relative polycythemia, which occurs when the red cell mass is normal but the plasma volume is decreased

Polycythemia vera is a rare disease. Five to 17 cases per million people are diagnosed each year in the United States with this disorder. There is a slight male predominance (1.2:1). The median age at diagnosis is 60 years, and the disease is rare in persons younger than 30. The incidence of secondary polycythemia is increased in smokers, patients with chronic obstructive lung disease who are persistently hypoxemic, and persons who live at high altitudes. The patients who develop relative polycythemia have an increased incidence of obesity, smoking, and hypertension and are often treated with diuretics, leading to decreased plasma volume.

Symptoms and Signs. The clinical presentation of polycythemia is directly related to increased concentration of red blood cells, which leads to increased blood viscosity. Neurologic symptoms are most common and include headache, weakness, and dizziness. If hyperviscosity is severe, confusion, paresthesias, and impaired visual acuity are frequent. Pruritus and associated peptic ulcer disease are due to increased histamine levels. Clinical signs include a ruddy complexion, plethora of conjunctival blood vessels, and dilated veins noted on funduscopic examination. Splenomegaly is found in 70% to 90% of patients with polycythemia vera. Thromboembolic complications occur in 40% to 60% of patients over a 10-year span. In general, patients with relative polycythemia do not have any of these findings.

Clinical Approach. If the hematocrit is greater than 60%, the red blood cell mass is almost certainly increased. If the hematocrit is between 55% and 60% and the patient has a normal PaO_2, the red blood cell mass should be determined by the chromium-51–labeled red blood cell assay. If the red cell mass is normal, the patient has relative polycythemia. If the red cell mass is elevated, the patient should be evaluated for polycythemia vera or secondary polycythemia. The presence of associated leukocytosis, basophilia, thrombocytosis, splenomegaly, and trilineage hyperplasia in the bone marrow is consistent with polycythemia vera. The serum erythropoietin level is normal in polycythemia vera.

If the hematologic workup is normal, the patient should be evaluated for secondary polycythemia. Conditions associated with secondary polycythemia

Table 198–1. DIFFERENTIAL EVALUATION OF POLYCYTHEMIA

Findings	Polycythemia Vera	Secondary Polycythemia	Relative Polycythemia
Red cell mass	Increased	Increased	Normal
Erythropoietin level	Decreased	Increased	Normal
Splenomegaly	Present	Absent	Absent
Leukocytosis	Present	Absent	Absent
PaO_2 saturation	Normal	Normal–decreased	Normal
Marrow	Trilineage hyperplasia	Erythroid hyperplasia	Normal

include chronic pulmonary disease with hypoxemia, smoking with elevated carboxyhemoglobin, hemoglobinopathies with increased oxygen affinity, and inappropriate erythropoietin secretion (usually associated with renal tumors). Consequently, evaluation should include arterial blood gas measurement with determination of the P_{50} to screen for impaired oxygen release (abnormal < 27 mm Hg) and an ultrasound evaluation of the kidneys to rule out a renal lesion. The serum erythropoietin level will usually be elevated in secondary polycythemia (>30 mU/mL). (See Table 198–1.)

Management. Relative polycythemia can usually be corrected by cessation of smoking or controlling the hypertension that is usually noted in these patients. Patients with secondary polycythemia from hypoxemia should undergo phlebotomy with removal of 250 to 500 mL of blood every other day until the hematocrit reaches less than 45% in men and 43% in women. Patients with underlying cardiovascular and cerebrovascular disease should be phlebotomized, using a reduced volume (100–200 mL) with simultaneous replacement with volume expanders to correct hyperviscosity that may occur. Although supplemental oxygen may benefit those with arterial PaO_2 less than 60 mm Hg, red cell mass will not decrease unless smoking is stopped. Secondary polycythemia due to erythropoietin-secreting tumors or cysts can be managed with phlebotomy or removal of the lesion.

The hematocrit of patients with polycythemia vera should be maintained at less than 44% to prevent thrombotic complications. Patients younger than 40 should be treated with phlebotomy. Because older patients have a much greater incidence of thrombotic complications, they should receive chemotherapy as well as phlebotomy. Options include phosphorus-32 intravenously every 3 months as necessary, hydroxyurea (500–1000 mg every day as blood cell counts permit), or interferon alfa. These interventions require consultation with a hematologist and close monitoring of blood cell counts to prevent marrow aplasia. Experimental approaches include bone marrow transplantation, which may be considered for patients younger than age 50 with an appropriate donor.

Follow-Up. Patients with relative polycythemia should be monitored for thromboembolic complications, which occur in 30% to 70% of patients. Follow-up of patients with secondary polycythemia includes serial hematocrit levels every 3 to 6 months as well as correction of the underlying disorder. The patient with polycythemia vera may suffer from thrombotic and hemorrhagic complications due to the hyperviscosity. In addition, acute leukemia evolves in 15% of patients with polycythemia vera, and 15% to 30% of patients develop myelofibrosis with myeloid metaplasia. The median survival for patients with polycythemia vera who have appropriate therapy is 10 years from diagnosis.

Cross-References: Smoking Cessation (Chapter 12), Pruritus (Chapter 23), Sleep Apnea Syndromes (Chapter 64), Asthma and Chronic Obstruction Pulmonary Disease (Chapter 68).

REFERENCES

1. Berk PD, Goldberg JD, Donovan PB, et al. Therapeutic recommendation in polycythemia vera based on the Polycythemia Vera Study Group Protocols. Semin Hematol 1986;23:132–143.
   A useful review of 10 years of clinical trials in polycythemia vera is presented.

2. Bilgrami S, Greenberg B. Polycythemia rubra vera. Semin Oncol 1995;22:307–326.

   This is an excellent review of treatment options including interferon and hydroxyurea.

3. Gruppo Italiano Studio Policitemia. Polycythemia vera: The natural history of 1213 patients followed for 20 years. Ann Intern Med 1995;123:656–664.

   The authors of this large retrospective review suggest that aggressive intervention to reduce thrombosis may increase the risk of secondary neoplasms.

4. Hocking WG, Golde DW. Polycythemia: Evaluation and management. Blood Rev 1989;3:57–65.

   Excellent algorithms are provided for evaluating patients with polycythemia.

199 Anemia

Problem

STEPHEN H. PETERSDORF

Epidemiology and Etiology. Anemia reflects an underlying pathologic process and is a common finding in a wide variety of acute and chronic diseases. It is defined as a hemoglobin concentration less than 12 g/dL in women and 13.5 g/dL in men. The common causes of anemia are iron deficiency (25% of patients), acute blood loss (25%), anemia of chronic inflammatory disorders (25%), hemolysis (10%), megaloblastic anemia (10%), and bone marrow failure or replacement (< 5%).

Symptoms and Signs. The anemic patient may present with nonspecific complaints such as lethargy, fatigue, weakness, or palpitations. Symptoms are more pronounced with rapidly developing anemia, more severe anemia, and underlying cardiovascular disease.

   Physical signs of anemia are nonspecific but may include pallor, tachycardia, postural hypotension, and a systolic murmur. Other findings provide clues to the cause of the anemia, such as jaundice (hemolysis), lymphadenopathy (marrow infiltrative process), hepatosplenomegaly (hemolysis, marrow infiltration), ecchymoses (blood loss), Hemoccult-positive stools (blood loss and/or iron deficiency), and neurologic findings (megaloblastic anemia).

Clinical Approach. After anemia is diagnosed by measuring a decreased red cell mass, hemoglobin concentration, and hematocrit, the specific cause should be determined. Once acute blood loss is excluded by history and physical examination, the initial evaluation includes a reticulocyte index to determine whether the anemia is secondary to decreased production or increased destruction of red blood cells. If the corrected reticulocyte index is less than 2% to 3%, the anemia is secondary to decreased production (Table 199–1). Additional studies should include review of the peripheral blood smear and red blood cell

Table 199-1. DIFFERENTIAL DIAGNOSIS OF ANEMIA

Diagnosis	Blood Smear	Diagnostic Test
Anemia secondary to decreased production (corrected reticulocyte count <2%; no maturation abnormality)		
Iron deficiency	Hypochromic, microcytic	Fe decreased; TIBC increased; Fe/TIBC <15%
		Marrow iron stores absent
Sideroblastic anemia	Hypochromic, microcytic	Fe increased, Fe/TIBC 60–95%, check lead level
	Basophilic stippling	
Anemia of chronic, renal, or endocrine diseases	Normochromic, normocytic	Fe and TIBC decreased
		Marrow iron present
Anemia secondary to marrow replacement or failure	Normochromic, normocytic	Marrow empty or replaced with leukemia or metastatic tumor
Anemia secondary to decreased production from maturation abnormality (corrected reticulocyte count <2%)		
Megaloblastic anemia	Macrocytic, macro-ovalocytes, hypersegmented neutrophils	Vitamin B_{12} or serum/red cell folate decreased
Refractory anemia	Dimorphic with macro- and microcytes	Ringed sideroblasts or ineffective erythropoiesis in marrow
Anemia secondary to increased destruction (corrected reticulocyte count >2%)		
Mechanical destruction	Red cell fragments	Increased bilirubin, LDH; decreased haptoglobin
Autoimmune hemolysis	Spherocytes	Positive Coombs' test
Hereditary membrane defects	Spherocytes, elliptocytes	
Hemoglobinopathy	Sickle cells present	Hemoglobin electrophoresis

Fe, iron; TIBC, total iron binding capacity; LDH, lactate dehydrogenase.

indices. When appropriate, measurement of iron, total iron-binding capacity, ferritin, folate, and vitamin B_{12} should be performed. If the reticulocyte count is greater than 3%, the patient should be evaluated for increased destruction of red cells. The peripheral blood smear should be examined for spherocytes (a sign of immune hemolytic anemia), fragmented cells (signifying microangiopathic anemia), and sickle cells. Bone marrow examination should be performed if there is an unexplained hypoproliferative anemia or if nucleated red blood cells or blasts are seen on the peripheral blood smear.

Management. Long-term correction of the anemia requires resolution of the underlying medical condition. The nutritional anemias (i.e., iron deficiency, folate deficiency) can be corrected by replacement therapy. Iron deficiency can usually be corrected by administering 300 mg of ferrous sulfate three times a day, which provides 10 mg of elemental iron daily. The reticulocyte count will peak 5 to 10 days after starting iron therapy. The hemoglobin level should reach normal within 2 months, and therapy should be continued for 6 months to replenish iron stores fully. Vitamin B_{12} deficiency can be corrected rapidly with 1000 μg cobalamin given intramuscularly every day for a week, followed by 1000 μg cobalamin intramuscularly weekly until the hematocrit normalizes and then 1000 μg monthly for life. Oral replacement with 1000 μg/d may be effective but requires close monitoring of response because absorption may be erratic. Folate deficiency can be corrected with 1 mg of folate once or twice daily for 1 to 4 months. Patients with hemolytic anemia should also receive folate supplementation.

Patients who are anemic secondary to chronic renal failure, cancer chemotherapy, and human immunodeficiency virus infection may benefit from the administration of recombinant human erythropoietin. The use of recombinant human erythropoietin in other chronic anemias is under study.

Transfusion of red cells should be performed when diminished tissue oxygenation is secondary to decreased red cell mass. Accepted indications include the presence of angina in a severely anemic patient or an acute blood loss of more than 750 to 1000 mL of blood (see Chapter 202, Transfusion Therapy).

Follow-Up. The patient should be monitored for resolution of the underlying disorder. Unless the cause of blood loss is obvious (e.g., menorrhagia), patients with iron deficiency should be evaluated for gastrointestinal sources of blood loss. Long-term management of other types of anemia depends on the underlying cause.

Cross-References: Fatigue (Chapter 21), Angina (Chapter 78), Congestive Heart Failure (Chapter 79), Colorectal Cancer Screening (Chapter 90), Sigmoidoscopy and Colonoscopy (Chapter 104), General Approach to Arthritic Symptoms (Chapter 106), Peripheral Neuropathy (Chapter 147), Abnormal Uterine Bleeding (Chapter 159), Chronic Renal Failure (Chapter 179), Transfusion Therapy (Chapter 202), Dyspnea in Patients with Cancer (Chapter 208), Preoperative Hematologic Problems (Chapter 219).

REFERENCES

1. Hillman RS, Finch CA. The Red Cell Manual, 6th ed. Philadelphia, FA Davis, 1992.
   A complete review of normal and abnormal pathophysiology is presented.

2. Colon-Otero G, Menke D, Hook CC, et al. A practical approach to the differential diagnosis and evaluation of the adult patient with macrocytic anemia. Med Clin North Am 1992;76:581–597.

   A clinical discussion of macrocytic anemia is provided.

3. Nardone DA, Roth KM, Mazur DJ, et al. Usefulness of physical examination in detection of the presence or absence of anemia. Arch Intern Med 1990;150:201–204.

   The authors evaluate the utility of physical findings in determining the presence of anemia.

4. Sears DA. Anemia of chronic disease. Med Clin North Am 1992;76:567–579.

   This is an excellent discussion of inflammatory block leading to anemia.

. . . .

200 Sickle Cell Disease

Problem

STEPHEN H. PETERSDORF

Epidemiology and Etiology. Sickle cell disease includes not only sickle cell anemia but also other disorders that result from interactions between hemoglobin S and other β-hemoglobin abnormalities, such as thalassemia or hemoglobin C. In the United States, approximately 8% of blacks carry a gene for sickle cell (Hb AS, sickle cell trait), and approximately 0.15% of black children have the disease (Hb SS). Other sickle cell syndromes such as Hb SC (1:2600 blacks) are less common. The relatively high incidence of sickle cell trait is due to the survival advantage of the heterozygote under the selective pressure of falciparum malaria infection.

Symptoms and Signs. Patients with sickle cell trait (Hb AS) are usually asymptomatic, although some experience painless hematuria that is typically mild and self-limiting.

Patients with sickle cell disease develop hemolytic anemia within a few months of birth. These infants typically present with systemic complications such as infection and growth retardation or complications from vaso-occlusive events. Infections are often due to encapsulated organisms (pneumococcus, *Haemophilus influenzae*, meningococcus) because splenic function is impaired. Osteomyelitis due to *Salmonella* species is relatively unique to sickle cell disease. Adults commonly present with pain from a vaso-occlusive crisis, the severity and frequency of which varies among patients. Pain occurs in 50% of patients, most often in the hips, shoulders, and long bones. Other acute presentations include priapism (40% of males), stroke, skin ulcers, and an acute chest syndrome secondary to a vaso-occlusive process in the lungs, which is characterized by pleuritic pain, fever, cough, and pulmonary infiltrates that may be difficult to distinguish from pneumonia.

Splenic sequestration crises may be seen in children with rapid onset of splenomegaly and a fall in hematocrit. An aplastic crisis is characterized by severe anemia due to infection with parvovirus, which inhibits erythropoiesis.

Physical examination may be notable for scleral icterus, cardiomegaly, hepatomegaly, and skin ulcers on the lower extremity.

Clinical Approach. The diagnosis of sickle cell disease is usually made in childhood. Evaluation of patients with sickle cell disease demonstrates a hemoglobin concentration of 7 to 9 g/dL, mild leukocytosis (12,000–15,000/mm³) from splenic atrophy, and a peripheral blood smear remarkable for sickled and nucleated red blood cells. Hemoglobin electrophoresis reveals 75% to 95% hemoglobin S; the remainder is hemoglobin A2 and F.

All patients with painful crises should be evaluated for underlying infection, a common inciting event. The chest radiograph may show an infiltrate reflecting a chest crisis or underlying pneumonia. If the patient has persistent bone pain, aseptic necrosis or osteomyelitis must be excluded by magnetic resonance imaging and other testing, as appropriate.

Management. Sickle cell disease is a chronic condition. Although there is no treatment to prevent sickling, certain measures may reduce the frequency of vaso-occlusive crises and complications, including good nutrition, folic acid supplementation, avoiding temperature extremes and dehydration, and immunization for pneumococcus and *H. influenzae*. Treatment of painful crises includes intravenous fluids for dehydration and analgesics. Narcotics may be required to alleviate severe pain. Transfusions should be performed only during an aplastic crisis, because they may precipitate a crisis by increasing blood viscosity. Direct exchange transfusion, however, is indicated to break the cycle of recurring vaso-occlusive events, to assist the healing of chronic leg ulcers, and to prevent complications during pregnancy or before surgery.

Hemoglobin F inhibits polymerization of deoxyhemoglobin S, so pharmacologic interventions to increase hemoglobin F may benefit these patients. Hydroxyurea, in doses sufficient to produce myelosuppression, may increase hemoglobin F levels to 20% to 30% and may decrease the frequency of painful crises.

Follow-Up. Sickle cell disease is a chronic disease that may lead to deterioration of several organ systems. Aseptic necrosis of the hips and shoulders, proliferative retinopathy, and leg ulcers are common complications. Health care maintenance of these patients dictates careful attention to neurologic, hepatic, cardiac, renal, pulmonary, orthopedic, and ophthalmologic symptoms at frequent intervals (every 3 to 6 months) with appropriate testing as indicated. Prenatal diagnosis of the disease can be made with chorionic villus sampling or amniocentesis.

Cross-References: Adult Immunizations (Chapter 11), Abdominal Pain (Chapter 94), Leg Ulcers (Chapter 133), Anemia (Chapter 199).

REFERENCES

1. Rodgers GP, Dover GJ, Noguchi CT, et al. Hematologic responses of patients with sickle cell disease to treatment with hydroxyurea. N Engl J Med 1990;322:1037–1045.
   The authors present the initial description of the use of hydroxyurea to increase hemoglobin F.

2. Steingart R. Management of patients with sickle cell disease. Med Clin North Am 1992;76:669–682.

This article is an excellent review of management of complications of sickle cell disease.

3. Wayne AS, Kevy SV, Nathan DG: Transfusion management of sickle cell disease. Blood 1993;81:1109–1123.

The role of exchange transfusion is reviewed.

201 Chronic Anticoagulation

Procedure

STEPHAN D. FIHN and NANCY J. ROBEN

Indications and Contraindications. Patients with extremely high risk of thromboembolism, such as those with mechanical cardiac valves or acute deep venous thrombosis, must be treated with anticoagulants. For patients with a lower risk of thromboembolism the decision to anticoagulate the patient must balance the potential benefit of preventing a thromboembolic event against the risk of a serious hemorrhagic complication.

Because it is administered orally, is relatively inexpensive ($0.50 per day), has been in use for 50 years, and is backed by extensive data on its efficacy from clinical trials, warfarin is the most commonly used agent for long-term anticoagulation. Contraindications to warfarin anticoagulation include active bleeding, recent cerebrovascular hemorrhage, severe congenital or acquired defect of hemostasis, major recent surgery of the central nervous system or eye, and pregnancy. (Warfarin crosses the placenta and may cause birth defects and fetal hemorrhage; optimal anticoagulation during pregnancy is controversial.)

Relative contraindications to the use of warfarin include severe hepatic or renal disease, chronic alcohol use, markedly elevated blood pressure (> 200/105 mm Hg), requirements for intensive salicylate or nonsteroidal anti-inflammatory agents, poor patient compliance, unstable gait, history of falling, and history of gastrointestinal, urologic, or intracranial hemorrhage. Advanced age, in and of itself, is not a contraindication to chronic anticoagulation, although the risk of serious bleeding may be higher in very elderly patients (those older than 80 years of age).

Thromboembolic events occurring in patients taking warfarin can sometimes be successfully managed using heparin. In addition to bleeding complications and the inconvenience of daily injections, problems with heparin include thrombocytopenia and osteoporosis, both of which can be profound. Low molecular weight heparin appears to be as effective as the unfractionated preparation but has several advantages. There is once- or twice-daily administration, standard dosing, no need for monitoring, and lower risk of complications, including bleeding, thrombocytopenia, and osteopenia. However, low molecular weight heparin must still be given by subcutaneous injection and it is very expensive (approximately $60.00 per day), so that its long-term administration is limited and will likely remain so.

Rationale. Warfarin interferes with the synthesis of vitamin K–dependent coagulation factors. Although the half-life of warfarin is less than 24 hours, 10 to 14 days of therapy may be required to achieve a stable state of anticoagulation because of the half-lives of the previously synthesized vitamin K–dependent clotting factors (factor VII = 6 hours; factor IX = 24 hours; factor X = 40 hours; factor II = 60–100 hours).

Warfarin therapy is monitored with the prothrombin time ratio (PTR) or, preferably, the International Normalized Ratio (INR), which standardizes variations in the PTR related to the use of varying reagents in different laboratories and facilitates the application of international guidelines for therapy. Lower (INR 2.0 to 3.0) and higher (INR 2.5 to 3.5) levels of intensity are recommended according to the reason for anticoagulation. The less intensive range is recommended for all patients except those with mechanical prosthetic valves or recurrent systemic embolism.

Methods. In hospitalized patients receiving intravenous heparin, warfarin is started using loading doses to hasten achievement of a therapeutic INR. In the outpatient setting, however, warfarin should be started at 2.5 to 5 mg daily because loading doses larger than this often lead to excessive anticoagulation and subsequent wide fluctuations of the INR. Patients who are elderly, medically unstable, or taking drugs that potentiate warfarin should receive the 2.5-mg dose. The INR should be monitored every 5 to 7 days in the same laboratory until it is stable. Dosage changes should generally be made in increments of 2.5 mg per week, or 5% to 15% of the total weekly dosage. Once stable, the INR is monitored every 4 to 8 weeks. Flow sheets or specialized computer programs that record warfarin dose, INR results, all drugs taken, and complications are of great value.

The simplest warfarin regimens are based on days of the week and use a single tablet size and drug manufacturer. The patient should receive some warfarin every day, even when only small doses (1–2 mg) are required. For example, a patient may take 5 mg on Monday, Wednesday, and Friday and 7.5 mg on all other days or 7.5 mg every Sunday and 5 mg all other days. Use of "even" and "odd" days leads to patient confusion and may result in unstable anticoagulation from week to week and during months with 31 days.

Patients vary widely in their warfarin requirements. Any change in the patient's disease process or medications may affect the INR results (Tables 201–1—201–3).

Warfarin is extensively protein bound and is susceptible to displacement by other, more strongly bound drugs (see Table 201–2). When any of these drugs is initiated, altered, or discontinued, the INR requires close monitoring. Drugs that affect platelet function (e.g., aspirin, sulfinpyrazone, certain antibiotics) or damage gastric mucosa (aspirin and other nonsteroidal agents) are best avoided. When the INR exceeds the therapeutic range, the clinician should

Table 201–1. QUESTIONS TO POSE WHEN AN UNEXPECTED INTERNATIONAL NORMALIZED RATIO VALUE IS ENCOUNTERED

1. Is the prescribed warfarin dosing regimen being followed? Have any doses been missed during the past week?
2. Is there confusion about the tablet strength?
3. Have any other drugs been added, changed, or stopped? If so, is any of them known to affect warfarin pharmacokinetics?
4. Has there been any evidence of bleeding or unusual bruising?
5. Has there been an acute illness during the past 10 days, such as diarrhea or fever?
6. Has there been an exacerbation of an underlying chronic illness, such as heart, liver, or kidney failure?
7. Have there been any dietary changes, such as more leafy green vegetables or diet preparations or formulas?
8. Has there been a change in alcohol consumption?
9. Could there be a laboratory error?

withhold one dose, substitute a lower maintenance dose, and monitor the INR every other week until it is stable. If the INR exceeds 10 to 12, vitamin K should be given either subcutaneously (1 or 2 mg) or orally (5–10 mg) and the warfarin withheld for 2 to 3 days. For extremely high INR values, such as more than 40 to 50, the patient should be hospitalized. Patients with active bleeding

Table 201–2. DRUGS KNOWN TO INTERACT WITH WARFARIN AND THEIR EFFECTS ON THE INTERNATIONAL NORMAL RATIO*

Drugs Known to Prolong the INR	Drugs Known to Shorten the INR	Drugs with Variable Effect on the INR
Allopurinol	Antacids	Alcohol
Amiodarone	Antihistamines	Chloral hydrate
Aspirin (high doses)	Barbiturates	Diuretics
Chlorpropamide	Carbamazapine	Phenytoin
Clofibrate	Chlordiazepoxide	Ranitidine
Disulfiram	Cholestyramine	
Ethacrynic acid	Colestipol	
Fenoprofen	Griseofulvin	
Gemfibrozil	Oral contraceptives	
Indomethacin	Rifampin	
Phenylbutazone	Vitamin K	
Piroxicam		
Quinidine		
Quinine		
Sulfonamides (long acting)		
Sulindac		
Thyroid drugs		
Tricyclic antidepressants		
Trimethoprim/sulfamethoxazole		
Fluoroquinolones (ofloxacin, enoxacin, ciprofloxacin, lomefloxacin)		

*This table does not represent a total list of known drug versus warfarin reactions. The drugs that are *italicized* often produce a dramatic effect. Each patient needs to be monitored carefully for individual differences.

Table 201-3. ADVICE TO PATIENTS

1. Report any unusual bleeding or bruising.
2. Check regularly for blood in urine or stools or black stools.
3. Report all medication changes within 3 days.
4. Limit alcohol use to occasional beer, wine, or 2 ounces of liquor.
5. Minimize exposure to possible injury in regular activities including work, sports, and hobbies.
6. Avoid all aspirin-containing drugs. Read labels of over-the-counter drugs carefully. Substitute acetaminophen, up to 2 g/d.
7. Take warfarin at the same time every day and never take extra doses to compensate for doses missed.
8. If menses are delayed more than 3 days and pregnancy is a possibility, notify provider.
9. Avoid sudden changes in diet.

or an extremely high INR may require vitamin K or fresh-frozen plasma to reverse the anticoagulation.

Patients should repeatedly receive the information that appears in Table 201-3. The decision for anticoagulation should be reevaluated at least annually. When the warfarin is discontinued, no tapering of the dose is necessary.

For the vast majority of patients, therapy with warfarin is successful. For the minority who must receive chronic therapy with unfractionated sodium heparin, it is generally administered subcutaneously twice daily in a dose that achieves a therapeutic activated partial thromboplastin time that is typically 12 to 22 times the control value.

Cost and Complications. Warfarin is available as a 1-mg (pink), 2-mg (lavender), 2.5-mg (green), 5-mg (peach), or 10-mg (white) scored tablet. The wholesale cost of 100 tablets of warfarin, 5 mg, averages $55.00. The cost of an INR test ranges from $12.00 to $25.00, often with an additional $5.00 blood drawing or handling charge. Portable monitors are available but expensive (approximately $1200 for the monitor and $5.00 for cassettes for each test).

The main complication of anticoagulation therapy is bleeding. The overall incidence of hemorrhage that requires some sort of medical attention is approximately 8 events per 100 patient-years. The incidence of life-threatening or fatal bleeding is approximately 1 event per 100 patient-years. Definite risk factors for major bleeding include hypertension; higher intensity of anticoagulation; presence of an underlying gastrointestinal or intracranial lesion that may bleed; a history of prior bleeding on anticoagulation; and duration of anticoagulation, with those just beginning anticoagulation at highest risk. Some studies have found that the risk of bleeding is higher among elderly patients, particularly those older than 75 to 80 years of age.

Warfarin-induced necrosis of the skin and subcutaneous tissue is rare; lesions appear, usually in women, on the lower half of the body within 3 to 10 days of initiation of therapy. The "purple toe syndrome," also rare, occurs early during therapy and causes bilateral, painful purplish discoloration of the toes.

Cross-References: Aortic Stenosis (Chapter 80), Other Valvular Disease (Chapter 81), Atrial Fibrillation (Chapter 82), Cerebrovascular Disease (Chapter 146), Preoperative Hematologic Problems (Chapter 219).

REFERENCES

1. Atrial Fibrillation Investigators. Risk factors for stroke and efficacy of antithrombotic therapy in atrial fibrillation: Analysis of pooled data from five randomized controlled trials. Arch Intern Med 1994;154:1449–1457.

   Combined data from five randomized controlled trials from five different countries convincingly demonstrate a 68% reduction in the incidence of stroke. Aspirin, on the other hand, reduced the risk of stroke by at most 15%.

2. Cannegieter SC, Rosendaal FR, Wintzen AR, van der Meer FJM, Vandenbroucke JP, Brint E. Optimal intensity of oral anticoagulation therapy in patients with mechanical heart valves. N Engl J Med 1995;331:11–17.

   The optimal intensity of anticoagulation for caged ball and tilting disk valves was an INR range of 4.0 to 4.9 whereas patients with bileaflet valves derived no additional benefit above an INR of 3.0. Patients with prostheses in the mitral or mitral and aortic positions also fared better with higher-intensity anticoagulation.

3. Fihn SD, Callahan CM, Henikoff JG, McDonell MB, Martin D. The risk and severity of bleeding complications in elderly patients treated with warfarin. Ann Intern Med 1996;124:337–341.

   Age was not an important determinant of the risk of bleeding among patients taking warfarin, except possibly among patients 80 years or older. The incidence of life-threatening or fatal complications ranged between 0.75 per 100 patient-years for patients younger than age 50 to 3.4 for those older than 80.

4. Hirsh J, Dalen JE, Deykin D, Poller L, Bussey HI. Oral anticoagulants: Mechanisms of action, clinical effectiveness, and optimal therapeutic range. Chest 1995;108:231S–246S.
5. Levine M, Raskob GE, Landefeld CS. Hemorrhagic complications of anticoagulant treatment. Chest 1995;108:276S–290S.

   Both of these articles are published in the Fourth ACCP Consensus Conference on Antithrombotic Therapy (Dalen JE, Hirsh J [eds]. Chest 1995;108[4 suppl]:225S–522S). In its third iteration, this supplement remains the single best resource on anticoagulant therapy. The article by Hirsh and colleagues sets forth the most recent recommendations for the indications for and intensity of warfarin therapy. The article by Levine and associates reviews the large and confusing literature related to the frequency of complications and risk factors.

202 Transfusion Therapy

Procedure

GERALD J. ROTH

Indications and Contraindications. Transfusion services, such as blood banks, fractionate whole blood from donors into red blood cells (RBCs), platelets, plasma, and cryoprecipitate. Each component is used for specific reasons, such as RBCs for severe chronic anemia or platelets for severe thrombocytopenia. Because of expense and potential complications (e.g., transfusion reactions, viral transmission), the use of blood components is monitored and controlled in most hospitals.

Rationale. The prevention or treatment of shock from hemorrhage is a major indication for transfusion. For example, surgery or trauma can result in acute blood loss that requires both volume and red cell replacement. In these instances, a combination of saline, packed RBCs, and whole blood is often indicated. In the absence of acute blood loss, blood components are used.

Red Blood Cells. The decision to transfuse packed (sedimented) RBC preparations is based on the hemoglobin/hematocrit value, the degree of symptoms (e.g., dyspnea, claudication, fatigue), and the expected benefit. The most common indication for RBC transfusion is anemia (hemoglobin < 7 g/dL). Patients who are transfused for less severe anemia (hemoglobin > 7 g/dL) may not benefit from additional oxygen-carrying capacity, although those with cardiopulmonary disease may respond to RBCs with improvement in angina or dyspnea. Clear guidelines do not exist concerning a single level of hemoglobin below which a chronically anemic, but stable, patient should be transfused with RBCs. A reasonable compromise is a hemoglobin value of 6 to 7 g/dL. Single-unit RBC transfusions are rarely indicated.

Platelets. The degree of thrombocytopenia that warrants platelet transfusion lies in the range of 10,000 to 20,000/mm^3, although some patients with platelet counts of 5000 to 10,000/mm^3 do not experience severe bleeding. A unit of transfused platelet concentrate can raise the circulating platelet count by approximately 10,000/mm^3, but antiplatelet antibodies, fever, infection, or drugs frequently blunt this ideal response. Although thrombocytopenia secondary to decreased platelet production or increased platelet loss is a common indication for transfusion, platelet concentrates can also provide functional platelets in patients whose endogenous platelets are numerically normal but functionally abnormal.

Plasma and Cryoprecipitate. Fresh-frozen plasma is a convenient but dilute source of plasma coagulation factors. Cryoprecipitate is enriched in both fibrinogen and von Willebrand factor and therefore is used to replace fibrinogen in patients with disseminated intravascular coagulation and to provide von Willebrand's factor for patients with von Willebrand's disease. Cryoprecipitate is also useful as replacement therapy in patients with factor VIII deficiency (hemophilia A).

Granulocytes. Granulocyte transfusion is reserved for severely neutropenic patients (absolute neutrophil count < 500/mm^3) with an identified microbial infection that is unresponsive to appropriate antibiotic therapy. However, granulocyte transfusions are rarely used because they seldom provide the quantity of white blood cells needed to alter the course of a significant systemic bacterial infection. Hematopoietic growth factors (e.g., granulocyte-colony stimulating factor) may blunt the severity of neutropenia seen in patients undergoing aggressive chemotherapy.

Methods. Medical personnel administering blood products must ascertain that the product is indeed intended for the recipient. Most problems arise from inaccurate labeling or from inadvertent administration of a correctly labeled product to the wrong recipient. In handling a transfusion accident, the clinician should first disconnect and discontinue the transfusion while obtaining new samples of blood and urine for laboratory testing. The original intravenous line is retained to facilitate later therapy.

Table 202–1. TRANSFUSION PRACTICE

Component	Indication	Benefit	Risk/Problem	Cost/Unit ($)*
Whole blood	Active bleeding	O₂ transport Replace volume	Volume overload Reactions to blood	96
Packed RBCs	Stable anemia	O₂ transport	Reactions to blood	96
Platelets	Bleeding secondary to platelet defects	Replace platelets	Reactions to blood	47
Fresh-frozen plasma	Bleeding secondary to factor defects	Replace factors	Dilute factor source Volume overload	57
Cryoprecipitate	Replace fibrinogen, von Willebrand factor, factor VIII	Replace factors	Limited indications: disseminated intravascular coagulation, von Willebrand's disease, factor VIII deficiency	30
Granulocytes	Sepsis with identified organism	Replace polymorphonuclear leukocytes	Limited number of cells, not often practical	400

*Puget Sound Blood Center, 1997.

Autologous blood donation adds to the expense of blood processing but avoids rare exposure to pathogens in donor blood (a rare circumstance).

Costs and Complications. Representative current costs for one unit of a blood component are given in Table 202–1. Many blood banks deplete all "whole" blood of platelets and cryoprecipitate. Simple cross-matching of blood (not transfused, later returned to the blood bank) may cost $30 to $35. Therefore, clinicians should avoid prophylactic "just-in-case" ordering of cross-matched RBCs and reserve such orders for patients likely to require actual transfusion.

Hazards of RBC transfusion include volume overload in patients with cardiopulmonary disease, acute and delayed hemolytic transfusion reactions, febrile and pulmonary hypersensitivity reactions, and transmission of infectious contaminants. Platelet transfusions can also cause febrile responses. Blood products are screened for markers of viral disease (human immunodeficiency virus types 1 and 2; hepatitis B and C); nevertheless, transmission of viral illness may occur despite these precautions.

Cross-References: Bleeding (Chapter 195), Thrombocytopenia (Chapter 197), Anemia (Chapter 199), Preoperative Hematologic Problems (Chapter 219).

REFERENCE

1. Schroeder ML, Rayner HL: Transfusion of blood and blood components. In Lee GR, Bithell TC, Foerster J, Athens JW, Lukens JN, eds. Wintrobe's Clinical Hematology, 9th ed. Philadelphia, Lea & Febiger, 1993:651–699.

   A detailed discussion of appropriate uses and risks of blood products is presented.

203 HIV Infection: Disease Prevention and Antiretroviral Therapy

Problem

ERNIE-PAUL BARRETTE

IMMUNIZATIONS

Immunizations in persons with human immunodeficiency virus (HIV) infection produce an attenuated response. Resulting antibody titers are highest early in HIV infection and in individuals with normal or mildly decreased CD4+ cell counts. Consequently, immunization is recommended as soon as possible after discovery of HIV infection. Because of the greatly increased risk of pneumococcal pneumonia and bacteremia, the Centers for Disease Control and Prevention (CDC) recommends the 23-valent *pneumococcal vaccine* followed by a booster every 6 years. Serologic response to this vaccine in asymptomatic HIV-positive patients is approximately 88%. Because there is reported to be a higher risk of *Haemophilus influenzae* pneumonia and invasive infections in persons with HIV infection and adverse effects are minimal, the CDC recommends *H. influenzae type b vaccine*. The polysaccharide-protein conjugate vaccine provides a better response in individuals with the acquired immunodeficiency syndrome (AIDS), whereas the polysaccharide vaccine has higher responses in earlier (asymptomatic) infection.

Influenza vaccination should be given annually during October or November. Patients with HIV are at higher risk of bacterial infections complicating influenza, and the vaccine may decrease the number of evaluations for pulmonary infections. Immunologic response to the vaccine is poor, and several early reports suggest that immunization may accelerate disease by transiently increasing HIV viral load after influenza immunization. These studies were small, however, and no adverse clinical outcomes were observed. Despite the contradictory evidence, most clinicians advise patients to receive the vaccine.

Because the risk groups overlap, many persons with HIV infection have also been exposed to hepatitis B. If antibody to hepatitis B is absent and lifestyle or occupation places the patient at risk, vaccination with the *recombinant hepatitis B virus (HBV) vaccine* is indicated (three intramuscular doses at 0, 1, and 6 months). Protective antibody to the surface antigen (anti-HBs) should be confirmed 1 to 6 months after the series. Anti-HBs greater than 10 mIU is adequate; lower values warrant a fourth dose.

Administration of a booster for *tetanus-diphtheria (TD)* every 10 years is standard. *Measles-mumps-rubella (MMR)* is a live vaccine and should be avoided in those with severe immunosuppression. However, because of increased mortality and atypical presentations of measles, those born after 1956 without documented vaccination or history of measles should receive MMR. Recipients of the killed virus vaccine used before 1967 should be revaccinated. In general, live vaccinations are contraindicated (e.g., live oral polio, bacille Calmette-Guérin [BCG], and yellow fever).

ANTIRETROVIRAL THERAPY

The list of available drugs to treat HIV infection has continued to grow. Eight drugs have been licensed, and the Food and Drug Administration (FDA) will be reviewing several more in the near future. The decision to approve drugs with early access has been based on surrogate markers (e.g., increase in CD4+ count and decrease in HIV viral load) as opposed to demonstration of improved survival or decreased morbidity. Early access has expanded the options for patients with advanced disease in whom other agents failed or were not tolerated. However, many questions remain, such as when to start therapy, what is the optimal initial regimen, when to change agents, and when to use monotherapy versus combination therapy. Because most trials have included only patients with no exposure to zidovudine (azidothymidine [AZT]) or other antiretroviral agents, the results may not be applicable to patients treated with several drugs.

Many patients will have opinions regarding antiretroviral therapy. These should be explored, because most patients will experience adverse symptoms with antiretroviral drugs. The expected benefits of the medications should be weighed against the potential decrement in quality of life, taking into account patient preferences in all decisions.

Zidovudine (AZT, Retrovir) was the first drug approved for HIV infection and was long considered the best drug for initial monotherapy. It is a nucleoside analogue that causes termination of the DNA chain produced by viral reverse transcriptase. The usual dose of zidovudine is 200 mg three times a day except when treating HIV dementia, in which a dose of 1 to 2 g/d is beneficial.

In an early placebo-controlled trial, patients with prior *Pneumocystis carinii* pneumonia (PCP) (mean CD4+ count = 66/mm^3) or symptomatic HIV infection (mean CD4+ count = 199/mm^3) treated with zidovudine exhibited a significant decrease in mortality, reduction in opportunistic infections, weight gain, increased CD4+ count, and decreased p24 antigen levels. In several studies of asymptomatic patients with a CD4+ count less than 500/mm^3, zidovudine has delayed the progression to AIDS or severe symptomatic disease, but this benefit lasts for only 1 to 2 years. Zidovudine also delays disease progression among symptomatic patients with a CD4+ count below $500/mm^3$, but without any improvement in survival. For asymptomatic patients with a CD4+ count greater than $500/mm^3$, no benefit has been noted.

Zidovudine received FDA approval in 1995 for use during pregnancy to decrease perinatal transmission. In women with a CD4+ count greater than $200/mm^3$, zidovudine started during weeks 14 through 34 in pregnancy, along with intravenous zidovudine during labor and delivery and zidovudine given to the newborn for 6 weeks, has reduced HIV transmission by 67.5% (8.3% with zidovudine vs. 25.5% with placebo, $P < .001$). The utility of zidovudine in pregnant women with lower CD4+ counts and the long-term risk to the infant are not known. The US Public Health Service has recommended that all pregnant women be offered zidovudine counseling and voluntary testing and, if HIV positive, be informed of the risks and benefits of zidovudine.

The use of this agent is limited by adverse effects. Bone marrow suppression causes anemia and, less often, granulocytopenia and thrombocytopenia. Macrocytic anemia is dose related and may respond to erythropoietin if serum levels of endogenous erythropoietin are less than 500 mU/mL^3. Headache, malaise, fatigue, nausea, and vomiting are common. Gradual dosage increases limit side effects. An attenuation of the side effects is seen with time. Rare adverse effects include proximal myopathy, hepatitis, and lactic acidosis.

Didanosine (DDI, Videx) is approved by the FDA for patients with advanced HIV infection who have received a prolonged course of zidovudine. Studies in patients treated for 4 or more months with zidovudine demonstrate that switching to didanosine delayed disease progression when compared with continued therapy with zidovudine. Changing drugs appears to be of benefit even if clinical deterioration has not occurred. The benefit of switching to didanosine is greatest when the CD4+ count was above $100/mm^3$.

Dosing of didanosine is weight based: 200-mg tablets or 250-mg powder for patients weighing more than 60 kg and 125-mg tablets or 167-mg powder for those weighing less than 60 kg given twice a day on an empty stomach. The buffered powder may be better tolerated. Food reduces absorption by 50%. The tablets contain a buffer. Each dose should include two tablets to provide an adequate amount of the buffer, to avoid degradation by gastric acid. Severe adverse effects of didanosine include peripheral neuropathy (12%) and pancreatitis (6%). The neuropathy is distal and symmetric and presents as a painful numbness or tingling in the hands or feet. It is dose related and occurs more frequently in patients with a history of neuropathy. Ten percent of patients require dose reduction because of the adverse effects. Clinical pancreatitis may be severe, and fatal cases have been reported. Patients with a history of pancreatitis should not receive didanosine. Diarrhea, abdominal pain, headaches, and elevated transaminase levels are also noted.

Zalcitabine (DDC, Hivid) has not been FDA approved for initial monotherapy because a higher mortality was seen in antiretroviral-naive patients (CD4+ count below $200/mm^3$) treated with zalcitabine compared with zidovudine. Zalcitabine in combination with zidovudine has been recommended after more than 6 months of zidovudine in patients in whom a delay in disease progression was observed and who had a CD4+ count greater than $150/mm^3$. Zalcitabine monotherapy for patients intolerant of zidovudine or with progression on zidovudine is likely to be replaced by therapy with newer agents.

Zalcitabine is given in a dose of 0.75 mg three times a day. Peripheral neuropathy is the major toxicity (22%–35%). Pancreatitis is less common than with didanosine. Patients with a history of pancreatitis should be observed closely. Oral, esophageal, and vaginal ulcers are reversible when the drug is stopped.

Stavudine (d4T, Zerit) has been approved for three patient groups: patients intolerant of therapies with proven clinical benefit (zidovudine, didanosine, zalcitabine); persons who experience disease progression on proven therapies; or those for whom previous agents are contraindicated. Studies have shown increased weight and improved quality of life with the use of this agent compared with continued therapy with zidovudine; yet approval was based on surrogate markers. Stavudine has increased CD4+ cell counts at 12 weeks compared with continued therapy with zidovudine in persons who have had more than 24 weeks of zidovudine. Peripheral neuropathy is the major adverse effect and is dose related (up to 21%). Other adverse effects include elevated levels of alanine transaminase, diarrhea, nausea, and minimal myelosuppression. The dosage regimen is 40 mg twice a day for persons weighing 60 kg or more and 30 mg for those weighing less than 60 kg.

Lamivudine (3TC, Epivir) is a nucleoside reverse transcriptase inhibitor; approval by the FDA is based on studies of surrogate markers. The effect of this agent on disease progression and survival is unknown. Studies in both zidovudine-naive and zidovudine-treated patients have shown significant increases in CD4+ cell counts and decreases in viral load for lamivudine/zidovudine combination therapy versus zidovudine monotherapy. Lamivudine is well tolerated, but monotherapy is associated with rapid development of viral resistance. The dosage regimen is 150 mg twice daily and is adjusted for impaired renal function. Patients weighing less than 50 kg receive an oral solution at 2 mg/kg twice daily.

The protease inhibitors are a new class of antiretroviral agents. Impressive results for these agents when combined with the nucleoside analogues far exceed those for monotherapy or combined therapy with nucleoside analogues (e.g., > 2 log, 100-fold, decrease in viral load). They inhibit HIV protease, which processes viral Gag-Pol polyproteins into functional units of Gag, nucleocapsid core proteins, and the viral enzymes protease and integrase. Blocking this step results in noninfectious virion particles. The FDA has approved three protease inhibitors in record time based on changes in CD4+ cell counts and HIV viral load. Although monotherapy with a protease inhibitor rapidly decreases viral load and increases CD4+ cell counts, viral resistance generally develops in several months.

Due to rapid approval, limited data on only a few combinations for each protease inhibitor are available. *Saquinavir (Invirase)* is approved by the FDA for advanced HIV infection in combination with nucleoside analogues. Saquinavir with zidovudine, zalcitabine, or both improved surrogate markers. This drug is limited by poor absorption, gastrointestinal side effects, and three-times-a-day dosing of three 200-mg capsules. *Ritonavir (Norvir)* received approval for both combination therapy with nucleoside analogues and monotherapy, though when used alone viral resistance likely appears sooner. A survival benefit was seen in patients with a CD4+ cell count less than 100/mm³ at 6 months in a randomized controlled trial in which patients continued their prior antiretroviral therapy (6-month cumulative mortality: ritonavir, 5.8%, vs. placebo, 10.1%). Combined with zidovudine or zidovudine/zalcitabine, ritonavir improves surrogate markers. Side effects include asthenia, gastrointestinal disturbances (25%), and circumoral and peripheral paresthesias. Significant increases in triglycerides (10% greater than 1500 mg/dL), transaminases (aspartate transaminase, alanine transaminase), and creatinine phosphokinase have been reported. The dosage is six 100-mg capsules twice daily. *Indinavir* (*Crixivan*) has been approved for use with nucleoside antiretroviral agents based on improvements in surrogate markers. Combinations of indinavir with zidovudine, zidovudine/lamivudine, and zidovudine/didanosine are reported. The dosage is two 400-mg capsules three times a day taken on an empty stomach. Side effects include gastrointestinal symptoms, headaches, nephrolithiasis (4%), and hyperbilirubinemia (10%).

Several drawbacks to these drugs exist. The just-discussed three protease inhibitors are potent inhibitors of the hepatic cytochrome enzymes and thus have the potential for adverse drug interactions. The approximate order of this effect is ritonavir > indinavir > saquinavir. Before initiating therapy with any of these, a review of all medications is needed. Many doses of drugs commonly used in HIV care (e.g., rifabutin and rifampin) may need to be reduced or discontinued. Concern exists that development of resistance to one of the protease inhibitors will confer cross-resistance to some, or possibly all, of the other protease inhibitors. The available protease inhibitors are also extremely expensive, costing $360 to $625 per month.

In late 1995 the results of AIDS Clinical Trials Group (ACTG) study 0175, the first of several large trials comparing combination and monotherapy regimens, were released in a National Institutes of Health bulletin. Patients with CD4+ cell counts between 200 and 500/mm^3 (median = 352/mm^3) were randomized into four treatment arms: (1) zidovudine, (2) didanosine, (3) zidovudine/didanosine, and (4) zidovudine/zalcitabine. For antiretroviral-naive patients, zidovudine/didanosine was significantly better than zidovudine alone when considering disease progression and deaths. In zidovudine-experienced patients, zidovudine/zalcitabine or didanosine alone proved better than zidovudine alone considering clinical endpoints. If a criterion of a greater than 50% decline in CD4+ cell count was also followed, then results with zidovudine/zalcitabine, zidovudine/didanosine, and didanosine alone were significantly better than with zidovudine alone in both populations.

Several excellent guidelines assist with clinical decisions. However, new information is being published rapidly. For patients with no prior antiretroviral experience and a CD4+ cell count below 500/mm^3, ziduvudine/zalcitabine, zidovudine/didanosine, or didanosine as initial therapy is better than that with zidovudine. The combination of a protease inhibitor and two nucleoside antiretroviral agents is the most potent available therapy. At what CD4+ cell count or viral load should this be instituted is uncertain. Experts do not presently agree on how best to use the available agents. Drug changes should be based on clinical progression or a progressive decline in the CD4+ cell count. Patients with a high viral load may benefit from antiretroviral therapy to reduce this. A patient's past experience and preferences, risk of serious adverse drug event (e.g., pancreatitis or neuropathy), and intercurrent illnesses often dictate which agents to use next.

PROPHYLAXIS AGAINST OPPORTUNISTIC INFECTIONS

When immune function declines, the risk of infections rises dramatically. Primary prophylaxis (i.e., prevention of first infection) and secondary prophylaxis (i.e., prevention of recurrent infection) are indicated when the risk outweighs the cost, inconvenience, and potential adverse effects of medications. Also when the infection is associated with serious morbidity and mortality or is difficult to treat, prevention may be prudent even if absolute risk is modest. However, if morbidity and mortality are low, treatment is efficacious, and prophylaxis is costly, continuous prophylaxis has not been recommended. Because prophylaxis is a lifelong recommendation, patient acceptance is essential. Tolerability, number and frequency of doses, and cost are important considerations. Oral medications are preferred and simpler regimens improve compliance.

Pneumocystis carinii **Pneumonia.** Before widespread use of primary prophylaxis, the risk of PCP was approximately 18% at 1 year, 25% at 2 years, and 33% at 3 years, when the CD4+ cell count had fallen below 200/mm^3. Despite advances that have dramatically reduced the mortality of PCP, 10% to 20% of patients still die of their initial PCP infection. Cohort studies suggest that prophylaxis against PCP delays the initial AIDS-defining illness for 6 to 12 months and increases the incidence of other diseases (i.e., *Mycobacterium avium-intracellulare* complex disease, wasting syndrome due to HIV, cytomegalovirus [CMV] disease, and esophageal candidiasis) that typically occur when immune function has further declined, as both the initial AIDS-related illness and subsequent AIDS-related illness. Early trials comparing trimethoprim-sulfamethoxazole (TMP-SMX) versus placebo and aerosolized pentamidine versus placebo showed significantly longer survival with prophylaxis.

Indications for PCP prophylaxis are CD4+ cell counts less than 200/mm^3; unexplained fevers (> 37.8°C [100°F]) or constitutional symptoms for 2 or more weeks; or oral candidiasis. The latter two are independent risk factors regardless of CD4+ cell count. Because PCP has been seen in patients whose CD4+ cell counts were greater than 200/mm^3 at their most recent visit, some have advocated instituting prophylaxis when the count falls below 250/mm^3. Finally, patients with PCP should receive secondary prophylaxis after treatment of the acute infection because recurrence rates of 70% in 1 year have been seen.

TMP-SMX is the drug of choice for primary prophylaxis because it results in fewer bouts of primary or recurrent PCP than the more expensive agents (i.e., aerosolized pentamidine or dapsone). The cumulative risk of developing PCP at 36 months on any of the three drugs is approximately 20%. Systemic prophylaxis, with TMP-SMX or dapsone, appears to be most effective in patients with a CD4+ cell count less than 100/mm^3 (19%–22%, compared with 33% with aerosolized pentamidine).

The advantages of TMP-SMX include prophylaxis against toxoplasmosis and bacterial infections. It is also substantially less expensive than aerosolized pentamidine. The CDC recommends one double-strength tablet a day, but one single-strength tablet a day or one double-strength tablet three times a week is effective. Up to 50% of those receiving TMP-SMX prophylaxis have adverse effects, including neutropenia, fever, rash, abdominal pain, nausea, hepatitis, pancreatitis, hyperkalemia, and, rarely, anaphylaxis. Patients with mild cutaneous reactions may continue TMP-SMX with symptomatic therapy because the rash may resolve.

Dapsone provides better protection than aerosolized pentamidine against PCP. Looking at on-drug failure rates, TMP-SMX is better than dapsone, and dapsone in a dose of 50 mg twice daily is better than 50 mg/d. Many smaller trials have shown protection with dapsone against PCP on various regimens of daily or intermittent dapsone usually with weekly pyrimethamine, but the current recommendation for dapsone is 50 mg twice a day for those intolerant to TMP-SMX. Dapsone is inexpensive but limited by adverse effects: rash, fever, nausea, neutropenia, methemoglobinemia, and hemolytic anemia in patients with glucose-6-phosphate dehydrogenase (G6PD) deficiency. Up to 40% of patients discontinue dapsone due to toxicity.

Aerosolized pentamidine is easily tolerated but expensive. Common adverse effects of coughing and bronchospasm can be prevented by pretreating with an inhaled β-adrenergic agonist (e.g., albuterol). Because transmission of tuberculosis in treatment centers is increased owing to frequent coughing, screening for active tuberculosis is necessary before beginning aerosolized pentamidine prophylaxis. There are reports of spontaneous pneumothoraces and a higher incidence of extrapulmonary pneumocystis in patients receiving aerosolized pentamidine, but these may be due to reporting bias.

Overall, when prophylaxis is indicated, initial therapy with TMP-SMX should be started. Mild adverse reactions can be treated symptomatically or by dose reduction if using greater than one double-strength tablet three times a week. Persons with a history of non–life-threatening reaction to TMP-SMX or sulfa drugs should be given TMP-SMX because of its efficacy and benefit in other conditions. Patients with a history of a more severe reaction to TMP-SMX may tolerate desensitization in a supervised setting. Fifty percent of patients will be able to tolerate this drug. When TMP-SMX cannot be used, dapsone is recommended, starting at 50 mg twice daily. Screening for G6PD deficiency before beginning dapsone therapy is important. Dose reduction may ameliorate adverse effects. If neither drug is tolerable, then aerosolized pentamidine should be started at 300 mg monthly through a Respirgard nebulizer. Other drugs and combinations have potential but cannot be recommended over aerosolized pentamidine. Some experts have advocated initial therapy with aerosolized pentamidine when the CD4+ cell count drops below $200/mm^3$ and switching to TMP-SMX when counts are below $100/mm^3$.

Toxoplasmosis. All HIV-positive patients should be tested for IgG antibody to *Toxoplasma* at the time of diagnosis because toxoplasmosis is the most common cause of central nervous system lesions in AIDS. Thirty percent to 40% of patients with HIV infection who have IgG antibodies to *Toxoplasma* will eventually develop active toxoplasmosis. The prevalence of individuals seropositive to *Toxoplasma gondii* is much greater in Europe, Haiti, and Latin America than in the United States. Individuals who are seronegative to *Toxoplasma* should be counseled on possible sources of exposure, including undercooked and raw meats, unwashed fruits and vegetables, or gardening. Cat litter boxes should be changed daily, preferably by an HIV-negative person. If this is done by an

HIV-positive person, careful hand washing afterward is recommended. Seronegative patients should be tested annually when their CD4+ cell count drops below 100/mm³.

In July 1995, the CDC began advising prophylaxis for all patients with a CD4+ cell count below 100/mm³ and antibodies against *Toxoplasma*. TMP-SMX is the drug of choice, and doses effective for PCP prophylaxis also protect against toxoplasmosis. For patients intolerant to TMP-SMX, dapsone (50 mg/d) with pyrimethamine (50 mg/wk) is effective. Intermittent therapy (dapsone, 100 mg, with pyrimethamine, 50 mg twice weekly) was protective in a randomized controlled trial. To decrease the hematologic toxicity of pyrimethamine, folinic acid (leucovorin), 25 mg/wk, should be added. Inexpensive folic acid cannot be substituted for expensive folinic acid. Pyrimethamine monotherapy is ineffective and possibly associated with increased mortality. Unfortunately, aerosolized pentamidine provides no protection for toxoplasmosis.

Tuberculosis. Reactivation of latent tuberculosis occurs in 2% to 10% of HIV-positive individuals per year, strikingly higher than the 10% lifetime reactivation rate in HIV-negative individuals. Reactions of 5 mm or greater induration to purified protein derivative (PPD) skin testing require chemoprophylaxis. Patients with a history of a positive PPD test who did not receive prophylaxis and those with chest radiographic abnormalities consistent with remote, untreated tuberculosis should also receive prophylaxis with isoniazid, 300 mg daily for 12 months. Because of the increased risk of peripheral neuropathy in HIV-positive patients, pyridoxine, 50 mg daily, is added. Active tuberculosis must be excluded before initiation of prophylaxis.

HIV-positive individuals exposed to active or infectious tuberculosis (i.e., smear-positive pulmonary disease) should be evaluated for active disease. Even if the PPD skin test is negative, prophylaxis with isoniazid should be started. In patients who are PPD negative, retesting in 3 months can guide decisions regarding continuing prophylaxis.

Anergic patients should be offered prophylaxis if they are from a group in which the prevalence of tuberculosis is known to be greater than 10%. In the United States, these include injection drug users, homeless persons, prisoners, migrant laborers, and persons from Asia, Africa, and Latin America. In addition, anergic patients exposed to infectious tuberculosis should receive prophylaxis after active disease is excluded. It is not known if individuals who become anergic are at less risk than those anergic on initial evaluation.

For HIV-positive patients from cities where multidrug-resistant tuberculosis is common, the choice of drug or drugs for prophylaxis is complicated and often based on local patterns of resistance. Consultation with the local health department or an infectious disease specialist is advisable.

***Mycobacterium Avium-Intracellulare* Complex.** Because of the success of the regimens to prevent PCP, approximately a third of HIV-positive patients will develop disseminated infection with *M. avium-intracellulare* complex, more than twice that seen before routine PCP prophylaxis. For 13% of HIV-positive persons this is the AIDS-defining illness. Disseminated *M. avium-intracellulare* complex is seen only in those with very low CD4+ cell counts (mean value less than 60/mm³). Untreated disseminated *M. avium-intracellulare* complex has a median survival of 3.5 to 4 months. Because treatment of disseminated *M. avium-*

intracellulare complex involves multiple drugs, high rates of failure, drug toxicity, and the need for lifelong suppressive therapy, preventive therapy for *M. avium-intracellulare* complex may be beneficial.

Rifabutin, 300 mg daily, decreases the rate of disseminated *M. avium-intracellulare* complex bacteremia by 50% (70% in compliant patients) compared with placebo in patients with a CD4+ cell count less than 100/mm³. Prophylactic treatment of 11 patients prevented one infection. No survival benefit was observed. Before a patient starts rifabutin, disseminated *M. avium-intracellulare* complex needs to be ruled out with one or more blood cultures. Persons with constitutional symptoms, fevers, and anemia are more likely to have active disease. Active tuberculosis must also be excluded because monotherapy with rifabutin can lead to rifampin-resistant tuberculosis. Rifabutin is generally well tolerated, but neutropenia, thrombocytopenia, rash, nausea, and uveitis do occur infrequently. Because rifabutin has liver enzyme–inducing properties, drug interactions may occur.

Clarithromycin, 500 mg twice daily, is also approved for prophylaxis against disseminated *M. avium-intracellulare* complex. Compared with placebo, clarithromycin decreased the risk of *M. avium-intracellulare* complex bacteremia by 69% in patients with a CD4+ cell count less than 100/mm³. A survival benefit was seen: 31% reduction at 12 months.

A US Public Health Service Task Force has recommended prophylaxis for persons with a CD4+ cell count below 75/mm³. This intervention is controversial because of its high cost (approximately $200/month for rifabutin and $175/month for clarithromycin), drug interactions, and potential for drug resistance.

Cytomegalovirus. Consistent use of PCP prophylaxis has increased the frequency of reactivated CMV disease from 25% to 45%. When the CD4+ cell count falls below 100/mm³, the 2-year probability of end-organ CMV disease is 21%. Homosexuals and injection drug users have high rates of past exposure and seropositivity for CMV. Persons outside these risk groups should be tested for the presence of antibodies to CMV. Seronegative individuals should receive CMV antibody–negative or leukocyte-reduced cellular blood products. CMV-seronegative persons should be warned about the risk of sexually acquiring CMV and advised to use latex condoms. HIV-positive persons may acquire CMV from children who attend day care facilities, and careful attention to hygiene, especially hand washing, may offer protection.

Two separate placebo-controlled trials of primary prophylaxis against CMV end-organ disease using oral ganciclovir, 1 g three times a day, in persons with a CD4+ cell count below 100/mm³ have been completed and have yielded conflicting results. The cost of oral ganciclovir is prohibitive, approximately $14,500 per year.

Valacyclovir offers much higher bioavailability than acyclovir. Data suggest that although valacyclovir may be more effective in preventing end-organ CMV disease than acyclovir, valacyclovir may be associated with increased mortality.

In the absence of a consensus regarding prophylaxis for CMV, most clinicians recommend annual screening examinations by an ophthalmologist when the CD4+ cell count is less than 100/mm³. Teaching patients the early symptoms of CMV retinitis (i.e., floaters, subtle flashes of light, visual field loss) may help identify early disease.

Fungal Infections. Mucocutaneous or esophageal candidiasis occurs in over 90% of AIDS patients. Significant morbidity is associated with esophageal disease. Fluconazole, 200 mg/d, reduces the incidence of esophageal candidiasis and superficial fungal infections, mostly thrush, when compared with clotrimazole troches, 10 mg five times a day. Primary prophylaxis is not recommended because initial episodes are easily treated, the risk of resistant fungal infections is increased, drug interactions are more likely, and it is expensive (approximately $5000 per year for fluconazole).

Invasive infection with *Cryptococcus neoformans*, primarily meningitis, occurs in 5% to 10% of AIDS patients. Untreated cryptococcal meningitis is fatal, and even with treatment mortality is still 20%. Patients should avoid places known to be potentially infected with *C. neoformans* (e.g., areas with pigeon droppings). Fluconazole afforded protection against cryptococcal infections compared with clotrimazole; the adjusted relative hazard was 8.5, but no survival benefit was seen. The benefit was greatest in patients with a CD4+ cell count less than $50/mm^3$. Prophylaxis is not uniformly recommended. The CDC recommends against uniform use of fluconazole for primary prophylaxis owing to low incidence of cryptococcal disease, the potential for drug resistance, increased drug interactions, and high cost.

In the endemic areas, primarily the central and south central regions of the United States, disseminated *Histoplasma capsulatum* infections represent 5% of the opportunistic infections in AIDS patients. In hyperendemic cities, where the incidence approaches 25%, prophylaxis may be beneficial but no data exist. Activities known to increase risk of exposure in endemic areas should be avoided (e.g., exploring caves, cleaning chicken coops, or disturbing soil beneath bird-roosting sites).

Severe coccidioidomycosis occurs in HIV-positive persons, usually when the CD4+ cell count is less than $250/mm^3$. *Coccidioides immitis* is endemic to the southwestern United States and northern Mexico. There are no studies of primary prophylaxis. Infection occurs by inhalation of spores, and patients should be warned when in endemic areas to avoid areas of increased exposure (e.g., construction projects, farms, and areas with dust storms).

Cross-References: Diagnosis and Management of Drug Abuse (Chapter 9), Adult Immunizations (Chapter 11), Fever (Chapter 16), Unintentional Weight Loss (Chapter 17), Dyspnea (Chapter 19), Fatigue (Chapter 21), Superficial Fungal Infections (Chapter 26), Tuberculosis Screening (Chapter 60), Diarrhea (Chapter 91), Peripheral Neuropathy (Chapter 147), Anemia (Chapter 199).

REFERENCES

1. Centers for Disease Control and Prevention. Recommendations of the U.S. Public Health Service Task Force on the use of zidovudine to reduce perinatal transmission of human immunodeficiency virus. MMWR 1994;43(RR-11):1–21.

   This announcement of evidence for significant prevention of perinatal transmission by zidovudine during pregnancy includes recommendations concerning counseling.

2. Centers for Disease Control and Prevention. USPHS/IDSA Guidelines for the prevention of opportunistic infections in persons infected with human immunodeficiency virus: A summary. MMWR 1995;44(RR-8):1–34.

This excellent clinical guideline utilizing a rating system for the evidence for prophylaxis against diseases in both adults and children includes specific recommendations for pregnancy. The full version was published in Clinical Infectious Diseases 1995;21:S1–S43.

3. Gallant JE, Moore RD, Chaisson RE. Prophylaxis for opportunistic infections in patients with HIV infection. Ann Intern Med 1994;120:932–944.

   Prophylaxis for HIV infection is reviewed and extensive references are provided.

4. Masur H, and the Public Health Service Task Force on Prophylaxis and Therapy for *Mycobacterium avium* Complex. Recommendations on prophylaxis and therapy for disseminated *Mycobacterium avium* complex disease in patients infected with the human immunodeficiency virus. N Engl J Med 1993;329:898–904.

   Disseminated M. avium-intracellulare complex is described in detail with discussion of clinical manifestations, prophylaxis, diagnosis, and therapy.

5. Sande MA, Carpenter CCJ, Cobbs CG, Holmes KK, Sanford JP. Antiviral therapy for adult HIV-infected patients: Recommendations from a state-of-the-art conference. JAMA 1993;270:2583–2589.

   Recommendations are given regarding use of zidovudine, didanosine, and zalcitabine based on clinical scenarios. Detailed analysis of early trials is provided. For more up-to-date data on newer antiretroviral agents the published clinical experience is lagging behind licensing and release. The Internet and World Wide Web has several AIDS-related pages, such as AIDS Clinical Trial Information Service (http://www.actis.org), HIV/AIDS Treatment Information Service (http://www.hivatis.org/), and JAMA HIV/AIDS Information Center (http://www.ama-assn.org/special/hiv/hivhome.htm).

· ·

204 HIV Infection: Office Evaluation

Problem

ERNIE-PAUL BARRETTE

Epidemiology. The reports of opportunistic pneumonias in young homosexual men in 1981 opened a new era in medicine. Since 1981, more than 300,000 deaths have been a result of the acquired immunodeficiency syndrome (AIDS), and more than 500,000 cases of AIDS have occurred in the United States. More than 1 million persons are living with human immunodeficiency virus (HIV) infection in the United States. In 1992, AIDS became the leading cause of death in men aged 25 to 44 years old and the fourth leading cause of death in women in the same age group.

Natural History. HIV infection has several distinct stages: primary infection, chronic infection, and AIDS. Patients in the chronic phase are initially without symptoms, but eventually most patients will develop constitutional symptoms as immune function declines. The 1993 Centers for Disease Control and Prevention (CDC) revised classification system for HIV (Table 204–1) makes use of this clinical separation along with the CD4+ cell count to generate nine possible stages. Clinical category A includes primary infection, asymptomatic infection, and persistent generalized lymphadenopathy. Category B defines patients with constitutional symptoms, thrush, vulvovaginal candidiases, bacillary angiomatosis, and other conditions. Clinical category C is reserved for opportunistic infections, recurrent bacterial pneumonias, lymphomas, wasting, Kaposi's sarcoma, and invasive cervical cancer. The clinical categories are further divided by the CD4+ count: 1 = greater than or equal to $500/mm^3$; 2 = $200–499/mm^3$; 3 = less than or equal to $200/mm^3$. AIDS is defined by all of category C (C1, C2, C3) or a CD4+ count less than $200/mm^3$ (A3 and B3).

Primary Infection. Symptoms of primary infection start 2 to 4 weeks after exposure. The illness is acute and lasts 1 to 3 weeks. Symptoms include fever (97%), adenopathy (77%), pharyngitis (73%), rash (70%), myalgia and arthralgia (58%), and headache (30%). However, asymptomatic seroconversion is not uncommon. Initially described as a mononucleosis-like syndrome, primary HIV infection can be distinguished from Epstein-Barr virus (EBV) mononucleosis. The latter involves significant tonsillar hypertrophy and exudative pharyngitis, which are not usually seen in primary HIV infection. Moreover, mucocutaneous ulcers, rash, and diarrhea are more often evident in primary HIV infection than in EBV infection. The differential diagnosis includes cytomegalovirus (CMV) infection, toxoplasmosis, rubella, viral hepatitis, secondary syphilis, disseminated gonococcal infection, primary herpes simplex virus (HSV) infection, other viral illnesses, and drug reactions. Laboratory features include transient lymphopenia followed by lymphocytosis (mainly CD8+ cells), thrombocytopenia, elevated transaminase levels, and, occasionally, atypical lymphocytosis. The diagnosis is confirmed by a positive p24 antigen assay along with a negative HIV enzyme-linked immunosorbent assay (ELISA). Several months later the antibody to HIV develops, and repeating the HIV ELISA and Western blot analysis will confirm seroconversion. Individuals with severe primary infection or prolonged episodes usually have shorter asymptomatic phases and progress to AIDS more quickly.

Chronic Phase. After seroconversion, patients enter a chronic phase marked by the absence of symptoms or signs. For the majority, this period is 7 to 10 years long. On average, the absolute CD4+ count declines 50 to 80 cells/mm³ per year, although persons with no evidence of disease progression (e.g., CD4+ cell count decline, lymphadenopathy, thrush) after 12 to 15 years have been described. A small number of patients progress to AIDS in less than 2 years.

Many laboratory markers have been used to follow disease progression and to assist in clinical decisions. The absolute and percentage CD4+ cell counts are the most widely used markers. Absolute values are often used in trials and clinical guidelines, but the percentage is less subject to variation. Many factors affect CD4+ counts: diurnal variation (lower in the morning and higher in the evening), age (decline after age 65), intercurrent infections (usually decrease), surgery (decrease), and delay in processing (increase). Strategies to avoid this variability include drawing samples at the same time of day, avoiding periods when infections or therapies may interfere, and following trends over time rather than single values when making clinical decisions. Some markers, such

Table 204–1. 1993 REVISED CDC HIV CLASSIFICATION SYSTEM AND EXPANDED AIDS SURVEILLANCE DEFINITION

CD4+ Cell Category*	Clinical Category		
	A	B	C (AIDS Indicator Condition)
	Primary HIV infection Asymptomatic HIV infection Persistent generalized lymphadenopathy	Symptomatic, not A or C conditions Examples include but are not limited to: Bacillary angiomatosis Candidiasis, oropharyngeal Candidiasis, vulvovaginal: persistent, frequent, poorly responsive to therapy Cervical dysplasia Constitutional symptoms (e.g., fever [38.5°C] or diarrhea) lasting > 1 month Oral hairy leukoplakia Peripheral neuropathy The above must be considered as due to HIV infection or have a clinical course or management complicated by HIV infection.	Candidiasis, esophageal or lungs Cervical cancer, invasive Coccidioidomycosis, extrapulmonary Cryptococcosis, extrapulmonary Cryptosporidiosis, chronic CMV disease other than liver, spleen, nodes CMV retinitis Encephalopathy, HIV-related Herpes simplex, chronic ulcer, bronchitis, pneumonitis, or esophagitis Histoplasmosis, extrapulmonary Isosporiasis, chronic Kaposi's sarcoma Lymphoma, Burkitt's or immunoblastic Lymphoma, primary in brain *Mycobacterium avium* complex, disseminated *M. tuberculosis* infection Mycobacterial infection, atypical species *Pneumocystis carinii* pneumonia Pneumonia, recurrent Progressive multifocal leukoencephalopathy *Salmonella* bacteremia, recurrent Toxoplasmosis, cerebral Wasting due to HIV
≥ 500/mm^3	A1	B1	C1
200–499/mm^3	A2	B2	C2
≤ 200/mm^3	A3	B3	C3

Adapted from Centers for Disease Control and Prevention. 1993 Revised classification system for HIV infection and expanded surveillance case definition for AIDS among adolescents and adults. MMWR 1992:41 (RR-17):1–19.

*AIDS is defined by all of category C (C1, C2, C3) or a CD4+ count less than 200/mm^3 (A3 and B3).

as the p24 antigen, are hindered by low sensitivity. Other markers such as β_2-microglobulin and neopterin are followed less frequently.

CD4+ cell counts correlate with survival: 1-year survival after a count of 200 to 499/mm^3 is approximately 90%, whereas the corresponding 1-year survival rates for lower CD4+ counts are 100 to 199/mm^3, 80%; 60 to 99/mm^3, 70%; and 40 to 59/mm^3, 60%. For CD4+ cell counts less than 50 cells/mm^3, the 1-year survival falls off logarithmically. Median survival when the CD4+ cell count falls below 50/mm^3 is 1 year.

Newer techniques to measure HIV viral load may add greatly to current methods of assessing disease progression. Multiple assays have been developed: quantitative polymerase chain reaction (PCR) to detect proviral DNA in cells, quantitative PCR to detect viral RNA in plasma and peripheral blood mononuclear cells (PBMC), and branched-chain DNA (bDNA) techniques to quantify viral RNA in plasma. The bDNA assay is somewhat less sensitive than the PCR assays. Low or undetectable HIV load predicts a stable CD4+ cell count and low risk of AIDS. Viral loads of greater than 100,000 HIV RNA copies/mL by bDNA measured within 6 months of seroconversion are strongly associated with development of AIDS (odds ratio 10.8). The use of measurements of HIV viral load is controversial. Stability of viral load, costs, and clinical significance need to be more fully evaluated before the routine use of these measurements can be recommended.

Initial Evaluation. The baseline history should include routine past medical history, medications, allergies, and family history. Specific questions regarding HIV risk factors are needed: exposure to blood products (particularly prior to March 1985), injection drug use (type of drug, site of injection, medical complications), and complete sexual history (number of partners; male, female, or both). Specific sexual practices and condom use are noted. Condoms are strongly encouraged because consistent use has been proven effective in decreasing disease transmission. Sexually transmitted disease history is important. Travel and residence history may indicate potential exposure to histoplasmosis or coccidioidomycosis. Because gynecologic abnormalities are more common in HIV-infected women, a careful review of menstrual history, infections, and Papanicolaou smear results is necessary. If advanced disease is present, a nutritional evaluation is indicated.

The first issue to be addressed in a patient who presents with a history of HIV is confirmation of the HIV test results. When documentation of HIV is lacking, then repeat testing to confirm HIV status is indicated, especially when risk factors seem minimal or when secondary gain is an issue. Further issues to be addressed include the use of antiretroviral medications (dose, response, reasons for starting and stopping, adverse effects), history of opportunistic infections (method of diagnosis, treatments, response to medications), CD4+ cell counts and trends, and prophylactic medications used (adverse effects). Specific inquiry regarding alternative, naturopathic, herbal, and experimental/protocol medications is necessary because high rates of usage of these types of treatments have been documented in HIV-positive patients.

Attention should be paid to the patient's social and emotional support system. A discussion of case management by a social worker familiar with HIV issues, community resources, and insurance concerns is essential. Legal and ethical issues related to ultimate disability and death should include an advance directive, a durable power of attorney, and a will. Often these patients have had friends who have died of AIDS and will have strong opinions regarding intensity of care, cessation of treatment, and withdrawal of support.

Review of Systems. Careful attention to a complete systems review is often useful owing to the high incidence of many diseases in HIV-positive individuals. *Constitutional symptoms* (fevers, chills, night sweats, weight loss, fatigue) may represent advance of HIV or systemic disease (lymphoma if the CD4+ cell count is 200 to 500/mm^3 or *Mycobacterium avium-intracellulare* complex if the CD4+ count is below 100/mm^3). High rates of treatable dermatologic conditions have been reported. The patient often benefits from a review of *skin changes:* papulosquamous conditions (seborrheic dermatitis, xerotic eczema, dermatophytosis, psoriasis, or crusted/Norwegian scabies), maculopapular disorders (primary HIV infection, drug reaction, secondary syphilis, candidiasis, pruritic insect bites, or disseminated fungal infections), plaques (if violaceous, consider Kaposi's sarcoma or bacillary angiomatosis), and pustules (staphylococcal folliculitis, eosinophilic folliculitis, HSV, varicella-zoster virus [VZV], typical scabies). Chronic ulcers are usually due to HSV or VZV, and viral cultures or direct fluorescent antibody testing will confirm the diagnosis. If these results are negative, biopsy is required to diagnose opportunistic infections.

A *head, eye, ear, nose, and throat* review must include eye symptoms. Floaters, flashes of light, and visual loss suggest retinal disease most often due to CMV (CD4+ cell count less than 100/mm^3). Sinus symptoms including facial pain or purulent drainage may explain a fever. Oral cavity disease is common and may be the first sign of advancing disease. Kaposi's sarcoma is frequently found in the mouth, most commonly on the hard palate. Both thrush and oral hairy leukoplakia predict progression to AIDS. Painful aphthous ulcers are more prolonged in HIV-positive patients. When an oral ulcer is nonhealing, a biopsy to rule out lymphoma and other opportunistic infections should be considered.

Lymphadenopathy is common. Diffuse involvement, with nodes less than or equal to 2 cm, suggests that HIV is the cause. When significant constitutional symptoms are present, alternative diagnoses need to be considered, especially non-Hodgkin's lymphoma, secondary syphilis, and tuberculosis. Focal lymph node enlargement is an indication for fine-needle or open biopsy unless a clinical explanation is obvious (e.g., local infection).

Pulmonary review of cough, dyspnea, sputum production, and hemoptysis is important. In older HIV patients who smoke, separation of chronic baseline pulmonary symptoms from early infections becomes more difficult. *Cardiovascular symptoms* are also reviewed. Cardiomyopathy due to HIV and zidovudine is well described. *Gastrointestinal symptoms* are extremely common. Odynophagia and dysphagia suggest an esophageal origin. Diarrhea, tenesmus, and frequent small-volume stools point to large bowel disease. Large-volume diarrhea, cramping, periumbilical pain, and weight loss suggest small bowel disease. Rectal symptoms in homosexual men need full evaluation because treatable sexually transmitted diseases and enteric pathogens are common.

A complete *neurologic* review is essential in both early asymptomatic and advanced disease. Headache, fever, and neck stiffness indicate meningeal inflammation, which can be aseptic or bacterial meningitis, seen at all CD4+ cell counts; or if CD4+ counts are low, an opportunistic infection, such as cryptococcal meningitis, tuberculous meningitis, or one of the endemic mycoses, may be the cause. When the CD4+ cell count is less than $100/mm^3$, focal neurologic deficits and seizures suggest a mass lesion. Most often the etiology is toxoplasmosis, central nervous system lymphoma, or progressive multifocal leukoencephalopathy, but a brain abscess is possible. Peripheral nerve symptoms occur both early and late. Many types have been described, but the most common is a predominately distal sensory neuropathy that manifests as painful burning sensation in the feet. Muscle pain and weakness may be due to either HIV myopathy or zidovudine myositis.

Cognitive complaints of inattention, forgetfulness, and poor concentration are sometimes noted first by friends and family. Neuropsychiatric testing may help document mild cognitive deficits. If clumsiness, ataxia, behavioral changes (typically apathy), and normal level of consciousness are present, then the AIDS-dementia complex is likely. However, treatable CNS infections (especially if the CD4+ cell count is less than $200/mm^3$) and mood disorders need to be considered. Because major depression is a readily treatable condition, mood disorders and neurovegetative symptoms need to be pursued. In addition, suicide is greatly increased in both HIV infection and major depression. Consequently, it is imperative to ask a patient about thoughts of suicide.

Physical Examination. A complete physical examination should be performed at the first visit. The patient's weight should be recorded with other vital signs. Attention should be paid to areas identified in the history and to systems known to be affected by immune compromise. A complete skin examination frequently yields easily treatable conditions. Careful lymph node palpation including cervical, supraclavicular, axillary, and inguinal nodes is important. A head, eye, ear, nose, and throat examination should focus on the funduscopic examination, the sinuses, and the oral cavity. Peripheral retinal lesions are not easily seen with the direct ophthalmoscope, but this should not discourage using this readily available tool. Oral cavity examination should include inspection of the hard and soft palates and the lateral margins of the tongue. White candidiasis plaques can be scraped off with a tongue blade, whereas oral hairy leukoplakia cannot be removed. Potassium hydroxide preparation of the plaque scrapings confirms the diagnosis of candidiasis. Pelvic, genital, and rectal examinations must be included. A careful neurologic examination greatly assists interpretation of subtle abnormalities later when trying to determine the presence of a central nervous system condition.

Baseline Laboratory Evaluation. T-cell subsets are done to assess immunosuppression. Most laboratories include absolute and percentage CD4+ cell counts, CD4+/CD8+ ratio, and absolute and percentage CD8+ counts. The absolute CD4+ count is most often used, but the percentage may prove to be less variable. Absolute CD4+ counts greater than $500/mm^3$ correspond to a CD4+ percentage of greater than 29%, and a CD4+ count less than $200/mm^3$ is equivalent to a percentage less than 14%.

Results of complete blood cell counts including platelet counts may be abnormal even in asymptomatic patients. Neutropenia (up to 50% of AIDS patients), thrombocytopenia (greater than 10% of AIDS patients), and anemia (up to 85% of AIDS patients) should be evaluated. Myelosuppression from drugs is particularly common. Zidovudine, ganciclovir, trimethoprim, foscarnet, pentamidine, and sulfonamides are the most common culprits. Screening for glucose-6-phosphate dehydrogenase deficiency is necessary before dapsone and primaquine therapy.

Baseline measurement of electrolytes, blood urea nitrogen, creatinine, liver function (transaminases, alkaline phosphatase, albumin), and amylase are useful. Recording baseline values before initiation of any chronic therapy (e.g., antiviral, antiretroviral, antibiotic, antiparasitic) will allow determination of whether drug toxicity is present.

Serologic testing for hepatitis documents past infection. Absent hepatitis B surface antibody is an indication for hepatitis B vaccine. Hepatitis C may explain chronic elevations in transaminase levels.

Serologic tests for syphilis are recommended yearly by the CDC. A Venereal Disease Research Laboratory (VDRL) or a rapid plasma reagin (RPR) test is preferred for screening. Early screening for syphilis is important because there is a high prevalence of syphilis in persons with HIV, the virulence of syphilis in persons with HIV may be greater, and treatment is more complicated in late syphilis.

Toxoplasma titers measuring IgG antibodies identify patients at risk for active disease. It is estimated that 30% of patients with evidence of past exposure to *Toxoplasma* will develop cerebral toxoplasmosis. Prevalence rates vary significantly by geographic region. A positive titer may prompt more aggressive evaluation of neurologic complaints. Prophylaxis is recommended for *Toxoplasma*-seropositive patients with a CD4+ cell count less than $100/mm^3$. *Toxoplasma*-seronegative patients whose CD4+ cell counts drop below $100/mm^3$ should be retested yearly.

CMV antibodies are present in more than 95% of persons with HIV infection. Initial measurement is important because seronegative patients should receive only CMV-negative blood products.

Tuberculin testing with intermediate-strength (5-TU) purified protein derivative (PPD) is recommended by the CDC in all HIV-infected persons except those who have a history of a positive PPD reaction. The Mantoux procedure involves injecting 0.1 mL of antigen intracutaneously on the forearm. The reaction is read at 48 to 72 hours. Those with a history of definite or probable bacille Calmette-Guérin (BCG) vaccination should be screened. Two or three controls, usually *Candida albicans*, mumps, or tetanus toxoid, are used at the time of the PPD test. As the CD4+ cell count falls, the delayed-type hypersensitivity (DTH) response also wanes. Fewer than 10% of HIV-infected persons with CD4+ cell counts greater than $500/mm^3$ do not display DTH, but this figure rises to 80% when the CD4+ cell count is less than $50/mm^3$. For this reason, PPD testing with two or more controls should not be delayed. The CDC recommends a cutoff of greater than 5 mm as positive, but some have argued that any induration is significant. For the controls, any amount of induration is considered positive but erythema alone is not read as a positive reaction. *Anergy* is defined as the absence of DTH reaction to both PPD and controls. Anergy has been observed more frequently in HIV-positive injection drug users than in HIV-positive individuals from other risk groups. Patients with a positive PPD test or who are anergic should be evaluated to rule out active tuberculosis.

For those who test PPD negative, repeat testing annually is the standard until the patient is anergic.

Baseline chest radiography is recommended by some experts to aid in the interpretation of films taken at a later date. Early pneumonia, especially that due to *Pneumocystis carinii,* may be subtle, and an older baseline radiograph may be helpful, although there are no studies confirming this.

Follow-Up Evaluations. Follow-up visits should focus on careful review of symptoms and investigations of new complaints. Repeated complete examinations are not useful. However, even in the asymptomatic individual, focused examination of the skin, fundi, oral cavity, and lymph nodes should be routine. Repeating the Papanicolaou test yearly is recommended by the CDC, although some have advised biannual testing.

Appropriate frequency of clinic visits has not been prospectively studied. If a person is seen soon after primary infection, visits every 3 months until resolution of symptoms and seroconversion are appropriate. Most patients' CD4+ cell counts return to the normal range and they can be seen every 6 months. Less frequent visits are reasonable for asymptomatic patients. When the CD4+ cell count is 200 to 500/mm^3, clinical follow-up every 3 to 4 months is usual. With a CD4+ count less than 200/mm^3, there are many issues of disease prophylaxis and a need for increased surveillance. Most clinicians observe these patients every 2 months.

Cross-References: Periodic Health Assessment (Chapter 8), Diagnosis and Management of Drug Abuse (Chapter 9), Adult Immunizations (Chapter 11), Fever (Chapter 16), Unintentional Weight Loss (Chapter 17), Anorexia (Chapter 18), Dyspnea (Chapter 19), Fatigue (Chapter 21), Principles of Dermatologic Diagnosis and Therapy (Chapter 22), Warts (Chapter 25), Superficial Fungal Infections (Chapter 26), Scabies and Lice (Chapter 27), Seborrheic Dermatitis (Chapter 29), Herpes Zoster (Chapter 30), Redness of the Eye (Chapter 37), Ophthalmoscopy (Chapter 46), Detection and Initial Management of Oral Cancer (Chapter 47), Tuberculosis Screening (Chapter 60), Cough and Sputum (Chapter 63), Diarrhea (Chapter 91), Dysphagia and Heartburn (Chapter 96), Viral Hepatitis (Chapter 100), Dementia (Chapter 140), Vaginitis (Chapter 164), Sexually Transmitted Diseases (Chapter 176), Screening for Depression (Chapter 185), Psychological Assessment (Chapter 193), Lymphadenopathy (Chapter 196), Thrombocytopenia (Chapter 197), Anemia (Chapter 199).

REFERENCES

1. Centers for Disease Control and Prevention. 1993 Revised classification system for HIV infection and expanded surveillance case definition for AIDS among adolescents and adults. MMWR 1992;41(RR-17):1–19.

   Details of the most current CDC case definition and classification system are provided, along with the definitive diagnostic methods for AIDS-defining illnesses.

2. Coopman SA, Johnson RA, Platt R, Stern RS. Cutaneous disease and drug reactions in HIV infection. N Engl J Med 1993;328:1670–1674.

   This study documents in a cohort of 684 HIV-infected members of a large health maintenance organization the increased rates of cutaneous diseases compared with non–HIV-infected members. Rates increased as immune function declined.

3. El-Sadr W, Oleske JM, Agins BD, Bauman KA, Brosgart CL, Brown GM, et al. Evaluation and Management of Early HIV Infection. Clinical Practice Guideline No. 7. AHCPR Publication No. 94-0572. Rockville, MD, Agency for Health Care Policy and Research, Public Health Service, US Department of Health and Human Services, January 1994.

This comprehensive handbook for care of the patient with early HIV infection includes an extensive discussion of tuberculosis, syphilis, and pregnancy.

4. Jewitt JF, Hecht FM. Preventive health care for adults with HIV infection. JAMA 1993;269:1144–1153.

Preventive care interventions are examined, including markers of disease progression, screening laboratory testing, immunizations, and prophylaxis of opportunistic infections.

5. Minkoff HL, DeHovitz JA. Care of women infected with the human immunodeficiency virus. JAMA 1991;266:2253–2258.

A gender-based discussion of HIV infection includes contraception, obstetric care, and evaluation of the HIV-infected female patient.

· ·

205 HIV Infection: Evaluation of Common Symptoms

Symptom

ERNIE-PAUL BARRETTE

Evaluation of any symptom in a patient with human immunodeficiency virus (HIV) infection must take into account the patient's immune status. Many conditions are exacerbated by HIV infection (e.g., psoriasis and sinusitis), whereas others are relatively unique to HIV-positive individuals (e.g., Kaposi's sarcoma and benign parotid lymphoepithelial lesions). The strength of the patient's immune system, reflected by the CD4+ cell count, helps to determine which pathogens are likely. However, even with relatively normal immune function, some diseases are seen more frequently (e.g., tuberculosis and aseptic meningitis). Acute HIV infection may be accompanied by complications rarely seen in other mononucleosis-like syndromes, especially neurologic complications. Medications used to treat HIV infection, prevent opportunistic infections, and treat symptoms have many adverse effects that complicate the evaluation of symptoms.

The most frequent symptoms are discussed and a general approach is presented. The most serious symptoms involve the pulmonary, gastrointestinal, and neurologic systems.

Pulmonary Manifestations. Pulmonary complications of HIV infection are extremely common. Although *Pneumocystis carinii* pneumonia (PCP) occurs in 30% of AIDS cases, other pathogens are too numerous to be treated empirically.

The CD4+ cell count and chest radiograph assist in the differential diagnosis. A CD4+ cell count greater than 250 to 300/mm^3 makes opportunistic infections unlikely and bacterial pneumonias, tuberculosis, or lymphoma more likely. Tuberculosis may occur at any CD4+ cell count. PCP, Kaposi's sarcoma, and nocardiosis occur when the CD4+ count is less than 200/mm^3. The endemic mycoses are seen when the CD4+ count is less than 100/mm^3, whereas aspergillosis and *Mycobacterium avium-intracellulare* complex occur when counts fall below 50/mm^3.

Clinical markers narrow the diagnostic possibilities, but histologic or microbiologic identification should be pursued. Acute cough and dyspnea suggest a bacterial pneumonia, usually caused by *Streptococcus pneumoniae* or *Haemophilus influenzae*. *Staphylococcus aureus* pneumonia may be seen in injection drug users. *Pseudomonas aeruginosa* pneumonia occurs when the CD4+ cell count is less than 50/mm^3. PCP may present acutely, but this and other opportunistic infections usually evolve over several weeks. Purulent sputum is seen in bacterial pneumonias and tuberculosis. Hemoptysis suggests Kaposi's sarcoma or tuberculosis.

After the history and physical examination, a chest radiograph is the first step in the evaluation. Several findings should suggest specific causes. *Pleural effusions* occur in tuberculosis, fungal and pyogenic pneumonias, lymphoma, Kaposi's sarcoma, or noninfectious conditions. *Hilar adenopathy* may occur in tuberculosis, in lymphoma, and less often in Kaposi's sarcoma but is rarely observed in PCP. *Cavitary lesions* are caused by tuberculosis, PCP, cryptococcosis, invasive aspergillosis, nocardiosis, *Rhodococcus equi, Pseudomonas* species, anaerobes, *Staphylococcus* species, and noninfectious causes. *Nodular lesions* suggest fungal infection, tuberculosis, PCP, Kaposi's sarcoma, or lymphoma. *Spontaneous pneumothoraces* and *pneumatoceles* are seen with PCP. Poorly defined *nodules with pleural effusions* are likely due to Kaposi's sarcoma. A *rapidly changing nodule* suggests either hemorrhage into a Kaposi's lesion or lymphoma. Predominately *upper lobe disease* is typical of reactivated tuberculosis but is also seen when PCP occurs in patients who have received aerosolized pentamidine.

The most common patterns on the chest radiograph are focal or diffuse infiltrates. Sputum examination is necessary to select empirical therapy. When focal infiltrates are present, sputum Gram stain, stain for acid-fast bacilli, sputum culture for pyogenic bacteria and mycobacteria, and blood cultures are routine. In patients at risk for tuberculosis, several first-morning sputum specimens should be collected for acid-fast bacilli. Isolation of patients suspected of having active tuberculosis is appropriate. Patients with smears positive for acid-fast bacilli may prove to have atypical mycobacteria, but treatment for tuberculosis should be initiated while awaiting final culture results. Initial therapy is based on the Gram stain and includes empirical coverage for bacterial pneumonias. When no organism is seen on Gram stain, therapy should cover atypical pneumonias and PCP. Patients with focal infiltrates that do not respond to therapy should undergo biopsy to rule out carcinoma, because primary lung cancers have been seen in younger (< 45 years old) HIV-positive smokers.

Diffuse infiltrates should be evaluated with an induced sputum specimen unless a productive cough is present. The specimen is tested for *P. carinii* (Giemsa stain and fluorescent antibody), bacteria, mycobacteria, and fungus.

When an induced sputum specimen is unrevealing, fiberoptic bronchoscopy with bronchoalveolar lavage and transbronchial biopsy is recommended. Initial therapy should cover PCP and possibly bacterial pneumonias. The results of the sputum studies will help narrow the choice of therapy. Inpatient treatment of PCP should be either intravenous trimethoprim-sulfamethoxazole or intravenous pentamidine. Adjunctive corticosteroids are added when treating PCP if either the room air PO_2 is less than 70 mm Hg or the alveolar-arterial gradient is greater than 35 mm Hg during the first 72 hours of hospitalization. Because corticosteroids may worsen other conditions, it is necessary to confirm a diagnosis of PCP.

When the chest radiograph is normal, further testing is warranted for the patient with a depressed CD4+ count because 5% to 10% of patients with PCP may have a normal chest film. Determination of oxygen saturation with and without exertion, arterial blood gas value, and diffusing capacity of the lung for carbon monoxide help separate individuals who should be further evaluated from those who may be observed clinically.

Gastrointestinal Manifestations. Swallowing disorders are common in AIDS patients and may occur during primary HIV infection. Gastroesophageal reflux disorder is infrequently a cause of dysphagia, presumably due to HIV-related achlorhydria, but should be considered. Drugs known to cause esophageal ulcers (zalcitabine, aspirin, and nonsteroidal anti-inflammatory drugs) may be the cause. Discontinuation may result in resolution, but if symptoms persist, further evaluation is warranted.

Dysphagia, difficulty swallowing, often described as food sticking when swallowing, is usually due to candidal esophagitis. The discomfort is moderate and poorly localized. If symptoms are severe, another diagnosis should be sought. When inspection of the oropharynx reveals the typical white plaques of thrush, diagnosis can be presumed. Treatment is with fluconazole, 200 mg/d for 2 weeks. Frequent recurrence may be prevented with fluconazole, 100 mg twice weekly, although fluconazole resistance may then occur. For those who fail an empirical course of antifungal medication, a second cause or a drug-resistant fungus may be present and endoscopy should be performed.

Odynophagia, pain on swallowing, or retrosternal pain unassociated with swallowing, is usually due to esophageal ulcers or erosions. Localized pain is the primary complaint, and dysphagia is minor. Endoscopy is recommended because ulcers may appear similar on barium esophagography and a tissue diagnosis enables directed therapy.

Cytomegalovirus (CMV) esophagitis associated with a median CD4+ cell count less than $15/mm^3$ is the most common finding. The typical appearance is a large single shallow ulcer in the distal esophagus. Biopsy specimens show cytomegalic inclusion cells (owl's eyes) and inflammation. Viral cultures are unreliable and may be contaminated by viremia from blood. In situ DNA hybridization may be more sensitive than histopathologic staining but does not distinguish between latent CMV infection and CMV disease. Intravenous ganciclovir at 5 mg/kg twice daily for 14 to 21 days is curative in 75% of patients. Neutropenia may limit therapy. Relapses are frequent, but the use of ganciclovir for maintenance is controversial. Those who do not respond to ganciclovir are treated with foscarnet, 60 mg/kg given intravenously every 8 hours for 14 to 21 days. The dose is adjusted for renal function, and adverse effects are common. Median survival after this diagnosis is reported to be 7.6 months.

Herpes simplex virus (HSV) esophagitis presents as severe odynophagia. Endoscopy reveals multiple ulcers. Biopsy demonstrates multinucleated giant cells with intranuclear inclusions. Response to acyclovir administered intravenously in a dose of 5 mg/kg every 8 hours is excellent. If this fails, treatment is with foscarnet.

Idiopathic esophageal ulcerations are increasingly being reported. The appearance at endoscopy is similar to that of CMV infection. Multiple biopsy specimens with histologic examination are needed to exclude viral esophagitis. Success with prednisone, 40 mg daily tapering 10 mg/wk for 4 weeks, for idiopathic esophageal ulcerations in small series has been reported. Trials with thalidomide are ongoing.

More than half of patients with AIDS experience significant *diarrhea*, which, if chronic, may cause weight loss, malabsorption, and social disability. Rehydration is often necessary. Antimotility agents (loperamide and diphenoxylate) are safe in the absence of bloody diarrhea, fecal leukocytes, or substantial abdominal pain. Although the optimal evaluation has not been determined, extensive testing uncovers an etiology in 75% of cases. However, some pathogens have no proven therapy (e.g., cryptosporidiosis and microsporidiosis).

A single stool culture followed by antimotility agents is a reasonable approach in patients with minimal to moderate diarrhea. Nonresponders are further tested with a stool culture for enteric pathogens and with a minimum of three fresh stool specimens for ova and parasite testing, including stains for *Cryptosporidium* and *Microsporidium*. If the patient has received antibiotics in the previous 3 months, a stool specimen is tested for *Clostridium difficile* toxin. A sensitive Giardia antigen stool assay is available. If the CD4+ cell count is less than 100/mm^3, infection with *Mycobacterium avium-intracellulare*, CMV, *Cryptosporidium*, *Microsporidium*, or *Isospora belli* may be present. Blood cultures for mycobacteria are done if the CD4+ cell count is less than 100/mm^3 and fever or constitutional symptoms are present. Eosinophilia is seen only with infection with *Isospora* and *Strongyloides stercoralis*.

When the diagnosis remains unclear, colonoscopy, endoscopy, or both are needed. The clinical picture may help determine which of these to pursue first. If large-volume diarrhea, cramping periumbilical pain, weight loss, or a positive Sudan stain for fecal fat is present, upper endoscopy should be performed. Duodenal biopsy specimens are cultured for CMV and mycobacteria and studied for histologic markers for viral, mycobacterial, and protozoal infection. When frequent small-volume stools, tenesmus, left lower quadrant pain, or fecal leukocytes are present, colonoscopy should be done. Colonic biopsy specimens are studied like duodenal specimens.

Neurologic Manifestations. In late HIV infection, neurologic complications become increasingly common. Presentations may be atypical and overlap.

Headache is frequently seen with zidovudine therapy as well as other systemic infections. Meningitis may be insidious, and typical signs may be lacking. Cryptococcal meningitis is the most common meningeal infection. Headache, fever, malaise, and nausea are usual, but nuchal rigidity and photophobia are not always present. Serum cryptococcal antigen should be positive. The diagnosis is confirmed by study of the cerebrospinal fluid (CSF) with India ink, cryptococcal antigen, and culture. CSF glucose, protein, and cell count values may be near normal. Elevated CSF pressure (> 350 mm Hg) is treated with daily lumbar punctures, shunting, or acetazolamide. Aseptic meningitis usually occurs when the CD4+ cell count is between 200 and 500/mm³. The headache may be severe, but cultures of the CSF are negative. There is typically a mild pleocytosis and elevated CSF protein level. Bacterial meningitis presents similarly as in immunocompetent patients. Meningitis from *Listeria monocytogenes* occurs more frequently in HIV-positive patients. Uncommon causes of meningitis include tuberculosis, syphilis, histoplasmosis, and coccidioidomycosis. Therefore, CSF analysis should always include the Venereal Disease Research Laboratory (VDRL) test, cultures, and stains for bacteria, acid-fast bacilli, and fungi.

A *focal neurologic deficit or seizure* suggests a structural neurologic lesion (e.g., toxoplasmosis), which may present in this manner in advanced HIV infection. Neuroimaging with magnetic resonance imaging is more sensitive, but computed tomography with and without contrast medium enhancement is less expensive. Multiple ring-enhancing lesions located in the basal ganglia or cortex with edema suggest toxoplasmosis. Most patients have a positive serology for anti-*Toxoplasma* antibodies. When the evidence supports a diagnosis of toxoplasmosis, empirical therapy with pyrimethamine and sulfadiazine should result in improvement in 2 to 3 weeks. Central nervous system (CNS) lymphoma, presenting as single or multiple weakly enhancing lesions in the periventricular white matter, may be confused with toxoplasmosis. Lymphoma progresses more slowly over weeks, and fever is absent. A biopsy is necessary for diagnosis. Although the prognosis is very poor, these lesions may respond to radiation therapy. Early biopsy is advocated for a single mass suggestive of CNS lymphoma with a negative *Toxoplasma* serology. Positron-emission tomography may identify contrast medium–enhancing lesions correctly as lymphoma or toxoplasmosis.

Progressive multifocal leukoencephalopathy (PML) presents over weeks with focal findings in alert patients with CD4+ cell counts less than 50/mm³. Imaging studies show multiple hypodense nonenhancing lesions in the subcortical white matter. A biopsy provides a definitive diagnosis but is not required unless the presentation is atypical. Most patients with PML survive less than 6 months, but remission and benign courses have been reported. Because many pathogens have been reported to cause CNS abscesses (e.g., cryptococcoma), an early biopsy is recommended for atypical lesions.

When there is depression in the level of consciousness, noninfectious causes to be considered include hypoxia, sepsis, and metabolic or adverse drug reaction. The causes of focal brain dysfunction discussed earlier may also present as *global disease*. CMV encephalitis, which is difficult to diagnose, presents subacutely and is seen most often with active CMV infection in another organ and a CD4+ cell count less than 50/mm³. Hydrocephalus and periventricular enhancement on imaging studies are suggestive, but CMV viremia and viruria are not diagnostic for end-organ disease. Median survival is only 5 weeks, and treatment is of unclear benefit. Herpes simplex virus encephalitis is definitively diagnosed by brain biopsy, but polymerase chain reaction testing of the CSF may prove to be useful.

Dementia due to HIV infection presents as a normal level of consciousness and progresses over months. A constellation of forgetfulness, inattention, clumsiness, and apathy occurs initially. Cognitive changes precede the motor and behavioral changes. Depression and early HIV dementia may mimic each other. Complete CSF analysis and neuroimaging studies are performed to exclude other treatable diagnoses. Treatment with zidovudine, 1000 mg/d, has proven beneficial.

Cross-References: Tuberculosis Screening (Chapter 60), Pleuritic Chest Pain (Chapter 61), Cough and Sputum (Chapter 63), Pleural Effusion (Chapter 65), Lower Respiratory Infection (Chapter 67), Thoracentesis (Chapter 70), Arterial Blood Sampling (Chapter 71), Diarrhea (Chapter 91), Dyspepsia (Chapter 95), Dysphagia and Heartburn (Chapter 96), Sigmoidoscopy and Colonoscopy (Chapter 104), Upper Gastrointestinal Endoscopy (Chapter 105), Tremor (Chapter 136), Muscular Weakness (Chapter 137), Headache (Chapter 138), Dementia (Chapter 140), Electroencephalography (Chapter 148).

REFERENCES

1. Barnes PF, Bloch AB, Davidson PT, Snider DE. Tuberculosis in patients with human immunodeficiency virus infection. N Engl J Med 1991;324:1644–1650.

   A review of this rapidly expanding disease is presented with regard to how it intersects with HIV infection.

2. Lane HC, Laughon BE, Falloon J, Kovacs JA, Davey RT, Polis MA, Masur H. Recent advances in the management of AIDS-related opportunistic infections. Ann Intern Med 1994;120:945–955.

   NIH conference discusses the most recent advances for treating Pneumocystis carinii *pneumonia, toxoplasmosis, tuberculosis,* Mycobacterium avium-intracellulare *complex infection, other mycobacterial diseases, and cytomegalovirus infections.*

3. Masur H. Prevention and treatment of *Pneumocystis* pneumonia. N Engl J Med 1992;327:1853–1860.

   The author succinctly reviews the prophylaxis and treatment of Pneumocystis carinii *pneumonia.*

4. Simpson DM, Tagliati M. Neurologic manifestations of HIV infection. Ann Intern Med 1994;121:769–785.

   A useful review of HIV dementia, focal lesions, and infections of the central nervous system, myelopathy, peripheral neuropathies, and myopathy is provided with extensive references.

5. Smith PD, Quinn TC, Strober W, Janoff EN, Masur H. Gastrointestinal infections in AIDS. Ann Intern Med 1992;116:63–77.

   This comprehensive review of viral, fungal, protozoan, and bacterial gastrointestinal infections includes diagnostic and therapeutic strategies.

SECTION XIX

The Patient with Known Cancer

· ·

206 Altered Mentation in the Patient with Cancer

Symptom

ANTHONY L. BACK

Epidemiology. Of the neurologic symptoms experienced by patients with cancer, altered mental status is second in frequency only to pain. Although an outpatient workup is often feasible, altered mental status was the presenting complaint in 13% of patients requiring hospitalization at one solid tumor inpatient service.

Etiology. Altered mental status in cancer patients can result from direct invasion of the central nervous system (CNS) by tumor, indirect effects of the tumor on the CNS, or complications of therapy (Table 206–1). Metabolic encephalopathy, brain metastases, and medication side effects (often opioid-related) are the most frequent neurologic diagnoses, followed by leptomeningeal metastases and infections. Hepatic encephalopathy secondary to hepatic metastases occurs only after extensive loss of normal liver parenchyma. Hyperviscosity syndrome is restricted, except in rare instances, to patients with Waldenström's macroglobulinemia (IgM myeloma). Up to 30% of patients who have received whole-brain irradiation, including prophylactic irradiation (e.g., small cell lung cancer), subsequently develop symptomatic cerebral dysfunction, presumably due to the radiation itself. CNS infections occur mostly in patients with chemotherapy-related neutropenia. In contrast to patients with acquired immunodeficiency syndrome, CNS toxoplasmosis is rare in cancer patients. Paraneoplastic syndromes rarely cause altered mental status. Several chemotherapy drugs have been reported to cause encephalopathy, and intracarotid chemotherapy infusions have caused strokes. Failure to define an etiology for altered mental status in a cancer patient is uncommon.

Clinical Approach. History and physical examination usually indicate the diagnosis. Headache is relatively nonspecific. Focal neurologic signs suggest intracerebral metastases or a stroke syndrome. Isolated cranial nerve palsies usually indicate leptomeningeal metastases. Meningeal signs are seen with leptomenin-

Table 206–1. ALTERED MENTATION IN CANCER PATIENTS

Metastases
  Brain metastases
  Leptomeningeal metastases
Stroke syndromes
  Embolic: nonbacterial thrombotic endocarditis
  Thrombotic: hypercoagulable states
  Hemorrhagic: metastasis related
Paraneoplastic syndromes
  Dementia
  Peripheral neuropathies
  Cerebellar degeneration
Metabolic derangements
  Hypercalcemia
  Hyponatremia (including syndrome of inappropriate secretion of antidiuretic hormone)
  Hepatic encephalopathy
  Uremia
  Hyperviscosity syndrome
Infection
  Sepsis
  Meningitis, especially that caused by *Listeria* and *Cryptococcus*
  Encephalitis, especially herpes
  Multifocal leukoencephalopathy
Depression
Therapy related
  Late toxicity after radiotherapy
  Medications, especially opioids

geal metastases as well as meningitis. Alterations in level of consciousness suggest metabolic derangements, infection, medications, or, rarely, as a diagnosis of exclusion, paraneoplastic dementia.

Diagnostic studies should include determination of serum electrolytes, creatinine, and calcium; liver function tests; complete blood cell count; absolute neutrophil count; prothrombin time; and activated partial thromboplastin time. Unenhanced computed tomography should precede lumbar puncture to exclude midline shift because mass lesions sometimes present without focal findings. To detect intracerebral metastases, magnetic resonance imaging is most sensitive, followed by contrast medium–enhanced computed tomography. Both multifocal leukoencephalopathy and herpes encephalitis have characteristic appearances on computed tomography and magnetic resonance studies. The sensitivity of cerebrospinal fluid (CSF) cytology for detecting leptomeningeal metastases is directly related to the volume of CSF collected; three CSF specimens of 10 mL each provide a sensitivity of approximately 80%. If the CSF is negative, magnetic resonance imaging may detect meningeal disease. Even when nonbacterial thrombotic endocarditis is suspected, echocardiograms are usually unrevealing because the valvular lesions are small (1 to 2 mm).

Management. Corticosteroids usually improve neurologic symptoms in patients with symptomatic brain metastases; the usual regimen is dexamethasone, 4 mg every 6 hours. Larger doses of dexamethasone may be used if neurologic progression occurs but have not proven superior in a randomized trial. Phenytoin does not benefit patients with brain metastases who have not experienced a seizure. In selected patients with solitary brain metastases and no other sites of cancer, surgical resection followed by radiotherapy provides a survival advantage over radiotherapy alone. For other patients with brain metastases, radiotherapy is standard care. Special radiotherapy techniques such as radiosurgery may be beneficial for selected patients. Over 60% of patients receiving radiotherapy for brain metastases experience some palliative benefit, but the median survival of patients with unresectable brain metastases is only 3 to 7 months, depending on the number of brain metastases, performance status, and control of cancer at other metastatic sites.

Patients with leptomeningeal metastases can be treated with intrathecal chemotherapy, although response rates and survival are poor except for patients with breast cancer. Paraneoplastic neurologic syndromes can be treated with chemotherapy, corticosteroids, and plasmapheresis, although responses may consist only of stabilization of symptoms. Hyperviscosity syndromes can respond dramatically to plasmapheresis.

Hypercalcemia may require admission for treatment with intravenous fluid and furosemide; treatment of the underlying cancer is the best therapy. Pamidronate, 90 mg given as a 4-hour infusion, is the best second-line treatment for tumor-associated hypercalcemia. If a patient is near death, treatment of hypercalcemia may not be appropriate.

Cross-References: Cirrhosis and Chronic Liver Failure (Chapter 99), Muscular Weakness (Chapter 137), Headache (Chapter 138), Seizures (Chapter 139), Dementia (Chapter 140), Electrolyte Abnormalities (Chapter 182), Management of Depression (Chapter 189), Management of Pain in Patients with Cancer (Chapter 207), End-of-Life Care for Patients with Cancer (Chapter 209).

REFERENCES

1. Cascino TL. Neurologic complications of systemic cancer. Med Clin North Am 1993;77:265–278.

    Neurologic complications of systemic cancer are common. This review provides a useful clinical description of common syndromes including toxic encephalopathy and complications of cancer treatment.

2. Clouston PD, DeAngelis LM, Posner JB. The spectrum of neurological disease in patients with systemic cancer. Ann Neurol 1992;31:268–273.

    This prospective study of patients at Memorial Sloan-Kettering Cancer Center summarizes the diagnoses of neurologic consultation. For cancer patients with altered mentation, the most common diagnosis was metabolic encephalopathy (61%), followed by intracranial metastases (a distant second at 15%).

3. Grant R, Naylor B, Greenberg HS, Junck L. Clinical outcome in aggressively treated meningeal carcinomatosis. Arch Neurol 1994;51:457–461.

    In this case series of 36 patients, median survival was only 9 weeks, although in patients with breast cancer who also received systemic chemotherapy it was 20 weeks. Symptoms improved in only 15% of treated patients.

4. Gucalp R, Theriault R, Gill I, et al. Treatment of cancer-associated hypercalcemia: Double-blind comparison of rapid and slow intravenous infusion regimens of pamidronate disodium and saline alone. Arch Intern Med 1994;154:1935–1944.

    Pamidronate given as a 4-hour infusion is as safe and effective as a 24-hour infusion. However, the median duration of complete response was only 7 days, emphasizing the need for clinicians and patients to consider more definitive therapy or end-of-life decisions.

207 Management of Pain in Patients with Cancer

Symptom

ANTHONY L. BACK

Epidemiology. Moderate to severe pain is reported by 33% of cancer patients receiving therapy and by 60% to 90% of patients with advanced cancer. Many patients are concerned that physicians undertreat their cancer pain.

Etiology. Approximately two thirds of pain syndromes in cancer outpatients result from direct tumor involvement (Table 207–1). For instance, metastases to vertebral bodies may result in spinal cord compression. Chemotherapy can result in oral mucositis or painful infections such as oral herpes simplex or fungal esophagitis. Radiotherapy can cause pain from acute skin toxicity or delayed radiation fibrosis. Approximately 10% of cancer outpatients have pain that is unrelated to their cancer or cancer therapy.

Clinical Approach. A careful pain history and directed physical examination are essential, with special attention to the neurologic examination. Use of a simple pain measurement scale helps measure the initial severity of pain and subsequent response to therapy ("Rate your pain on a scale of 1 to 10, where 1 is pain you can barely feel and 10 is the worst pain imaginable."). The status of the patient's cancer will help determine whether specific cancer therapy will be useful in relieving the pain syndrome. These therapies include local radiation, hormonal manipulation, palliative surgical procedures, and palliative chemotherapy.

Table 207–1. TYPES OF CANCER-RELATED PAIN

Bone pain
  Bone metastases
  Pathologic fractures
Abdominal pain
  Liver metastases
  Bowel obstruction
  Malignant ascites
Neurogenic pain
  Peripheral nerve compression or infiltration
  Nerve root compression or infiltration
  Spinal cord compression
Therapy-related pain
  Mucositis
  Radiation skin toxicity
  Radiation fibrosis syndromes
  Corticosteroid osteonecrosis

Certain pain complaints require prompt diagnostic evaluation. Bone pain in weight-bearing areas may require surgical stabilization and radiotherapy to prevent pathologic fracture. Headache should prompt evaluation for intracerebral metastases.

Back pain is usually the first symptom of spinal cord compression, and early recognition of this syndrome is critical to avoid paralysis and institutionalization. The back pain of cord compression is often nonmechanical (i.e., unrelated to strain and unchanged with rest), although this does not reliably differentiate malignant from benign processes. This pain is usually local but may be radicular, referred, or diffuse due to uneven compression of nerve roots. Neurologic examination should include assessment of motor strength, a search for a sensory level, and reflexes including cremasteric and anal wink in patients with bladder or bowel incontinence. Cancer patients presenting with severe, mild, or equivocal symptoms of metastatic cord compression should undergo spinal magnetic resonance imaging or myelography. Those patients with marked neurologic signs or rapidly progressive deterioration should be admitted for intravenous corticosteroids and rapid evaluation.

Because psychological distress may contribute to pain, patients often benefit from evaluation by a psychiatrist, psychologist, or social worker.

Management. Oral analgesics provide relief to most patients and facilitate the workup, but severe pain may require immediate hospitalization and intravenous analgesics. Early consideration should be given to specialized pain management techniques beyond oral medications (e.g., an epidural nerve block for a patient with metastatic disease involving the sacrum).

For mild pain, acetaminophen and nonsteroidal anti-inflammatory drugs (NSAIDs: aspirin, ibuprofen, and others) are the drugs of choice. The gastrointestinal and hematologic side effects of NSAIDs may be dose limiting, especially in patients with platelet counts less than $100,000/mm^3$. If pain relief is not obtained or the pain presents at the moderate to severe level, opioid analgesics should be used. NSAIDs alone are inadequate for most patients with cancer-related pain.

For those with moderate to severe pain or pain unrelieved by NSAIDs, the second level of pain medication is the "weak" opioids, such as codeine and oxycodone (Table 207–2). These are most often prescribed in fixed-dose combinations with aspirin or acetaminophen (e.g., acetaminophen plus codeine) but can be given as single agents when aspirin and acetaminophen are contraindicated. For the fixed-dose combinations, dose-limiting toxicities are usually the gastrointestinal, hepatic, or renal effects of aspirin or acetaminophen.

The third level of pain medication is the "strong" opioids, such as mor-

Table 207–2. COMMONLY USED OPIOID ANALGESICS

Drug	Starting Dose Range
Codeine	15–30 mg q3–4h
Oxycodone	5–10 mg q3–4h
Morphine SR (sustained release)	15–30 mg q8–12h
Morphine IR (immediate release)	10–30 mg PO q1–2h prn breakthrough pain
Fentanyl	25 μg every 3 days transdermally

phine or fentanyl. For patients with severe cancer pain, strong opioids should be given on standing schedules, not on an as-needed basis. For most patients, sustained-release morphine administered around the clock every 8 or 12 hours should be the first choice among agents in this class. When initiating therapy, the dose of sustained-release morphine should rapidly be titrated based on the patient's pain relief and need for breakthrough morphine. All patients who take a long-acting opioid should have available a short-acting opioid to take for breakthrough pain, usually immediate-release oral morphine. The break-through dose should be at least 50% of the sustained-release dose, and patients should be instructed to use it as often as necessary. For patients who cannot take oral medications, transdermal fentanyl every 3 days also provides excellent analgesia. Because the pharmacokinetics of transdermal fentanyl are quite variable, some patients will require every-other-day dosing. The dose ceiling for transdermal fentanyl is related to the transdermal delivery system, and a patient who requires more than 300 μg transdermal fentanyl every 3 days will often need to switch to a subcutaneous or intravenous opioid. Sublingual morphine is useful nonoral medication for breakthrough pain but is erratically absorbed.

Many opioids are not recommended for cancer pain. Methadone is difficult to manage because of its long half-life (average 24 hours) and because sedating side effects outlast its analgesic action. Meperidine is poorly absorbed when given orally and has a short half-life (3–4 hours); its metabolite normeperidine has a long half-life (12–16 hours) and causes seizures at high levels. Mixed agonist-antagonist drugs (e.g., pentazocine) are of limited use because of psychotomimetic side effects (e.g., hallucinations) that occur with dose escalation; these drugs also precipitate opioid withdrawal in patients who are dependent on morphine agonists.

Combinations of opioids and acetaminophen or NSAIDs can often provide additive analgesia. The clinician should avoid combinations of opioids with other drugs that increase sedation (e.g., opioids and benzodiazepines).

Neurologic deafferentation pain, such as postherpetic neuralgia, is often opioid resistant. Treatment of neurogenic pain syndromes often requires individualized sequential drug trials, usually starting with amitriptyline. Other useful medications include carbamazepine, mexiletine, and clonidine; phenytoin is not particularly useful.

When oral medications produce insufficient analgesia or excessive sedation, specialized techniques may be useful, including continuous infusion, epidural or intrathecal infusions, nerve blocks, and neurosurgical ablative procedures.

Patients with metastatic cord compression should be treated with corticosteroids, generally dexamethasone, 4 mg every 6 hours. However, based on laboratory studies, some cancer centers routinely use doses as high as dexamethasone, 100 mg, followed by 24 mg every 6 hours, especially for patients with profound or rapid neurologic deterioration. Radiotherapy is the most common definitive therapy. Because the patient's degree of neurologic function at the time radiotherapy is begun is the most important prognostic factor, cord compression represents a genuine oncologic emergency. For selected patients, neurosurgical anterior decompression may have results superior to radiotherapy.

Follow-Up. Side effects of opioids are common. Patients starting opioids should receive stool softeners and be advised about cathartics. Sedation can be minimized by avoiding interactions with other drugs (e.g., cimetidine, barbiturates, and benzodiazepines) and using psychostimulants such as methylphenidate or pemoline. Nausea and vomiting can be treated with antiemetics or a different opioid, although many patients become tolerant to this side effect. Intentional overdose in cancer patients is uncommon, and when a patient on a stable drug regimen suddenly develops signs of overdose (excessive sedation and respiratory depression), the most common reason is medical deterioration with superimposed metabolic encephalopathy.

Many cancer patients fear addiction, but these patients rarely exhibit hallmarks of addictive behaviors such as psychological dependence or opioid use despite harm. However, tolerance develops in all patients chronically taking opioids: over time a dose increase may be necessary to maintain a stable level of analgesia; and patients are at risk for withdrawal syndromes if opioids are abruptly discontinued. Signs of withdrawal commonly include increased salivation, lacrimation, and diaphoresis and may include nausea, vomiting, abdominal cramps, and myoclonus. Importantly, fear of tolerance should not lead physicians to limit opioid use because patients may "need it later"; the most common reason for increased opioid dosing is progressive cancer, and increased pain should be addressed with escalated doses of opioids or specialized pain techniques.

Cross-References: Death of Clinic Patients (Chapter 6), Abdominal Pain (Chapter 94), Low Back Pain (Chapter 107), Management of Depression (Chapter 189), Altered Mentation in the Patient with Cancer (Chapter 206).

REFERENCES

1. Byrne TN. Spinal cord compression from epidural metastases. N Engl J Med 1992;327:614–619.

   A concise summary of a large literature review concludes that magnetic resonance imaging (MRI) has made earlier diagnostic algorithms obsolete, and no prospective data are available to risk-stratify patients to allow for a more conservative approach in patients with back pain and possible metastases.

2. Cleeland CS, Gonin R, Hatfield AK, et al. Pain and its treatment in outpatients with metastatic cancer. N Engl J Med 1994;330:592–596.

   In this study of outpatients with cancer, 42% of those with pain were not given adequate analgesic therapy by their physicians. A discrepancy between patient and physician in judging the severity of the patient's pain was predictive of inadequate pain management. Incomplete physician assessment is one of the most important barriers to adequate pain management.

3. Elliott K, Foley KM. Neurologic pain syndromes in patients with cancer. Crit Care Clin 1990;6:393–420.

   This is a comprehensive review with a wealth of clinical detail especially helpful in that it is not written for neurologists. It emphasizes clinical recognition and the neurologic examination.

4. Jacox A, Carr DB, Payne R. New clinical-practice guidelines for the management of pain in patients with cancer. N Engl J Med 1994;330:651–655.

   These guidelines are easy to read yet comprehensive and extensively referenced; they are incredibly valuable to the practicing physician. Their major limitation is that recommendations in the algorithms that are not backed by study data are not always clearly identified.

208 Dyspnea in Patients with Cancer

Symptom

ANTHONY L. BACK

Epidemiology. Dyspnea is the subjective sensation of uncomfortable respiration—being "short of breath." In patients with known cancer, early recognition and treatment of pulmonary complications can avert respiratory failure, which carries a grim prognosis. For cancer patients with respiratory failure requiring mechanical ventilation, the overall mortality is at least 75%.

Etiology. In adult primary care clinics, dyspnea most commonly results from congestive heart failure or chronic obstructive pulmonary disease (see Chapter 19, Dyspnea). In patients with cancer, however, there are additional diagnostic considerations. Dyspnea can be caused directly by tumor. *Bronchial obstruction* is most often due to primary or metastatic lung cancer but can be produced by metastatic renal cell carcinoma and melanoma. *Lymphangitic tumor* commonly results from metastatic breast, lung, or head and neck carcinoma. *Superior vena cava syndrome* is most often produced by lymphoma or lung cancer (small cell more often than non–small cell). *Malignant pleural effusions* and *cardiac tamponade* are frequent complications of lung and breast carcinoma.

Dyspnea can also represent a toxic effect of cancer therapy. Up to 15% of patients undergoing radiation therapy to the chest develop *radiation pneumonitis,* which is usually evident as an infiltrate in the shape of the radiation therapy port developing 6 weeks to 6 months after therapy has been completed. Less commonly, pulmonary toxicity is due to chemotherapy; bleomycin, methotrexate, and carmustine are most frequently implicated. *Chemotherapy-induced pneumonitis* can occur within hours of administration as a hypersensitivity-induced drug effect or can develop over weeks. *Anthracycline cardiotoxicity,* which occurs as a dose-dependent side effect after treatment with doxorubicin or daunorubicin (most often for breast cancer or sarcomas), presents as congestive cardiomyopathy but is uncommon when a patient has received a cumulative doxorubicin dose of less than 400 mg/M^2.

Infectious pneumonitis most commonly presents as dyspnea. Patients receiving chemotherapy are at greatest risk, particularly during periods of neutropenia (absolute neutrophil count < 1000/mm^3). *Pulmonary emboli* also occur because of cancer-related hypercoagulable states, inactivity, thrombus formation associated with indwelling catheters, or chemotherapy-related vascular toxicity.

Clinical Approach. Review of recent treatment may suggest chemotherapy or radiation toxicity. Physical examination may disclose pulsus paradoxus (tamponade), unilateral wheezing (bronchial obstruction), dilated chest wall veins (superior vena cava syndrome), dullness to percussion (pleural effusion), S3 heart sound (congestive heart failure), elevated neck veins, or pathologic lymph nodes. Evaluation should be guided by clinical suspicion based on history, physical examination, and chest radiograph. A hematocrit, absolute neutrophil count, and platelet count are required for patients receiving chemotherapy or with advanced cancer. In diagnosing superior vena cava syndrome, computed tomography of the chest with contrast medium enhancement is more useful than angiography. Echocardiography may support the diagnosis of tamponade in cases where physical signs are inconclusive. An ultrasound examination of the lower extremities and a ventilation-perfusion scan are useful when pulmonary embolus is suggested. Pulmonary function tests may be helpful when chemotherapy toxicity is suggested. A radionuclide ejection fraction is useful in suspected anthracycline cardiotoxicity.

Management. Patients with mild, slowly progressive dyspnea can often be managed as outpatients. Pulmonary toxicity secondary to radiation therapy and chemotherapy is treated with corticosteroids, usually prednisone, 1 mg/kg for 2 weeks followed by a slow taper. Anthracycline cardiotoxicity is treated with diuretics, digoxin, and angiotensin-converting enzyme inhibitors (e.g., enalapril or lisinopril). Malignant pulmonary effusions may be drained initially in the outpatient department. Hospital admission is usually necessary for patients with recurrent malignant effusions requiring chest tube placement or pleurodesis. Clinically evident tamponade requires immediate hospitalization for a surgical pericardial window or for pericardiocentesis followed by catheter drainage. Superior vena cava syndrome often requires admission for rapid diagnostic biopsy and initiation of therapy. If caused by lymphoma or small cell lung cancer, superior vena cava syndrome is treated with chemotherapy alone. Other causes of superior vena cava syndrome are treated with radiation therapy, which is delivered emergently if upper airway obstruction is present. Bronchoscopy-guided laser therapy can relieve selected cases of bronchial obstruction. Patients with neutropenia (absolute neutrophil count 1000/mm³) and fever (temperature 38.3°C [101°F]) should be admitted for empirical therapy with broad-spectrum antibiotics. Especially for patients who are terminally ill, codeine or morphine and oxygen are useful palliative treatments for dyspnea.

Cross-References: Death of Clinic Patients (Chapter 6), Dyspnea (Chapter 19), Pleural Effusion (Chapter 65), Lower Respiratory Infection (Chapter 67), Thoracentesis (Chapter 70), Arterial Blood Sampling (Chapter 71), Congestive Heart Failure (Chapter 79), Echocardiographic and Nuclear Assessment of Cardiac Function (Chapter 86), Echocardiography (Chapter 89), Anemia (Chapter 199), End-of-Life Care for Patients with Cancer (Chapter 209).

REFERENCES

1. Ahmedzai S. Palliation of respiratory symptoms. In Doyle D, Hanks GW, Macdonald N, eds. The Oxford Textbook of Palliative Medicine. New York, Oxford University Press, 1993.
   This is the most comprehensive review of treatments for dyspnea, especially regarding the use of oral and inhaled opioids.

2. Pizzo PA. Management of fever in patients with cancer and treatment-induced neutropenia. N Engl J Med 1993;328:1323–1332.

This review contains practical clinical tips on the infections that can evolve from neutropenic fever, as well as guidelines for managing suspected central venous catheter infections.

3. Ruckdeschel JC. Management of malignant pleural effusions. Semin Oncol 1995;22(2 Suppl 3):58–63.

   This review concludes that the most cost-effective and efficacious therapy is still tube thoracostomy and pleurodesis. However, newer techniques including soft catheters and thoracoscopy may become standard therapy.

4. Vaitkus PT, Herrmann HC, LeWinter MM. Treatment of malignant pericardial effusion. JAMA 1994;272:59–64.

   In many cases, pericardial drainage for several days with an indwelling catheter alleviates the effusion without subsequent recurrence. Systemic antitumor therapy with chemotherapy or radiation therapy is effective in controlling malignant effusions in cases of sensitive tumors such as lymphomas, leukemias, and breast cancer.

• •

209 End-of-Life Care for Patients with Cancer

Problem

ANTHONY L. BACK

Epidemiology. End-of-life care for patients with advanced cancer is managed mostly with outpatient care and home care. For patients with access to home care or hospice services, about 90% of their terminal care can be managed at home. During their last 6 months of life, about half of these patients are admitted for evaluation or symptom control, and 30% to 70% actually die at home. Clinical issues include advance care planning, withdrawing or withholding therapy, do not resuscitate orders, and futility. The most common clinical problems are pain, dyspnea, and depression.

Clinical Approach. Although the elements of a "good" death probably vary considerably among individuals, many would agree that the following are important: relative physical comfort, a chance to reconnect with important people, and a sense of closure. Truthful discussions about medical conditions are extremely important and enable patients to plan. Bad news should be delivered with empathy, privacy, and respect for what the patient already knows, as well as what level of detail he or she wishes to know. Care plans should include explicit definitions of expectations and goals, and goals may be nonmedical, such as a chance to visit with a particular friend. Many patients wish to die at home, but other patients prefer the security of a care institution, and occasional patients will want to receive aggressive therapy, including chemotherapy and intensive care, until death. These patient preferences should be formalized in advance directives to allow physicians and surrogate decision-makers to respect patient wishes. Organ donation is not possible for patients with cancer.

Medical interventions such as cardiopulmonary resuscitation can be withheld based on patient preference or a judgment of medical futility. However, medical orders to withhold cardiopulmonary resuscitation do not imply that other interventions, such as therapies to control symptoms, should also be withheld. An individualized care plan based on a patient's overall goals (for instance, wanting to die at home) can clarify caregiver roles and emphasize caring rather than withholding of "high-tech" interventions.

Symptom control is the part of terminal care that falls naturally to physicians, but end-of-life care is best performed by a multidisciplinary team that also includes nurses, social workers, psychologists, and chaplains. Home caregivers may need training in basic care and may suffer grief, strain, and personal health problems that must be addressed separately.

Patient requests for physician-assisted suicide or euthanasia should prompt an exploration for the reasons underlying the request, which may include inadequate symptom control or inadequately treated psychological problems such as depression. In particular, a request for barbiturates (especially for secobarbital, which is recommended by the Hemlock Society) may constitute an indirect request for physician-assisted suicide. Some patients making requests for physician-assisted death simply wish to explore the topic or signal their distress, and these patients should not be referred to advocacy groups prematurely.

The assurance that a physician will be available throughout the period of terminal illness and that the patient will not be abandoned can be a powerful component of care. When patients become too ill to come into a clinic, physicians must rely on assessments made by home care nurses, but it is valuable for physicians to retain direct contact with the patient and home caregiver by phone.

Management. Hospice services can be arranged with a phone call to a local service and provide patients with 24-hour nursing coverage. Most patients are referred to a hospice only when death is imminent, but a hospice can provide many medical and psychological benefits and will not be discontinued should a patient live longer than 6 months.

Pain should be managed aggressively; oral analgesics can be rapidly titrated over hours to days, and hospitalization should be considered for poorly controlled pain. For patients who become too weak to swallow, transdermal fentanyl is useful, and subcutaneous or intravenous morphine can be managed by most home care services. Although caregivers often voice concern about respiratory depression from opioids, it is ethically desirable to provide pain relief for these patients even if death is hastened as a secondary result. Provision of adequate pain relief for a patient dying of cancer does not constitute euthanasia.

Dyspnea can be managed initially with oxygen and low doses of opioids (15 mg morphine sustained release (SR) every 12 hours). Supplemental oxygen should be humidified because a dry mouth will exacerbate the sensation of dyspnea. For refractory air hunger, chlorpromazine, 25 mg per rectum q6–12 hours or 12.5 mg intravenously every 4 hours, can be useful. As with the treatment of pain, it is ethically desirable to relieve dyspnea in patients who are dying even if death is hastened as a secondary result.

For depression, psychostimulants can be especially helpful because their onset of action is faster than other antidepressants and because they can counteract opioid-related sedation (methylphenidate [Ritalin] 5–10 mg at 8 AM and noon; or pemoline (Cylert) 18.5–37.5 mg at 8 AM and noon).

For patients who do complain of hunger, thirst, or dry mouth, these symptoms can usually be treated with oral feeding, ice chips, or mouth swabs.

Excessive secretions can be treated with transdermal scopolamine or atropine, 0.2–0.4 mg subcutaneously every 4 hours as needed.

Terminal restlessness or agitation can be treated with lorazepam, 0.5–1.0 mg orally or intravenously every 4 to 6 hours, or chlorpromazine, 25 mg per rectum q6–12 hours or 12.5 mg intravenously every 4 hours. If pain has been present, a trial of increasing pain medication may be useful.

Artificial hydration and nutrition are not routinely indicated because most dying patients do not complain of hunger or thirst. For a patient who is dying of cancer, nonprovision of artificial hydration should not be equated with starving the patient to death. Artificial hydration generally increases oral secretions and consequently increases discomfort for many dying patients.

The final hours or days of life are marked by fluctuating consciousness and increasing detachment. However, some patients remain conscious until they are within 15 minutes of death. Noisy or moist breathing (sometimes called a "death rattle") occurs in over 50% of patients during the last 48 hours of life.

A phone call from a physician after death is usually of great comfort to the patient's bereaved family or friends and may be used to direct them to grief counseling.

Cross-References: Ethics in Outpatient Medicine (Chapter 3), Death of Clinic Patients (Chapter 6).

REFERENCES

1. Block SD, Billings JA. Patient requests to hasten death: Evaluation and management in terminal care. Arch Intern Med 1994;154:2039–2047.

   The authors present a thoughtful approach to a controversial topic; this article focuses on evaluating the patient rather than on moral arguments for or against these practices.

2. Gavrin J, Chapman R. Clinical management of dying patients. West J Med 1995;1663:268–277.

   This useful short summary covers physical and psychological aspects of end-of-life care. Its shortcoming is lack of specific doses for recommended medications—the most comprehensive source for doses is the Oxford Textbook of Palliative Medicine.

3. McCann RM, Hall WJ, Groth-Juncker A. Comfort care for terminally ill patients: The appropriate use of nutrition and hydration. JAMA 1994;272:1263–1266.

   In this series, patients terminally ill with cancer generally did not experience hunger or thirst, and their symptoms were relieved with small amounts of food, liquid, and mouth care. Thus, forced feeding, routine intravenous hydration, and parenteral nutrition probably play a minimal role in comfort care.

4. Quill TE, Brody RV. "You promised me I wouldn't die like this!" A bad death as a medical emergency. Arch Intern Med 1995;155:1250–1254.

   The authors put forth a thought-provoking reflection intended to reframe medical priorities for patients near the end of life.

210 Diagnosis of Pregnancy

Screening

DIANE L. ELLIOT

Epidemiology. The prevalence of unsuspected pregnancy is unknown, although one study reported that 2 of 110 women hospitalized for nonobstetric reasons were found to have unsuspected pregnancies.

Rationale. The patient interview (e.g., sexual activity, contraceptive practices, last menses) does not reliably exclude pregnancy. Because history and physical examination are neither sensitive nor specific for the early diagnosis of pregnancy, laboratory tests are needed.

The urine latex or hemagglutination tests detect only high levels of human chorionic gonadotropin (hCG) (500–3500 mIU/mL) and have been replaced by monoclonal antibody tests for the intact molecule or its beta subunit. Two weeks after conception, the hCG level is approximately 80 mIU/mL, and it doubles each 2 days thereafter. The hCG levels in serum and concentrated urine are comparable. Serum testing detects a lower hCG level and is generally slightly more expensive. Both the urine and monoclonal serum assays are more than 90% sensitive at the time of the first missed menses. Several home urine tests, using monoclonal antibodies, are available and cost approximately $10. Although manufacturers claim these tests are accurate at the time of the first missed menses, the accuracy in actual use is several percentage points lower.

Transabdominal ultrasonography can detect a gestational sac at 5 to 6 weeks and a fetal heartbeat at 7 to 8 weeks. Fetal heart tones are heard by Doppler at 10 to 12 weeks and by fetoscope at 16 to 20 weeks. Quickening, perception of fetal movement by the mother, occurs between 16 and 20 weeks.

Although ectopic pregnancies result in lower hCG levels, more than 95% of women with proven ectopic pregnancy have a serum hCG value in excess of 40 mIU/mL. Prior to the sixth week, both an ectopic and an intrauterine pregnancy can result in a positive qualitative pregnancy test and a negative ultrasound. In that circumstance, quantitative hCG levels help to distinguish the two situations. An intrauterine pregnancy should be associated with an hCG level doubling every 2 days; and when the serum hCG exceeds 6500 mIU/mL, an intrauterine gestational sac should be seen by transabdominal ultrasonography.

Not all hCG elevations indicate a viable pregnancy. More than 20% of conceptions result in a subclinical abortion. After a miscarriage, low and declining hCG levels may persist for 2 months. Detectable levels also can occur with choriocarcinoma and breast cancer.

Strategy. Laboratory tests are appropriate for women with amenorrhea, suspected pregnancy, pelvic pain, and scheduled radiographic studies. After the first missed menses, serum and urine monoclonal tests have comparable sensitivity; the choice of tests depends on considerations of cost and convenience. Serum tests are preferred when evaluating a suspected ectopic pregnancy.

Action. A positive pregnancy test leads to review of the implications and limitations of the test. Ultrasonography may be required when evaluating pelvic pain or a suspected ectopic pregnancy (see Chapter 160, Pelvic Pain in Women) and to date the pregnancy. In established intrauterine pregnancy, the clinician should discuss the woman's feelings about the pregnancy and emphasize the importance of early and continuous prenatal care. The clinician should assess the patient's diet, review her medications for contraindicated drugs, and emphasize discontinuation of cigarette smoking and alcohol use. Laboratory tests (e.g., complete blood cell count, Rh antibody screen, Papanicolaou smear, and vaginal cultures) are usually deferred until the first visit with the health care provider who will care for the woman during her pregnancy.

Cross-References: Abdominal Pain (Chapter 94), Pelvic Pain in Women (Chapter 160).

REFERENCES

1. Bluestern D. Should I trust office pregnancy tests? Postgrad Med 1990;87(6):57–68.

   The author reviews test characteristics for urine, serum, and home kits and use of these tests in women with early and ectopic pregnancies.

2. Ramoska EA, Sacchetti AD, Nepp M. Reliability of patient history in determining the possibility of pregnancy. Ann Emerg Med 1986;18:48–50.

   Historical features do not exclude pregnancy.

211 Bacteriuria in Pregnancy

Screening

STEPHAN D. FIHN

Epidemiology. The prevalence of bacteriuria in pregnancy is 4% to 7%, similar to that among young, sexually active women in general. Bacteriuria is more common among women of low socioeconomic status and black women with sickle cell trait.

Rationale. Twenty percent to 40% of pregnant women with asymptomatic bacteriuria detected in the first trimester will develop acute pyelonephritis if left untreated. This infection is associated with a substantial risk of prematurity and perinatal morbidity. Placebo-controlled trials have shown that treatment of asymptomatic bacteriuria can reduce the incidence of pyelonephritis by 80% to 90%.

Group B streptococcus is the leading cause of life-threatening perinatal infections among both infants and mothers. These infections usually arise from colonization of the vagina with this organism, but group B streptococcus can also cause bacteriuria.

Strategy. Screening all pregnant women for bacteriuria in early pregnancy will detect 40% to 70% of those who would otherwise develop symptomatic infections; the remainder develop bacteriuria later in pregnancy. For most patients, one screening should be performed at the first prenatal visit using either a urine culture or a leukocyte esterase/nitrate dipstick. Cultures growing 10^5 bacteria/mL or more should be considered positive. Both positive screening cultures and positive dipsticks should be confirmed with a quantitative, mid-stream culture. Women who test negative at the first screening but have a history of recurrent urinary tract infection should be screened again at the beginning of the third trimester.

Action. The safest oral drugs for treating asymptomatic bacteriuria or cystitis in pregnancy are the β-lactams, amoxicillin, ampicillin, and the oral cephalosporins, but antimicrobial resistance of typical infecting organisms to these agents has been steadily increasing. Single-dose therapy with amoxicillin eradicates bacteriuria in approximately 80% of women. A single dose of amoxicillin produces higher cure rates, but its safety during pregnancy remains in question. Nitrofurantoin, trimethoprim-sulfamethoxazole, and the fluoroquinolones have been used in pregnancy, but because their safety in pregnancy is less well established, they should be reserved for women who have organisms resistant to or who fail treatment with β-lactam antibiotics. Women with symptomatic urinary tract infections should be treated with antibiotics for 3 days. Infection due to group B streptococcus is readily treated with penicillin VK. Tetracycline should be avoided.

All of the material in Chapter 211 is in the public domain, with the exception of any borrowed figures and tables.

Follow-Up. Follow-up cultures should be obtained to ascertain the effectiveness of treatment because up to 25% of bacteriuric women develop recurrent bacteriuria.

Cross-References: Principles of Screening (Chapter 7), Dysuria (Chapter 170), Urinary Tract Infections in Women (Chapter 175).

REFERENCES

1. Andriole VT, Patterson TF. Epidemiology, natural history, and management of urinary tract infections in pregnancy. Med Clin North Am 1991;75:359–373.

   The authors present a thoughtful review.

2. Etherington IJ, James DK. Reagent strip testing of antenatal urine specimens for infection. Br J Obstet Gynaecol 1993;100:806–808.

   This study supports use of leukocyte esterase/nitrite strips, although serial testing was more accurate.

3. Rouse DJ, Andrews WW, Goldenberg RL, Owen J. Screening and treatment of asymptomatic bacteriuria of pregnancy to prevent pyelonephritis: A cost-effectiveness and cost-benefit analysis. Obstet Gynecol 1995;86:119–123.

   In a decision analytic model, no screening resulted in 23 cases of pyelonephritis per 1000 pregnancies, versus 16 cases using dipsticks and 11 using cultures. The dipstick approach appeared to be more cost-effective, particularly when the prevalence of bacteriuria was low.

4. Stenqvist K, Dahlen-Nilsson I, Liden-Janson G, et al. Bacteriuria in pregnancy. Am J Epidemiol 1989;129:372.

   A study of over 3000 women found a steady increase in the incidence of bacteriuria from 0.8% at the 12th gestational week to 1.9% before delivery. The authors suggest that a single screening performed at 16 weeks might be the most efficient strategy.

5. Vercaigne LM, Zhanel GG. Recommended treatment for urinary tract infection in pregnancy. Ann Pharmacother 1994;28:248–251.

   Rates of cure with different agents and durations of therapy are reviewed, and missing data in the literature are pointed out.

212 Diabetes Mellitus in Pregnancy

Problem

DIANE L. ELLIOT

Epidemiology. Most women with type I diabetes do well during pregnancy, although maternal risk, perinatal mortality, and the risk of congenital malformations are increased. Risk factors for maternal morbidity and relative contraindications to pregnancy include established renal disease (creatinine > 2.0 mg/dL or proteinuria > 2 g/24 h), uncontrolled hypertension, severe gastroparesis, and atherosclerotic vascular disease.

Management. Organogenesis occurs early in the first trimester. Because tight blood glucose control during this interval appears to decrease the risk of congenital malformations, optimal control is especially appropriate when women are considering pregnancy and early in gestation. Women taking oral hypoglycemic agents should be switched to insulin before conception. Management includes patient education, nutrition, close self-monitoring, and insulin therapy.

The recommended diet is 30 to 35 kcal/kg per day (60% carbohydrates, 15% to 20% protein, and 20% to 25% fat), and weight gain during pregnancy should be approximately 25 pounds. Calories are divided as three meals and two snacks a day: 20% breakfast; 30% lunch; 35% dinner; 10% evening snack; 5% midmorning snack.

Women must be able to monitor their blood glucose level and obtain several values per day (fasting, after breakfast, late afternoon, and evenings). In addition, women should check morning ketone levels at least once a week or more frequently if the blood glucose value fluctuates unduly or remains over 150 mg/dL.

Insulin is administered in multiple injections per day, adjusted to maintain a fasting glucose level of approximately 80 mg/dL and less than 130 mg/dL during the remainder of the day. Insulin requirements increase during pregnancy, but actual adjustments are variable. The physician should emphasize the need for early recognition of hypoglycemia, with management using oral glucose and, when needed, intramuscular glucagon.

Hospitalization for intense patient education and glucose control may be appropriate early in gestation. Additional indications for hospitalization include nausea and vomiting, poor glucose control that is unresponsive to insulin adjustments, and persistent ketonuria.

Follow-Up. The obstetrician coordinates care with the internist and the pediatrician near delivery, and appointments are scheduled for every 1 to 2 weeks and weekly after 30 weeks. Women with diabetes are at increased risk for urinary tract infections and preeclampsia. Weight, blood pressure, and renal function should be assessed every 2 weeks; and monthly glycated hemoglobin levels may reflect problems with glucose control if information from daily self-monitoring of blood glucose is unreliable or inadequate. Because retinopathy can progress rapidly during pregnancy, patients should be examined by an ophthalmologist each trimester. Insulin requirements decrease by approximately 50% 1 week after delivery.

Cross-References: Diabetic Retinopathy (Chapter 44), Diabetes Mellitus (Chapter 154), Bacteriuria in Pregnancy (Chapter 211), Pregnancy and Hypertension (Chapter 214).

REFERENCES

1. Hollingsworth DR. Pregnancy, Diabetes and Birth: A Management Guide. Baltimore, Williams & Wilkins, 1984.

   Detailed information is presented on all aspects of care.

2. Kitzmiller JL, Gavin LA, Gin GD, et al. Preconception care of diabetes: Glycemic control prevents congenital anomalies. JAMA 1989;254:731–736.

   Animal studies and clinical reports support the importance of normalizing glycated hemoglobin before conception to reduce spontaneous abortions and congenital malformations.

3. Miller EH. Metabolic management of diabetes in pregnancy. Semin Perinatol 1994;18:414–431.

   The author provides an extensive review of the consequences of diabetes during pregnancy, with explicit management recommendations.

· ·

213 Gestational Diabetes Mellitus

Problem

DIANE L. ELLIOT

Epidemiology. Gestational diabetes develops in 1% to 6% of pregnant women. Risk factors include obesity, age older than 35, family history of type II diabetes, and prior delivery of a large (> 9 lb) infant.

Symptoms and Signs. Gestational diabetes is asymptomatic when diagnosed.

Clinical Approach. Because control of an elevated blood glucose level decreases maternal and infant morbidity, the Centers for Disease Control and Prevention recommends screening all pregnant women at 24 to 28 weeks with a glucose measurement obtained 1 hour after ingestion of 50 g of oral glucose. A serum glucose concentration higher than 140 mg/dL or a whole blood glucose value higher than 170 mg/dL is considered positive. This screen is 90% sensitive and 80% specific. A 100-g 3-hour glucose tolerance test confirms gestational diabetes.

Management. Diet should include 30 to 35 kcal/kg/d (based on desirable body weight), with 50% carbohydrates and 100 g of protein per day. Women should avoid "concentrated" sweets and non-nutritive artificial sweeteners. Low-intensity aerobic exercise is being studied for its management benefits, and obese women may be advised to use a mild caloric restriction (e.g., 25 kcal/kg/d). Ketonuria adversely affects the fetus, and care must be taken to prevent starvation ketosis and weight loss.

Oral hypoglycemic agents are contraindicated during pregnancy. Depending on the criteria used, 15% to 30% of women with gestational diabetes require insulin therapy. Insulin is usually initiated when the fasting glucose level exceeds 105 mg/dL or the 2-hour postprandial glucose value exceeds 120 mg/dL on two occasions within 2 weeks. The initial human insulin dose is 0.3 to 0.7 unit/kg (based on pre-pregnancy weight). Management is the same as that for women with type I diabetes mellitus (see Chapter 212, Diabetes Mellitus in Pregnancy).

Follow-Up. The obstetrician coordinates the patient's care. Women are usually followed at 2-week intervals until 32 weeks, when visits are scheduled weekly. Fasting and 2-hour postprandial blood glucose levels are obtained at each visit. The blood glucose concentration usually becomes normal immediately after delivery. However, two thirds of the women will have gestational diabetes in subsequent pregnancies, and up to 50% will develop diabetes over the next 15 years.

Cross-References: Diabetes Mellitus (Chapter 154), Diabetes Mellitus in Pregnancy (Chapter 212).

REFERENCES

1. Fagen C, King JD, Erick M. Nutritional management in women with gestational diabetes mellitus: A review by ADA's Diabetes Care and Education dietetic practice group. J Am Diet Assoc 1995;95:460–467.
   Explicit recommendations and a helpful listing of patient education materials are presented.

2. Langer O. Management of gestational diabetes. Clin Perinatol 1993;20:603–617.
   The author reviews pathogenesis and management, including calorie restriction, exercise, and insulin therapy.

3. Thompson DM, Dansereau J, Creed M, Ridell L. Tight glucose control results in normal perinatal outcome in 150 patients with gestational diabetes. Obstet Gynecol 1994;83:362–366.
   Tight glucose control resulted in normal perinatal outcomes.

214 Pregnancy and Hypertension

Problem

DIANE L. ELLIOT

Epidemiology. Hypertension during pregnancy is diagnosed when blood pressure is greater than 140/90 mm Hg or increases more than 30/15 mm Hg from preconception or first-trimester values. It is classified as preeclampsia, pregnancy-induced hypertension, or essential hypertension.

The prevalence of hypertension during pregnancy is 10% to 20%; most cases are pregnancy-induced hypertension (hypertension without other features of preeclampsia). Because blood pressure normally decreases during the first trimester, distinguishing essential from pregnancy-induced hypertension is difficult when blood pressure readings before pregnancy are not known. Risk factors for preeclampsia include the first pregnancy, underlying renal disease, previous hypertension, twin pregnancies, and a family history of preeclampsia.

Symptoms and Signs. Preeclampsia usually develops during the third trimester and produces rapid weight gain (> 2 lb/wk), proteinuria (> 0.5 g/24 h), and hypertension. Diastolic pressure increases more than systolic pressure, and systolic levels are often less than 160 mm Hg (which should not be considered reassuring). Severe organ system dysfunction can occur with what would be only moderate hypertension among nonpregnant women. Additional findings of preeclampsia can include headache, epigastric pain, or diffuse edema. The spectrum of manifestations varies, and the presence of all features is not required for diagnosis.

Clinical Approach. Physicians should order a urinalysis for all women with an elevated blood pressure, rapid weight gain, or edema. If proteinuria is present, a 24-hour urine quantitation is appropriate.

Although there are fewer than 200 reported cases, pheochromocytoma during pregnancy produces significant morbidity and mortality. Its symptoms (headache, excessive perspiration, and palpitations) overlap with those of pregnancy, and evaluation with urinary catecholamines is indicated for all women newly diagnosed with elevated blood pressure before 34 weeks of pregnancy. To screen for coarctation of the aorta, arm and leg blood pressures should be measured.

Management. Pregnancy-induced hypertension usually is treated with bed rest and medications. Exactly when to initiate drug treatment is controversial, but most authorities recommend medications when the blood pressure, monitored by the patient at home, persistently exceeds 140/90 mm Hg. The goal of

Table 214–1. SAFETY OF ANTIHYPERTENSIVE DRUGS DURING PREGNANCY*

Drug	Comment
Safe	
Methyldopa	Extensive use; no adverse effects
β-Blockers	Extensive use; rare anecdotal report of neonatal bradycardia and hypoglycemia
Hydralazine	Extensive use; no adverse effects; used in combination with methyldopa or β-blocker
Controversial†	
Calcium channel blockers	Probably safe for treatment of hypertension; also have tocolytic effects
Diuretics	Use controversial; if used before pregnancy, they can be continued or discontinued; they should not be initiated for treatment of hypertension during pregnancy
Contraindicated	
Angiotensin-converting enzyme inhibitors	Reports of neonatal renal failure

*Drugs with limited use during pregnancy (e.g., clonidine or prazosin) should be switched to agents with established safety.

†Consult an expert before use.

treatment of blood pressure is 120–135/75–95 mm Hg. The experience with antihypertensive medications in pregnancy appears in Table 214–1.

Preeclampsia is a multisystemic disorder usually managed by the obstetrician. Because the woman's condition may deteriorate rapidly, patients require immediate hospitalization, medical therapy, and delivery of the infant.

In women who were hypertensive before pregnancy, the usual blood pressure decrease during the first trimester may allow gradual discontinuation of antihypertensive medications. Pharmacologic treatment resumes during the third trimester, if indicated, with methyldopa or a β-blocker.

Follow-Up. The obstetrician closely follows women with hypertension, with consultation from an internist. Visits are scheduled every 2 to 3 weeks until approximately week 32, when they occur weekly. During each encounter, the physician assesses symptoms, blood pressure, weight, edema, and proteinuria.

Pregnancy-induced hypertension resolves post partum. Chronic hypertension, newly diagnosed during pregnancy, can be identified by the persistent need for therapy at 3 months post partum.

Cross-References: Essential Hypertension (Chapter 85), Proteinuria (Chapter 181).

REFERENCES

1. Ferris TF. Pregnancy complicated by hypertension and renal disease. Adv Intern Med 1990;35:269–288.

   The author discusses drug therapy of hypertension during pregnancy, including its use in patients with underlying renal disease.

2. Gallery EDM. Hypertension in pregnancy. Drugs 1995;49:S55–S62.

   This is a practical review structured around the typical questions that occur when caring for pregnant women with hypertension.

3. Sibai BM. Preeclampsia-eclampsia. Curr Probl Obstet Gynecol Fertil 1990;13:1–45.

   A thorough discussion of pathophysiology, multisystemic problems, and management is presented.

215 Asthma in Pregnancy

Problem

DIANE L. ELLIOT

Epidemiology. Asthma is the most common chronic respiratory disease during pregnancy, with a prevalence of approximately 1.0%.

Symptoms and Signs. The course of asthma during pregnancy is variable and cannot be predicted from patient characteristics. In general, in approximately one third of women asthma remains stable, in one third it improves, and in one third it worsens. Dyspnea is a nonspecific symptom during pregnancy and occurs in 50% of nonasthmatic women during the first and second trimesters. The signs and symptoms of asthma exacerbations are no different in pregnant and nonpregnant women.

Clinical Approach. Because pregnancy results in minimal alterations in pulmonary function, changes in spirometry are reliable indicators of the patient's asthma. The clinical assessment of asthma symptoms is confounded by pregnancy-associated dyspnea; therefore, monitoring peak flow provides the best method of following the status of patients with asthma during pregnancy. Chest radiography should be avoided; if it is absolutely necessary, special shielding is indicated.

Management. Management is similar to that of asthma in nonpregnant individuals, and pharmacologic treatment is not altered by pregnancy. Inhaled and oral β₂-agonists can be used during pregnancy. They are tocolytic agents and rarely have been reported to inhibit labor. Inhaled cromolyn sodium can be continued. Aminophylline crosses the placenta but, other than causing newborn jitteriness in rare cases, is safe during pregnancy. Its clearance is reduced in the third trimester, and levels should be monitored. Few data on inhaled ipratropium during pregnancy are available, although it is probably safe. Control of environmental triggers remains important; immunotherapy can be continued but should not be initiated during pregnancy.

Prednisone is metabolized by the placenta, which limits fetal exposure to the active drug. Corticosteroids, both inhaled and systemically administered, can be used during pregnancy. Among inhaled corticosteroids, beclomethasone has been used most extensively and is the preferred agent.

The risk of an asthma exacerbation compromising pregnancy far outweighs any potential corticosteroid risk. Maternal hypoxia, hypocapnia, and alkalemia are detrimental to the fetus. Exacerbations should be treated early and aggressively; oxygen is needed if the partial pressure of oxygen in arterial blood (PaO₂) is less than 75 mm Hg.

Most exacerbations are associated with respiratory infections, which may require antibiotic treatment. Erythromycin (avoiding the estolate esters), penicillins, and first- and second-generation cephalosporins can be used during pregnancy. Tetracycline and trimethoprim-sulfamethoxozole are contraindicated. Other antibiotics are used less commonly and should be reviewed for safety during pregnancy.

Follow-Up. Depending on severity, women are seen every 1 to 4 weeks, in addition to self-monitoring their peak flows.

Cross-References: Upper Respiratory Infection (Chapter 66), Asthma and Chronic Obstructive Pulmonary Disease (Chapter 68), Pulmonary Function Testing (Chapter 69).

REFERENCES

1. Greenberger PA. Asthma in pregnancy. Clin Chest Med 1992;13:597–605.
   This is a useful review article from a volume concerning pulmonary disease and pregnancy.
2. Mays M, Leiner S. Asthma: A comprehensive review. J Nurse Midwifery 1995;40:256–268.
   This review includes basic information on management and highlights how asthma interacts with pregnancy.

· ·

216 Thyroid Disorders in Pregnancy

Problem

DIANE L. ELLIOT

Epidemiology. Hyperthyroidism develops during 0.02% to 0.3% of pregnancies. Because hypothyroidism is often associated with anovulation, the coexistence of hypothyroidism and pregnancy is rare. Postpartum thyroid dysfunction has an incidence of approximately 5%. Risk factors include a family or personal history of postpartum thyroid dysfunction and the presence of antimicrosomal antibodies. Postpartum hyperthyroidism occurs 4 to 6 weeks after delivery and is usually followed by hypothyroidism, with return of normal thyroid function by 6 months post partum.

Symptoms and Signs. Certain findings of hyperthyroidism (e.g., tachycardia, sensations of warmth, fatigue) are features of a normal pregnancy. Rather than causing the traditional weight loss, hyperthyroidism during pregnancy can cause an inappropriately low weight gain.

Clinical Approach. Because treating hyperthyroidism improves pregnancy outcome, the clinician should have a low threshold for obtaining thyroid function tests. Thyroid-binding globulin increases during pregnancy, leading to an elevation of total thyroxine and a decreased triiodothyronine resin uptake. However, free thyroxine and the calculated thyroid index accurately reflect thyroid function during pregnancy. Thyroid-stimulating hormone (TSH) remains a useful screening test for hypothyroidism and for assessing the adequacy of thyroid hormone replacement.

Hyperthyroid pregnant women are presumed to have Graves' disease, and thyroid scanning is contraindicated during pregnancy. The rare molar pregnancy that produces large amounts of hCG, a hormone that weakly cross-reacts with TSH, can also cause hyperthyroidism.

Management. The hyperthyroid pregnant woman should be treated medically with propylthiouracil, 100 mg three times a day. β-blockers may be necessary transiently to control initial symptoms. Radioactive iodine is absolutely contraindicated during pregnancy. Surgery is reserved for the unusual individual with complications from medical therapy. Hypothyroid pregnant women should begin full replacement doses of thyroxine.

Follow-Up. Propylthiouracil treatment usually reduces the thyroid hormone level within 3 to 4 weeks, at which time the dose is tapered to 50 mg three times a day. Thyroid function is monitored every 3 to 4 weeks. Because propylthiouracil crosses the placenta, whereas thyroid hormones and TSH do not, the therapeutic goal is to use the lowest effective dose, maintaining the woman's thyroid hormone in the high-normal range and thereby minimizing fetal exposure to propylthiouracil. Because Graves' disease may worsen post partum and because fetal exposure is no longer a consideration, many clinicians empirically increase the propylthiouracil dose after delivery.

Approximately 20% of women on thyroid replacement require a dose increase during pregnancy, and the physician should monitor TSH levels each trimester and adjust the replacement dose as appropriate.

Postpartum hyperthyroidism is transient and symptoms are treated with β-blockers. Hypothyroidism is also usually transient and can be managed with several months of thyroid replacement, with a subsequent attempt to discontinue therapy.

Cross-References: Common Thyroid Disorders (Chapter 153).

REFERENCES

1. Burrow GN. Thyroid disease. In Burrow GN, Ferris TF, eds. Medical Complications During Pregnancy. Philadelphia, WB Saunders, 1988:224–253.

   The author presents a thorough review from an extremely useful text.

2. Gerstein HC. How common is postpartum thyroiditis? Arch Intern Med 1990;150:1397–1400.

   Meta-analysis of postpartum thyroiditis indicates that the incidence in unselected cohorts is 4.9%.

3. Mandel SJ, Larsen R, Seeley EW, et al. Increased need for thyroxine during pregnancy in women with primary hypothyroidism. N Engl J Med 1990;323:91–96.

   Nine of 12 women needed increased replacement dose of thyroxine, based on elevation of thyroid-stimulating hormone during pregnancy.

SECTION XXI

The Preoperative and Postoperative Patient

217 Preoperative Evaluation

DOMINIC REILLY

Epidemiology. More than 25 million patients undergo surgery in the United States each year. Many of these patients have significant medical problems that complicate their surgical course. The successful management of these patients requires attention to their medical problems and coordination of their care with the other members of the surgical team.

Clinical Approach. The preoperative evaluation consists of four components: (1) a thorough history and physical examination, (2) appropriate testing, (3) risk assessment, and (4) planning the perioperative medical management. The history and physical examination should include the information outlined in Table 217–1. It is particularly important to determine the patient's exercise tolerance and to document any previous surgical complications.

Extensive testing of otherwise healthy individuals before surgery is generally not indicated. Most centers have guidelines for preoperative testing based on the patient's age and concomitant medical illnesses (Table 217–2). Other testing should be performed as clinically indicated (e.g., coagulation studies/

Table 217–1. COMPONENTS OF A COMPLETE PREOPERATIVE ASSESSMENT

Identifying data
Brief synopsis of reason for surgery
Past medical history
Past surgical history, including complications
Medications and allergies
Habits
Family history
Social history
Exercise tolerance
Review of systems, particularly for cardiac and pulmonary problems
Physical examination, especially cardiovascular, pulmonary, neurologic
Laboratory data
Assessment and plan by problem

Table 217–2. PREOPERATIVE TESTING REQUIREMENTS

	Age			Illness	
	< 40	40–60	> 60	Diabetes/Hypertension	Cardiac/Pulmonary
Hematocrit	Yes	Yes	Yes	Yes	Yes
SMA-6 chemistry panel	No	No	Yes	Yes	Yes
Electrocardiogram	No	Yes	Yes	Yes	Yes
Chest radiograph	No	No	No	No	Yes

*Minimum requirements; other tests should be ordered as clinically indicated.

platelet count in patients with liver disease or a bleeding disorder). The following tests should be considered: pregnancy testing, electrolytes/renal panel, complete blood cell count, urinalysis, liver function tests, coagulation studies, chest radiography, electrocardiography, and measurement of therapeutic drug levels. Indications for specific preoperative cardiac and pulmonary testing are discussed in Chapters 218 and 221, respectively.

The potential risks of surgery should be reviewed with the patient. Risk factors for perioperative complications include increasing age (> 65), the number and severity of medical problems, the type and duration of surgery, the patient's exercise tolerance, and the history of previous complications. The risk of complications is highest in patients undergoing vascular, thoracic, abdominal, and orthopedic procedures. Patients who cannot walk two blocks or climb one to two flights of stairs without symptoms (Canadian classification III or IV) are at increased risk.

The American Society of Anesthesiology (ASA) classification is a commonly used method of assessing a patient's general risk of perioperative mortality. The patient's ASA class is based on the presence and severity of medical problems (Table 217–3). Specific risk factors for cardiac and pulmonary complications are reviewed in Chapters 218 and 221, respectively. Relative contraindications to elective surgery include poorly controlled medical problems, recent myocardial infarction, active infections, and acute metabolic derangements.

The plan for managing the patient's medical problems postoperatively should include consideration of the type and severity of medical problems and the patient's ability to take medications by mouth postoperatively. Most medications should be continued perioperatively if possible, substituting intra-

Table 217–3. AMERICAN SOCIETY OF ANESTHESIOLOGY (ASA) CLASSIFICATION

ASA Class	Disease State	Surgical Mortality
1	Healthy	Very low (0.01%)
2	Mild/moderate systemic illness (hypertension, anemia)	Low (0.1%)
3	Severe systemic illness (angina, poorly controlled diabetes)	Moderate (0.66%)
4	Severe, life-threatening illness (unstable angina, sepsis)	High (4.6%)
5	Moribund	Very high (9.2%)

venous or topical agents when necessary. Patients taking physiologic doses of corticosteroids should receive stress-dose corticosteroids perioperatively (see Chapter 220). The plan for postoperative care should always include efforts to maximize the patient's pulmonary function, including incentive spirometry and early mobilization postoperatively. Recommendations for deep venous thrombosis and endocarditis prophylaxis (see Chapters 218 and 219) should be made when appropriate.

Some medications should be discontinued preoperatively. Aspirin should be stopped approximately 2 weeks before surgery if possible, and other nonsteroidal agents should generally be discontinued for 3 or 4 days before surgery. Some authors recommend discontinuing monoamine oxidase inhibitors and guanethidine 2 weeks before surgery to minimize potential drug interactions. The oral hypoglycemic agent metformin should be discontinued 48 hours before surgery to minimize the risk of lactic acidosis.

Follow-Up. Patients with significant medical problems should be observed closely postoperatively. Particular attention should be paid to therapy for medical problems, pain control, nutrition, pulmonary toilet, and deep venous thrombosis prophylaxis. Careful attention to the patient's medications and allergies is essential. Patients should be seen in the clinic shortly after discharge to reassess their medical condition.

Cross-References: Assessment of Physical Activity (Chapter 72), Angina (Chapter 78), Essential Hypertension (Chapter 85), Bleeding (Chapter 195), Preoperative Cardiovascular Problems (Chapter 218), Preoperative Hematologic Problems (Chapter 219), Preoperative Endocrine Problems (Chapter 220), Preoperative Pulmonary Problems (Chapter 221).

REFERENCES

1. Choi J. An anesthesiologist's philosophy on "medical clearance" for surgical patients. Arch Intern Med 1987;147:2900–2902.

   The author writes an editorial discussing the appropriate medical evaluation from the anesthesia perspective.

2. Cygan R, Waitzkin H. Stopping and restarting medications in the perioperative period. J Gen Intern Med 1987;2:270–283.

   This is an excellent summary of perioperative medical management.

3. Dripps RD, Lamont A, Eckenhoff JE. The role of anesthesia in surgical mortality. JAMA 1961;778:261.

   The authors assess the risk associated with the ASA classification.

4. Kroenke K. Preoperative evaluation, the assessment and management of surgical risk. J Gen Intern Med 1987;2:257–269.

   A comprehensive review of preoperative evaluation and risk assessment is presented.

218 Preoperative Cardiovascular Problems

Problem

DOMINIC REILLY

Epidemiology. More than 20% of patients undergoing elective surgery have some form of cardiovascular disease. Postoperative cardiac complications represent a major source of morbidity and mortality in this population.

Clinical Approach. Evaluation of the cardiovascular risk requires a thorough history and physical examination. The cardiac review of systems should include exercise tolerance, dyspnea, chest pain, orthopnea, palpitations, edema, stroke, transient ischemic attacks, claudication, and cardiac risk factors.

Patients with cardiovascular illness or diuretic use should have their serum electrolyte levels checked and have an electrocardiogram and chest radiograph performed preoperatively. Echocardiography may be used to evaluate suspicious murmurs, measure left ventricular function, and assess wall motion abnormalities or hypertrophy.

The value of preoperative cardiac stress testing (exercise or pharmacologic) is debatable. Patients who can achieve 85% of their maximum predicted heart rate during standard exercise testing or who have no evidence of reversible ischemia by pharmacologic stress testing are at low risk for perioperative cardiac complications (< 5%). Unfortunately, abnormal stress tests have a poor predictive value. Patients with evidence of ischemia on pharmacologic stress testing have approximately a 15% chance of developing a cardiac complication after vascular surgery. The poor predictive value of these studies limits their usefulness as screening tools preoperatively.

In general, patients with good exercise tolerance (able to walk four blocks and climb two flights of stairs without symptoms) do not need any further cardiac evaluation. Patients with poor exercise tolerance who have symptoms, physical findings, or laboratory studies consistent with coronary disease may benefit from preoperative stress testing. However, such testing should be performed only when the results will be used to modify the surgical procedure, medical therapy, or perioperative monitoring. Patients with positive stress tests may benefit from preoperative cardiology consultation.

Goldman and colleagues developed a risk index to help predict cardiac complications in patients undergoing noncardiac surgery (Table 218–1). Points are assigned on the basis of the patient's history and physical findings. The points are totaled, and the patient's approximate risk of cardiac complications may be assessed.

Table 218-1. RISK OF CARDIAC COMPLICATIONS IN PATIENTS UNDERGOING NONCARDIAC SURGERY

Factor	Points
Myocardial infarction within 6 mo	10
Age > 70 y	5
S3 gallop or jugular venous distention	11
Significant aortic stenosis	3
Rhythm other than normal sinus rhythm with premature atrial contractions	7
Premature ventricular contractions of more than 5 min	7
Poor medical condition	3
Potassium < 3.0 mEq/L, HCO_3 < 20 mEq/L	
Blood urea nitrogen > 50 mg/dL, creatinine > 3.0 mg/dL	
PO_2 < 60 mm Hg, PCO_2 > 50 mm Hg	
Liver disease, bedridden	
Abdominal, thoracic, or aortic surgery	3
Emergency operation	4
Total	53

Class	Points	Cardiac Complication	Death
I	0–5	1%	0.2%
II	6–12	5%	2%
III	13–25	11%	2%
IV	>25	22%	56%

From Goldman L, et al. Multifactorial index of cardiac risk in noncardiac surgical procedures. N Engl J Med 1977;297:845–850. Copyright 1977, Massachusetts Medical Society. All rights reserved.

Management

CORONARY ARTERY DISEASE. All patients should be counseled about their risk of surgery. Elective surgery should be delayed, or reconsidered, in patients with poorly controlled illness or recent myocardial infarction (< 6 months). Patients with severe coronary artery disease who are candidates for invasive therapy (angioplasty or coronary revascularization) should undergo these procedures before elective surgery. Revascularization should be performed only when clinically indicated on the basis of coronary anatomy, left ventricular function, and response to medical management (see Chapter 73, Acute Chest Pain, and Chapter 78, Angina). There is no evidence that prophylactic preoperative revascularization reduces mortality.

Unless otherwise contraindicated, one should consider adding a β-blocker perioperatively (e.g., metoprolol, 25 to 50 mg orally twice daily). Cardiac medications should be taken on the day of surgery and continued postoperatively when possible. Intravenous and topical agents should be substituted when patients are unable to take medications orally. It is wise to write orders for appropriate "hold" parameters because many patients are transiently hypotensive postoperatively.

The primary goals of therapy are to control blood pressure, heart rate, and pain. The hematocrit, electrolytes, ventilation, and oxygenation must be monitored closely. Patients with known (or suspected) coronary artery disease should have an electrocardiogram postoperatively. Patients with perioperative arrhythmias, hypotension, or ischemic changes on their electrocardiogram should be monitored on telemetry. These patients should also have serial measurement of their creatine phosphokinase isoenzymes (every 8 hours for 24 hours) and monitoring of their electrocardiogram for evidence of myocardial infarction or ischemia.

HYPERTENSION. Hypertension does not represent a significant risk for surgery unless it is poorly controlled. A preoperative diastolic pressure over 110 mm Hg has been associated with an increased perioperative morbidity. Elective surgery should be delayed until the blood pressure has been well controlled for at least 2 weeks. Surgery must be delayed in patients with a suspected pheochromocytoma or other secondary causes of hypertension until an evaluation is complete and appropriate therapy is instituted.

Most antihypertensive agents should be continued perioperatively, with two exceptions. Diuretics are frequently held after surgery and used only as needed in the initial postoperative period. Some authors recommend discontinuing guanethidine (Ismelin) 2 weeks before surgery because of potential drug interactions.

Blood pressure tends to fall postoperatively as a result of phlebotomy, bed rest, and narcotic analgesia. Consequently, it is wise to write "hold" parameters (e.g., hold for systolic blood pressure < 120) for antihypertensive medications. β-Blockers and clonidine should be continued postoperatively (when possible) to avoid rebound tachycardia and hypertension. Intravenous and topical agents may be used when patients are unable to take their medications orally (Table 218–2). Transdermal clonidine requires 2 to 3 days to take effect.

VALVULAR HEART DISEASE. Patients with valvular heart disease have special risks associated with surgery. These patients require antibiotic prophylaxis for nonsterile procedures (see Chapter 222, Preoperative Infectious Disease Problems). In most cases, those taking anticoagulants must discontinue them preoperatively (see Chapter 219). Patients with valvular heart disease are frequently predisposed to atrial arrhythmias, and fluid management may pose significant challenges. Echocardiography should be considered in patients with symptomatic valvular heart disease (if not performed recently), particularly if there has been a change in symptoms or exercise tolerance.

Patients with mild or moderate disease need antibiotic prophylaxis and close attention to fluid management and monitoring for arrhythmias. Patients with severe disease who are candidates for valvular repair/replacement should strongly consider undergoing those procedures before elective surgery. Other-

Table 218–2. ALTERNATIVE CARDIOVASCULAR AGENTS FOR PERIOPERATIVE USE

Drug	Dose
Topical	
Nitroglycerine ointment	0.5–2 in. q4–6h
Clonidine transdermal	TTS—1 is equivalent to 0.1 mg/d (begin 2–3 days prior)
Intravenous*	
Labetalol	10–20 mg IV q10 min, repeat prn
Nitroglycerin	5–10 μg/min titrate to response
Diltiazem	0.25 mg/kg IV bolus over 2 min, followed by a 10-mg/hr infusion
Hydralazaine	10–20 mg, repeat prn

*Use caution and appropriate monitoring when using intravenous agents.

wise they may be managed with close (invasive) monitoring and cardiology consultation. The primary goals of perioperative management of specific problems are listed below:

Aortic stenosis: avoid hypovolemia, hypotension, and tachycardia.

Aortic insufficiency: avoid negative inotropes; maintain afterload reduction.

Mitral stenosis: maintain normal to low filling pressures; monitor pulmonary status closely; avoid tachycardia.

Mitral insufficiency: maintain afterload reduction; avoid volume overload and negative inotropes; monitor pulmonary status and hepatic function.

ARRHYTHMIAS. In general, one must assume that patients with known paroxysmal arrhythmias will go into that rhythm perioperatively and must be prepared to treat that rhythm when it occurs. Patients with atrial arrhythmias should have adequate rate control and have medications at therapeutic levels. Serum electrolytes and pulmonary status are monitored closely, and other medical problems are treated aggressively. Patients with hemodynamically significant arrhythmias may benefit from cardiologic consultation.

PACEMAKERS AND DEFIBRILLATORS. Pacemakers and defibrillators may be affected by the electrocautery equipment in the operating room. Defibrillators should be inactivated before surgery, because electrocautery bursts may result in inadvertent firing of the device. Pacemakers may be inhibited or reprogrammed by electrocautery. Appropriate pacemaker precautions may include the following:

1. Performing preoperative pacemaker assessment.
2. Placing the electrocautery ground pad as far from the pacemaker as possible.
3. Using only very short bursts with the cautery.
4. Having chronotropic agents available in the operating room.
5. Considering temporary or external pacemaker placement.
6. Performing postoperative pacemaker assessment.

Patients with these devices should generally have cardiologic consultation.

Cross-References: Acute Chest Pain (Chapter 73), Recurrent Chest Pain (Chapter 74), Angina (Chapter 78), Congestive Heart Failure (Chapter 79), Aortic Stenosis (Chapter 80), Other Valvular Disease (Chapter 81), Atrial Fibrillation (Chapter 82), Supraventricular Arrhythmias (Chapter 84), Echocardiographic and Nuclear Assessment of Cardiac Function (Chapter 86), Exercise Tolerance Testing (Chapter 88), Echocardiography (Chapter 89), Preoperative Evaluation (Chapter 217), Preoperative Infectious Disease Problems (Chapter 222).

REFERENCES

1. Detsky AS, Abrams HB, McLaughlin JR, Drucker DJ, Sasson Z, et al. Predicting cardiac complications in patients undergoing non-cardiac surgery. J Gen Intern Med 1986;1:211–219.

   These researchers confirmed the findings of Goldman and associates and further identified the risks associated with severe or unstable angina.

2. Goldman L, Caldera DL, Nussbaum SR, Southwick FS, Krogstad D, et al. Multifactorial index of cardiac risk in noncardiac surgical procedures. N Engl J Med 1977;297:845–850.

   This is the classic article describing clinical risk factors in 1001 patients undergoing elective surgery.

3. Granieri R. Surgery in the hypertensive patient. In Goldmann DR, Brown FH, Guarnieri DM, eds. Perioperative Medicine, 2nd ed. New York, McGraw-Hill Book Company, 1994:175–184.

   A comprehensive review is presented of the risks and management of perioperative hypertension, including 131 references.

4. Leppo JA. Preoperative cardiac risk assessment for noncardiac surgery. Am J Cardiol 1995;75:42D–51D.

   This is an excellent and timely review of risk assessment and the use of perioperative stress testing (including stress echocardiography).

5. Mangano DT, Goldman L. Preoperative assessment of patients with known or suspected coronary disease. N Engl J Med 1995;333:1750–1756.

   This article is an excellent summary of clinical indexes and testing available for assessing perioperative cardiac risk.

· ·

219   Preoperative Hematologic Problems

Problem

MARC W. MORA

HEMATOLOGIC LABORATORY SCREENING

Epidemiology. Indiscriminate preoperative laboratory testing is often wasteful. For example, 50% or more of routine hematologic tests have no recognizable indications, and less than 0.25% uncover abnormalities that might influence perioperative management.

Clinical Approach and Management. A complete health history and physical examination are the two most important tools in helping physicians identify patients at high risk for specific conditions. Laboratory testing can then be used to verify suspected disease or to optimize medical management. Table 219–1 lists the indications for various hematologic screening tests.

DISCONTINUING CHRONIC ANTICOAGULATION THERAPY PERIOPERATIVELY

Epidemiology. As many as 2 million persons are on long-term anticoagulation therapy in the United States, and many will require surgery. There are no well-

Table 219–1. INDICATIONS FOR HEMATOLOGIC SCREENING TESTS

Indication	Type/Screen	Hemoglobin	PT/PTT	Platelet	White Blood Cell Count
Procedure with blood loss	+	+			
Procedure without blood loss		Women of any age Men > 65 y			
Hematologic malignancy		+	+	+	+
Hepatic disease			+		
Renal disease		+			
History of bleeding*			+	+	
Anticoagulant use		+	+		
History of chemotherapy/ immunosuppression		+	+		+
Radiation therapy					+
Malnutrition/malabsorption		+	+		

PT/PTT, prothrombin time/partial thromboplastin time.
*Order bleeding time.

designed comparative studies on the management of chronic anticoagulation in the perioperative setting.

Management. In deciding on a reasonable management strategy, one must weigh the risk of perioperative hemorrhage against the likelihood of thromboembolism when effective anticoagulation is discontinued. These vary according to the type of surgery and the underlying indication for anticoagulation. Table 219–2 outlines one approach to the management of preoperative anticoagulation. In most situations, warfarin can be discontinued in the outpatient setting at considerable cost advantage without appreciable increase in risk to the patient. Preoperative heparin therapy should be reserved for patients with high thromboembolic risk undergoing major surgical procedures. The timing of heparin therapy, preoperative discontinuation, and postoperative resumption should be carefully discussed with the surgeon and will vary depending on the type of surgery performed. If reversal of anticoagulation needs to be achieved in a timely manner, small parenteral doses of vitamin K (e.g., 1 to 2 mg) may be administered. Small doses make resumption of oral anticoagulation postoperatively less problematic.

PROPHYLAXIS FOR VENOUS THROMBOEMBOLISM

Epidemiology. Fatal pulmonary embolism (PE) may be the most common cause of preventable hospital death in the United States. In hospitalized patients, PE causes or contributes to the death of 200,000 patients annually.

The rationale for prophylaxis of venous thromboembolism is based on the clinically silent nature of the disease and the significant morbidity and mortality caused by PE. Both deep venous thrombosis (DVT) and PE manifest few specific symptoms, and the clinical diagnosis is insensitive and unreliable. To rely on the diagnosis and treatment of established venous thrombosis may expose susceptible patients to unacceptable risks.

Clinical risk factors for venous thrombosis are reviewed in Table 219–3.

Table 219–2. PERIOPERATIVE MANAGEMENT OF PATIENTS ON CHRONIC ANTICOAGULATION

Thromboembolic Risk	Hemorrhagic Risk		
	Low (dental extraction, soft tissue biopsy)	Intermediate (most surgeries)	High (neurosurgery, ophthalmologic surgery)*
High			
Any caged ball valve; any mechanical valve in the mitral position; dialysis patients with previous shunt or graft thrombosis; recent embolus in the setting of chronic atrial fibrillation	No modification of anticoagulation	Tight Control†: heparin off 6–12 h preoperatively; resume heparin postoperatively	Tight Control†: heparin off 6–12 h preoperatively; resume heparin postoperatively
Intermediate			
Tilting disk valves in the aortic position; atrial fibrillation in the setting of valvular heart disease	No modification of anticoagulation	Intermediate Control‡: to OR when PT within 2–3 s of control; resume heparin postoperatively	Intermediate Control‡: to OR when PT normal; resume heparin postoperatively
Low			
Previous deep venous thrombosis/pulmonary embolus; transient ischemic attack/ cerebrovascular accident; myocardial infarction; nonvalvular chronic atrial fibrillation	No modification of anticoagulation	Loose Control§: to OR when PT 2–3 s of control	Loose Control§: to OR when PT normal

OR, operating room; PT, prothrombin time; PTT, partial thromboplastin time; INR, International Normalized Ratio.

*Many authorities do not discontinue warfarin in the setting of routine cataract surgery.

†Tight Control:
  1. Stop warfarin 2 days preoperatively. Admit 1 day before surgery and start heparin to achieve a therapeutic PTT.
  2. Check PT on admission; if INR > 1.5, give 0.5 to 1 mg vitamin K; if INR > 2.0, give 1 to 5 mg vitamin K.
  3. Stop heparin preoperatively; check PT/PTT before surgery. Resume heparin postoperatively.
  4. Resume warfarin when patient is tolerating oral medications.
  5. After the PT is therapeutic, overlap heparin and warfarin for 24 to 48 h.
  6. If bleeding problems occur, consider using low molecular weight dextran for 2 to 3 days to minimize thrombosis.

‡Intermediate Control:
  1. Stop warfarin 3 to 4 days preoperatively as an outpatient.
  2. Proceed to surgery when PT is at desired level.
  3. Start heparin postoperatively.
  4–6. As for "Tight Control."

§Loose Control:
  1. Stop warfarin 3 to 4 days preoperatively.
  2. Proceed to surgery when PT is at desired level.
  3. Resume warfarin 1 to 2 days postoperatively or when tolerating oral medications.

Table 219–3. CLINICAL RISK FACTORS FOR VENOUS THROMBOEMBOLISM

Advanced age*	Prolonged immobility or paralysis
Prior venous thromboembolism	Malignancy
Major surgery†	Obesity
Varicose veins	Stroke
Fractures of the pelvis, hip, or leg	High-dose estrogen use
Congestive heart failure or recent myocardial infarction	Congenital or acquired aberrations in hemostasis‡

*Clinically becomes important by 40 years and increases with further aging.

†Particularly operations involving the abdomen, pelvis, and lower extremity.

‡For example, protein C or S deficiency, activated protein C resistance (factor V mutation), antithrombin III deficiency, the lupus anticoagulant, or myeloproliferative disorders.

Table 219–4. INCIDENCE OF PROXIMAL DEEP VEIN THROMBOSIS (DVT) AND PULMONARY EMBOLISM (PE) IN UNTREATED CONTROL PATIENTS AND SUGGESTED DVT PROPHYLAXIS

Patient Group	Proximal Vein Thrombosis (%)	Clinical PE (%)	Suggested DVT Prophylaxis
*General Surgery**			
Low risk—uncomplicated minor surgery in patients younger than 40 y and with no clinical risk factors	0.4	0.2	No specific measures Early ambulation
Moderate risk—major surgery in patients older than 40 y with no other clinical risk factors	2–4	1–2	Elastic stockings, LDUH† 5000 units SQ bid or IPC‡
High risk—major surgery in patients older than 40 y who have additional risk factors	4–8	2–4	LDUH 5000 units SQ tid, LMWH,§ or IPC. In selected very high risk patients, combine IPC with LDUH or LMWH.
Orthopedic Surgery			
Total hip replacement	23–36	7–30	Oral anticoagulants started preoperatively or immediately postoperatively to achieve an INR of 2.0–3.0, LMWH, or adjusted dose heparin‖
Total knee replacement	9–20	2–7	IPC or LMWH
Hip fracture surgery	17–36	4–24	Oral anticoagulants or LMWH

INR, International Normalized Ratio.

*Includes individuals undergoing gynecologic, urologic, thoracic, and vascular operations.

†LDUH, low-dose unfractionated heparin: an increased incidence of wound hematomas, but not major bleeding, is associated with the use of this agent.

‡IPC, intermittent pneumatic compression: an attractive measure with no risk of hemorrhagic complications.

§LMWH, low molecular weight heparin: dosed twice daily and begun preoperatively or immediately postoperatively and also associated with a higher risk of wound hematomas.

‖Adjusted-dose heparin must be started preoperatively and administered subcutaneously three times a day to keep the partial thromboplastin time 6 h after dosing at 30–40 s.

Because these risk factors are additive, postoperative patients are particularly at risk for the development of DVT.

Management. An appropriate preventive strategy in an individual patient takes into account the risk of venous thromboembolism, the potential benefits of prophylaxis, and the associated expense and possible complications.

The overall incidence of DVT in general surgery patients is approximately 25%. Patients at highest risk for DVT are elderly patients; general surgery patients with multiple clinical risk factors; patients with a recent spinal cord injury; or patients undergoing major lower extremity orthopedic surgery of the hip or knee. The incidence of DVT in these groups is more than 50%. This includes both calf and proximal vein thromboses. Although the development of an isolated calf vein thrombus is not an indication for anticoagulation, it represents an important clinical finding. Calf vein thrombi require sequential imaging with either ultrasonography or impedance plethysmography to identify the 10% to 20% of patients who will develop proximal extension.

With appropriate prophylaxis the incidence of DVT can be reduced by 50% to 80%. The incidence of proximal DVT and PE in untreated control patients is outlined in Table 219–4, and suggestions are provided for prophylaxis in selected situations.

In very high risk patients the choice among low molecular weight heparin (LMWH), low-intensity oral anticoagulation, or adjusted-dose heparin prophylaxis should depend on cost and convenience because they all appear to be equal in efficacy. Although the cost of LWMH is currently high, with the anticipated approval of several other preparations by the Food and Drug Administration cost is likely to decrease.

Cross-References: Pleuritic Chest Pain (Chapter 61), Bleeding (Chapter 195), Thrombocytopenia (Chapter 197), Chronic Anticoagulation (Chapter 201), Preoperative Cardiovascular Problems (Chapter 218).

REFERENCES

1. Clagett GP, Anderson FA, Heit J, et al. Prevention of venous thromboembolism. Chest 1995;108:312s–334s.

    This is an important article that was presented before the Fourth American College of Chest Physicians Consensus Conference on Antithrombotic Therapy.

2. Kaplan EB, Sheiner LB, Boeckmann AJ, et al. The usefulness of preoperative laboratory screening. JAMA 1985;253:3576–3581.

    This is a good review of the indications for many laboratory tests.

3. Littin SC, Gastineau DA. Current concepts in anticoagulation therapy. Mayo Clin Proc 1995;70:266–272.

    The authors present an excellent overall review for the primary care physician.

4. Roizen MF. Cost-effective preoperative laboratory testing. JAMA 1994;271:319–320.

    A short summary of recommended preoperative tests is provided.

5. Stein PD, Alpert JS, Dalen JE, et al. Antithrombotic therapy in patients with mechanical and biological prosthetic heart valves. Chest 1995;108:371s–379s.

    This review of the risks and benefits of anticoagulation is based on the most recent data.

220 Preoperative Endocrine Problems

Problem

C. SCOTT SMITH

DIABETES MELLITUS

Epidemiology. Diabetes is present in 5% to 10% of all adults, with a higher prevalence among the elderly. Cardiovascular mortality is two to four times more common in diabetics. Clinically significant renal dysfunction, present in nearly half of patients with more than 10 years of diabetes, may complicate postoperative care. Autonomic neuropathy, also common, may be associated with respiratory depression or wide fluctuations of blood pressure perioperatively. Moreover, diabetics have delayed wound healing and are more susceptible to wound infections, particularly when the blood glucose concentration continuously exceeds 250 mg/dL in the weeks preceding surgery.

Symptoms and Signs. See Chapter 154 (Diabetes Mellitus).

Clinical Approach. Because myocardial infarctions may be asymptomatic in diabetics, an electrocardiogram should be obtained before and after major surgery. The clinician should carefully monitor the patient's electrolytes and renal function. Radiologic procedures involving intravenous contrast materials should be avoided if possible, but if the procedure is absolutely necessary, it should be performed only after adequate hydration.

Uncontrolled hyperglycemia (blood glucose > 350 mg/dL) or ketoacidosis should be reversed for at least 48 hours before elective surgery.

Management. The stress of surgery causes an unpredictable release of counter-regulatory hormones, including catecholamines, glucagon, cortisol, and growth hormone. In the perioperative period, most diabetics are relatively unstable and even those who do not normally use insulin may require it. During this time, the goal is to maintain the serum glucose between 150 and 250 mg/dL, avoiding hypoglycemia while minimizing poor wound healing and any possible immunologic dysfunction. Specific recommendations appear in Table 220–1.

Follow-Up. For 24 hours to 48 hours postoperatively, the patient should be followed closely, with finger-stick blood glucose determinations at least every 4 hours. Scrupulous care to avoid wound and urinary tract infections is required, and Foley catheters should be discontinued as soon as possible.

THYROID DISEASE

Epidemiology. Operating on thyrotoxic patients carries a 10% to 30% risk of thyroid storm, with an operative mortality of up to 60%.

Table 220–1. PERIOPERATIVE MANAGEMENT OF DIABETES

Disease Controlled with Oral Agents

1. Stop agents before surgery.
   a. Short-acting (tolbutamide, tolazemide, acetohexamide, glyburide, metformin, glypizide) 1 to 2 days before surgery.
   b. Long-acting (chlorproamide) 3 days before surgery.
2. Cover with finger-stick glucose determinations four times a day and subcutaneous or intravenous insulin while NPO (see below).
3. Resume usual medication when tolerating oral intake.

Disease Controlled with Insulin

1. Previously well controlled, not seriously ill, minor procedure: "no insulin, no glucose."
2. Previously well controlled, major procedure:
   a. 5% dextrose in water (D5W) 1–2 mL/kg/h and insulin drip 1–2 units/h* *or*
   b. D5W 1–2 mL/kg/h and one-half usual morning dose of insulin; supplemental regular or lispro insulin while NPO.
   c. Finger-stick or serum glucose determinations q1–2h for the first day.
3. Very ill or brittle
   a. D5W 1–2 mL/kg/h and insulin drip 1–2 units/h.
   b. Finger-stick glucose determinations q1–2h the first day.

*Some studies demonstrate reduced mortality and morbidity with this regimen.

Hypothyroid patients exhibit minimally increased perioperative mortality but have increased sensitivity to digitalis, anesthetics, and analgesics. In addition, hypothyroid patients are known to have decreased hypoxic ventilatory drive and impaired free water excretion, which may lead to carbon dioxide retention or hyponatremia.

Clinical Approach. Elective surgery on hyperthyroid patients should be postponed until they are euthyroid (usually at least 1 month of treatment). Any patient with suspected hyperthyroidism or hypothyroidism should receive screening (determination of thyroid-stimulating hormone level) before surgery.

Patients with autoimmune thyroid disorders (Graves' disease or Hashimoto's thyroiditis) should be screened for coexisting conditions, such as diabetes mellitus, Addison's disease, pernicious anemia, and myasthenia gravis.

Management. The appropriate management of hyperthyroid patients during urgent or emergent surgery is shown in Table 220–2. In patients with hyperthy-

Table 220–2. MANAGEMENT OF HYPERTHYROIDISM IN EMERGENCY SURGERY

1. Propiothiouracil (PTU), 200–400 mg PO/NG q6h
2. Iodide
   a. Start 1–2 h after propiothiouracil
   b. Saturated solution of potassium iodide 5 drops PO/NG q8h
      or
      sodium iodide, 1 g IV over 12 h q12–24h.
3. Propranolol, 20–120 mg PO/NG q4–8h.
   or
   1–3 mg IV q15min as needed until desired effect, appearance of toxicity, or total dose of 0.15 mg/kg is reached; may repeat in 6–8 h.
4. Dexamethasone, 2 mg PO/IV q6h.

roidism and atrial fibrillation, propranolol should be administered to control the heart rate if there are no contraindications (e.g., congestive heart failure, asthma).

When hypothyroidism is diagnosed, elective surgery is best postponed until a stable replacement dose is achieved (usually 2 to 3 months). Replacement hormone is generally not started immediately before urgent surgery unless the patient has myxedema coma, when delay in therapy leads to a poorer prognosis. In these patients, an initial dose of 300 μg of L-thyroxine should be administered slowly intravenously, followed by 50 μg/d given intravenously. Moreover, hypothyroid patients often lack adrenal reserve and, if surgery cannot be delayed, require treatment with hydrocortisone, 100 mg intravenously every 8 hours starting the night before surgery and tapering rapidly the day after surgery (usually stopping within 72 hours).

Follow-Up. In the perioperative period, hyperthyroid patients should be monitored closely for fever, tachyarrhythmias, mental status changes, or dehydration, all signs that herald thyroid storm.

Hypothyroid patients should receive small doses of analgesics and be monitored closely for hyponatremia and, if they are not intubated, hypercapnia.

ADRENAL INSUFFICIENCY

Etiology. The most common cause of adrenal insufficiency is suppression of the hypothalamic-pituitary-adrenal axis with exogenous glucocorticoids, followed in frequency by Addison's disease, pituitary dysfunction, and bilateral adrenalectomy.

Symptoms and Signs. Signs of previous or current exogenous glucocorticoids are thinning of the skin, purple striae, truncal obesity, "moon" facies, plethoric cheeks, prominent fat pad of the posterior neck, and proximal muscle weakness. Symptoms of adrenal insufficiency include weakness, anorexia, weight loss, and postural light-headedness. Signs include postural hypotension and, in Addison's disease, hyperpigmentation (especially of skin creases and pressure points).

Clinical Approach. Patients who have received corticosteroids in doses greater than 7.5 mg of prednisone or its equivalent per day for at least 4 weeks should be considered potentially adrenally suppressed. These patients, as well as those suspected of adrenal insufficiency from other causes, should receive empirical corticosteroids perioperatively or undergo a cosyntropin (ACTH) stimulation test of adrenal reserve.

Management. The usual cosyntropin stimulation test involves a baseline and a 60-minute plasma cortisol sample after the intramuscular or intravenous administration of 0.25 mg of cosyntropin. A normal response is a 60-minute level of at least 18 μg/dL with an increment from baseline of at least 7 μg/dL.

Perioperative corticosteroid coverage for adrenal insufficiency is the same as for hypothyroid patients.

Follow-Up. During withdrawal of corticosteroid coverage, patients should be observed closely for findings that suggest too rapid a taper, such as hypotension, nausea, or anorexia.

Cross-References: Common Thyroid Disorders (Chapter 153), Diabetes Mellitus (Chapter 154).

REFERENCES

1. Gavin LA. Management of diabetes mellitus during surgery. West J Med 1989;151:525–529.
   This is an excellent review of the continuous intravenous insulin approach.
2. Goldman DR, Brown FH, Levy WK, et al. Medical Care of the Surgical Patient: A Problem-Oriented Approach to Management. Philadelphia, JB Lippincott, 1982.
   The authors provide one of the best reviews of the subject.
3. White VA, Kumagai LF. Preoperative endocrine and metabolic considerations. Med Clin North Am 1979;63:1321–1334.
   This article is a good general review of perioperative endocrine problems.

221 Preoperative Pulmonary Problems

Problem

C. SCOTT SMITH and DOMINIC REILLY

Epidemiology. Although definitions vary, pulmonary complications develop in 10% to 40% of patients after general surgery.

Clinical Approach. The basic approach to the preoperative evaluation and testing is outlined in Chapter 217. Evaluation of pulmonary risks requires a thorough history and physical examination. The pulmonary review of systems should include evaluation for cough, dyspnea, chest pain, smoking history, previous pulmonary complications, and exercise tolerance.

Risk factors for pulmonary complications (Table 221–1) include cigarette smoking, obstructive lung disease, advanced age, active pulmonary infection, morbid obesity, low serum albumin (< 3.0 mg/dL), long preoperative stay (> 4 days), residual intra-abdominal infection, and duration of anesthesia for more than 4 hours. The site of surgery also affects the complication rate, with the highest incidence for thoracic surgery (40%), followed by surgery of the upper abdomen, lower abdomen, and extremities. A maximal voluntary ventilation (MVV) less than 50% predicted and forced expiratory volume in 1 second (FEV_1) less than 2 L are predictors of pulmonary complications in thoracic and upper abdominal procedures. Arterial hypoxemia (PaO_2 < 50 mm Hg) or hypercapnia ($PaCO_2$ > 45 mm Hg) also predicts increased perioperative complications.

Table 221–1. **RISK FACTORS FOR POSTOPERATIVE PULMONARY COMPLICATIONS**

Risk Factor	Likelihood Ratio
Definite	
Obstructive lung disease	3–4
Age > 70	3
Smoker	2–6
Probable	
Anesthesia > 3 h	2
Obesity	?
Respiratory tract infection	?

A baseline chest radiograph is recommended in all patients having abdominal or thoracic procedures, in those with pulmonary risk factors, and in those with an abnormal examination. Measurement of pulmonary function and arterial blood gas analysis are advisable when multiple risk factors are present or if the chest radiograph is abnormal.

Pulmonary consultation should be considered for patients with established pulmonary disease undergoing lung resection. Preoperative pulmonary function tests are helpful in predicting outcome in this group. Patients with an FEV_1 of more than 2 L and an MVV of more than 50% of their predicted value may generally proceed to surgery. If the FEV_1 is less than 2 L or the MVV is less than 50% of the predicted value, a lung ventilation-perfusion scan is obtained to estimate the postresection FEV_1 (postoperative FEV_1 = the preoperative FEV_1 multiplied by the percentage of perfusion or ventilation to the lung that will remain after surgery). If the predicted postresection FEV_1 is greater than 800 mL, the surgery may proceed, although the risk of perioperative mortality is approximately 15%; if it is less than 800 mL, resection is contraindicated.

Management. Measures that reduce perioperative pulmonary complications include smoking cessation (for at least 8 weeks), intensive use of bronchodilators perioperatively, chest physical therapy (including postural drainage), incentive spirometry, and early mobilization. Patients with corticosteroid-responsive obstructive lung disease may benefit from preoperative corticosteroids (e.g., prednisone, 20 to 40 mg/d orally PO for 1 week before surgery). Corticosteroids should be continued postoperatively but tapered rapidly over the first few days after surgery (50% per day) to preoperative doses, as tolerated. Patients with active pulmonary infections should have their surgery delayed while they undergo therapy.

Cross-References: Smoking Cessation (Chapter 12), Obesity (Chapter 15), Dyspnea (Chapter 19), Pleuritic Chest Pain (Chapter 61), Cough and Sputum (Chapter 63), Lower Respiratory Infection (Chapter 67), Asthma and Chronic Obstructive Pulmonary Disease (Chapter 68), Pulmonary Function Testing (Chapter 69), Arterial Blood Sampling (Chapter 71).

REFERENCES

1. DeLisser HM, Grippi MA. Preoperative evaluation and preparation of patients with pulmonary disease. In Goldmann DR, Brown FH, Guarnieri DM, eds. Perioperative Medicine, 2nd ed. New York, McGraw-Hill Book Company, 1994:223–235.

A comprehensive review of the subject is presented including 165 references.

2. Hall JC, Tarala RA, Hall JL, Mander J. A multivariate analysis of the risk of pulmonary complications after laparotomy. Chest 99:923–927, 1991.

   The authors present a descriptive study of pulmonary complications in 1000 patients admitted for abdominal surgery.

3. Jackson CV. Preoperative pulmonary evaluation. Arch Intern Med 1988;148:2120–2127.

   This article is a good review of effects of surgery on pulmonary function, pulmonary risk assessment, and perioperative management.

· ·

222 Preoperative Infectious Disease Problems

Problem

MARC W. MORA

PROPHYLAXIS OF POSTOPERATIVE INFECTION

Epidemiology. Some bacterial contamination of the surgical incision occurs with every operation. Postoperative surgical wound infections, more appropriately labeled surgical site infections, should be defined as superficial, deep incisional, or organ/space. Extremes of age, a higher American Society of Anesthesiology (ASA) preoperative assessment score, and increasing length of operation are all associated with an increased incidence of postoperative infection. A standardized surgical classification system, based on the degree of intraoperative bacterial contamination, is a reasonable approach in estimating the risk of postoperative infection (Table 222–1).

Table 222–1. INCIDENCE OF POSTOPERATIVE SURGICAL-SITE INFECTIONS

Type of Surgery	Percentage
Clean—Elective operation, no acute inflammation encountered, and no entrance of normally or frequently colonized body cavity	< 2
Clean contaminated—Nonelective case that is otherwise a clean, controlled opening of a normally colonized body cavity, with minimal spillage or break in sterile technique	8
Contaminated—Acute nonpurulent inflammation encountered due to major break in technique, spill from hollow organ, or penetrating trauma less than 4 hours old	15
Dirty—Purulence or abscess encountered or drained, preoperative perforation of colonized body cavity, penetrating trauma more than 4 hours old	40

Clinical Approach. Careful surgical technique, along with conscientious infection control procedures that include tracking wound infection rates, have long been recognized as the best way to decrease surgical site infection rates. Although antibiotics do not substitute for good surgical practices, when used appropriately they reduce the risk of postoperative infection by about 50%. The principles of antibiotic prophylaxis before surgery are as follows:

1. Choose an effective antibiotic that targets the flora most likely to cause postoperative infection (i.e., do not try to cover all possible organisms).
2. Time the antibiotics to achieve maximal tissue levels at the time of surgery.
3. Administer antibiotics for a short period. Antibiotics routinely administered longer than 24 hours promote resistance and increase the likelihood of side effects such as pseudomembranous colitis.
4. Follow antimicrobial susceptibilities of wound isolates to detect shifts in patterns of resistance.

Antibiotic prophylaxis is indicated in "clean" surgical procedures that use foreign materials, grafts, or prosthetic devices. Although routinely used by many surgeons, the benefit of prophylaxis in other "clean" (i.e., soft tissue, orthopedic, cardiovascular) procedures is still being investigated.

Patients undergoing "clean contaminated" and "contaminated" surgical procedures appear to benefit most from antimicrobial prophylaxis. For example, the postoperative surgical site infection rate in appendicitis may be as low as 3% with optimal prophylaxis.

"Dirty" surgery requires broad-spectrum antibiotic coverage for longer periods of time and should more appropriately be considered treatment rather than prophylaxis.

Management. The first dose of parenteral prophylactic antibiotics should be given in sufficient dosage within 30 minutes preceding incision (typically by the anesthesiologist when starting the intravenous line). This ensures maximal therapeutic tissue levels in the wound but does not allow time for the emergence of antibiotic-resistant bacteria. In general, a single preoperative dose of antibiotic is adequate unless surgery is prolonged or there is major blood loss, in which case a second dose may be advisable. Table 222–2 outlines some guidelines for prophylactic antibiotic use.

Follow-Up. The patient's vital signs and wounds are monitored several times during the first 1 to 2 days after the operation. Slight serosanguineous drainage and redness surrounding the incision and sutures are common. Purulent or foul-smelling drainage requires culture, careful observation, and consideration of therapeutic antibiotics and surgical drainage.

PROPHYLAXIS OF BACTERIAL ENDOCARDITIS

Epidemiology. The frequency of bacteremia after health care procedures varies greatly; generally it is highest for dental and oral procedures, intermediate for procedures involving the genitourinary tract, and low for gastrointestinal diagnostic procedures. The relative frequency of endocarditis associated with

Table 222–2. GUIDELINES FOR PROPHYLACTIC ANTIBIOTIC USE

Type of Surgery	Drug	Dose	Cost ($)*
Clean	Cefazolin or	1 g IV	3.00
	vancomycin†	1 g IV	15.60
Contaminated (including clean contaminated)			
Head and neck	Cefazolin or	2 g IV	6.00
	clindamycin	600 mg IV	10.00
Colon or appendectomy‡	Cefoxitin	2 g IV	18.40
Other	Cefazolin	1 g IV	3.00

*Average wholesale price, 1995 *Drug Topics Red Book*; may be less with the purchase of large quantities.

†Use in hospitals where infection with methicillin-resistant *Staphylococcus aureus* or *S. epidermidis* are common.

‡Many authorities recommend elective colorectal preparation using oral neomycin and erythromycin, which is as effective as parenteral antibiotics.

these procedures follows the same order. Very few cases of endocarditis are attributable to health care procedures, and no prospective trial in humans has proven antibiotic prophylaxis effective in preventing valvular infection. However, because the morbidity and mortality of endocarditis is so great, the current standard of care is to give patients with high- and intermediate-risk cardiac lesions prophylactic antibiotic therapy when undergoing procedures associated with high rates of bacteremia.

Clinical Approach. Table 222–3 outlines the cardiac lesions and procedures for which endocarditis prophylaxis is recommended. In general, any cardiac lesion resulting in a pressure gradient or turbulent flow poses a risk for endocarditis. Left-sided cardiac lesions tend to have the highest risk. Right-sided, or low-flow, lesions (e.g., previous coronary artery bypass grafts, isolated secundum atrial septal defect, physiologic or functional heart murmurs) have low risk. Procedures that generally do not require prophylaxis include flexible bronchoscopy, cardiac catheterization, upper gastrointestinal endoscopy, intrauterine device

Table 222–3. BACTERIAL ENDOCARDITIS PROPHYLAXIS*

Cardiac Conditions in Which Prophylaxis is Recommended

Prosthetic valves (including bioprosthetic valves)
Mitral valve prolapse with regurgitation (murmur on examination)
Rheumatic and other acquired valvular dysfunction (including both aortic and mitral regurgitation and stenosis)
Most left-sided congenital defects
Idiopathic hypertrophic subaortic stenosis
Prior endocarditis

Procedures in Which Prophylaxis is Recommended

Any dental or surgery procedure/instrumentation of the respiratory tract likely to result in bleeding
Any surgery or instrumentation of the gastrointestinal or genitourinary tract (except as noted under clinical approach)
Incision and drainage of infected tissue

*Specific guidelines appear in Dajani AS, et al. Prevention of bacterial endocarditis: Recommendations by the American Heart Association. JAMA 1990;264:2919–2922.

Table 222–4. RECOMMENDED ENDOCARDITIS PROPHYLAXIS

Group	Drug
Oral/Respiratory Tract Procedures	
Low risk	Amoxicillin, 3 g PO 1 h before; then 1.5 g PO 6 h later
Penicillin allergic	Erythromycin, 1 g PO 2 h before; then 500 mg PO 6 h later
High risk*	Ampicillin, 2 g IM/IV plus gentamicin, 1.5 mg/kg (not to exceed 80 mg) 30 min before; then amoxicillin, 1.5 g PO 6 h later
Pencillin allergic	Vancomycin, 1 g IV starting 1 h before procedure
Gastrointestinal or Genitourinary Procedures	
Any risk†	Ampicillin, 2 g IM/IV plus gentamicin, 1.5 mg/kg (not to exceed 80 mg) 30 min before; then amoxicillin, 1.5 g PO 6 h later
Penicillin allergic	Substitute vancomycin, 1 g IV for ampicillin; give gentamicin as above

*Prosthetic valve, prior endocarditis.
†Some authorities use oral amoxicillin in low-risk patients.

insertion and removal, and urethral catheterization in the absence of infection. In high-risk patients (e.g., cardiac prosthesis, prior endocarditis), however, many physicians choose to administer antibiotics before even these low-risk procedures.

Management. Specific recommendations are listed in Table 222–4.

Follow-Up. Because endocarditis may occur in spite of appropriate antibiotic prophylaxis, physicians should be alert to unusual symptoms 1 to 2 weeks after procedures in patients at risk. During the immediate postoperative period, intravenous devices and urinary catheters should be discontinued as soon as possible.

Cross-References: Aortic Stenosis (Chapter 80), Other Valvular Disease (Chapter 81), Echocardiography (Chapter 89).

REFERENCES

1. Antibiotic prophylaxis in surgery. Med Lett 1995;37:79–82.
   Specific recommendations for prophylaxis are based on surgical site.

2. Durack DT. Prevention of infective endocarditis. N Engl J Med 1995;332:38–44.
   In this critical review the author suggests only modest benefit from antibiotic prophylaxis.

3. Nichols RL. Surgical antibiotic prophylaxis. Med Clin North Am 1995;79:509–522.
   Risk factors for infection for discussed by surgical site.

4. Sawyer RG, Pruett TL. Wound infections. Surg Clin North Am 1994;74:519–536.
   A complete review of risk factors for surgical-site infections is presented.

5. Ulualp K, Condon RE. Antibiotic prophylaxis for scheduled operative procedures. Infect Dis Clin North Am 1992;6:613–625.
   The authors present an excellent overview.

Index